MEDICAL

SECRETS

Fifth Edition

Mary P. Harward, MD
Staff Physician
Department of Medicine
St. Joseph Hospital
Orange, California

ELSEVIER
MOSBY

ELSEVIER
MOSBY

1600 John F. Kennedy Blvd.
Ste 1800
Philadelphia, PA 19103-2899

MEDICAL SECRETS, FIFTH EDITION   ISBN: 978-0-323-06398-2

Notices

Previous editions copyrighted 2005, 2001, 1996, 1991.

Library of Congress Cataloging-in-Publication Data

Medical secrets. – 5th ed. / [edited by] Mary P. Harward.
   p. ; cm.
   Rev. ed. of: Medical secrets / [edited by] Anthony J. Zollo, Jr. 4th ed. c2005.
   Includes bibliographical references and index.
   ISBN 978-0-323-06398-2 (pbk.)
   1. Internal medicine–Examinations, questions, etc. I. Harward, Mary P.
   [DNLM: 1. Internal Medicine–Examination Questions. WB 18.2]
   RC58.M43 2012
   616.0076–dc22   2011006144

Acquisitions Editor: James Merritt
Developmental Editor: Andrea Vosburgh
Publishing Services Manager: Pat Joiner-Myers
Senior Project Manager: Joy Moore
Marketing Manager: Jason Oberacker
Design Direction: Steven Stave

Printed in the United States of America

Last digit is the print number: 9 8 7 6 5 4 3 2 1

CONTENTS

CONTRIBUTORS

William L. Allen, MDiv, JD
Associate Professor, Program in Bioethics, Law, and Medical Professionalism, Department of Community Health and Family Medicine, University of Florida College of Medicine, Gainesville, Florida
Medical Ethics

Holly H. Birdsall, MD, PhD
Professor, Departments of Otorhinolaryngology and Immunology, Baylor College of Medicine, Houston, Texas; Acting Deputy, Chief Research and Development Officer, Veterans Health Administration, Washington, DC
Allergy and Immunology

Joseph Caperna, MD, MPH
Clinical Professor of Medicine, Department of Medicine, University of California, San Diego, Attending Physician, University of California San Diego Medical Center, San Diego, California
AIDS and HIV Infection

Rhonda A. Cole, MD
Associate Professor, Division of Gastroenterology, Department of Internal Medicine, Baylor College of Medicine; Chief, GI Endoscopy, Digestive Diseases Section, Department of Medicine, Michael E. DeBakey VA Medical Center, Houston, Texas
Gastroenterology

Kathryn H. Dao, MD, FACP, FACR
Associate Director of Rheumatology Research, Department of Rheumatology, Baylor Research Institute, Dallas, Texas
Rheumatology

Gabriel Habib, Sr., MS, MD, FACC, FCCP, FAHA
Professor of Medicine, Departments of Medicine and Cardiology, Baylor College of Medicine; Director of Education and Associate Chief, Section of Cardiology, Michael E. DeBakey VA Medical Center, Houston, Texas
Cardiology

Eloise M. Harman, MD
Professor and Clinical Division Chief, Department of Pulmonary, Critical Care and Sleep Medicine, University of Florida College of Medicine; Attending Physician, Medical Intensive Care Unit, Shands Hospital at the University of Florida, Gainesville, Florida
Pulmonary Medicine

Mary P. Harward, MD
Staff Physician, Department of Medicine, St. Joseph Hospital, Orange, California
General Medicine and Ambulatory Care

Timothy R.S. Harward, MD
Medical Staff, Department of Surgery, Medical Director, Wound Care Center, St. Joseph Hospital, Orange, California
Vascular Medicine

Teresa G. Hayes, MD, PhD
Associate Professor, Hematology-Oncology, Department of Internal Medicine, Baylor College of Medicine; Chief, Hematology-Oncology Section, Michael E. DeBakey VA Medical Center, Houston, Texas
Oncology

Henrique Elias Kallas, MD, CMD
Assistant Professor, Departments of Internal Medicine and Geriatrics, University of Florida, Gainesville, Florida
Geriatrics

Roger Kornu, MD
Attending Physician, Departments of Internal Medicine and Rheumatology, St. Joseph Hospital, Orange, California
Rheumatology

Harrinarine Madhosingh, MD
Assistant Professor, Department of Medicine, University of Central Florida College of Medicine, Orlando, Florida; Attending Physician, Infectious Disease Consultants, Altamonte Springs, Florida
Infectious Diseases

Ara D. Metjian, MD
Instructor, Department of Medicine, Division of Hematology, Duke University, Durham, North Carolina
Hematology

John Meuleman, MD
Associate Professor, Department of Aging, University of Florida College of Medicine; Clinical Director, Geriatric Research, Education and Clinical Center, Gainesville Veterans Affairs Medical Center, Gainesville, Florida
Geriatrics

Dang M. Nguyen, MD
Senior Gastroenterology Fellow, Department of Gastroenterology, Baylor College of Medicine, Houston, Texas
Gastroenterology

Catalina Orozco, MD
Physician, Rheumatology Associates, Dallas, Texas
Rheumatology

Rahul K. Patel, MD
Assistant Professor, Department of Rheumatology, UNT Health Science Center, Fort Worth, Texas
Rheumatology

Leslye C. Pennypacker, MD
Assistant Professor of Medicine, Department of Internal Medicine, University of Florida College of Medicine; Medical Director, Palliative Care Program, North Florida/South Georgia Veterans Health System, Gainesville, Florida
Palliative Medicine

Sharma S. Prabhakar, MD, MBA, FACP, FASN
Professor of Medicine and Cell Physiology, Chief, Nephrology Division, and Vice Chairman, Department of Medicine, Texas Tech University Health Sciences Center; Director of Nephrology and Dialysis Services, Department of Medicine, University Medical Center, Lubbock, Texas
Nephrology; Acid-Base and Electrolytes

Eric I. Rosenberg, MD, MSPH, FACP
Clinical Associate Professor and Interim Chief, Division of Internal Medicine, Department of Medicine, University of Florida College of Medicine, Gainesville, Florida
Medical Consultation

Roger D. Rossen, MD
Professor, Departments of Immunology and Internal Medicine, Baylor College of Medicine; Acting Associate Chief of Staff for Research, Immunology, Allergy and Rheumatology Section, Michael E. DeBakey VA Medical Center, Houston, Texas
Allergy and Immunology

Damian Silbermins, MD
Assistant Professor, Departments of Hematology and Oncology, Duke University, Durham, North Carolina
Hematology

Amy M. Sitapati, MD
Associate Clinical Professor, Department of Medicine, University of California, San Diego; Associate Director, Owen Clinic, University of California San Diego Medical Center, San Diego, California
AIDS and HIV Infection

David B. Sommer, MD, MPH
Staff Physician, Department of Neurology, Fallon Clinic, Worcester, Massachusetts
Neurology

Frederick S. Southwick, MD
Professor of Medicine and Chief of Infectious Diseases, Department of Medicine, University of Florida; Infectious Diseases Consultant, Department of Medicine, University of Florida and Shands Medical Center, Gainesville, Florida
Infectious Diseases

Susan E. Spratt, MD
Assistant Professor, Department of Medicine, Duke University Medical Center, Durham, North Carolina
Endocrinology

Alfredo Tiu, DO, FACP, FASN
Assistant Clinical Professor, Department of Medicine, University of California, San Diego; Department of Medicine, Owen Clinic, University of California San Diego Medical Center, San Diego, California
AIDS and HIV Infection

Adriano R. Tonelli, MD
Pulmonary Fellow, Department of Pulmonary, Critical Care and Sleep Medicine, University of Florida, Gainesville, Florida; Staff, Respiratory Institute, Cleveland Clinic, Cleveland, Ohio
Pulmonary Medicine

Whitney W. Woodmansee, MD
Assistant Professor, Department of Medicine, Harvard Medical School; Director, Clinical Neuroendocrine Program, Division of Endocrinology, Diabetes and Hypertension, Brigham and Women's Hospital, Boston, Massachusetts
Endocrinology

PREFACE

Doctors constantly question. We question our patients, our colleagues, ourselves, and our students. We know that in order to accurately diagnose and treat our patients, we must first ask the right questions. For the students reading this book, you may feel that you are constantly on the receiving end of the questions, only expected to provide the answers. The purpose of this book is to give you access to some of those answers. Additionally, we hope this book reveals the questions that experienced clinicians ask themselves (and not just the student on attending rounds). We hope that our questions will stimulate your intellect and generate more queries that you can independently research and answer. The Neurology chapter contributor, David B. Sommer, expressed the purpose of his chapter exceedingly well when he wrote, "By necessity, this is a non-comprehensive discussion. We were asked to write a chapter, not a book! The most important thing is to keep asking questions and seeking answers. We hope this chapter will help you know some of the more important questions to ask."

This book is an extensive collection of ideas from many physicians, all of whom are dedicated to sharing their knowledge. We hope this book will continue to be a source of reference not just for students but also for teachers, practitioners, and those in all levels of medical training. Most importantly, we hope this book fulfills the primary role of the doctor and reminds us that the simple word *doctor* derives from the Latin, *doceo*—to teach.

Mary P. Harward, MD

TOP 100 SECRETS

These secrets are 100 of the top board alerts. They summarize the most important concepts, principles, and salient details of internal medicine.

1. Informed consent is not merely a signature on a form, but a process by which the patient and physician discuss and deliberate the indications, risks, and benefits of a test, therapy, or procedure and the patient's outcome goals.

2. Patients should participate in informed consent whenever they have sufficient decision-making capacity.

3. Decision-making capacity is determined by assessing the patient's ability to (1) comprehend the indications, risks, and benefits of the intervention; (2) understand the significance of the underlying medical condition; (3) deliberate the provided information; and (4) communicate a decision.

4. Some patients with impaired memory or communication skills may retain decision-making capacity.

5. Closely examine the feet and pedal pulses of diabetic patients regularly, looking for ulcerations, significant callous formation, injury, and joint deformities that could lead to ulceration, and reduced blood flow.

6. Patients aged 19 to 64 years should receive at least one dose of tetanus, diphtheria, pertussis (Tdap) vaccine in place of a booster dose of tetanus-diphtheria (Td) vaccine to improve adult immunity to pertussis (whooping cough).

7. Adolescent girls and women aged 11 to 26 years should receive three doses of human papillomavirus (HPV) vaccine to prevent HPV infection and reduce cervical cancer risk.

8. Subclavian artery stenosis should be suspected in patients with a blood pressure (BP) difference between the right and the left arms of > 10 mmHg.

9. Antibiotic prophylaxis before dental procedures is recommended only for patients with (1) significant congenital heart disease; (2) previous history of endocarditis; (3) cardiac transplantation, and, (4) prosthetic valve.

10. The effectiveness of clopidogrel can be altered by medications such as proton pump inhibitors and inherited mechanisms of clopidogrel metabolism.

11. Patients should be closely assessed during the preoperative consultation for risk factors for postoperative venous thromboembolism and treated appropriately.

12. Patients receiving current or previous (within the past year) glucocorticoid therapy may need additional stress doses during surgery owing to suppression of the hypothalamic pituitary axis.

13. Beta blockers may be helpful to reduce perioperative cardiac risk in patients with peripheral vascular disease and known coronary disease.

14. Metformin should be held and renal function closely monitored for patients undergoing surgery or imaging procedures involving contrast.

15. Asking the patient about personal and family history of bleeding episodes associated with minor procedures or injury is as effective in identifying bleeding diatheses as measuring coagulation studies.

16. Noninvasive stress testing has the best predictive value for detecting coronary artery disease (CAD) in patients with an intermediate (30–80%) pretest likelihood of CAD and is of limited value in patients with very low (<30%) or very high (>80%) likelihood of CAD.

17. Routine use of daily low-dose aspirin (81–325 mg) can reduce the likelihood of cardiovascular disease in high-risk patients with known CAD, diabetes, or peripheral vascular disease.

18. Routine daily low-dose aspirin use is associated with an increased risk of gastrointestinal bleeding, which can be reduced through the use of proton pump inhibitors.

19. Right ventricular infarction should also be considered in any patient with signs and symptoms of inferior wall myocardial infarction.

20. Diabetes is considered an equivalent of known CAD and treatment and prevention guidelines for diabetic patients are similar to those for patients with CAD.

21. Renovascular stenosis should be considered in patients with the new onset of hypertension at a younger (<20 yr) or older (>70 yr) age.

22. Consider aortic dissection in the differential diagnosis of all patients presenting with acute chest or upper back pain.

23. Increasing size of an abdominal aortic aneurysm (AAA) increases the risk of rupture. Patients with AAA greater than 5 cm or aneurysmal symptoms should have endovascular or surgical repair. Smaller aneurysms should be followed closely every 6 to 12 months by computed tomography (CT) scan.

24. Patients presenting with pulselessness, pallor, pain, paralysis, and paresthesias of a limb likely have acute limb ischemia due to an embolus and require emergent evaluation for thrombolytic therapy or revascularization.

25. Patients presenting with symptoms of transient ischemic attack are at high risk of stroke and require urgent evaluation for symptomatic carotid artery disease and treatment that may include antiplatelet agents, carotid endartectomy, statin drugs, antihypertensive agents, and anticoagulation.

26. All patients with peripheral arterial disease and cerebrovascular disease should stop smoking.

27. Asthma, chronic obstructive pulmonary disease (COPD), congestive heart failure (CHF), and upper airway cough syndrome (UACS) can all cause wheezing.

28. Inhaled corticosteroid therapy should be considered for asthmatic patients with symptoms that are more than mild and intermittent.

29. Pulmonary embolism cannot by diagnosed by history, physical examination, and chest x-ray alone. Additional testing such as D-dimer level, spiral chest CT scan, angiography, or a combination of these tests will be needed to effectively rule in or rule out the disease.

30. Sarcoidosis is a multisystem disorder that frequently presents with pulmonary findings of abnormal chest x-ray, cough, dyspnea, or chest pain.

31. Hepatitis C virus infection can lead to cirrhosis, hepatocellular carcinoma, and severe liver disease requiring transplantation.

32. Travelers to areas with endemic hepatitis A infection should receive hepatitis A vaccine.

33. Celiac sprue should be considered in patients with unexplained iron-deficiency anemia or osteoporosis.

34. In the United States, gallstones are common among American Indians and Mexican Americans.

35. Esophageal manometry may be needed to complete the evaluation of patients with noncardiac chest pain that may be due to esophageal motility disorders.

36. The estimated glomerular filtration rate (eGFR) is now frequently routinely reported when chemistry panels are ordered and can provide a useful estimate of renal function.

37. Angiotensin-converting enzyme (ACE) inhibitor use should be evaluated for all diabetics, even those with normotension, for their renoprotective effects.

38. Diabetes is the most common cause of chronic kidney disease (CKD) in the United States.

39. When erythrocyte-stimulating agents are used for the treatment of anemia associated with chronic kidney disease (CKD) and end-stage renal disease, the hemoglobin should *not* be normalized, but maintained at a level of 11 to 12 g/dL.

40. Low-dose dopamine may not prevent acute kidney injury in critically ill patients, but may cause tachycardia and digital, bowel, and myocardial ischemia.

41. Hyponatremia can commonly occur after transurethral resection of the prostate.

42. Thrombocytosis, leukocytosis, and specimen hemolysis can falsely elevate serum potassium levels.

43. Intravenous calcium should be given immediately for patients with acute hyperkalemia and electrocardiographic changes.

44. Hypoalbuminemia lowers the serum total calcium level but does not affect the ionized calcium.

45. Hypokalemia, hypophosphatemia, and hypomagnesemia are common findings in alcoholics who require hospitalization.

46. Lupus mortality is bimodal in distribution—patients who die early die from the disease or infection; patients who die later in life tend to die from cardiovascular diseases.

47. In a patient who is a smoker and presents with what looks like Raynaud's phenomenon, think of Buerger's disease (thromboangiitis obliterans).

48. Patients with autoimmune disorders who smoke should be counseled to quit because tobacco has recently been linked to precipitation of symptoms and poorer prognosis.

49. Antinuclear antibody (ANA) titers are not associated with disease activity.

50. Early, aggressive intervention with disease-modifying antirheumatic drugs reduces the morbidity (deformity leading to reduced functionality and disability) and mortality associated with rheumatoid arthritis.

51. Packed red cells in freshly acquired blood may include lymphocytes that can mount a graft-versus-host reaction in patients who are immunocompromised.

52. Intranasal steroids are the single most effective drug for treatment of allergic rhinitis. Decongestion with topical adrenergic agents may be needed initially to allow corticosteroids access to the deeper nasal mucosa.

53. ACE inhibitors can cause dry cough and angioedema.

54. Beta blockers should be avoided whenever possible in patients with asthma because they may accentuate the severity of anaphylaxis, prolong its cardiovascular and pulmonary manifestations, and greatly decrease the effectiveness of epinephrine and albuterol in reversing the life-threatening manifestations of anaphylaxis.

55. Patients with persistent fever of unknown origin should first be evaluated for infections, malignancies, and autoimmune diseases.

56. Viruses are the most common causes of acute sinusitis; therefore, antibiotics are ineffective.

57. Most cases of Rocky Mountain spotted fever (RMSF) do not occur in the Rocky Mountain region but in the south Atlantic and south central regions. Patients with febrile illnesses and a rash who have been in these regions in the summer (May to September) should receive empirical doxycycline therapy for presumptive RMSF.

58. Asplenic patients (either anatomic or functional) are susceptible to infections with encapsulated organisms (*Streptococcus pneumoniae, Haemophilus influenzae,* and *Neisseria meningitides*) and should receive appropriate vaccinations.

59. Allergic bronchopulmonary aspergillosis (ABPA) occurs in asthmatics and is evident by recurrent wheezing, eosinophilia, transient infiltrates on chest x-ray, and positive serum antibodies to aspergillus.

60. Chagas' disease, caused by *Trypanosoma cruzi,* can cause cardiomyopathy and conduction abnormalities.

61. Human immunodeficiency virus (HIV) infection is preventable and treatable but not curable.

62. Routine HIV testing should be considered for all patients older than 13 years.

63. Nucleic acid–based testing (NAT) is needed for diagnosis of acute primary HIV infection.

64. HIV-infected patients with undetectable viral loads can still transmit HIV.

65. HIV-infected patients with tuberculosis are more likely to have atypical symptoms and present with extrapulmonary disease.

66. All patients with HIV infection should be tested for syphilis, and all patients diagnosed with syphilis (and any other sexually transmitted disease) should be tested for HIV.

67. The presence of thrush (oropharyngeal candidiasis) indicates significant immunosuppression in an HIV-infected patient.

68. Ferritin is an effective screening test for hemochromatosis.

69. Methylmalonic acid can be helpful in the diagnosis of vitamin B_{12} deficiency in patients with low normal B_{12} levels.

70. Pneumococcal polysaccharide, *Haemophilius influenzae* B (HiB), and meningococcal vaccines should be given to patients before elective splenectomy, preferably 14 days before the procedure.

71. Chronic lymphocytic leukemia is the most common leukemia in adults and is often found in those older than 70 years.

72. Patients with antiphospholipid syndrome have an antiphospholipid antibody and the clinical occurrence of arterial or venous thromboses or both, recurrent pregnancy losses, or thrombocytopenia.

73. Mesothelioma, a pleural malignancy associated with asbestosis exposure, is not associated with smoking.

74. The preferred treatment for esophageal cancer is resection.

75. Renal cell carcinomas frequently present with symptoms of multiple other organs, making its diagnosis difficult.

76. Tobacco and alcohol use are significant risk factors for head and neck cancers.

77. Aggressive cervical cancer is found in women with HIV infection. Invasive cervical cancer is an acquired immunodeficiency syndrome (AIDS)–defining condition.

78. The best initial screening test for evaluation of thyroid status is the thyroid-stimulating hormone (TSH), because it is the most sensitive measure of thyroid function in the majority of patients. The one exception is patients with pituitary and hypothalamic dysfunction in whom TSH cannot reliably assess thyroid function.

79. Patients with type 1 and type 2 diabetes should be screened at regular intervals for the microvascular complications of retinopathy, neuropathy, and nephropathy.

80. Some patients with subclinical thyroid disease (elevated TSH in the absence of hypothyroidism symptoms) do have mild thyroid disease and may benefit from treatment.

81. Erectile dysfunction and decreased libido in men and amenorrhea and infertility in women are the most common symptoms of hypogonadism.

82. Hyperparathyroidism is the most common cause of hypercalcemia.

83. Ataxia can be localized to the cerebellum.

84. Gait dysfunction, urinary dysfunction, and memory impairment are symptoms of normal-pressure hydrocephalus.

85. In the appropriate setting, thrombolysis can markedly improve the outcome of stroke. Prompt initiation of thrombolytic therapy is essential.

86. The sudden onset of a severe headache may indicate an intracranial hemorrhage.

87. Optic neuritis can be an early sign of multiple sclerosis.

88. Vitamin D deficiency is common in older adults and can contribute to osteoporosis, fractures, and falls. Vitamin D levels are measured by the 25-OH vitamin D.

89. Older adults are particularly susceptible to the anticholinergic effects of multiple medications, including over-the-counter antihistamines.

90. Anemia is not a normal part of aging, and hemoglobin abnormalities should be investigated.

91. Decisions regarding screening for malignancies in the elderly should be based not on the age alone, but on the patient's life expectancy, functional status, and personal goals.

92. Systolic murmurs in the elderly may be due to aortic stenosis or aortic sclerosis.

93. Delirium in hospitalized patients is associated with an increased mortality.

94. When delirium occurs, the underlying etiology should be thoroughly evaluated and treated.

95. Pneumonia is the most common infectious cause of death in the elderly.

96. Discussion and preparations for palliative care should begin at the time of diagnosis of a terminal illness.

97. Medications to prevent constipation should be prescribed at the same time as the initial prescription of chronic opioid therapy.

98. Patients can discontinue hospice care if their symptoms improve or their end-of-life goals change.

99. Opioids are the safest, most effective medications for pain control at the end of life.

100. Opioid analgesics are available in many forms including tablets to swallow, tablets for buccal application, oral solutions, lozenges for transmucosal absorption, injection, transdermal, intramuscular, and rectal suppositories.

MEDICAL ETHICS

William L. Allen, M.Div., J.D.

> *I will use treatment to help the sick according to my ability and judgment, but I will never use it to injure or wrong them.*
>
> Attributed to Hippocrates
> 4th-Century Greek Physician

ETHICAL PRINCIPLES AND CONCEPTS

1. **Define the following terms in relation to the patient and physician-patient relationship: "beneficence," "nonmaleficence," and "respect for autonomy."**
   - **Beneficence:** The concept that the physician will contribute to the welfare of the patient through the recommended medical interventions
   - **Nonmaleficence:** An obligation for the physician not to inflict harm upon the patient
   - **Autonomy:** The obligation of the physician to honor the patient's right to accept or refuse a recommended treatment, based on respect for persons

2. **What is fiduciary duty?**
   A duty of trust imposed upon physicians requiring them to place their patients' best interests ahead of their own interests.

3. **What is conflict of interest?**
   A situation in which one or more of a professional's duties to a client or patient conflicts with the professional's self interests, or when a professional's roles or duties to more than one patient or organization are in tension or conflict.

4. **How should conflicts of interest be addressed?**
   - Avoided, if possible
   - Disclosed to institutional officials or to patients affected
   - Managed by disinterested parties outside the conflicted roles or relationships

5. **What is conscientious objection?**
   Objection to participation in or performance of a procedure or test grounded on a person's sincere and deeply held belief that it is morally wrong.

6. **What is a conscience clause?**
   A provision in law or policy that allows providers with conscientious objections to decline participation in activities to which they have moral objections, under certain conditions and limitations.

7. **Describe futility.**
   The doctrine that physicians are not required to attempt treatment if there will be no medical benefit from it. This has become a very controversial term in recent times, in part because of inconsistency in definition and usage. In its clearest sense, it is not so controversial. For example, when the substance laetrile, derived from apricot pits, was rumored to be a cure for cancer in the early 1970s, desperate cancer patients besieged their physicians to give them

this drug. Most physicians in this country declined to do so on the grounds that such a treatment would be futile and the exercise of professional autonomy warranted refusal of their patients' requests in this case. Futility is sometimes inappropriately invoked when the chance of a treatment's efficacy is significantly limited, but not zero, and the physician determines that minimal chance of efficacy to be "futile."

INFORMED CONSENT

8. How should one request "consent" from a patient?
   Consent is not a transitive verb. Sometimes a medical student or resident is instructed to "go consent the patient." This implies that consent is an act that a health professional performs upon a passive recipient who has no role in the action other than passive acceptance. A health professional seeking consent from a patient should be asking the patient for either an affirmative endorsement of an offered intervention or a decision to decline the proposed intervention.

9. What is consent or mere consent?
   Consent alone, without a sufficiently robust level of information to justify the adjective "informed." Although "mere consent" may avoid a finding of battery (which is defined as physical contact with a person without that person's consent), it is usually insufficient permission for the physician to proceed with a procedure or treatment.

10. What is informed consent?
    Consent from a patient that is preceded by and based on the patient's understanding of the proposed intervention at a level that enables the patient to make a meaningful decision about endorsement or refusal of the proposed intervention.

11. What are the necessary conditions for valid informed consent?
    - Disclosure of relevant medical information by health care providers
    - Comprehension of relevant medical information by patient (or authorized representative)
    - Voluntariness (absence of coercion by medical personnel or institutional pressure)

12. What topics should always be addressed in the discussion regarding informed consent (or informed refusal)?
    - Risks and benefits of the recommended intervention (examination, test, or treatment)
    - Reasonable alternatives to the proposed intervention and the risks and benefits of such alternatives
    - The option of no intervention and the risks and benefits of no intervention

KEY POINTS: INFORMED CONSENT ✔

1. Informed consent involves more than a signature on a document.

2. Before beginning the informed consent process, the physician should assess the patient's capacity to understand the information provided.

3. The physician should make the effort to present the information in a way the patient can comprehend and not just assume the patient is "incompetent" because of difficulty in understanding a complex medical issue.

4. The patient's goals and values are also considered in the informed consent process.

13. What are the different standards for the scope of disclosure in informed consent?
- **Full disclosure:** Disclosure of everything the physician knows. This standard is impractical, if not impossible, and is not legally or ethically required.
- **Reasonable person** (sometimes called "prudent person standard"): Patient-centered standard of disclosure of the information necessary for a reasonable person to make a meaningful decision about whether to accept or to refuse medical testing or treatment. This standard is the legal minimum in some states.
- **Professional practice** (also called "customary practice"): Physician-centered standard of disclosure of the information typically practiced by other practitioners in similar contexts. Sometimes the professional practice standard is the legal minimum in states that do not acknowledge the reasonable person standard.
- **Subjective standard:** Disclosure of information a particular patient may want or need beyond what a reasonable person may want to know. This is not a legally required minimum, but is ethically desirable if the physician can determine what additional information the particular patient might find important.

14. What are the exceptions to the obligation of informed consent?
- **Implied consent:** For routine aspects of medical examinations, such as blood pressure, temperature, or stethoscopic examinations, explicit informed consent is not generally required, because presentation for care plausibly implies that the patient expects these measures and consent may be reasonably inferred by the physician. Implied consent does not extend to invasive examinations or physical examination of private or sensitive areas without explicit oral permission and explanation of purpose.
- **Presumed consent:** Presentation in the emergency room does not necessarily mean that emergency interventions are routine or that the patient's consent is implied. The justification for some exception to informed consent is that most persons would agree to necessary emergency interventions; therefore, consent may be presumed, even though this presumption may turn out to be incorrect in some instances for some patients. Such treatment is limited to stabilizing the patient and deferring other decisions until the patient regains capacity or an authorized decision maker has been contacted.

15. What should you do when a patient requests the physician to make the decision without providing informed consent?
When a patient seems to be saying in one way or another, "Doctor, just do what you think is best," it is appropriate to make a professional recommendation based on what the physician believes to be in the patient's best medical interests. This does not mean, however, that the patient does not need to understand the risks, benefits, and expected outcomes of the recommended intervention. This type of request is sometimes referred to as requested paternalism or waiver of informed consent. It is best in this situation to explain, in terms of risks and benefits of a recommended intervention, the reasons why you recommend the intervention and why it would seem to be in the patient's best medical interest and ask the patient to endorse it or to decline it.

16. What is a physician's obligation to veracity (truthful disclosure) to patients?
In order for patients to have an accurate picture of their medical situation and what clinical alternatives may best meet their goals in choosing among various medical tests or treatments or to decline medical intervention, patients must have a truthful description of their medical condition. Such truthful disclosure is also essential for maintaining patient trust in the physican-patient relationship. Truthful disclosure, especially of "bad news," however, does not mean that the bearer of bad news must be brutal or insensitive in the timing and manner of disclosure.

17. **Define "therapeutic privilege."**
    A traditional exception to the obligation of truthful disclosure to the patient, in which disclosures that were thought to be harmful to the patient were withheld for the benefit of the patient. In recent decades, this exception has narrowed almost to the vanishing point from the recognition that most patients want to know the truth and make decisions accordingly, even if the truth entails bad news. Nevertheless, some disclosures may justifiably be withheld temporarily, such as when a patient is acutely depressed and at risk of suicide. Ultimately, however, with appropriate medical and social support, the patient whose decisional capacity can be restored should be told the information that had been temporarily withheld for her or his benefit.

CONFIDENTIALITY

18. **What is medical confidentiality?**
    The confidential maintenance of information relating to a patient's medical and personal data. Maintaining the confidential status of patient medical information is crucial not only to trust in the physician-patient relationship but also to physician's ability to elicit sensitive information from patients that is crucial to adequate medical management and treatment. The Health Information Portability and Accountability Act (HIPAA, a federal statute) as well as most state statutes provide legal protections for patients' personally identifiable health information (PHI), but the professional ethical obligation of confidentiality may exceed these minimal protections or apply in situations not clearly addressed by HIPAA or state statutes.

19. **What are recognized exceptions to patient medical confidentiality?**
    - Duty to warn (Tarasoff duty): A basis for justifying a limited exception to the rule of patient confidentiality when a patient of a psychiatrist makes an explicit, serious threat of grave bodily harm to an identifiable person(s) in the imminent future. The scope of this warning is limited to the potential victim(s) or appropriate law enforcement agency, and the health-care provider may divulge only enough information to convey the threat of harm.
    - Reporting of communicable disease to public health authorities.
    - Reporting of injuries from violence to law enforcement.

20. **What is the obligation to veracity to nonpatients?**
    Physicians are not obligated to lie to persons who inquire about a patient's confidential information, but they may be required simply to decline to address such requests from persons to whom the patient has not granted access.

DECISION-MAKING CAPACITY

21. **How do physicians assess decision-making capacity in patients?**
    Whereas most adult patients should be presumed to have intact decisional capacity, some patients may be totally incapacitated for making their own medical decisions. Totally incapacitated patients will generally be obvious cases. But decisional capacity is not an all-or-nothing category, so it is not uncommon for patients to have variable capacity depending on the status of their condition and the complexity of the particular decision at hand. Thus, one crucial aspect of assessing decisional capacity is to determine whether the patient can comprehend the elements required for valid informed consent to the particular decision that needs to be made.

22. **What are common pitfalls in assessing patient decisional capacity or competence?**
    If one uses the **outcome approach,** the patient's capacity is determined based on the outcome of the patient's acceptance of the physician's recommendation. The physician may

incorrectly assume that the refusal of a recommended treatment indicates incapacity. Refusal of a recommended treatment is not adequate grounds to conclude patient incapacity. Nor is patient acceptance of the physician's recommendation an adequate means of assessing patient capacity. An incapacitated patient may acquiesce to recommended treatment, whereas a capacitated patient may refuse the physician's best medical advice. If one uses the **status approach,** patients with a history of a mental illness or memory impairment may be considered incapacitated. Psychiatric conditions or other medical conditions that can result in incapacity may have resolved or may be under control with appropriate therapy that mitigates the condition's impact on patient capacity for decision making. Patients with memory impairment or dementia may also be able to express wishes regarding treatment.

23. **What is the best approach to assessing patient capacity?**
    The **functional approach,** which determines the patient's ability to function in a particular context to make decisions that are authentic expressions of the patient's own values and goals. Determining whether a patient is capacitated for a particular medical decision entails assessing whether the patient is able to:
    - Comprehend the risks and benefits of the recommended intervention, risks and benefits of reasonable alternative intervention, and the risks and benefits of no intervention.
    - Manifest appreciation of the significance of his or her medical condition.
    - Reason about the consequences of available treatment options (including no treatment).
    - Communicate a stable choice in light of his or her personal values.

    Appelbaum PS: Clinical practice. Assessment of patients' competence to consent to treatment, *N Engl J Med* 357:1834–1840, 2007.

24. **What is involuntary commitment?**
    Assignment of a person to an inpatient psychiatric facility without patient consent when the appropriate criteria are met. The patient must be unable to provide informed consent owing to a mental illness *and,* owing to the same mental illness, pose a danger to themselves or to others.

25. **What is assent?**
    The obligation prospectively to explain medical interventions in language and concepts the patient can comprehend even if the patient is deemed to be not capable of full informed consent, such as children or mentally impaired adults. The patient's agreement is elicited, even though the final decision requires parental, guardian, or other legally authorized decision maker's permission.

ADVANCE DIRECTIVES

26. **What is an advance directive?**
    A generic term for any of several types of patient instructions, oral or written, for providing guidance and direction in advance of a person's potential incapacity. The instructions and authorization in an advance directive do not take effect until the person loses decisional capacity and the advance directive ceases to be in effect if or when the patient regains capacity.

27. **What are the types of advance directives?**
    Designation by a capacitated patient of the person the patient chooses to make medical decisions during any period when the patient is incapacitated, whether during surgery, temporary unconsciousness or mental condition, as well as irreversible condition of lost decisional capacity. The decisions the designated person can make include withholding or withdrawal of treatment in life-limiting circumstances. These may variously be called a

"durable power of attorney for health care," a "surrogate health-care decision maker," or a "proxy health-care decision maker."

A **living will** is a formal expression of a patient's choices about end-of-life care and specifications or limitations of treatment, either with or without the naming of a person to reinforce, interpret, or apply what is expressed to the patient's current circumstances.

28. **Who are statutorily authorized next of kin decision makers?**
    If a patient has not made a living will or designated a person to make decisions during periods of patient incapacity, state statutes determine the order of priority for persons related to or close to the patient to assume the role of making medical decisions on the patient's behalf. These are typically called "surrogates" or "proxies," but they differ from decision makers designated by the patient in the way they are selected, and in many cases, they bear a greater burden of demonstrating that they know what the patient would want.

29. **What are the standards of decision making for those chosen either by the patient or by statute to make decisions for the incapacitated patient?**
    - **Substituted judgment:** The decision the patient would have made if she or he had not been incapacitated. In some cases, this will not be the same as what others may think is in the patient's best interest.
    - **Best interest:** Choosing what is considered most appropriate for the patient. If there is substantial uncertainty about what the patient would have chosen for herself or himself, then the traditional best interest standard is the appropriate basis for decision making.

END-OF-LIFE ISSUES

30. **What are end-of-life care physician orders?**
    Orders that give direction regarding interventions at the time of death or cardiopulmonary arrest. Patient-directed measures such as advance directives or statutory next of kin decisions should be the basis for underlying medical decisions that entail informed consent or refusal issues at the end of life.

KEY POINTS: END OF LIFE ISSUES ✔

1. Patients should be encouraged to discuss their wishes for end-of-life care with family members or close friends and physicians while still able to clearly express these wishes.

2. Forms such as Preferences of Life-Sustaining Treatment can designate the patient's specific requests to accept or decline therapies at the end of life.

3. Patients are frequently unaware of the numerous, complex therapies related to end-of-life care and may not be able to write down what is wanted. Designation of a surrogate decision maker with whom the patient discusses her or his values and goals related to end-of-life care and also ensure the patient's wishes will be respected.

31. **How are end-of-life care orders written?**
    - **Do not resuscitate (DNR) or do not attempt resuscitation (DNAR):** An order written by the attending physician to prevent emergency cardiopulmonary resuscitation (CPR) for a patient who has refused CPR as a form of unwanted treatment. The decision of an incapacitated patient's authorized decision maker may also be a basis for a written DNR order by the physician.

- **Physician Orders for Life-Sustaining Treatment (POLST):** Similar to the concept of DNR, but broadened to include all aspects of end-of-life care based on the choices of the patient or authorized decision maker, including withholding or withdrawal of care and palliative measures. Many states now have statutory acknowledgment that a properly executed POLST form, signed by a physician, should be followed by all health-care providers for the patient.

  Available at www.polst.org.

32. **What is brain death?**
The term used to replace the traditional definition of death by cessation of heartbeat and respiration. In the most conservative definition of this term, it refers to whole brain death, cessation not only of higher cortical function but of brainstem function as well.

33. **What is physician-assisted suicide?**
The provision of a lethal amount of a medication that the patient voluntarily takes to end his or her life. Oregon and Washington established legislation to allow these prescriptions, and other states are considering the issue.

BIBLIOGRAPHY

1. Beauchamp TL, Childress JF: *Principles of Biomedical Ethics*, ed 6, Oxford, 2008, Oxford University Press.
2. Jonsen A, Siegler M, Winslade W: *Clinical Ethics: A Practical Approach to Ethical Decisions in Clinical Medicine*, ed 6, New York, 2006, McGraw-Hill Medical.
3. Lo B: *Resolving Ethical Dilemmas. A Guide for Clinicians*, ed 4, Philadelphia, 2009, Lippincott Williams & Wilkins.

CHAPTER 2

GENERAL MEDICINE
AND AMBULATORY CARE

Mary P. Harward, M.D.

When I see a new patient, I find it valuable, at the first meeting, <u>consciously</u> to look at the hands. Clues to diseases in the nervous system, heart, lung, liver, and other organs can be found there.... In medicine, a hand is never merely a hand; symbolically it is much more. That is why the "laying on of hands" is so important for the physician and patient.

John Stone (1936–2008)
"Telltale Hands" from
In the Country of Hearts: Journeys in the Art of Medicine, 1990

It's the humdrum, day-in, day-out everyday work that is the real satisfaction of the practice of medicine; ... the actual calling on people, at all times and under all conditions, the coming to grips with the intimate conditions of their lives, when they were being born, when they were dying, watching them die, watching them get well when they were ill, has always absorbed me.

William Carlos Williams (1883–1963)
"The Practice" from
The Autobiography of William Carlos Williams, 1951

LISTENING TO THE PATIENT

1. **What interviewing skills can help the physician identify all the significant issues to the patient during the visit?**
    Remaining open-ended and encouraging the patient to "go on" until all the pertinent issues have been expressed by the patient. Other facilitative techniques to keep the patient talking include a simple head nod or saying, "and," or "what else?" Continue these facilitative techniques until the patient says, "nothing else." During the opening of the interview, the physician should listen to the patient's "list" of the concerns for that visit, without focusing on specific signs and symptoms at that time. Physicians too often interrupt the patient and direct the remaining interview, only focusing on what the physician deems important.
    A patient may have other, significant issues that are not immediately expressed, and the physician may miss this "hidden agenda" if the patient is interrupted. Once the patient has listed the concerns, the patient and physician can then decide which ones will be addressed.

2. **How can the physician understand more clearly what the patient is trying to describe?**
    By rephrasing the response in the physician's words or simply restating what the patient said. Sometimes the physician simply needs to ask, "Can you find other words to describe your pain?" Emotional responses and pain are particularly difficult to put into words.

3. **What questions help characterize a symptom?**
    - Where does the symptom occur?
    - What does it feel like?
    - When does the symptom occur?
    - How is it affected by other things you do?
    - Why does the symptom occur (what brings the symptom on)?
    - What makes the symptom better?

EVALUATING THE TESTS

4. **Define "sensitivity" and "specificity" of tests.**
   - **Sensitivity:** The percentage of patients who have the disease that is being tested and have a positive test result
   - **Specificity:** The percentage of patients who do not have the disease and have a negative test result

5. **What are the positive and negative predictive values of tests?**
   - **Positive predictive value:** The percentage of patients who have a positive test and have the disease that is being tested
   - **Negative predictive value:** The percentage of patients who have a negative test and do not have the disease

6. **How are these values calculated?**
   See Figure 2-1.

		Disease: Present	Disease: Absent
Test result	+	a	b
	–	c	d

a = True positive

b = False positive

c = False negative

d = True negative

Sensitivity = $\frac{a}{a+c}$ = Percentage of patients who have the disease and test positive

Specificity = $\frac{d}{b+d}$ = Percentage of persons who do not have the disease and test negative (True-Negative).

Positive predictive value = $\frac{a}{a+b}$ = Percentage of patients who test positive and actually do have the disease.

Negative predictive value = $\frac{d}{c+d}$ = Percentage of patients who test negative and really do not have the disease.

Figure 2-1. Calculation of sensitivity, specificity, and predictive value.

7. **What is the NNT?**
   The number needed to treat that quantifies the number of patients who will require treatment with a therapy (and who will have no benefit) in order to ensure that at least one of the adverse events that the therapy should prevent does not occur. Most publications now include this number. There is no absolute NNT that is appropriate for all therapeutic decisions, but it will depend on the risks of the therapy, the benefits of treatment, and the patient's goals for treatment.

SCREENING FOR MALIGNANCIES

8. **What are the recommendations for colon cancer screening?**
   The U.S. Preventive Services Task Force (USPSTF) recommends one of three screening procedures beginning at age 50–75 years. For patients of *average risk:*

- Annual fecal occult blood test (FOBT) with a sensitive test
- Flexible sigmoidoscopy every 5 years, with sensitive FOBT every 3 years
- Colonoscopy every 10 years

Screening should end at age 85 years, and it is recommended on an individual basis for patients aged 76–84 years. Immunochemical tests are now currently available for FOBT screening. Other organizations such as the American Cancer Society and American Gastroenterology Association have different recommendations.

Levin B, Lieberman DA, McFarland B, et al: Screening and surveillance for the early detection of colorectal cancer and adenomatous polyps, 2008: A joint guideline from the American Cancer Society, the U.S. Multi-Society Task Force on Colorectal Cancer, and the American College of Radiology, *CA Cancer J Clin* 58:130–160, 2008.

U.S. Preventive Services Task Force: Screening for colorectal cancer: U.S. Preventive Services Task Force recommendation statement, *Ann Intern Med* 149:627–637, 2008.

Rex DK, Johnson DA, Anderson JC, et al: American College of Gastroenterology guidelines for colorectal cancer screening 2008, *Am J Gastroenterol* 104:739–750, 2009.

9. **What are the guidelines for breast cancer screening?**
In 2009, the guidelines for mammography screening from the USPSTF were changed to allow for more patient and physician discretion for patient selection for breast cancer screening in women of *average risk.* The Task Force recommended against routine screening in women aged 40-49 years and suggested biennial screening (if appropriate and desired by the patient) for patients aged 50–74 years. The benefits of screening in women > 75 years old are unknown owing to lack of evidence. Other groups have suggested that women of average risk continue to receive annual mammograms, starting at an earlier age.

American Cancer Society responds to changes to USPSTF mammography guidelines: *The American Cancer Society guidelines will not change; annual mammography recommended for women 40 and over.* Available at www.cancer.org/docroot/med/content/med_2_1x_american_cancer_society_responds_to_changes_to_uspstf_mammography_guidelines.asp. Accessed June 12, 2010.

U.S. Preventive Services Task Force: Screening for breast cancer: U.S. Preventive Services Task Force Recommendation Statement, *Ann Intern Med* 151:716–726, 2009.

10. **How should childhood cancer survivors be screened for breast cancer?**
For this group who likely received chest radiation, mammography should begin at age 25 years or 8 years after chest radiation exposure, whichever is earlier. Mammograms should be continued annually.

Oeffinger KC, Ford JS, Mokowitz CS, et al: Breast cancer surveillance practices among women previously treated with chest radiation for a childhood cancer, *JAMA* 301:404–414, 2009.

11. **What are the controversies related to prostate cancer screening?**
The prostate-specific antigen (PSA) currently used for prostate cancer screening does not have sufficient evidence to support its routine use in men of *average risk* for prostate cancer. False-positive and false-negative PSA tests occur. The evidence is also unclear as to whether treatment of prostate cancer, when discovered, prolongs life. Prostate cancer screening decisions should be made on an individual basis. As with mammograms, not all expert groups concur with the USPSTF recommendations. Currently trials are under way to try to more clearly identify appropriate prostate cancer screening tests.

Screening for Prostate Cancer, Topic Page. *U.S. Preventive Services Task Force*, Rockville, MD, 2008, Agency for Healthcare Research and Quality. Available at http://www.ahrq.gov/clinic/uspstf/uspsprca.htm.

12. **When should screening begin for cervical cancer?**
At age 21 years or within 3 years after the onset of sexual activity, whichever is sooner. A Papanicolaou (Pap) smear is the appropriate screening test. After two or three negative

Pap smears, the screening interval may be lengthened to every 3 years. The USPSTF recommends ending screening in women after age 65 years if they have had appropriate routine screening.

Screening for Cervical Cancer, Topic Page. *U.S. Preventive Services Task Force*, Rockville, MD, 2003, Agency for Healthcare Research and Quality. Available at www.ahrq.gov/clinic/uspstf/uspscerv.htm.

13. **Do women who have had a total hysterectomy (with cervix removal) for nonmalignant reasons need Pap smears?**
No. The yield of finding significant disease in this population is low.

14. **Is there an effective screening test for ovarian cancer?**
No, not at this time, although this is an area of active research. Although the pelvic examination, transvaginal ultrasound, and the tumor marker CA-125 have all been used as screening tests, none has been shown to reduce death from the disease.

15. **What is the role of chest x-rays and computed tomography (CT) scans in lung cancer screening?**
The National Cancer Institute is currently sponsoring the National Lung Screening Trial (NLST) to evaluate this question. Early results suggest that screening may reduce lung cancer mortality by 20%. CT scanning is probably helpful. Early results from the NLST suggest a 20% reduction in lung cancer mortality in subjects screened with CT scans. The NLST compares the efficacy of chest x-ray and CT scan in early cancer detection. The data are currently undergoing further analysis.

Available at: http://www.cancer.gov/nlst/updates

CARDIOLOGY

16. **What is the first step to evaluate a patient with an initial blood pressure (BP) reading of 150/90 mmHg?**
Confirm that the BP was measured under the right conditions with:
- The patient seated comfortably in a chair
- The patient's legs uncrossed
- Support of patient's back and arm for BP measurement
- All clothing removed that covers the area of the cuff placement
- Middle of the cuff on the upper arm at the midpoint of the sternum
- Allowance of approximately 5 minutes after the patient is seated comfortably before measuring the BP
- Adequate cuff size for the patient's arm (cuff bladder length is 80% and width is 40% of the patient's arm circumference)
- Measurement of the BP in both arms if initial visit

Pickering TG, Hall JE, Appel LJ, et al: Recommendations for blood pressure measurement in humans and experimental animals: Part 1: Blood pressure measurement in humans: A statement for professionals from the Subcommittee of Professional and Public Education of the AHA Council on HBP, *Circulation* 111:697–716, 2005.

17. **What can cause a difference in BP between the right and the left arm?**
Arterial occlusion in the arm with the lower BP. "Normal" BP difference should be < 10 mmHg. The arm with the higher reading should be used for future measurements.

18. **Should systolic BP between 120 and 139 and/or diastolic BP between 80 and 89 be treated?**
Yes, with lifestyle modification. BP readings such as these are called "prehypertension" and are associated with increased risk of cardiovascular events. Pharmacologic therapy should be initiated if the BP increases to the hypertensive range (systolic ≥ 140 or diastolic ≥ 90).

Chobanian AV, Bakris GL, Black HR, et al: The Seventh Report of the Joint National Committee on Prevention, Detection, Evaluation, and Treatment of High Blood Pressure: The JNC 7 Report, *JAMA* 289:2560, 2003.

19. **What lifestyle modifications are helpful for reducing BP?**
   - Weight loss (to body mass index [BMI] of 18.5–24.9)
   - Salt restriction (<6 g sodium chloride or <2.5 g sodium)
   - Limited alcohol use (12 oz of beer, 5 oz of wine, 1.5 oz of 80-proof whiskey)
   - Stress management
   - Smoking cessation
   - Regular aerobic exercise
   - Low–saturated fat diet rich in fruits and vegetables

U.S. Department of Health and Human Services: Your guide to lowering your blood pressure with DASH. National Heart, Lung, and Blood Institute. NIH Publication No. 06-4082. Originally printed 1998. Revised April 2006. Available at: www.nhlbi.nih.gov/health/public/heart/hbp/dash/new_dash.pdf.

20. **What are the risks of prehypertension?**
   Coronary artery disease, myocardial infarction, and death from a cardiovascular event.

21. **What is the initial laboratory evaluation of newly diagnosed hypertension (HTN)?**
   - Glucose
   - Hematocrit
   - Fasting lipid panel
   - Potassium
   - Creatinine
   - Calcium
   - Electrocardiogram

22. **How can the patient's history identify secondary HTN due to medications and other substance use?**
   Ask the patient about use of:
   - **Over-the-counter medications:** decongestants, stimulants, appetite suppressants, nonsteroidal anti-inflammatory drugs (NSAIDs), and caffeine
   - **Prescription medications:** NSAIDs, corticosteroids, antidepressants (venlafaxine, desvenlafaxine, bupropion), cyclosporine, oral contraceptive pills (OCPs)
   - **Illicit drug use (acute and chronic):** cocaine, amphetamines, stimulants, MDMA (3,4-methylenedioxymethamphetamine or ecstasy), PCP (phencyclidine), cannabis (marijuana), and herbal designer drugs
   - **Alcoholism:** alcohol history, CAGE questionnaire (see Question 155), family history of alcoholism

23. **How can the patient's history identify secondary HTN due to an endocrine disorder?**
   Ask the patient about:
   - **Cushing's syndrome:** weight gain, central obesity, easy bruising, "moon" facies, abdominal striae.
   - **Hyperthyrodism:** weight loss, tachycardia, nervousness
   - **Hypothyroidism:** weight gain, fatigue, constipation, dry skin
   - **Pheochromocytoma:** labile HTN, sweating, headache, palpitations
   - **Hyperaldosteronism:** fatigue, muscle weakness due to low potassium

24. **List two elements in the history that may suggest secondary HTN due to sleep apnea.**
   Snoring and daytime sleepiness. (See also Chapter 6, Pulmonary Medicine.)

KEY POINTS: RISK FACTORS FOR CORONARY ARTERY DISEASE IN PATIENTS WITH HYPERLIPIDEMIA ✔

1. Cigarette smoking

2. Hypertension

3. Low HDL (<40 mg/dL)

4. Family history of premature CAD (father or brother < 55 yr; mother or sister < 65 yr)

5. Age ≥ 45 yr (men) and ≥ 55 yr (women)

CAD = coronary artery disease; HDL = high-density lipoprotein.

25. **What findings suggest renal artery stenosis?**
    - Presence of peripheral vascular disease
    - Periumbilical bruit
    - HTN resistant to multiple drug therapy
    - Worsening of renal function after initiation of angiotensin-converting enzyme (ACE) inhibitor or angiotensin receptor blocker (ARB)
    - Initial diagnosis of HTN in patient < 35 years of age or > 65 years of age
    - Sudden onset of pulmonary edema

26. **Which patients should be screened for primary aldosteronism?**
    Those with:
    - HTN associated with unexplained hypokalemia or hypokalemia associated with low-dose diuretic therapy
    - HTN resistant to multidrug (three-drug) therapy
    - HTN associated with adrenal incidentaloma (adrenal lesion noted on imaging study done for another reason)

    Funder JW, Carey RM, Fardella C, et al: Case detection, diagnosis, and treatment of patients with primary aldosteronism: An Endocrine Society clinical practice guideline, *J Clin Endocrinol Metab* 93:3266–3281, 2008.

27. **What do paroxysmal and postural HTN suggest?**
    Pheochromocytoma, which is a rare tumor of the adrenal gland that produces excess adrenaline and arises from the central portion of the adrenal gland.

28. **What are the signs and symptoms of pheochromocytoma?**
    - Paroxysmal HTN
    - Excessive sweating
    - Palpitations
    - Anxiety
    - Nervousness
    - Tremulousness
    - Heat intolerance
    - Resistant HTN

29. **What causes of secondary HTN can be detected by physical examination?**
    - **Aortic insufficiency:** diastolic murmur
    - **Aortic coarctation:** diminished femoral pulses and bruit best heard over the back
    - **Renovascular disease:** periumbilical bruit
    - **Subclavian stenosis:** BP difference > 10 mmHg between right and left arms

- **Cushing's syndrome:** abdominal striae, "buffalo hump," "moon" facies
- **Hyperthyroidism:** thyroid nodularity or tenderness
- **Sleep apnea:** obesity, particularly of neck
- **Alcoholism:** spider angiomata, hepatomegaly, gynecomastia

30. **Can licorice ingestion elevate the BP?**
Yes, although glycyrrhizic acid is found only in confectioner's black licorice. Most commercially sold licorice in the United States does not contain significant amounts, although glycyrrhizic acid may be found in chewing tobacco.

31. **What is the target BP for HTN treatment?**
In general, <140/90 mmHg. Lower target levels may be indicated for patients with significant risk factors for cardiovascular complications. More recent studies suggest that, although intensive BP control in diabetics reduce cardiovascular risk, there may be an increased risk of serious adverse events.

   The ACCORD Study Group: Effects of intensive blood-pressure control in type 2 diabetes mellitus, *N Engl J Med* 362:1575–1581, 2010.

32. **What antihypertensives are useful for patients at risk of recurrent stroke?**
Thiazide diuretics and ACE inhibitors.

33. **Which lipids can be measured without fasting?**
Total cholesterol and high-density lipoprotein (HDL) cholesterol. Low-density lipoprotein (LDL) cholesterol is calculated from the fasting triglyceride level, and total and HDL cholesterol levels are calculated by the following formula:

$$\text{LDL cholesterol} = \text{Total cholesterol} - (\text{HDL cholesterol} + \text{Triglycerides}/5)$$

34. **What are the guidelines for treating cholesterol?**
Treatment initiation values and treatment goals are based on the patient's underlying risk factors (age, tobacco use, HTN, family history, and low HDL) and coronary artery disease (CAD) risk equivalents. (CAD risk equivalents are symptomatic heart disease, known atherosclerotic disease in other vessels, and diabetes mellitus [DM].) See Table 2-1.

TABLE 2-1. TREATMENT GUIDELINES AND GOALS FOR ELEVATED CHOLESTEROL		
No. of Risk Factors* or CAD Risk Equivalents[†]	LDL Goal (mg/dL)	LDL Level for Initiation of Drug Therapy (mg/dL)
Known CAD or CAD risk equivalent	<100	≥130 (100–129: drug optional)
2+	<130	≥130 if 10-yr risk 10–20% ≥160 if 10-yr risk < 10%
0–1	<160	≥190 (160–189: drug optional)

CAD = coronary artery disease; HDL = high-density lipoprotein; LDL = low-density lipoprotein.
*Tobacco use, hypertension, low HDL cholesterol, family history of premature CAD, and age ≥ 45 yr (men) and ≥ 55 yr (women).
[†]Diabetes mellitus, symptomatic heart disease, known atherosclerotic disease, and abdominal aortic aneurysm.
From Grundy SM, Cleeman JI, Bairey Merz CN: Implications of recent clinical trials for the National Cholesterol Education Program Adult Treatment Panel III Guidelines. Circulation 110:227–239, 2004.

KEY POINTS: ATHEROSCLEROTIC DISEASES ASSOCIATED WITH HIGH RISK OF CORONARY ARTERY DISEASE ✓

1. Symptomatic carotid artery disease

2. Peripheral arterial disease

3. Abdominal aortic aneurysm

35. **How is the risk of a cardiac event calculated?**
    The risk assessment tool from the Framingham Heart Study can be calculated online and includes assessment based on sex, age, total cholesterol, tobacco use, HDL cholesterol level, and systolic BP (treated or untreated).

    Available at http://hp2010.nhlbihin.net/atpiii/calculator.asp?usertype=prof.

36. **List the lipid-lowering agents.**
    See Table 2-2.

37. **What is the New York Heart Association (NYHA) classification of congestive heart failure?**
    The NYHA classifies patients with known cardiac disease into four classes based on functional capacity and objective assessment (Table 2-3).

38. **What is Takotsubo cardiomyopathy?**
    Acute, reversible left ventricular dysfunction occurring in postmenopausal women after sudden and unexpected emotional or physical stress. The syndrome is also called "apical ballooning" or "stress cardiomyopathy." The syndrome likely results from high levels of catecholamines related to the acute stress.

    Akashi YJ, Goldstein DS, Barbaro G, et al: Takotsubo cardiomyopathy. A new form of acute, reversible heart failure, *Circulation* 118:2754–2762, 2008.

39. **What are the characteristics of an innocent heart murmur? Mitral valve prolapse (MVP) murmur?**
    See Table 2-4.

40. **List the cardiac conditions that require prophylactic antibiotics when a patient has a dental procedure.**
    - Prosthetic cardiac valve or presence of prosthetic material used for cardiac valve repair
    - Previous infectious endocarditis (IE)
    - Congenital heart disease (CHD)
      - Unrepaired cyanotic CHD
      - Completely repaired congenital heart defect with prosthetic material or device during the first 6 months after the procedure (either surgery or catheterization)
      - Repaired CHD with residual defects
    - Cardiac transplantation recipients who develop valvular disease

    These recommendations were updated in 2007, and antibiotic prophylaxis is no longer recommended for other cardiac conditions.

    Wilson W, Taubert KA, Gewitz M, et al: Prevention of infective endocarditis: Guidelines from the American Heart Association: From the American Heart Association Rheumatic Fever, Endocarditis, and Kawasaki Disease Committee, Council on Cardiovascular Disease in the Young, and the Council on Clinical Cardiology, Council on Cardiovascular Surgery and Anesthesia, and the Quality of Care and Outcomes research Interdisciplinary Working Group, *Circulation* 116:1736–1754, 2007.

TABLE 2-2. LIPID-LOWERING AGENTS

Class	Drugs	Mechanism	TG	LDL	HDL	Side Effects
HMG-CoA reductase inhibitors or "statins" (drugs of choice for lowering LDL)	Fluvastatin Pravastatin Lovastatin Simvastatin Atorvastatin Rosuvastatin (in order of ↑ potency)	Inhibits HMG-CoA reductase (rate-limiting enzyme in cholesterol synthesis) ↑ LDL receptor activity	↓, ↓↓ (dose-related)	↓↓↓	↑	Overall well-tolerated ↑ LFTs Rhabdomyolysis Myositis Drug interactions
Cholesterol absorption inhibitor	Ezetamibe	Inhibits cholesterol absorption from gut	↔	↓↓	↔	↑ LFTs (w/statins) GI upset/bloating
Bile acid resins	Colestipol Cholestyramine Colesevelam	Bind bile acids ↑ Hepatic LDL receptor activity	↔, ↑	↓↓	↑	Constipation Steatorrhea Bloating Bind other drugs
Fibrates (drugs of choice for lowering TG)	Clofibrate Gemfibrozil Fenofibrate	↓ VLDL synthesis ↑ VLDL clearance	↓↓↓	↔, ↓*	↑	Overall well-tolerated Gallstones Myopathy Drug interactions
Bile acid resins	Colestipol Cholestyramine Colesevelam	Bind bile acids ↑ Hepatic LDL receptor activity	↔, ↑	↓↓	↑	Constipation Steatorrhea Bloating Bind other drugs

(continued)

TABLE 2-2. LIPID-LOWERING AGENTS— *(continued)*

Class	Drugs	Mechanism	TG	LDL	HDL	Side Effects
Nicotinic acid (drug of choice for raising HDL)	Crystalline niacin Niaspan (long-acting niacin)	↓ VLDL secretion ↓ Adipose lipolysis	↓↓	↓	↑↑	Flushing with short-acting form ↑ LFTs Glucose intolerance Hyperuricemia Rash
Omega 3 fatty acids	Fish oils	↓ VLDL synthesis and secretion	↓↓	?	?	Glucose intolerance Smell like fish

GI = gastrointestinal; HDL = high-density lipoprotein; HMG-CoA = 3-hydroxy-3-methylglutaryl coenzyme A; LDL = low-density lipoprotein; LFTs = liver function tests; TG = triglyceride; VLDL = very low density lipoprotein.
*Fenofibrate has more LDL-lowering effect than gemfibrozil.

TABLE 2-3. NEW YORK HEART ASSOCIATION CLASSIFICATION OF CONGESTIVE HEART FAILURE

Class	Functional Capacity (Limitation of Physical Activity)	Objective Assessment (Evidence of Cardiovascular Disease)
I	None	None
II	Slight	Minimal
III	Marked	Moderately severe
IV	Inability to carry on any activity without symptoms	Severe

TABLE 2-4. INNOCENT HEART MURMUR VERSUS MURMUR DUE TO MITRAL VALVE PROLAPSE

Characteristic	Innocent Murmur	MVP Murmur
Location	Base	Apex
Intensity	<3/6	>2/6
Timing in cardiac cycle	Early systole	Mid-to-late systole
Response to standing	Decreased	Begins earlier in systole
Response to Valsalva	Decreases	May increase
Associated findings	None	Midsystolic click

41. **What other procedures require antibiotic prophylaxis for high-risk patients?**
    - Upper respiratory procedures that require incision or biopsy (tonsillectomy and adenoidectomy)
    - Procedures on infected skin and musculoskeletal tissue

42. **Is antibiotic prophylaxis indicated for procedures such as cystoscopy, prostate surgery, intestinal surgery, and colonoscopy in high-risk patients?**
    No.

    Wilson W, Taubert KA, Gewitz M, et al: Prevention of infective endocarditis: Guidelines from the American Heart Association: From the American Heart Association Rheumatic Fever, Endocarditis, and Kawasaki Disease Committee, Council on Cardiovascular Disease in the Young, and the Council on Clinical Cardiology, Council on Cardiovascular Surgery and Anesthesia, and the Quality of Care and Outcomes research Interdisciplinary Working Group, *Circulation* 116:1736–1754, 2007.

43. **Which dental procedures require endocarditis prophylaxis?**
    Those that involve manipulation of gingival tissues or periapical region of the teeth or any perforation of the oral mucosa.

44. **What antibiotics are used for prophylaxis for endocarditis?**
    See Table 2-5.

TABLE 2-5. ANTIMICROBIAL PROPHYLAXIS FOR THE PREVENTION OF BACTERIAL ENDOCARDITIS IN PATIENTS WITH UNDERLYING HIGH-RISK CARDIAC CONDITIONS UNDERGOING DENTAL PROCEDURES

Able to Take Oral Medications?	Allergic to Penicillin or Ampicillin?	Antibiotic	Dosage*
Yes	No	Amoxicillin	2 g
No	No	Ampicillin OR	2 g IM or IV
		Cefazoline or ceftriaxone	2 g
Yes	Yes	Cephalaxin[†‡] OR	2 g
		Clindamycin OR	600 mg
		Azithromycin or clarithromycin	500 mg
No	Yes	Cefazolin or ceftriaxone[†]	1 g IM or IV
		Clindamycin	600 mg IM or IV

IM = intramuscular; IV = intravenous.
*Given as single dose 30–60 min before procedure.
[†]Or another first- or second-generation oral cephalosporin.
[‡]Do not use a cephalosporin in a patient with a history of anaphylactic-, uriticarial-, or angioedema-type reaction to penicillin.
From Wilson W, Taubert KA, Gewitz M, et al: Prevention of infective endocarditis: guidelines from the American Heart Association: from the American Heart Association Rheumatic Fever, Endocarditis, and Kawasaki Disease Committee, Council on Cardiovascular Disease in the Young, and the Council on Clinical Cardiology, Council on Cardiovascular Surgery and Anesthesia, and the Quality of Care and Outcomes research Interdisciplinary Working Group. Circulation 116:1736–1754, 2007.

45. **What are the common causes of atrial fibrillation?**
Alcohol use (especially binge drinking), thyrotoxicosis, congestive heart failure, myocardial ischemia or infarction, pulmonary embolism, illicit or over-the-counter stimulant use, mitral valve disease, Wolff-Parkinson-White (WPW) syndrome, hypertensive cardiomyopathy, digoxin toxicity.

46. **What range of the International Normalized Ratio (INR) is the target treatment for most patients receiving anticoagulation for atrial fibrillation?**
2.0–3.0.

47. **If medications are taken with grapefruit juice, the absorption and blood level of the medication may be increased, resulting in toxicity. Which medications show this effect?**

Alprazolam	Buspirone	Dextromethorphan
Amiodarone	Carbamazepine	Diltiazem
Benzodiazepines	Cyclosporine	Erythromycin

Estrogens	Itraconazole	Sildenafil
Felodipine	Methylprednisone	Theophylline
Fexofenadine	Nicardipine	Verapamil
Fluoxetine	Nifedipine	Warfarin
3-hydroxy-3-methylglutaryl coenzyme A (HMG-CoA reductase inhibitors)	Nimodipine	
	Nisoldipine	
	Quinidine	
	Saquinavir	
	Sertraline	

48. **How much grapefruit juice can be consumed by patients on these medications?**
One cup of juice or ½ grapefruit is probably safe if taken at a different time from the medication.

Drug interactions with grapefruit juice. *Med Lett* 46:2–3, 2004.

49. **Which is a greater risk factor for cardiovascular disease: cigarette smoking or obesity?**
Cigarette smoking.

DERMATOLOGY

50. **List your treatment recommendations to an adolescent with mild, mixed noninflammatory acne (primarily comedones or "blackheads" and inflammatory acne [pustules and papules]).**
- Avoid oily cosmetics.
- Do not rub the face.
- Use sunscreen.
- Use mild cleansing soap.
- Apply topical retinoic acid cream (or gel).
- Apply topical antimicrobials.
- Consider topical benzoyl peroxide with topical antimicrobial to limit antibiotic resistance.
- Can use salicylic acid as alternative to topical retinoid.

51. **What OCPs are approved for acne treatment?**
- Norgestimate and ethinyl estradiol (Ortho Tri-Cyclen)
- Ethinyl estradiol 20 μg/drospirenone 3 mg (Yaz)
- Ethinyl estradiol and norethindrone (Estrostep)

52. **Define "hidradenitis suppurativa" and "erythrasma."**
- **Hidradenitis suppurativa:** An apocrine sweat gland infection of the axilla, groin, breasts, or buttocks that can cause inflammation and scarring
- **Erythrasma**: A skin infection caused by *Corynebacterium minutissimum* that occurs in the axilla or groin or sometimes between the toes

53. **How do you recognize tinea versicolor (pityriasis)?**
As macular lesions of various colors such as red, pink, or brown. Slight scale may be present. Involved areas do not tan and are hypopigmented.

54. **How do you treat pityriasis?**
With topical corticosteroids for severe itching. Usually no treatment is needed, but acyclovir may be helpful for severe itching or cosmetic reasons.

Drago F, Veechio F, Rebora A: Use of high-dose acyclovir in pityriasis rosea, *J Am Acad Dermatol* 54:82–85, 2006.

55. **What is the ABCDE rule for melanoma?**
    Skin lesions are likely melanoma if these characteristics are present:
    - **A**symmetry
    - **B**order irregularity
    - **C**olor variation (usually purple or black)
    - **D**iameter > 6 mm
    - **E**nlargement of volution of color change, shape, or symptoms

    Abbasi NR, Shaw HM, Rigel DS, et al: Early diagnosis of cutaneous melanoma: revisiting the ABCD criteria, *JAMA* 292:2771–2776, 2004.

ENDOCRINOLOGY

56. **Describe the typical follow-up examination for a patient with non–insulin-dependent DM.**
    - **History:** Ask about the frequency, cause, and severity of hypoglycemic or hyperglycemic episodes. Review home glucose monitoring records if used. Update medication list. Ask about any recent illnesses. Review diet and life stressors. Review contraception choices for women of child-bearing potential.
    - **Physical examination:** Weight, BP, annual foot examination (including inspection for lesions and callouses, assessment of sensation, and palpation of pedal pulses). Confirm annual ophthalmologic examination. Confirm annual dental examination.

57. **What laboratory testing should be ordered during follow-up visits?**
    - Glycohemoglobin (HgbA$_1$C) quarterly
    - Lipids, including triglycerides, total cholesterol, HDL cholesterol, LDL cholesterol
    - Liver function tests if taking statin or thiazolidinedione drugs
    - Urinalysis with annual testing for protein or microalbumin if proteinuria is absent

58. **What immunizations do diabetics need?**
    - Pneumococcal vaccine every 5 years
    - Annual influenza vaccination
    - Tetanus booster every 10 years (see Question 114 for specific vaccine choice)

KEY POINTS: COUNSELING FOR PATIENTS WITH DIABETES ✓

1. Exercise

2. Diet

3. Foot care

4. Medication adjustment when ill

5. Regular ophthalmologic follow-up

6. Regular dental follow-up

7. Up-to-date immunizations

8. Smoking cessation

9. Management of hypoglycemic and hyperglycemic episodes

59. **What test is most useful for monitoring thyroid replacement therapy?**
    Thyroid-stimulating hormone (TSH).

60. **List the skin findings of hyperthyroidism.**
    - Warm, moist, "velvety" texture of skin
    - Increased palmar or dorsal sweating
    - Facial flushing
    - Palmar erythema
    - Vitiligo
    - Altered hair texture
    - Alopecia
    - Pretibial myxedema

61. **What are the skin findings in hypothyroidism?**
    - Decreased sweating
    - Color changes to skin
    - Coarse hair or hair loss
    - Brittle nails
    - Pretibial myxedema (due to hypothyroidism resulting from treatment of Graves' disease)
    - Generalized nonpitting edema (myxedema)
    - Periorbital edema

62. **When should thyroid antibodies be ordered?**
    To distinguish Hashimoto's thyroiditis (and likely permanent hypothyroidism) from subclinical hypothyroidism, painless thyroiditis, or postpartum thyroiditis.

63. **What thyroid antibody test is ordered?**
    Thyroid peroxidase antibody.

64. **What are the thyroid effects of lithium?**
    - Goiter
    - Hypothyroidism
    - Chronic autoimmune thyroiditis
    - Hyperthyroidism (uncommon)

65. **How is hypothyroidism due to lithium detected?**
    By an elevated TSH. Hypothyroidism is most likely to occur in the first 2 years of therapy and is more common in women > 45 years of age.

66. **What are the risk factors for osteoporosis?**
    Women ≥ 65 years old, men ≥ 70 years old, postmenopausal state, medication use (glucocorticoids, chronic heparin, vitamin A, cyclosporine, methotrexate, anticonvulsants, thyroid replacement, and anxiolytics), chronic illnesses (systemic lupus erythematosus, rheumatoid arthritis, psoriatic arthritis, cancer treatment, cystic fibrosis, inflammatory bowel disease, celiac disease, hyperthyroidism, hypogonadism, vitamin D deficiency, and chronic liver disease), positive family history, cigarette smoking, excessive caffeine, low body weight, above average height, and lack of exercise.

67. **What is the role of estrogen-progesterone therapy in prevention and treatment of osteoporosis?**
    Although estrogen-progesterone therapy has been shown to reduce fracture risk in postmenopausal women, recent data from the Women's Health Initiative (WHI) suggest that the risks of cardiac events, breast cancer, and stroke are increased in treated women and outweigh potential benefit.

68. **How should you instruct patients to take a biphosphonate?**
    - Take weekly or monthly preparation.
    - Take the pill first thing in the morning with a full glass of water.
    - Do not take with other pills or food.
    - Do not eat, drink, or swallow any other pills for 30 minutes.
    - Maintain upright posture (either sitting or standing) for 30 minutes.

69. **What are some of the side effects of biphosphonate therapy?**
    - Esophageal ulceration, gastritis, and gastroesophageal reflux disease
    - Joint and muscle pain and long bone fracture (mid-shaft)
    - Osteonecrosis of the jaw
    - Increased risk of atrial fibrillation

70. **Which medications are associated with an increased risk of fracture?**
    - Glucocorticoids
    - Thiazolidinediones (rosiglitazone and pioglitazone)
    - Annual high-dose oral vitamin D (500,000 IU)

    Loke YK, Singh S, Furberg CD, et al: Long-term use of thiazolidinediones and fractures in type 2 diabetes: A meta-analysis, *CMAJ* 280:32–39, 2009.

    Yu-Xiao Y, Lewis JD, Epstein S, et al: Long-term proton pump inhibitor therapy and risk of hip fracture, *JAMA* 296:2947–2953, 2006.

71. **What is the BMI?**
    Body mass index. The BMI gives an estimate of risk of complications of obesity because it relates weight to height. It can be obtained from tables or normograms. Ideal BMI is < 25.

72. **List the complications of morbid obesity.**
    - HTN
    - Coronary artery disease
    - Impaired glucose tolerance (metabolic syndrome)
    - DM
    - Increased mortality from all causes, including cancer
    - Sleep apnea
    - Osteoarthritis
    - Depression
    - Recurrent skin infections (particularly intertriginous areas)

73. **Are gastric bypass procedures effective for treatment of morbid obesity?**
    Yes. Bariatric surgery has been shown to reduce the complications of obesity including DM, sleep apnea, HTN, and hyperlipidemia. The procedures are most effective with patients with BMI > 40, but may also be beneficial in those with significant complications of obesity and BMI > 35.

    Maggared MA, Shugarman LR, Suttopr M, et al: Meta-analysis: Surgical treatment of obesity, *Ann Intern Med* 142:547–559, 2005.

74. **What initial tests should be done to evaluate involuntary weight loss?**
    - Thorough interview to identify underlying depression or eating disorder
    - Complete blood count (CBC)
    - Electrolytes, glucose, calcium, liver function tests, blood urea nitrogen (BUN), and creatinine
    - TSH
    - Human immunodeficiency virus (HIV)
    - Erythrocyte sedimentation rate (ESR) or C-reactive protein (CRP)
    - Chest x-ray

    Additional testing will be guided by the results of additional history, physical examination, and these tests.

GASTROENTEROLOGY

75. **What medications can cause chronic constipation?**

   Calcium channel blockers
   Antihistamines
   Opiates
   Iron
   Tricyclic antidepressants
   Anticholinergics
   Aluminum- and calcium-based antacids
   Calcium supplements
   Sucralfate
   Disopyramide
   Laxatives (if abused)

76. **What is the treatment of chronic constipation?**
   - Regular exercise.
   - Establishment of regular bowel schedules. The gastrocolic reflex and urge to have a bowel movement are greatest about 30 minutes after breakfast.
   - Adjustment of dose or discontinuance of medications that contribute to constipation, if possible.
   - Bulk-forming agents (psyllium, methylcellulose, and polycarbophil) that should be taken with adequate fluids.
   - Hyperosmolar agents (lactulose, sorbitol, and polyethylene glycol).
   - Stimulant laxatives (senna and bisacodyl) as needed.

   Lubiprostone is an approved medicine for the treatment of women with irritable bowel syndrome who have constipation as the main symptom and can also be used for chronic constipation. Lubiprostone improves the frequency of bowel movements and reduces straining and bloating. Side effects include nausea, headache, abdominal pain, and diarrhea.

KEY POINTS: SYMPTOMS OF IRRITABLE BOWEL SYNDROME DISEASE ✔

1. Abdominal pain

2. Altered bowel habits (diarrhea or constipation)

3. Abdominal bloating

4. Excessive belching or flatulence

5. Dyspepsia

6. Early satiety

7. Nausea

8. Heartburn

9. Noncardiac pain

77. **Define "proctalgia fugax."**
   A fleeting, deep pain in the rectum, possibly caused by muscle spasm. Tenderness is found on digital rectal examination.

78. **What NSAIDs have the greatest risk of gastrointestinal (GI) symptoms?**
   Piroxicam and ketorolac. Ibuprofen has a low risk of GI bleeding, and cyclooxygenase-2 (COX-2) inhibitors have the lowest risk.

Gonzalez EM, Patrignani P, Tacconelli S, et al: Variability among nonsteroidal antiinflammatory drugs in risk of upper gastrointestinal bleeding, *Arthritis Rheum* 62:1592–1601, 2010.

79. **How can the risk of gastric and duodenal ulcers with the use of NSAIDs be decreased?**
    By testing for and treating *Helicobacter pylori* infection in patients with history of peptic ulcer disease and use of proton pump inhibitors.

    Bhatt DL, Scheiman J, Abraham NS, et al: ACCF/ACG/AHA 2008 Expert Consensus Document on Reducing the Gastrointestinal Risks of Antiplatelet Therapy and NSAID Use, *Am J Gastroenterol* 103:1–18, 2008.

80. **What is the effect of omeprazole on clopidogrel?**
    Concurrent use of omeprazole and clopidogrel may result in decreased effectiveness of clopidogrel in reducing thrombotic events.

GYNECOLOGY

81. **What topics should you cover in the history of a 20-year-old, sexually active woman with the complaint of acute dysuria?**
    Ask about hematuria; vaginal discharge; flank pain; fever; chills; last menses; previous medical history including DM, gynecologic surgeries, urologic procedures, pregnancy, and recent antibiotic use; current sexual activity; use of barrier contraception; use of OCPs; illness or symptoms in sexual partner; recent new sexual partner; previous sexually transmitted diseases (STDs); and HIV test results, if done.

82. **What should the physical examination include in the same patient?**
    Temperature, pulse, BP, abdominal examination, evaluation for flank tenderness, and bimanual examination if cervicitis or vaginitis or both likely by history.

83. **What laboratory tests should you order for this patient?**
    Urinalysis (dipstick) to examine for leukocyte esterase and hematuris, wet mount of any vaginal discharge and testing for *Chlamydia* spp. and *Neisseria gonorrhoeae* if cervical or adnexal tenderness is present. If the history and examination suggest acute cystitis without complications, empirical treatment can be started with trimethaprim-sulfamethaxole (TMP-SMX), nitrofurantoin, or fosfamycin for 3 days. If the known local *Escherichia coli* resistance > 20%, a fluoroquinolone should be used. If there are risk factors for STDs, doxycycline for 7 days or single-dose azithromycin is the appropriate choice. Urine culture is not necessary for young healthy women without history of recent antibiotic use or recurrent urinary tract infections (UTIs). Older women with underlying medical problems are at greater risk of complications and should have urine culture and antibiotic treatment for 7 days' duration.

84. **List the common causes of abnormal vaginal bleeding in premenopausal women.**

Threatened or complete abortion	Vulvar infection, laceration, or tumor	Uterine infection, polyp, fibroids, or carcinoma
Ectopic pregnancy	Vaginal laceration, tumor, or foreign body	Ovarian infection
Hypothyroidism		Intrauterine device
Hypercortisolism	Cervical infection, erosion, polyp, or carcinoma	Idiopathic
Polycystic ovary syndrome		
Thrombocytopenia		
Bleeding diathesis		

85. **How do you manage a woman with postmenopausal vaginal bleeding?**
With referral to a gynecologist for consideration of diagnostic studies to detect endometrial carcinoma.

86. **What is the interpretation of ASC-US result on Pap smear?**
Atypical squamous cells of uncertain insignificance. Women > 20 years should have testing for human papillomavirus (HPV) and referral for colposcopy and treatment if positive for HPV.

Wright TC Jr, Massad LS, Dunton CJ, et al: 2006 consensus guidelines for the management of women with abnormal cervical cancer screening tests, *Am J Obstet Gynecol* 197:346–355, 2007.

87. **What is the interpretation of ASC-H result on Pap smear?**
Atypical squamous cells in which a high-grade squamous intraepithelial lesion (HSIL) cannot be excluded. These women should be referred for colposcopy and treatment.

88. **List the characteristic vaginal discharges caused by *Candida albicans*, *N. gonorrhoeae*, *Gardnerella vaginalis*, and *Trichomonas vaginalis*.**
See Table 2-6.

TABLE 2-6. CHARACTERISTIC VAGINAL DISEASES OF COMMON INFECTIONS

Organism	Discharge Characteristics
Candida albicans	Thick, white, curdlike, adherent to vaginal wall with satellite lesions and erythema on perineum
Neisseria gonorrhoeae	Mucopurulent with cervicitis
Gardnerella vaginalis (and other organisms)	Foul-smelling ("fishy" with KOH), thin, scanty, white, frothy, and adherent to vaginal wall pH >3.5 and <4.5
Trichomonas vaginalis	Copious, yellow-green, frothy

KOH = potassium hydroxide.

89. **What are clue cells?**
Epithelial cells covered with coccobacilli or curved rods. Clue cells are found in the vaginal discharge of patients with bacterial vaginosis *G*.

90. **What is atrophic vaginitis?**
Symptoms of vaginal burning, pruritus, discharge, bleeding, and dyspareunia in postmenopausal women due to estrogen loss. Topical, intravaginal estrogen can help with symptoms.

91. **What are the absolute contraindications to the use of OCPs?**
- Pregnancy
- Lactation
- Thrombophlebitis
- History of stroke
- History of thromboembolic event
- History of estrogen-dependent tumor (breast and endometrium)

- Active liver disease
- Uterine bleeding of unknown cause
- Hypertriglyceridemia
- Heavy smoking (>15 cigarettes/day) in women > 35 years

92. **What conditions are associated with an increased risk of complications from OCPs?**
    - Uncontrolled HTN
    - DM (may require adjustment of insulin dose)
    - Migraine headaches
    - Use of anticonvulsants (may reduce effectiveness of OCPs)

93. **What are the preventive measures for cervical carcinoma?**
    Safer sex practices and immunization with HPV vaccine. HPV vaccination should begin at age 11–12 years, preferably before sexual activity and HPV exposure. Sexually active females can begin vaccination, and "catch-up" vaccinations can be given during ages 13–26. Males aged 9–26 years can also receive HPV vaccine, if desired. A complete series includes three doses over 8 months.

94. **Describe the evaluation of a new breast nodule discovered in a 50-year-old woman during routine examination.**
    - **History:** Personal history of breast disorders and biopsies; family history of breast, ovarian, or colon cancer; use of hormone replacement therapy; and use of OCPs
    - **Physical examination:** Location, size, mobility, and consistency of nodule; presence or absence of nipple discharge; presence or absence of axillary adenopathy; and complete examination of contralateral breast and axilla
    - **X-ray:** Mammogram with appropriate needle aspiration or biopsy of suspicious lesions
    Most importantly, a new solitary nodule should always be biopsied even if a mammogram is normal.

95. **What is the role of genetic testing in the risk assessment for breast cancer?**
    The gene mutations associated with an increased risk of breast and ovarian cancer (*BRAC1* and *BRAC2*) have been identified and can be commercially tested. The results may be difficult to interpret and women may be unduly concerned or relieved about their breast cancer risk if improperly interpreted. If a woman requests genetic testing because of a perceived increased family risk, she should be referred to a genetic counseling center or specialists where a thorough family history can be obtained and appropriate counseling and testing provided.

96. **What is premenstrual syndrome (PMS)?**
    A group of physical and psychological symptoms that occur approximately 5 days prior to menses consistently during a woman's menstrual cycle and lead to significant social and occupational functioning. Physical symptoms include abdominal bloating, fatigue, breast tenderness, and headaches. Emotional symptoms include depression, irritability, confusion, and feelings of isolation.

97. **What are the treatments for PMS?**
    Selective serotonin reuptake inhibitors (SSRIs) such as fluoxetine, sertraline, paroxetine, and citalopram have the most clinical efficacy when taken daily, as do alprazalom and danazole. Gonadotropin-releasing hormone agonists are helpful, too, but may have significant side effects.

98. **What is PMDD?**
    Premenstrual dysphoric disorder with symptoms of PMS in addition to at least one affective symptom such as anger, irritability, or emotional tension.

HEMATOLOGY

99. Which medications and supplements affect the effects of warfarin?
See Table 2-7.

TABLE 2-7. EFFECTS OF MEDICATIONS AND SUPPLEMENTS ON ANTICOAGULATION EFFECTS OF WARFARIN

Anticoagulant Effect	
Increased (Increased INR)	Decreased (Decreased INR)
Acetaminophen	Antithyroid agents
Allopurinol	Barbiturates
Amiodarone	Bile acid sequestrants
Clopidogrel	Carbamezepine
Cranberry (including juice)	Coenzyme Q10
5-FU	Dicloxacillin
Fenofibrate	Ginseng
Fluconazole	Nafcillin
Fluoroquinolones	Oral contraceptives
Fluvoxamine	St. John's wort
Gingko balboa	Sucralfate
Green tea	
H_2 receptor blockers	
HMG-CoA reductase inhibitors (except atorvastatin)	
Ketoconazole	
Metronidazole	
NSAIDs (COX-2 inhibitors)	
NSAIDs (nonselective)	
Omega 3 fatty acids	
Orlistat	
Phenytoin	
Proton pump inhibitors	
SSRIs	
Trimethoprim-sulfamethoxazole	
Tetracyclines	
Tricyclic antidepressant	
Venlafaxine	
Vitamin A	
Vitamin E	

COX-2 = cyclooxygenase-2; 5-FU = fluorouracil; HMG-CoA = 3-hydroxy-3-methylglutaryl coenzyme A; INR = International Normalized Ratio; NSAIDs = nonsteroidal anti-inflammatory drugs; SSRIs = selective serotonin reuptake inhibitors.

INFECTIOUS DISEASES AND IMMUNIZATION

100. **List the high-risk factors that indicate the need for the pneumococcal polysaccharide vaccine (PPSV).**
   - Age $\geq$ 65 years
   - Chronic cardiovascular disease such as congestive heart failure and cardiomyopathies
   - Chronic pulmonary disease (including asthma, emphysema, and COPD)
   - DM
   - Alcoholism
   - Chronic liver disease, including cirrhosis
   - Cerebrospinal fluid (CSF) leaks
   - Asplenia, either functional or anatomic
   - Immunosuppression including hematologic and generalized malignancy, multiple myeloma, renal failure, organ transplants, chronic corticosteroid use, and HIV infection
   - Cochlear implant
   - Cigarette smoking

101. **Who should receive revaccination with PPSV 5 years after the first dose?**
   Those with:
   - Functional (sickle cell disease) or anatomic (splenectomy) asplenia
   - Immunosuppression
   - Initial vaccination occurring > 5 years previously and aged < 65 years at the time

102. **List the symptoms of influenza.**

Sudden onset of high fever*	Myalgia Headache Malaise	Coryza Sore throat

103. **What are the complications of influenza?**
   - Pneumonia (either primary influenza pneumonia or secondary bacterial pneumonia)
   - Encephalitis and myelitis
   - Hepatitis and pancreatitis
   - Myositis and rhabdomyolysis
   - Asthenia and prolonged fatigue
   - Reye's syndrome (in children and adolescents)

104. **How do you diagnose influenza?**
   By clinical findings supported by community epidemiologic data and confirmed by laboratory testing. Influenza A or B is very likely when a patient presents with the symptoms described in Question 102 during the time when influenza is known to circulate in your community. The Centers for Disease Control and Prevention publishes influenza updates October through May on its website (http://www.cdc.gov/flu/weekly/fluactivitysurv.htm). Local health departments also publish data from the local community. The suspicion of influenza can be confirmed through rapid tests done in the office from nasal or throat swabs. Some rapid tests may only detect influenza A or detect influenza A and B but not distinguish between the two strains.

105. **Briefly describe some of the characteristics of the 2009 H1N1 influenza pandemic.**
   Children < 2 years of age were at increased risk and the highest hospitalization rates occurred among children < 1 year. Pregnant women with H1N1 influenza had a markedly

---

*Although influenza infection may present with mild upper respiratory tract symptoms without fever.

increased rate of hospitalization compared with nonpregnant women. Patient $\geq$ 65 years had the lowest rates of infection, but the highest case fatality rate. The clinical symptoms included influenza-like illness with fever, cough, sore throat, and rhinorrhea. GI symptoms, including diarrhea, nausea, and vomiting, were seen more frequently than in seasonal influenza viral infections.

Writing Committee for the WHO Consultation on Clinical Aspects of Pandemic (H1N1) 2009 Influenza: Clinical aspects of pandemic 2009 influenza A (H1N1) virus infection, *N Engl J Med* 362:1708–1719, 2010.

106. **What are the treatments for influenza?**
The symptoms may be relieved by cough suppressants and acetaminophen. Aspirin should not be used during influenza epidemics. Antiviral agents that reduce the duration and severity of influenza are also indicated for severe disease. Amantadine and rimantadine were the first agents available to treat influenza but are effective only against influenza A and have central nervous system (CNS) side effects, particularly in the elderly. Newer neuroaminadase inhibitors (zanamivir and oseltamivir) are effective against both influenza A and B. Zanamivir is given as an inhaled powder. All of these drugs should be given within the first 48 hours from the onset of symptoms and reduce the symptomatic phase by about 1 day. These treatments may not be effective in severe influenza. Some oseltamivir resistance was noted during the H1N1 pandemic. Intravenous antiviral agents are currently in trial for treatment of patients with severe influenza and were available under compassionate use during the 2009 pandemic.

107. **How do you prevent influenza?**
With seasonal influenza virus vaccine, given annually in the fall in physicians' offices, at the time of hospital discharge, and in local health departments. Many community groups, churches, pharmacies, and groceries also sponsor opportunities to receive vaccine. The vaccine is reformulated each year and should be given annually to ensure protection against the current year's circulating virus. An intranasal preparation was first available for the 2003–2004 influenza season but is recommended at this time only for adults < 50 years who are not contacts of high-risk patients, nonpregnant women < 50 years, children, and patients who are not at high risk for influenza complications. Amantadine, rimantadine, and zanamivir may also be used for prevention in those exposed to influenza before receiving the vaccine or those unable to receive the vaccine.

108. **Which groups at high risk for complications of influenza should receive the seasonal vaccine?**
- Patients with chronic pulmonary disease (including asthma)
- Patients with chronic cardiovascular disease
- Residents of nursing homes or long-term care facilities
- Those $\geq$ 50 years
- Those with chronic medical conditions such as DM, renal dysfunction, hepatic dysfunction, hemoglobinopathies, and immunosuppression (including medication-induced)
- Those with HIV infection
- Those with cognitive, neurologic, or neuromuscular disorders
- Adolescents on long-term aspirin therapy
- Women who are pregnant during influenza season (usually late November to early March)
- Those with asplenia (because of high risk of secondary bacterial infections after influenza viral infection)

109. **Who should receive the seasonal influenza vaccine because of high likelihood of transmitting the virus to high-risk groups?**
- Physicians and allied health professionals, nurses, health professions students with patient contacts, and office and hospital staff with direct patient contact
- Emergency medical personnel

- Home caregivers of high-risk groups including caregivers of children aged < 5 years
- Employees of nursing homes and long-term care facilities
- Household contacts (including children)

110. **What other groups should receive the seasonal influenza vaccine?**
Everyone over 6 months of age who does not have a contraindication to influenza vaccine.

    Prevention and Control of Influenza: Recommendations of the Immunization Practices Advisory
    Committee (ACIP). *MMWR Morb Mortal Wkly Rep* 59:1-62, 2010.

111. **Who should not receive seasonal influenza virus vaccine?**
- People with documented severe reaction to egg (i.e., anaphylaxis)
- People with a history of Guillain-Barré syndrome after previous influenza virus vaccination

112. **Who can receive intranasally administered live, attenuated seasonal influenza vaccine?**
Healthy, nonpregnant adults < 50 years without high-risk conditions and who do not have contact with severely immunocompromised individuals.

113. **Which patients with wounds should receive tetanus immune globulin (TIG) in addition to Td?**
- Those who have received < three previous doses of Td
- Those with wounds contaminated with dirt, feces, or saliva
- Those with injuries caused by puncture, sharp object penetration, frostbite, or burns

114. **When is tetanus, diphtheria, and pertussis (Tdap) vaccine indicated?**
As a replacement dose for Td toxoid in adults aged 19–64 years who have not received a previous Tdap dose and for those >64 years living in areas with epidemic pertussis.

115. **Which adults should receive the measles-mumps-rubella (MMR) vaccine if they were born after 1957 and not previously immunized or did not have clinical childhood illness?**
- Women of childbearing age
- College students
- Health-care workers who may transmit infection to women of child-bearing age
- International travelers
    At least two doses of MMR are required to obtain full immunity.

116. **Is MMR a live vaccine?**
Yes, and therefore should not be given to pregnant women and patients with HIV infection or other immunosuppression.

117. **Who should receive meningococcal vaccine?**
- College students
- New entrants to institutions with residential living (e.g., dormitories, military barracks)
- Those with anatomic or functional asplenia

118. **What preparations of meningococcal vaccine are available?**
- Meningococcal conjugate vaccine (MCV_4): adults ≤ 55 years
- Meningococcal polysaccharide vaccine ($MPSV_4$): adults ≥ 56 years
    Patients with anatomic or functional asplenia who received MCV_4 or $MPSV_4$ should be revaccinated with MCV_4 after 5 years.

119. **Who should receive hepatitis A virus (HAV) vaccine?**
    - Frequent travelers to Mexico, the Caribbean, Asia (excluding Japan), Eastern Europe, South America, and Africa
    - Patients with chronic liver disease
    - Anticipated close household or babysitting contact with an international adoptee from a country of high or intermediate endemicity
    - Residents of U.S. states with high prevalence (e.g., California)
    - Illegal drug users
    - Men who have sex with men
    - Day care center staff
    - Adults who receive clotting factor replacement
    - Food handlers
    - Research staff who work with HAV-infected primates or HAV in a laboratory

120. **Which immunizations should a person who has had a splenectomy or functional asplenia (i.e., sickle cell disease) receive?**
    - Pneumococcal
    - Meningococcal
    - *Haemophilus influenza* type B (HiB)

121. **What causes Lyme disease? How does it present?**
    Borrelia burgdorferi, a tick-borne spirochete. A rash, followed in weeks to months by involvement of other organ systems (including cardiovascular and neurologic systems and joints) often accompanies the initial infection.

122. **Who should receive prophylactic treatment for latent tuberculosis (TB)?**
    Anyone with recent conversion of purified protein derivative (PPD) skin test to positive classified on the size of the induration:
    - **≥5 mm:** Immunosuppression due to medications, HIV infection, and recent contacts of TB cases
    - **≥10 mm:** Health-care workers, recent immigrants from high-prevalence countries, mycobacteriology laboratory personnel, and injection drug users
    - **≥15 mm:** Low risk

123. **What organisms commonly cause nongonococcal urethritis (NGU) in men?**
    - *Chlamydia trachomatis*
    - *Mycoplasma genitalium*
    - *Trichomonas vaginalis*
    - *Ureaplasma urealyticum*

124. **What organisms commonly cause epididymitis?**
    - *C. trachomatis*
    - *N. gonorrhoeae*
    - *U. urealyticum*
    - Gram-negative organisms (older men)

NEUROLOGY

125. **What are the prodromal symptoms of herpes zoster (shingles)?**
    Headache, malaise, pain, and paresthesias (in the involved dermatome).

126. **What is meralgia paresthetica?**
    The entrapment of the lateral femoral cutaneous nerve producing pain and numbness over the anterolateral thigh.

127. **What causes meralgia paresthetica?**
   - DM
   - Pregnancy
   - Obesity
   - Sudden weight loss
   - Girdles, guns, belts, and other tight-fitting accessories

128. **List the typical symptoms of migraine, tension, and cluster headaches.**
   See Table 2-8.

TABLE 2-8. SYMPTOMS OF MIGRAINE, TENSION, AND CLUSTER HEADACHES			
Symptom	Migraine	Tension	Cluster
Location	Hemicranial	Entire head or bitemporal	Unilateral
Pain quality	Throbbing	Aching	Burning
Duration	2–6 hr	Days	1–2 hr
Frequency	Episodic	Daily	Flurry of attacks for several weeks
Associated symptoms	Prodrome	Neck and shoulder aching	Ipsilateral sweating, flushing, lacrimation, and rhinorrhea

129. **What are the prodromal symptoms of migraine headache?**
   Scotoma, paresthesias, confusion, and behavioral changes.

130. **What is amaurosis fugax?**
   Sudden loss of vision in one eye associated with transient ischemic attack (TIA). It may be described as a "shade" coming down over the eye.

131. **List the symptom triad of Ménière's syndrome.**
   Paroxysmal vertigo, hearing loss, and tinnitus.

132. **What are the frequent causes of acute loss or impairment of smell?**
   Head trauma and viral infection.

133. **What is Phalen's maneuver?**
   Forced flexion (hyperextension) of the wrist. If carpal tunnel syndrome is present, the symptoms of pain and paresthesia are reproduced.

134. **Compare the neurologic findings in a patient with the following nerve root compressions: L4, L5, and S1.**
   See Table 2-9.

ORTHOPEDICS

135. **What are the common causes of knee pain?**
   - Osteoarthritis
   - Inflammatory arthritis (rheumatoid, reactive, and psoriatic arthritis and gout)
   - Chondromalacia

TABLE 2-9. FINDINGS IN NERVE ROOT COMPRESSIONS AT L4, L5, AND S1

Root	Disc	Muscle Weakness	Sensory Loss	Absent Reflex
L4	L3–4	Leg extensors (quadriceps)	Anterolateral thigh, medial lower leg	Patellar
L5	L4–5	First toe dorsiflexion (extensor hallicus longus), heel walking (tibialis anterior)	Dorsum of foot	None
S1	L5–S1	Toe walking (gastrocnemius)	Lateral foot and fifth toe	Ankle

- Chondrocalcinosis (pseudogout)
- Baker's cyst
- Septic arthritis
- Trauma (ligamental and meniscal injuries)
- Bursitis
- Iliotibial band syndrome
- Patellofemoral syndrome

136. **What is trochanteric bursitis?**
A painful inflammation of the bursa superficial to the greater trochanter of the femur. Symptoms include lateral pain described as the "hip," although the hip joint itself is not involved. The most classic finding is point tenderness over the greater trochanter.

137. **Can hip pads prevent hip fractures?**
Yes. Commercially available, small, lightweight pads can be easily worn daily and prevent hip fractures after falls.

138. **Which toe fracture should be referred to an orthopedist?**
Fractures of the proximal phalanx of the first toe. A fracture that involves the distal phalanx and extends into the interphalangeal joint also should be referred.

139. **How do you treat a coccygeal fracture?**
Conservatively with analgesics and seating cushions. Inflatable "donut" cushions should not be used because they can lead to pressure ulcers. Coccygeal fractures usually result from a fall.

140. **How do you manage a patient with acute low back pain?**
If a patient has no signs of nerve root compression and mild-to-moderate pain, usual activity should be encouraged. Ice to the area of pain may be useful for the first 24 hours, but moist or dry heat is helpful later if used for 20 minutes 3–4 times/day. Pain can usually be controlled with regularly scheduled doses of acetaminophen, aspirin, or NSAIDs. Tramadol can be given by prescription. Muscle relaxants such as diazepam and cyclobenzaprine are needed only for patients with severe muscle spasm.

141. **What should be done if the patient has severe pain or signs of nerve root compression?**
Bed rest may be needed but should be limited to only 2 days. Once a patient can sit comfortably, increasing exercise levels is warranted. Patients with occupations that require prolonged sitting or standing, bending, or lifting will need evaluation and counseling to prevent future back injury.

142. **What are the rotator cuff muscles?**
- Supraspinatus
- Infraspinatus
- Teres minor
- Subscapularis

143. **What syndromes are associated with rotator cuff injury or dysfunction?**
Impingement syndrome and rotator cuff tendinitis. Impingement syndrome occurs when the supraspinatus tendon is injured through repetitive motions and is "caught." Pain worsens with overhead arm movement and internal rotation. Symptoms of tendinitis are usually acute.

144. **What is Tietze's syndrome?**
Mild inflammation of the costochondral junction that produces localized warmth, swelling, erythema, and pain. The symptoms are reproduced by palpation of the involved area.

PSYCHIATRY

145. **What are the diagnostic criteria for major depression?**
At least five of these symptoms must have been present nearly every day for 2 weeks:
- Depressed mood most of the day
- Diminished interest or pleasure in nearly all activities (anhedonia)
- Weight loss or gain or decrease or increase in appetite
- Insomnia or hypersomnia
- Psychomotor agitation or retardation
- Feelings of worthlessness or inappropriate guilt
- Decreased ability to think or concentrate
- Recurrent thoughts of death, suicidal ideation, or suicide attempt

American Psychiatric Association: *Diagnostic and Statistical Manual of Mental Disorders*, ed 4, Primary Care Version (DSM-IV-PC). Washington, DC, 1995, American Psychiatric Association Press.

146. **Which medical illnesses can also present with symptoms of depression?**
- **Endocrine disorders:** hyperthyroidism, hypothyroidism, Cushing's syndrome, Addison's disease, hypercalcemia, hyperparathyroidism
- **Rheumatic disorders:** rheumatoid arthritis, systemic lupus erythematosus, fibromyalgia
- **Neurologic disorders:** temporal lobe epilepsy, chronic intracranial hematoma, cerebrovascular accident, multiple sclerosis, frontal lobe tumor, Alzheimer's disease, vascular dementia
- **Infections:** hepatitis, infectious mononucleosis, Lyme disease, HIV infection, TB, syphilis, influenza, viral illnesses
- **Nutritional deficiency:** vitamin B_{12}

147. **Which antidepressant causes priapism?**
Trazodone (Desyrel).

148. **List the risk factors for suicide.**
- Male sex
- Single or widowed status
- Unemployment
- Social isolation
- Urban residence

- Recent loss of health
- Recent surgery
- History of impulsive behaviors
- History of suicide attempts
- History of chronic illness such as chronic pain, depression, organic brain syndromes, or psychosis
- History of alcoholism or substance abuse
- Family history of suicide

149. **What is an anniversary reaction?**

Occurrence of symptoms of depressed mood or undefined somatic symptoms as the anniversary of the death of a spouse, relative, or close friend approaches. An anniversary reaction may also occur after any significant loss such as that of a job, limb, health, or divorce.

150. **What is agoraphobia?**

Fear of being in public places. People with agoraphobia may live a reclusive life. Women are most often affected, and symptoms may present in adolescence or the early 20s. If panic attacks accompany agoraphobia, the patient has at least four of these symptoms when in a public place:

Dyspnea	Dizziness, faintness	Sweating
Palpitations	Feelings of unreality	Trembling
Chest discomfort	Paresthesias	Feeling of doom or
Choking sensation	Hot and cold flashes	fear of death

151. **What is bipolar disorder, type II?**

The bipolar syndrome characterized by at least one episode of major depression and at least one hypomanic episode. The hypomania is characterized by an abnormally elevated mood (for that individual) but the mood change does not impair function or require hospitalization. Type II bipolar disorder also requires maintenance medication therapy.

152. **Are antipsychotic drugs associated with an increased risk of sudden cardiac death?**

Yes, particularly in patients with dementia in whom these medications are frequently used for behavior management.

Ray WA, Chung CP, Murray KT: Atypical antipsychotic drugs and the risk of sudden cardiac death, *N Engl J Med* 360:225–235, 2009.

153. **What are some of the early signs and symptoms of anorexia nervosa?**

- Amenorrhea
- Weight loss
- Distorted body image (feeling "fat" even though clearly emaciated)

154. **What skin finding is associated with anorexia nervosa?**

Lanugo (abnormal fine hair growth on the arms and legs).

155. **What is the CAGE test?**

A reliable screening test for alcoholism. A positive answer to at least two of the questions warrants further evaluation for possible alcoholism.

C = Have you every felt the need to **c**ut down on drinking?
A = Have you ever felt **a**nnoyed by criticism of your drinking?
G = Have you ever felt **g**uilty about your drinking?
E = Have you ever taken a morning **e**ye-opener?

Johnson B, Clark W: Alcoholism: A challenging physician-patient encounter, *J Gen Intern Med* 4:445–452, 1989.

156. **Describe the stages of alcohol withdrawal and how soon after the last drink they occur.**
   - **Minor withdrawal syndromes** (6–36 hr): tremulousness, diaphoresis, tachycardia without mental status changes
   - **Seizures** (6–48 hr): grand mal
   - *Alcoholic halluconisis* (12–48 hr): tactile, auditory, or visual hallucinations or combination with normal orientation
   - **Delirium tremens** (48–96 hr): delirium, agitation, HTN, fever, diaphoresis that can be fatal

   Isbell H, Fraser HF, Wikler A, et al: An experimental study of the etiology of rum fits and delirium tremens, *Q J Stud Alcohol* 16:1–33, 1955.

PULMONARY MEDICINE

157. **What is Kartagener's syndrome?**
   The triad of:
   - Recurrent sinus and respiratory infections
   - Bronchiectasis
   - Situs inversus (occasionally)
   Male patients may also have immotile spermatozoa. Kartagener's syndrome should be considered in patients with recurrent sinusitis and bronchitis that are resistant to treatment.

158. **What causes Kartagener's syndrome?**
   An autosomal recessive disorder that leads to dysfunction of airways cilia. The dysfunctional cilia are unable to effectively clear and move mucous secretions of the respiratory tract.

   Eliasson R, Mossberg B, Camner P, et al: The immotile cilia syndrome, *N Engl J Med* 297:1–6, 1977.

MISCELLANEOUS

159. **Compare the characteristics of bacterial, viral, and allergic conjunctivitis.**
   See Table 2-10.

TABLE 2-10. CHARACTERISTICS OF BACTERIAL, VIRAL, AND ALLERGIC CONJUNCTIVITIS			
Characteristic	Bacterial	Viral	Allergic
Foreign body sensation	−	±	−
Itching	±	±	++
Tearing	+	++	+
Discharge	Mucopurulent	Mucoid	−
Preauricular adenopathy	−	+	−

Adapted from Goroll AH, Mulley HG: Primary Care Medicine: Office Evaluation and Management of the Adult Patient, 4th ed. Philadelphia, Lippincott Williams & Wilkins, 2000, p 1079.

160. **Define "complex regional pain syndrome (CRPS)."**
   A syndrome of severe pain, edema, vasomotor abnormalities with accompanying bone, muscle, and skin atrophy in the arms, hands, legs, or feet. The pain is usually out of proportion to the inciting event. CRPS was previously referred to as "reflex sympathetic dystrophy" and "Sudek's atrophy."

161. **What conditions are associated with Dupuytren's contractures?**
    - DM
    - Chronic liver disease
    - Epilepsy
    - Plantar fasciitis
    - Carpal tunnel syndrome
    - Rheumatoid arthritis
    - Hand trauma
    - Pulmonary TB
    - Alcoholism

162. **Are antidepressants effective for treating fibromyalgia?**
    Yes. Tricyclic antidepressants appear to be most effective for reduction of pain, fatigue, and sleep disturbances, although duloxetine (a selective norepinephrine reuptake inhibitor) is the only antidepressant approved for fibromyalgia treatment.

    Hauser W, Bernady K, Uceyle N, et al: Treatment of fibromyalgia syndrome with antidepressants: A meta-analysis, *JAMA* 301:198–209, 2009.

WEBSITE

1. www.UpToDate.com

BIBLIOGRAPHY

1. Barker LR, Fiebach NH, Kern DE, et al, editors: *Principles of Ambulatory Medicine*, ed 7, Philadelphia, 2006, Lippincott Williams & Wilkins.
2. Cassell EJ: *Talking with Patients*, Cambridge, MA, 1985, MIT Press.
3. Couhelan JL, Block MR: *The Medical Interview: A Primer for Students of the Art*, ed 2, Philadelphia, 2005, FA Davis.
4. Fletcher RH, Fletcher SW: *Clinical Epidemiology. The Essentials*, ed 4, Philadelphia, 2005, Lippincott Williams & Wilkins.
5. Goroll AH, Mulley AG, editors: *Primary Care Medicine. Office Evaluation and Management of the Adult Patient*, ed 6, Philadelphia, 2009, Lippincott Williams & Wilkins.
6. Nabel EG, editor: *ACP Medicine*, Hamilton, Ontario, Canada, 2009, BC Decker.
7. Stone J: *In the Country of Hearts. Journeys in the Art of Medicine*, New York, 1990, Delacorte Press.
8. Wallach J: *Interpretation of Diagnostic Tests*, ed 8, Philadelphia, 2006, Lippincott Williams & Wilkins.

CHAPTER 3

MEDICAL CONSULTATION

Eric I. Rosenberg, M.D., M.S.P.H., F.A.C.P.

Physicians who meet in consultation must never quarrel or jeer at one another.

Hippocrates
Precepts VIII

Whenever he [Thomas Jefferson] saw three physicians together, he looked up to discover whether there was not a turkey buzzard in the neighborhood.

Quoted by Dr. Everett,
Private Secretary to James Monroe

GENERAL ISSUES

1. **Why do physicians request medical consultation?**
   - For assistance in making a diagnosis in a patient with symptoms and signs suggestive of an unknown disease or syndrome
   - To obtain advice on specific disease management (such as diabetes or hypertension)
   - To obtain a procedure usually performed by a subspecialist (e.g., coronary angiogram in a patient with persistent angina)
   - To evaluate a patient's ability to safely undergo surgical procedures

2. **How can one assess the effectiveness of medical consultation?**
   - Is the consultation question answered?
   - Does the patient benefit from disease improvement or promotion of better long-term health?
   - Are the consultant's recommendations actually implemented?

3. **What factors increase the likelihood that the consultant's recommendations will be ignored by the referring physician?**
   - Poor communication between the requesting physician and the consultant (occurring 12–24% of the time in some studies)
   - Delayed response to the consultation request
   - Failure to address the requesting physician's key clinical question
   - Prematurely ending the consultant's involvement in the patient's care
   - Infrequent follow-up visits

   Goldman L, Lee T, Rudd P: Ten commandments for effective consultation, *Arch Intern Med* 143: 1753–1755, 1983.

   Horwitz RI, Henes CG, Horwitz SM: Developing strategies for improving the diagnostic and management efficacy of medical consultations, *J Chronic Dis* 36:213–218, 1983.

4. **What are the 10 commandments for effective consultation?**
   A classic list of principles that Goldman proposed in an effort to improve the quality of medical consultation, including:
   - Determine the question asked by the referring physician.
   - Establish the urgency of the consultation request.

- "Look for yourself" (always see patients and personally review data before providing recommendations).
- "Be as brief as appropriate."
- "Be specific" (including specific dosages and durations of medications).
- "Provide contingency plans" (including suggestions for evaluation likely problems should they occur).
- "Honor thy turf" (keep the patient's primary physicians updated on new information and support their role).
- "Teach …with tact."
- "Talk is cheap and effective" (direct conversation with requesting physicians increases the likelihood that your recommendations will be followed).
- Follow up.

Goldman L, Lee T, Rudd P: Ten commandments for effective consultation, *Arch Intern Med* 143:1753–1755, 1983.

5. **What is a curbside consult and why should it be avoided?**
The practice of giving an impression and recommendation to a physician without actually interviewing and examining the patient and reviewing the laboratory, radiographic, and medical records data. "Curbsides" are sometimes appropriately requested to determine whether a consultant feels a full consultation is needed. Consultants should avoid giving recommendations without having seen a patient because the premise for the curbside may be in error. For example, if a consultant is asked what dosage of warfarin a patient should receive when the International Normalized Ratio (INR) is 4.5, a review of the record might reveal that the patient has no medical indication to be on warfarin, and the proper recommendation is to discontinue the medication rather than to reduce its dosage.

6. **What are some examples of common and appropriate areas of consultation for the internist?**
   - Chest pain
   - Uncontrolled hypertension
   - Uncontrolled diabetes (hyper- or hypoglycemia)
   - Newly diagnosed thyroid disease
   - Electrolyte abnormalities (hypo-/hypernatremia; hypo-/hyperkalemia)
   - Unstable vital signs (fever, hypoxia, tachycardia, tachypnea)
   - Edema
   - Delirium
   - Management of alcohol withdrawal
   - Malnutrition
   - Preoperative evaluation
   - Medication reconciliation and polypharmacy
   - "Second opinions"

7. **How does an internist perform a consultation for "multiple medical problems"?**
By initially focusing on the most significant problem for the patient and referring physician. Most patients with "multiple problems" actually have an extensive, sometimes inactive past medical history. By setting the priorities, the internist can then focus care toward the acute, active, or neglected medical issues that can be effectively treated during the patient's hospitalization. The consultant may also help return (or start if necessary) the care to a primary care physician in the outpatient setting.

8. **What are key issues that a consultant should review prior to seeing a patient in consultation?**
   - **The patient's most important underlying diagnosis.** A patient with advanced Alzheimer's disease or other terminal diagnosis will most likely need supportive care instead of extended testing or new medical or surgical interventions. A patient with a fractured hip is more

likely in urgent need of repair instead of surgical delay to diagnose a possible history of asymptomatic chronic obstructive lung disease. The most important diagnosis may not be the reason the consultation was requested.

- **Reconciliation of home and hospital medications.** Is this patient receiving his or her customary medications? Uncontrolled hypertension or diabetes in the hospital is often because the patient is not receiving the usual prescriptions.
- **Previous care by a primary care physician.**
- **Any previous evaluation of this medical problem.**

9. **What are the ways of succinctly documenting the findings of a medical consultation?**
   A consultation report should not read as an unfocused history and physical examination or generic progress note, but should answer the question(s) posed by the requesting physician and provide clear and specific recommendations.
   - Example of appropriate initial consultation note:
     - Impression: A 72-year-old diabetic man with probable sepsis s/p recent amputation for gangrene now with recurrent fevers, leukocytosis. Leg wound with foul, purulent exudate. Already on empirical antibiotics given history of resistant pseudomonas and methicillin-resistant *Staphylococcus aureus* (MRSA) bacteremia. Hypoxemia and crackles on lung examination concerning for possible pneumonia. Sugars are suboptimally controlled, contributing to infection.
     - Recommendations
       - Will likely need drainage of leg wound tonight.
       - Repeat blood cultures × 2 sets.
       - Urinalysis (UA) with culture and sensitivity (C&S) today.
       - Chest x-ray (CXR) today.
       - Increase neutral protamine Hagedorn (NPH) insulin to 35 units.
         (These were discussed with Dr. Cutsalot and orders were written by me.)
   - Example of appropriate follow-up consultation note:
     - Impression
       - Fever: Resolved after drainage of massive abscess from stump wound. Cultures growing MRSA. CXR showed no evidence of pneumonia, still hypoxic.
       - Delirium: Improving. Likely secondary to sepsis.
       - Hypoxemia: Need to consider pulmonary embolism in patient at prolonged bed rest, s/p surgery.
       - Hyperglycemia: Diabetes control improving on increased NPH.
     - Recommendations
       - Can likely discontinue imipenem (will discuss with Infectious Disease consultant).
       - Ventilation-perfusion ratio ($\dot{V}/\dot{Q}$) scan today to evaluate for pulmonary embolism (PE).
       - Continue present dose insulin.

PREOPERATIVE ASSESSMENT: GENERAL

10. **In general, how risky is surgery?**
    Overall mortality rates are highest for emergent, vascular surgery procedures such as repair of a ruptured abdominal aortic aneurysm (AAA), where mortality rates may exceed 40%. Vascular surgery overall is associated with the highest risk of death; rates for elective procedures such as repair of an asymptomatic AAA are as high as 5% in highest-risk patients. Most nonvascular hospital surgery mortality rates are 1% or less. Mortality rates are lowest for ambulatory surgery and approach less than 0.01%. Operative risk can also be described in terms of invasiveness and bleeding risk. Procedures with the highest invasiveness and greatest risk of bleeding (>1500 mL) are cardiothoracic, intracranial, major orthopedic and spinal

reconstruction procedures, major gastrointestinal (pancreatic resection) and genitourinary surgery (radical prostatectomy and cystectomy), and vascular procedures. Procedures with mild-to-moderate invasiveness and bleeding of typically 500–1500 mL include arthroscopies, laparoscopic cholecystectomies, inguinal herniorrhaphies, hysterectomies, and hip and knee replacements. Procedures with minimal invasiveness and little to no associated bleeding risk are cystoscopies, breast biopsies, and bronchoscopic procedures.

11. **What are the three phases of general anesthesia (GA)?**
Induction, maintenance, and emergence.

12. **What are the complications associated with each phase?**
   - **Induction:** hypotension, bradycardia, nausea, and vomiting
   - **Maintenance:** hepatic necrosis with some volatile anesthestics (halothane) and vitamin B_{12} inactivation with use of nitrous oxide
   - **Emergence:** hypertension, tachycardia, bronchospasm, and laryngospasm

13. **What is monitored anesthesia care (MAC)?**
Monitoring and appropriate treatment by an anesthesiologist of a patient during a procedure that usually uses a local anesthetic. The patient is not fully sedated and may have some awareness of the procedure.

14. **Is spinal or epidural anesthesia safer than GA?**
Probably not. In spinal anesthesia, the anesthetic agent is inserted into the subarachnoid space, and in epidural anesthesia, into the epidural space. There still may be complications of hypotension and respiratory depression with these techniques, and there is less airway control because the patients are not intubated. Both can be combined with GA for lower extremity procedures.

15. **What tests are routinely indicated prior to surgery?**
None. Routinely ordered tests fail to help physicians predict perioperative complications, are expensive, can delay needed surgery, and can result in further morbidity if additional unnecessary and invasive confirmatory testing is performed. Preoperative tests should be ordered to address the acuity or stability of a medical problem or to investigate an abnormal symptom or physical sign detected during the preoperative assessment of a patient's fitness for surgery. Approximately $30 billion is spent yearly in the United States on "routine" preoperative testing alone; 60–70% of this testing is unnecessary because it rarely changes preoperative management.

   Roisen MF: More preoperative assessment by physicians and less by laboratory tests, *N Engl J Med* 342:204–205, 2000.

16. **How do internists assess patients in preparation for surgery?**
By assessing the patient's risk factors and identifying those risk factors that require modification prior to the scheduled procedure. The internists also determine the likelihood and nature of specific complications that may occur around the time of surgery.

17. **What are the specific goals of preoperative assessment?**
To reduce perioperative morbidity, mortality, and unnecessary evaluations by:
   - Optimizing chronic diseases such as chronic obstructive pulmonary disease (COPD), diabetes, and congestive heart failure.
   - Describing specific, modifiable risks and interventions including thromboembolic disease, pneumonia, and infection.
   - Correcting medication errors in the hospital record.
   - Reducing delays and costs of unnecessary testing and referral through expeditious referral to subspecialists and avoidance of unnecessary referral in cases in which patients show no signs of medical decompensation.

18. **Which physicians should play a role in preoperative assessment?**
    - Primary care physician
      - Provides the best source of information regarding patient's baseline health status.
      - Can address comorbidities prior to making a referral for elective surgery and incorporate them into the consultation request.
    - Surgeon
      - Assesses whether or not the procedure is indicated.
      - Discusses risks and benefits with the patient.
    - Anesthesiologist
      - Synthesizes medical and surgical management to assess risks of anesthesia.
      - Decides between general and regional anesthetic agents.
      - Detects recent changes in chronic illness.
    - Consultant (internist, cardiologist, or pulmonologist): Answers specific questions about the patient's risks for surgery.

19. **Which patients are most likely to benefit from preoperative assessment?**
    Those who:
    - Appear to be medically unstable.
    - Are likely to have a complicated postoperative course.
    - Are likely to require medical consultation perioperatively to assist in managing significant cardiopulmonary diseases or other disorders that could directly impact upon postoperative infection risk or wound healing (e.g., diabetes).
    - Have a "past medical history" that in reality describes a suboptimally treated active problem list. This is particularly important to recognize in patients awaiting elective or cosmetic surgical procedures.
    - Have symptoms, signs, or current and past illnesses that are known to be associated with increased risk for myocardial infarction (MI), pneumonia, thromboembolic event, stroke, infection, delirium, and uncontrolled bleeding

20. **Which medical conditions are most important to identify preoperatively because they may be contraindications to surgery?**
    - Cardiac
      - Unstable angina
      - MI within the past 30 days with persistent chest pain
      - Recurrent pulmonary edema with associated ischemic cardiomyopathy
      - Symptomatic ventricular arrhythmias such as ventricular tachycardia
      - Second- or third-degree atrioventricular (AV) block
      - Severe aortic or mitral stenosis or other severe valvular disease
      - Bradycardia associated with syncope
      - Unexplained chest pain
    - Pulmonary
      - Pneumonia
      - COPD or asthma exacerbation
      - Recent PE
      - Unexplained dyspnea
    - Miscellaneous
      - Recent stroke
      - Uncontrolled diabetes
      - Cellulitis
      - Endovascular infections
      - Thyrotoxicosis

KEY POINTS: PREOPERATIVE ASSESSMENT ✓

1. There are no laboratory tests that should be done before all surgeries. Preoperative testing should be based on an individual patient's risk factors.

2. The patient and family history is the best predictor of potential bleeding risk during surgery.

3. Much of the preoperative consultation involves identifying and managing acute illness or exacerbations of chronic illness.

4. Patients with unstable or significant underlying disease (particularly cardiac, pulmonary, and diabetes) are most likely to benefit from preoperative assessment.

21. **How does a preoperative medical interview differ from a conventional medical interview?**

The preoperative interview is an example of focused, targeted history taking. The physician should identify specific medical conditions or symptoms that may be associated with perioperative morbidity. The internist then documents how these conditions were diagnosed, what records substantiate the diagnosis, what treatments have been effective (or ineffective), and whether further diagnostic or follow-up testing is needed to better clarify these diagnoses. The interview usually does not focus on the illness requiring surgery; rather, the "history of present illness" becomes a discussion of concomitant or chronic illnesses that impact upon the perioperative period. The consultant does not simply document that a patient has hypertension and diabetes; instead, she or he documents the chronicity of the hypertension diagnosis, the presence of any end-organ damage (i.e., congestive heart failure, retinopathy, and nephropathy), the patient's baseline blood pressure (BP), the medication regimen, and the presence of any symptoms of decompensation (i.e., edema, dyspnea, curtailment of physical activity, unusual headaches, and chest pain). The consultant should focus on:

- Medication reconciliation by recording the names and dosages of prescription and nonprescription medications taken by the patient, particularly nonsteroidal anti-inflammatory drug (NSAIDs) and complementary or alternative supplements and medications. An accurate medication record is crucial to reduce the likelihood of medication errors of omission (a chronically prescribed medication that is omitted during the perioperative period) or commission (an incorrect dosage of a medication that is prescribed during the hospitalization).

- Any history of abnormal bleeding, particularly difficult-to-control bleeding during previous surgical or dental procedures. Excessive bleeding may indicate an undiagnosed inherited disorder of hemostasis (such as von Willebrand's disease). (See Chapter 14, Hematology.)

- Any history of adverse reactions to anesthesia. If a patient has never undergone prior surgery, the consultant can inquire about a family history of unexplained or sudden intraoperative death or muscle disorders. Unexpected death or muscle disorders associated in the patient or patient's family suggests malignant hyperthermia, a genetic, autosomal dominant skeletal muscle disorder in which patients develop severe fever and organ damage when exposed to anesthetic agents. The incidence of malignant hyperthermia is estimated at 1:50,000 adults and 1:15,000 children and is fatal in 10% of patients. If necessary, genetic testing and a skeletal muscle contracture test can be used for diagnosis in asymptomatic patients with an appropriate family history.

- The patient's baseline functional status. Instead of inquiring about theoretical functional limits (e.g., "Could you climb a flight of stairs if you needed to?") or questions about ability to perform activities that require minimal effort (e.g., "Can you dress yourself?"), physicians should instead ask a patient about his or her daily physical routine to detect physical limitations brought on by dyspnea, chest pain, or other signs of decompensated disease.

- A detailed cardiopulmonary review of systems including history of chest pain, angina with description of typical pattern, shortness of breath, dyspnea on exertion, orthopnea, paroxysmsal nocturnal dyspnea, wheezing, and peripheral edema. Most adult patients referred to an internist for preoperative assessment will have some degree of chronic organ impairment. In the United States, ischemic heart disease and COPD are common and viewed by surgeons as impediments to a successful operative course.

22. **What are some appropriate indications for tests that can be ordered as part of a preoperative assessment?**
See Table 3-1.

TABLE 3-1. INDICATIONS FOR PREOPERATIVE TESTS

Test	Suggested Indication in Asymptomatic Patients Awaiting Surgery	Common Indications in Symptomatic Patients or those with Chronic Disease
Electrocardiogram	Age $\geq$ 40 yr; diabetes, hypertension	Chest pain, coronary artery disease, dysrhythmia
Creatinine	Age > 65 yr	Prescribed diuretics, ACE inhibitors, potassium supplements, chronic kidney disease, hypertension
Glucose	Age > 65 yr	Prescribed steroids; diabetes (consider hemoglobin A_1c as better verification of diabetic control)
Serum electrolytes	Not routinely indicated	Prescribed diuretics, ACE inhibitors, potassium supplements; chronic kidney disease, hypertension
Hemoglobin or hematocrit	Age > 65 yr	Prescribed warfarin, NSAIDs; estimated blood loss with surgery > 500 mL; menstruating
Urine human chorionic gonadotropin (hCG)	Childbearing age	Uncertain menstrual history
Prothrombin time	Not routinely indicated	Prescribed warfarin; chronic liver disease, metastatic cancer, alcoholism, neurosurgical procedures
Liver function tests	Not routinely indicated	Prescribed warfarin; chronic liver disease, metastatic cancer, alcoholism
Chest x-ray	Age > 65 yr and never performed	Dyspnea, cough, fever

(continued)

TABLE 3-1. INDICATIONS FOR PREOPERATIVE TESTS—*(continued)*

Test	Suggested Indication in Asymptomatic Patients Awaiting Surgery	Common Indications in Symptomatic Patients or those with Chronic Disease
Urinalysis	Not routinely indicated	Genitourinary procedures, joint prostheses
Pulmonary function tests	Not routinely indicated	Thoracic or upper abdominal surgery; questionable history of COPD/asthma; unexplained dyspnea
Echocardiogram	Not routinely indicated	Unexplained dyspnea, orthopnea, or other features suggestive of heart failure: heart murmur suggesting significant valvular disease

ACE = angiotensin-converting enzyme; COPD = chronic obstructive pulmonary disease; NSAIDs = nonsteroidal anti-inflammatory disease.

23. **Which medications can be safely continued preoperatively?**
Most medications are safely taken with a small amount of water the morning of surgery. Patients with severe hypertension or recurrent angina are advised to take their usual medications as scheduled before surgery. Abrupt withdrawal of antihypertensive or antianginal medications could lead to unstable BP or chest pain. Diuretics such as furosemide and hydrochlorothiazide are customarily discontinued while the patient is fasting owing to concerns about dehydration or hypokalemia, but the evidence supporting this practice is limited. Aspirin, warfarin, and heparin are often discontinued preoperatively, but it is crucial that physicians understand the specific diagnosis that led to patients being prescribed these medications. For patients at high risk of perioperative deep venous thrombosis (DVT), PE, or stroke, anticoagulation should be discontinued for the minimum time possible. For patients at high risk for intracoronary thrombotic events but at low risk for catastrophic surgical bleeding, it may be advisable to continue antiplatelet medications (such as aspirin) perioperatively. Subspecialty consultation with the patient's cardiologist, hematologist, or neurologist (depending upon the diagnosis prompting anticoagulation) is recommended. Diabetic patients who are insulin-dependent or require insulin to maintain glucose control should continue to receive basal (long-acting) insulin while fasting, but at lower dose, with more frequent monitoring and with hydration to prevent hypoglycemia. Diabetic patients who are non–insulin-requiring should avoid taking sulfonylureas the morning of surgery because these could precipitate hypoglycemia while fasting.

PERIOPERATIVE MANAGEMENT: CARDIAC DISEASE

24. **Should BP achieve target goals in patients with known or newly diagnosed hypertension prior to scheduled surgery?**
No. Consistently elevated BP in a patient without symptoms of malignant hypertension is consistent with a chronically undertreated hypertension. Rapid correction with medication may induce myocardial and cerebral ischemia and is of no proven benefit. Diastolic BPs of > 100 mmHg are probably a contraindication to surgery.

25. **How can you stratify risk of cardiac death or nonfatal MI based on the type of noncardiac procedure?**
    - **Low** (<1%): endoscopic and superficial procedures, cataracts, breast procedures, and ambulatory surgery
    - **Intermediate** (1–5%): intraperitoneal, intrathoracic, head and neck, orthopedic, and prostate surgeries and carotid endarterectomy
    - **High** (>5%): vascular surgeries

    Fleisher LA, Beckman JA, Brown KA, et al: ACC/AHA 2007 guidelines on perioperative cardiovascular evaluation and care for noncardiac surgery, *Circulation* 116:e418–e500, 2007.

26. **Which patients should undergo preoperative cardiac testing?**
    Those with historical and physical findings suggesting a high likelihood of serious coronary artery disease (CAD) that may require prompt intervention, regardless of whether or not the patient is expected to undergo a surgical procedure in the near future (Table 3-2). Specific syndromes include:
    - Unstable coronary syndrome
    - Decompensated heart failure or new-onset heart failure
    - Significant arrhythmias
    - Severe valvular disease

    Fleisher LA, Beckman JA, Brown KA, et al: ACC/AHA 2007 guidelines on perioperative cardiovascular evaluation and care for noncardiac surgery, *Circulation* 116:e418–e500, 2007.

TABLE 3-2. RISK FACTORS FOR CARDIOVASCULAR PERIOPERATIVE CARDIOVASCULAR EVENTS (MYOCARDIAL INFARCTION, HEART FAILURE, AND DEATH)

Major	Intermediate	Minor
■ Unstable coronary syndrome	■ Mild angina pectoris	■ Advanced age
■ Acute or MI within past 7–30 days and evidence of ischemia by symptoms or noninvasive testing	■ Previous MI by history of pathologic Q wave on ECG	■ Abnormal ECG
■ Decompensated heart failure	■ Compensated or prior heart failure	■ Rhythm other than sinus
■ Significant arrhythmias	■ Diabetes mellitus (particularly if insulin-dependent)	■ Low functional capacity
■ High-grade atrioventricular block	■ Renal insufficiency	■ History of stroke
■ Symptomatic ventricular arrhythmia in patients with heart disease		■ Uncontrolled hypertension
■ SVT with uncontrolled ventricular rate		
■ Severe valvular disease		

ECG = electrocardiogram; MI = myocardial infarction; SVT = supraventricular tachycardia.
Adapted from Fleisher LA, Beckman JA, Brown KA, et al: ACC/AHA 2006 guideline update on perioperative cardiovascular evaluation for noncardiac surgery: Focused update on perioperative beta-blocker therapy. A report of the American College of Cardiology/American Heart Association Task Force on Practice Guidelines (Writing Committee to Update the 2002 Guidelines on Perioperative Cardiovascular Evaluation for Noncardiac Surgery). J Am Coll Cardiol 47:2347, 2006.

27. **What are the risks of preoperative cardiac testing?**
    Unnecessarily delayed urgent surgery or complications caused by invasive procedures. Performing routine cardiac "stress tests" on patients does not improve perioperative morbidity or mortality.

28. **Which patients should receive evaluation for preoperative revascularization?**
    Those who have angina or other symptoms likely due to CAD.

    Fleisher LA, Beckman JA, Brown KA, et al: ACC/AHA 2007 guidelines on perioperative cardiovascular evaluation and care for noncardiac surgery, *Circulation* 116:e418–e500, 2007.

29. **What specific perioperative complications may develop in patients with aortic stenosis (AS)?**
    - Hypotension
    - Pulmonary edema
    - MI
    - Arrhythmia

30. **In what situations does the current evidence most clearly support use of beta blockers for patients in the perioperative period?**
    For patients already taking beta blockers and those undergoing vascular surgery with high cardiac risk as identified by ischemia on preoperative testing.

31. **In what other situations might perioperative beta blocker use be considered?**
    In patients undergoing vascular surgery who have known, stable CAD identified on preoperative testing or multiple clinical risk factors for CAD. The role of perioperative beta blocker use continues to be closely reviewed and recommendations are likely to be modified.

    Fleisher LA, Beckman JA, Brown KA, et al: ACC/AHA 2006 guideline update on perioperative cardiovascular evaluation for noncardiac surgery: Focused update on perioperative beta-blocker therapy. A report of the American College of Cardiology/American Heart Association Task Force on Practice Guidelines (Writing Committee to Update the 2002 Guidelines on Perioperative Cardiovascular Evaluation for Noncardiac Surgery), *J Am Coll Cardiol* 47:2343–2366, 2006. Available at www.jacc.org. Accessed June 7, 2010.

PERIOPERATIVE MANAGEMENT: PULMONARY DISORDERS

32. **Which factors are commonly associated with perioperative pulmonary complications?**
    - Cigarette smoking
    - Upper abdominal or thoracic surgery
    - Surgery lasting > 3 hours
    - Active respiratory tract infection
    - Chronic sleep apnea

33. **What are the goals of preoperative assessment of a patient with chronic lung disease?**
    - Evaluate and stabilize acute exacerbations.
    - Smoking cessation.
    - Review and verify that the patient is receiving appropriate maintenance therapy.
    - Review any use of corticosteroids within the previous year.

34. **What degree of impairment from pulmonary function tests precludes safe surgical intervention?**
   None, unless a patient is being considered for partial lung resection. Pulmonary function tests, no matter how abnormal, do not preclude surgery. Forced expiratory volume in 1 second (FEV_1) or forced vital capacity (FVC) < 70%, FEV_1/FVC < 65%, and arterial carbon dioxide pressure ($PaCO_2$) > 45 mmHg suggest that patients are at higher risk for pulmonary complications, but there is no prohibitive threshold for surgery.

35. **What are some specific ways to lower the risk of perioperative pulmonary complications in patients with chronic lung diseases?**
   - Stop smoking 8 weeks preoperatively.
   - Continue bronchodilators and/or steroids throughout the perioperative period.
   - Treat respiratory infection and postpone elective surgery if possible until resolved.
   - Prescribe *lung expansion maneuvers* (preoperative education for either deep breathing or incentive spirometry, which are equally effective).
   - Initiate or continue continuous positive airway pressure (CPAP) for patients with known or suspected sleep apnea.
   - Prescribe perioperative venous thromboembolism (VTE) prophylaxis to prevent DVT and PE, if indicated.

36. **Which patients are at high risk for postoperative VTE?**
   Those with:
   - Major orthopedic procedures such as repair of pelvic, hip, or leg fractures
   - Multiple major trauma
   - Spinal cord injury
   - Abdominal or pelvic malignancy undergoing resection (e.g., colectomy for colorectal cancer; hysterectomy for endometrial or ovarian cancer)
   - Prior history of DVT and PE
   - Known thrombophilia (such as Factor V Leiden, lupus anticoagulant, and antiphospholipid antibody syndrome)
   - Critical illness with major comorbidities (decompensated heart failure, pneumonia requiring intubation sepsis, and burns)
   - Prolonged periods of immobilization before or after surgery

37. **Which patients should receive VTE prophylaxis?**
   Most undergoing procedures with a moderate-to-high risk of VTE, including general surgical, open gynecologic and urologic procedures, knee or hip arthroplasty, hip fracture surgery, trauma, and spinal cord surgery.

38. **What are the methods of VTE prophylaxis?**
   - Early and frequent ambulation when appropriate
   - Graduated elastic compression stockings
   - Sequential compression devices
   - Low-molecular-weight heparin (LMWH)
   - Low-dose unfractionated heparin (LDUH)
   - Vitamin K antagonists to maintain INR between 2 and 3
   - Fondaparinux
   - Inferior vena cava filter

39. **How does one choose the appropriate method of VTE prophylaxis?**
   The exact method of prophylaxis will depend on the patient's risk factors for VTE, the VTE risk associated with the procedure, and the risk of postoperative bleeding. Current guidelines from the American College of Chest Physicians recommend that institutions establish clearly

written thromboprophylaxis policies for all patients. Physicians should first identify whether their hospital has such guidelines. A complete description of the indications of the methods is available in the reference. See Table 3-3 for general guidelines.

Geerts WH, Bergqvist D, Piineo GF, et al: Prevention of venous thromboembolism. American College of Chest Physicians Evidence-Based Clinical Practice Guidelines (8th ed), *Chest* 133:381S–453S, 2006.

Risk of DVT	Pharmacologic Prophylaxis				Mechanical Prophylaxis[†]
	LMWH	LDUH	VKA	Fondaparinux*	
Low	No	No	No	No	None, but early and frequent ambulation
Moderate	Yes	Yes	No	Yes	Yes, if bleeding risk is high
High	Yes	No	Yes	Yes	Yes, if bleeding risk or as adjunctive therapy

TABLE 3-3. GENERAL GUIDELINES FOR POSTOPERATIVE PREVENTION OF VENOUS THROMBOEMBOLISM

DVT = deep venous thrombosis; LDUH = low-dose unfractionated heparin; LMWH = low-molecular-weight heparin; VKA = vitamin K antagonists.
*Not U.S. Food and Drug Administration (FDA) approved for nonorthopedic procedures.
[†]Includes graduated compression stockings and intermittent compression devices.
From Geerts WH, Bergqvist D, Piineo GF, et al: Prevention of venous thromboembolism. American College of Chest Physicians Evidence-Based Clinical Practice Guidelines (8th ed). Chest 133: 381S–453S, 2006.

40. **If a patient is on warfarin, how long before surgery is warfarin stopped to allow normalization of the INR?**
   5 days.

41. **When can warfarin be restarted after surgery?**
   Within 12–24 hours if there are no bleeding complications.

42. **How is perioperative warfarin managed in outpatients at high risk of an embolic event if the warfarin is stopped?**
   "Bridging" therapy is prescribed consisting of LMWH administered subcutaneously. LMWH should be started 3 days before surgery. The last dose is given 24 hours before surgery as one half of the total daily dose. The postoperative resumption of LMWH depends on the bleeding risks.

   Douketis JD, Berger PB, Dunn AS, et al: The perioperative management of antithrombotic therapy: American College of Chest Physicians Evidence-Based Clinical Practice Guidelines (8th ed), *Chest* 133:299S–339S, 2008.

43. **What antithrombotic drugs require adjustment for renal function?**
   LMWH and fondaparinux.

44. **How soon before surgery should aspirin and other antiplatelet agents (i.e., clopidogrel and prasugel) be stopped?**
   Usually 7–10 days, but patients at risk for thrombotic events may need to continue the antiplatelet agent.

PERIOPERATIVE MANAGEMENT: ENDOCRINOLOGY

45. **How should diabetes be treated during the perioperative period? Is "tight control" important?**
    - Patients with well-controlled diabetes should continue to receive their customary regimen as soon as they are able to eat normally.
    - Patients with type 1 (insulin-dependent) diabetes must continue to receive basal (long-acting) insulin even while fasting in order to protect them from developing diabetic ketoacidosis. These patients require frequent monitoring with blood glucose checks at least every 4 hours while fasting. The dose of their insulin is customarily reduced by 50% while fasting while at the same time hydration with parenteral dextrose and normal saline is provided to protect against dehydration and hypoglycemia.
    - Patients with poorly controlled type 2 diabetes are probably best managed with long-acting insulin.
    - "Tight" control of glucose (80–110 mg/dL) has been shown in some studies to reduce the risk of perioperative infection, wound healing, and cardiovascular complications. This remains controversial, however, because subsequent studies have failed to replicate these results.
    - Do NOT use "sliding scales" or "correction" doses of regular (short-acting) insulin to treat patients with poorly controlled diabetes, even while patients are fasting.

46. **How are patients taking metformin managed when undergoing imaging studies or procedures that involve iodinated contrast media?**
    By discontinuing the medication before or at the time of the procedure and not resuming until normal renal function is confirmed by laboratory testing 48 hours later. Patients can develop acute renal failure in this setting.

47. **Is metformin also withheld during surgery?**
    Yes. Metformin should be stopped before surgery and not restarted until the patient has usual oral intake and normal renal function is confirmed by laboratory testing.

48. **How are patients taking chronic glucocorticoids managed in the perioperative period?**
    By monitoring closely for signs of adrenal insufficiency postoperatively. The routine use of "stress doses" of glucocorticoids perioperatively is questionable. Those patients at high risk for adrenal suppression during major surgery should probably receive stress doses, though. (See Chapter 16, Endocrinology.)

49. **When indicated, how are stress doses of glucocorticoids given?**
    See Table 3-4.

TABLE 3-4. PERIOPERATIVE STRESS DOSES OF GLUCOCORTICOIDS		
	Intravenous Hydrocortisone Dose (mg)	
Procedure Risk	Preoperative	Postoperative
Minor	None	None
Moderate	50	25 q8h × 1–2 days
Major	100	50 q8h × 2–3 days

50. **What are the risks of surgery in patients with thyroid disease?**
    Patients with **hypothyroidism** on stable thyroid replacement doses should continue the medication perioperatively. Patients with newly diagnosed severe hypothyroidism or myxedema should have surgery delayed if possible. Patients with **hyperthyroidism** should have this adequately treated before surgery.

PERIOPERATIVE MANAGEMENT: MISCELLANEOUS

51. **When should dialysis patients be dialyzed?**
    Generally the day before surgery with nephrology consultation for post-operative dialysis.

52. **Do all patients with anemia need to be transfused before elective surgery?**
    Not for mild anemia, but those with hemoglobin < 8 mg/dL may benefit from transfusion, depending on the etiology of the anemia. Anemia is associated with increased risk of perioperative complications.

53. **Which patients with liver disease are at highest risk of complications?**
    Those with:
    - Acute viral hepatitis
    - Acute alcoholic hepatitis
    - Cirrhosis

54. **What are the complications of liver disease associated with surgery?**
    Bleeding, encephalopathy, hypotension, sepsis, and worsening of liver dysfunction.

55. **How can these complications be prevented?**
    With preoperative endoscopy, if indicated for possible variceal bleeding; correction of abnormal prothrombin time (PT) with vitamin K or fresh frozen plasma; replacement of electrolytes when indicated; cessation of alcohol use; ascites treatment as appropriate; postponement of elective surgery in unstable patients; and, minimal sedative use.

BIBLIOGRAPHY

1. Gross RJ, Caputo JM, editors: *Kammerer and Gross' Medical Consultation: The Internist on Surgical, Obstetric, and Psychiatric Services*, Philadelphia, 1998, Lippincott Williams & Wilkins.

CHAPTER 4

CARDIOLOGY

Gabriel Habib, Sr., M.S., M.D., F.A.C.C., F.C.C.P., F.A.H.A.

> *Her blood pressure was on the low side. I felt her pulse in the carotid artery in her neck; it was weak, difficult to detect. Unlike the usual thumping carotid artery, her pulse rose only reluctantly to the examining finger. At the base of her neck, on the chest wall, there was an easily felt shudder, a rough vibration with each pulse, like a cat's purr. When I listened to her heart, ... I heard a gruff, harsh sound like the clearing of a throat. ... It was no great Oslerian feat of diagnosis on my part to suspect that she had severe <u>aortic stenosis</u>.*
>
> John Stone (1936–2008)
> "The Long House Calls" from
> *In the Country of Hearts: Journeys in the Art of Medicine,* 1990

PHYSICAL EXAMINATION

1. **Explain normal splitting of the second heart sound (S_2).**
   S_2 is normally split into aortic (A_2) and pulmonic (P_2) components caused by the closing of the two respective valves. The degree of splitting varies with the respiratory cycle or physiologic splitting. With inspiration, the negative intrathoracic pressure leads to increased venous return to the right side of the heart and a decrease to the left side. The increased venous return to the right atrium (RA) causes P_2 to occur slightly later and A_2 to occur slightly earlier, leading to a widening of the S_2 split. With expiration, the negative intrathoracic pressure is eliminated and A_2 and P_2 occur almost simultaneously. The largest contributor to the physiologic third heart sound (S_3) split is the respiratory variation in the timing of the pulmonic closure sound.

2. **What is paradoxical splitting of S_2?**
   A widening of the split of A_2 and P_2 with expiration and shortening of the split with inspiration (the opposite of normal).

3. **What causes paradoxical splitting of S_2?**
   It is usually seen with aortic insufficiency, aortic stenosis, and hypertrophic cardiomyopathy (HCM). In paradoxical splitting, P_2 precedes A_2 during expiration and is usually due to conditions that delay A_2 by delaying ejection of blood from the left ventricle (LV) and, therefore, aortic valve closure. Causes include HCM, myocardial infarction (MI), left bundle branch block (LBBB), and a right ventricular (RV) pacemaker.

4. **What causes fixed and wide splitting of S_2?**
   Atrial septal defects (ASDs), RV dysfunction, or both, resulting in an interval between A_2 and P_2 that is wider than normal and does *not* change with the respiratory cycle. The wide and fixed S_2 split occurs because:
   - A_2–P_2 is wider than normal owing to shunting of blood from the left atrium (LA) to the RA, resulting in a greater RV filling and a resulting delay in the timing of the pulmonic closure sound P_2; and,

- A_2–P_2 splitting is fixed and does *not* increase with inspiration. The fixed splitting occurs because the extra filling of the RV that normally occurs during inspiration is small relative to the above-described increase in RV filling due to interatrial shunting and thus does *not* significantly delay P_2.

5. **Explain the significance of a loud P_2.**
   It usually indicates the presence of pulmonary hypertension (HTN), whether primary or secondary to chronic pulmonary disease.

6. **What is S_3?**
   A low-frequency sound heard just after S_2; also called a "ventricular gallop."

7. **What is a physiologic S_3?**
   An S_3 found in young patients without cardiac disease.

8. **How is S_3 best heard?**
   With the stethoscope bell. Unlike a physiologically split A_2–P_2, the A_2–S_3 interval does not change during respiration. Associated physical findings of congestive heart failure (CHF), such as pulmonary rales, distended neck veins, or edema are usually present along with an S_3.

9. **What is a pathologic S_3?**
   An S_3 occurring in a variety of pathologic conditions including CHF, mitral valve prolapse (MVP), thyrotoxicosis, coronary artery disease (CAD), cardiomyopathies, pericardial constriction, mitral or aortic insufficiency, and left-to-right shunts.

10. **Describe the mechanism behind an S_3.**
    The mechanism behind an S_3 is controversial, but it may be due to an increase in the velocity of blood entering the ventricles (rapid ventricular filling). When present, an S_3 usually represents myocardial decompensation associated with heart disease.

11. **What is the fourth heart sound (S_4)?**
    A sound occurring just before S_1; also called an "atrial gallop." An S_4 reflects decreased ventricular compliance (a stiff ventricle) and is associated with CAD, pulmonic or aortic valvular stenosis, HTN, and ventricular hypertrophy from any cause.

12. **What is an opening snap (OS)?**
    A high-frequency early diastolic sound associated with mitral or tricuspid valve opening. A diastolic rumble at the apex confirms the physical diagnosis of mitral stenosis.

13. **Summarize the pathophysiology and significance of an OS in patients with mitral stenosis.**
    An OS is typically present only when the mitral valve leaflets are pliable, and it is, therefore, usually accompanied by an accentuated first heart sound (S_1). Diffuse calcification of the mitral valve can be expected when an OS is absent. If calcification is confined to the tip of the mitral valve, an OS is still commonly present. The interval between the aortic closure sound and the OS (A_2–OS) is inversely related to the mean LA pressure. A short A_2–OS interval is a reliable indicator of severe mitral stenosis; however, the converse is not necessarily true.

14. **What is the differential diagnosis of an abnormal early diastolic sound heard at the apex and lower left sternal border?**
    - Loud P_2
    - S_3 gallop

- OS
- Pericardial knock
- Tumor plop (atrial myxoma)

An early diastolic sound may be due to wide splitting of S_2, with or without a loud pulmonic closure sound. An ASD causes wide and fixed splitting of S_2.

15. **What causes a pericardial knock?**
The sudden slowing of LV filling in early diastole associated with the restriction of a rigid pericardium acting as a "rigid shell" such as in chronic constrictive pericarditis.

16. **What is a tumor plop?**
The sound heard with cardiac auscultation caused by obstruction of blood flow by an atrial myxoma protruding through the mitral valve during diastole leading to sudden cessation of LV filling. Cardiac auscultation in various positions helps to detect a tumor plop; likewise, cardiac symptoms in these patients are often related to body position.

17. **What is a hyperdynamic precordial impulse?**
A thrust of exaggerated height that falls away immediately from the palpating fingers and is typically found in patients with a large stroke volume. The clinical conditions with a large stroke volume include thyrotoxicosis, anemia, beriberi, atrioventricular (AV) shunts or grafts, exercise, or mitral regurgitation (MR). (Stroke volume is the amount of blood ejected with each contraction.) A hyperdynamic precordial impulse should be differentiated from the sustained apical impulse, a graphic equivalent of a heave, detected in the presence of LV hypertrophy due to HTN or aortic stenosis.

18. **What are the classifications of and physical findings associated with heart murmurs?**
See Table 4-1. Systolic murmurs are classified from grade 1 to grade 6. Diastolic murmurs are classified from grade 1 to grade 4. Murmurs rarely exceed grade 4. Systolic murmurs grade 3 or greater are more likely to be clinically significant.

TABLE 4-1. CLASSIFICATION OF HEART MURMURS	
Grade (Classification)	Physical Examination Findings
1	Heard only with concentration in a quiet room
2	Soft, low-intensity audible murmur
3	Loud murmur
4	Loud murmur with a palpable chest vibration ("thrill")
5	Loudest murmur heard with stethoscope touching the chest
6	Murmur loud enough to be heard with the stethoscope off the chest

19. **What is the likely cause of a systolic ejection murmur, best heard at the second right intercostal space, in an 82-year-old asymptomatic man?**
Aortic **sclerosis**, not aortic **stenosis**. Aortic sclerosis is characterized by thickening and/or calcification of the aortic valve and, unlike valvular aortic stenosis, is typically *not* associated with any significant transvalvular systolic pressure gradient.

20. **How is aortic stenosis differentiated from aortic sclerosis by physical examination?**
The following clinical findings are **present** in patients with **aortic stenosis** but **absent** with **aortic sclerosis**:
- Diminished carotid arterial upstroke (i.e., the rate of rise of the carotid pulse is less steep)
- Diminished peripheral arterial pulses (a finding consistent with moderate-to-severe aortic stenosis)
- Late peaking of systolic murmur (as aortic stenosis worsens in severity, the systolic murmur peak becomes more delayed)
- Loud or audible (or both) S_4
- Syncope, angina, or heart failure signs or symptoms
- Loud systolic murmur associated with a systolic thrill

21. **How do standing, squatting, and leg-raising affect the intensity and duration of the systolic murmur heard on dynamic auscultation in a patient with HCM?**
Standing increases the murmur intensity, and leg-raising and squatting decrease the murmur intensity. In HCM, a decrease in the size of the LV increases the dynamic LV outflow obstruction, leading to an increased intensity of the murmur. A decrease in LV volume occurs on standing. In contrast, leg-raising and squatting increase venous return and thereby increase LV volume, decreasing the dynamic LV obstruction and the murmur intensity.

22. **What are the physical examination findings in MR?**
- An apical holosystolic murmur with variation of intensity and radiation depending on the cause and severity of the MR
- S_3
- Quick upstroke and short duration of peripheral pulses
- Widened pulse pressure
- Hyperdynamic precordium

23. **List the peripheral arterial signs of chronic aortic regurgitation (AR).**
- **de Musset's sign:** bobbing of the head with each heartbeat
- **Corrigan's pulse:** abrupt distention and quick collapse of femoral pulses (also called "water-hammer pulse")
- **Traube's sign:** booming, "pistol-shot" systolic and diastolic sounds heard over the femoral pulse
- **Müller's sign:** systolic pulsations of the uvula
- **Duroziez's sign:** systolic murmur over the femoral artery when compressed proximally and diastolic murmur when compressed distally
- **Quincke's sign:** capillary pulsations of the fingertips
- **Hill's sign:** popliteal cuff systolic pressure exceeding brachial cuff pressure by > 60 mmHg

24. **How do you measure the jugular venous pulse (JVP) as an estimate of central venous pressure (CVP) at the bedside?**
- Elevate the head of the bed until the patient's chest is at the point at which the venous pulsations are maximally visualized (usually 30–45°).
- Measure the height of this oscillating venous column above the sternal angle (angle of Louis) (Fig. 4-1).
- Estimate the CVP by adding 5 cm to the measurement.
  The sternal angle is about 5 cm from the RA regardless of the elevation angle.
  Normal CVP is 5–9 cmH_2O.

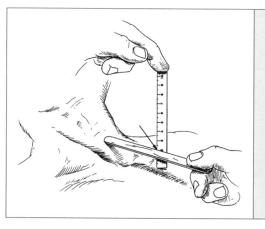

Figure 4-1. Measurement of venous jugular pressure at the bedside. (From Adair OV, Havranek EP: Cardiology Secrets. Philadelphia, Hanley & Belfus, 1995, p 6.)

25. **Name the three waves composing the JVP.**
  - **A wave:** produced by RA contraction, occurring just before S_1
  - **C wave:** caused by bulging upward of the closed tricuspid valve during RV contraction (often difficult to see)
  - **V wave:** caused by RA filling just before opening of the tricuspid valve

26. **What are "cannon" A waves?**
  Very large and prominent A waves occurring when the atria contract against a closed tricuspid valve. Irregular "cannon" A waves are seen in AV dissociation or ectopic atrial beats. Regular "cannon" A waves are seen in a junctional or ventricular rhythm in which the atria are depolarized by retrograde conduction.

27. **Define "pulsus paradoxus."**
  A decrease of > 10 mmHg in the systolic blood pressure (BP) during normal inspiration, first described by Adolf Kussmaul in 1873. Kussmaul originally described the disappearance of the pulse during inspiration, though.

28. **Describe the mechanism of a pulsus paradoxus.**
  Pulsus paradoxus can occur when the fall in intrathoracic pressure during inspiration is rapidly transmitted through a pericardial effusion, resulting in an exaggerated increase in venous return to the right side of the heart. The increased venous return causes bulging of the interventricular septum toward the LV, resulting in a smaller LV volume and a smaller LV stroke volume. The decreased LV stroke volume results in a lower cardiac output and lower systolic BP during inspiration. A drop in systolic BP is a normal physiologic finding as long as this drop does *not* exceed 10 mmHg. In contrast, an exaggerated drop in systolic BP > 10 mmHg is a pathologic finding characteristic of cardiac tamponade.

29. **What medical diseases present with pulsus paradoxus?**
  - Cardiac tamponade (classic finding but may be absent with severe volume contraction, dehydration, or hypotension)
  - Severe chronic obstructive pulmonary disease (COPD)
  - Chronic constrictive pericarditis (very rarely)

30. **Describe the Y descent of the JVP waveform tracing in chronic constrictive pericarditis.**

    The Y descent of the JVP waveform tracing corresponds to the rapid early RA emptying phase or the rapid early ventricular filling phase. In patients with chronic constrictive pericarditis, early ventricular filling is unimpeded. During the very early filling, the RV is very small and its filling is enhanced by the sudden "pouring" of blood as the tricuspid valve opens. During this early filling phase, the ventricle is too small and has not yet "perceived" the constricting effect of the calcified or thickened pericardium and, thus, filling is unimpeded. Once the ventricle meets the thick or calcified "noncompliant" pericardium, ventricular filling suddenly slows and corresponds to the "pericardial knock" sound. Although found in chronic constrictive pericarditis, the steep Y descent rarely occurs in cardiac tamponade. At the same time that the steep Y descent occurs, the RV early filling occurs and there is a "dip" or sudden decrease in RV pressure. Once the ventricular filling is suddenly slowed or halted by the thick or calcified noncompliant pericardium, the RV pressure rises to a plateau. The "dip-and-plateau" RV pressure waveform, just like the steep Y descent of the RA pressure waveform, is a distinctive finding in chronic constrictive pericarditis and helps to differentiate chronic constrictive pericarditis from cardiac tamponade.

31. **What is cardiac tamponade?**

    The sudden accumulation of fluid within the pericardial sac under pressure. When the clinical triad of cardiac tamponade was first described by Claude Beck in 1935, he noted hypotension, elevated systemic venous pressure, and a small, quiet heart. The condition was commonly due to penetrating cardiac injuries, aortic dissection, or intrapericardial rupture of an aortic or cardiac aneurysm. Today, the most common causes are neoplastic disease, idiopathic pericarditis, acute MI, and uremia.

32. **Summarize the physical examination findings in cardiac tamponade.**

    - **Jugular venous distention:** Almost universally present except in patients with severe hypovolemia.
    - **Pulsus paradoxus:** Defined as a decrease in systolic BP > 10 mmHg during quiet inspiration. Pulsus paradoxus is difficult to elicit in volume-depleted patients.
    - **Tachycardia with a thready peripheral pulse:** Sometimes severe cardiac tamponade may restrict LV and RV filling enough to cause hypotension, but a thready and rapid pulse is almost invariably present.

33. **What is Kussmaul's sign?**

    An inspiratory increase in systemic venous pressure commonly present in chronic constrictive pericarditis but rarely detected in acute cardiac tamponade.

ELECTROCARDIOGRAPHY

34. **What is the normal range for PR and QT intervals on a 12-lead electrocardiogram (ECG)? Do these intervals vary with heart rate or age?**

    - **PR interval:** 0.12–0.20 sec with no variation due to heart rate or age.
    - **QT interval:** Varies with heart rate but not with age. As the heart rate increases, the QT interval shortens. To help evaluate a QT interval independent of heart rate, the corrected QT interval (QTc) can be calculated:

    QTc (in msec) = measured QT (in msec)/square root of the R − R interval (in sec)

    The normal range for the **QTc** is 0.36–0.44 sec. A prolonged QTc is defined as QTc > 0.44 sec.

35. **What are the congenital causes of a prolonged QT interval?**
   - **With deafness:** Jervell and Lange-Nielsen syndrome
   - **Without deafness:** Romano-Ward syndrome

36. **List the acquired causes of a prolonged QT interval.**
   - Electrolyte abnormalities: low K^+, low Ca^{2+}, low Mg^{2+}. In clinical practice, the most common electrolyte abnormality causing a prolonged QT interval is hypokalemia often in a patient receiving a thiazide or loop diuretic.
   - Drugs: class IA/IC antiarrhythmics, tricyclic antidepressants, and phenothiazines.
   - Hypothermia.
   - CAD.
   - Cardiomyopathy.
   - Central nervous system injury (least common cause).

37. **Why is a prolonged QT interval clinically significant?**
   Because a prolonged QT interval is associated with an increased risk of sudden cardiac death due to a ventricular tachyarrhythmia such as ventricular tachycardia (VT) or ventricular fibrillation (VF). A distinctive type of VT associated with a prolonged QT interval is "Torsades-de-Pointes" (turning of the points) or more descriptively called "polymorphic VT."

38. **In the frontal plane, is a QRS axis of $+120°$ compatible with a diagnosis of left anterior hemiblock (LAHB)?**
   No. The diagnosis of LAHB requires the presence of a QRS of $-60°$ to $-90°$ in the frontal plane. A frontal plane QRS axis of $+120°$ is consistent with right axis deviation and is, therefore, not compatible with a diagnosis of LAHB (left anterior fascicular block).

39. **List the diagnostic criteria for left anterior fascicular block.**
   - QRS axis $-60°$ to $-90°$
   - Small Q wave in lead I
   - Small R wave in lead III

40. **Describe the ECG manifestations of RV hypertrophy.**
   - R wave > S wave in V_1 or V_2
   - R wave > 5 mm in V_1 or V_2
   - Right axis deviation
   - Persistent rS pattern (V_1–V_6)
   - Normal QRS duration

41. **Describe the three phases of the ECG evolution of an acute MI.**
   - **Tall upright or inverted T waves:** Typically seen in the first hour or two of MI evolution and are thus called "hyperacute T waves" but are not a common ECG presentation in patients with MI. Inverted T waves are more frequent and usually appear after the first 8 to 12 hours of MI symptom onset and may persist for an indeterminate length of time (days, weeks, or years). Thus, an ECG characterized by pathologic Q waves and inverted T waves is called "MI, age indeterminate."
   - **ST-segment elevations:** Found in ECG leads facing the infarcted myocardial wall and reciprocal **ST depressions** in opposite ECG leads. ST segment changes are the most common acute ECG signs of MI. ST segment elevations appear immediately at onset of a MI and usually resolve after the first 2–3 days and rarely persist longer than 2 weeks except in patients with a ventricular aneurysm.
   - **New pathologic Q waves:** Usually starting anywhere from 8–12 hours to several days after MI symptom onset. Some patients may not develop pathologic Q waves but develop a significant > 25% decrease in R wave amplitude (Fig. 4-2).

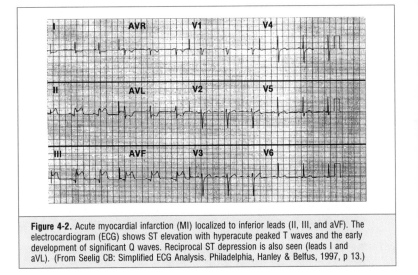

Figure 4-2. Acute myocardial infarction (MI) localized to inferior leads (II, III, and aVF). The electrocardiogram (ECG) shows ST elevation with hyperacute peaked T waves and the early development of significant Q waves. Reciprocal ST depression is also seen (leads I and aVL). (From Seelig CB: Simplified ECG Analysis. Philadelphia, Hanley & Belfus, 1997, p 13.)

42. **What is a pseudoinfarction? What is its differential diagnosis?**
An ECG pattern with changes similar to a MI without definitive evidence of ischemia. The differential diagnosis includes:

LV or RV hypertrophy	Wolff-Parkinson-	HCM
Hyperkalemia	White syndrome	Intracranial hemorrhage
LBBB	Cardiac sarcoid or	
Early repolarization	amyloid	

43. **What are the ECG manifestations of atrial infarction?**
Depressed or elevated PR segment and atrial arrhythmias such as atrial flutter, atrial fibrillation (AF), or AV nodal rhythms.

44. **Which arrhythmias can be detected by 24-hr ECG monitoring in young patients without apparent heart disease?**
 - Severe sinus bradycardia ($\leq$40 beats per minute [bpm])
 - Sinus pauses of up to 2 sec
 - Nocturnal AV nodal block
   Frequent premature atrial or ventricular beats were not commonly found.

   Brodsky M, Wu D, Denes P, et al: Arrhythmias documented by 24-hour continuous electrocardiographic monitoring in 50 male medical students without apparent heart disease, *Am J Cardiol* 39:390–395, 1977.

45. **What ECG findings help distinguish AF from other supraventricular tachycardias (SVTs)?**
AF differs from all other SVTs by having totally disorganized atrial depolarization without effective atrial contractions. An ECG may occasionally show fine or coarse irregular waves of variable amplitude and morphology, occurring at a rate of 350–600/min, but these are often difficult to recognize on a routine 12-lead ECG. A distinctive finding in AF is an irregular ventricular rhythm resulting from random and erratic transmission of the wave of depolarization from the atria to the ventricles via the AV conduction system. When untreated, patients with AF will usually have fast ventricular rates > 100 bpm, often in the 150–200 bpm

range. The finding of AF with a slow ventricular rate < 60 bpm in a patient *not* receiving any AV nodal blocking drugs is suggestive of severe AV nodal structural disease (due to degenerative or calcific disease or due to CAD) and prompts immediate cardiology consultation for possible pacemaker placement.

46. **How do you differentiate atrial tachycardia and atrial flutter from AF?**
Unlike AF, atrial tachycardia (or paroxysmal atrial tachycardia [PAT]) and atrial flutter demonstrate a regular ventricular rhythm and are characterized by regular and slower atrial rhythms (Table 4-2). The flutter rate (i.e., the atrial rate) in atrial flutter ranges between 250 and 350 bpm. The most common flutter rate is 300 bpm, and the most common ventricular rates are 150 and 75 bpm, respectively. Atrial tachycardias have slower atrial rates, ranging from 150 to 250 bpm. The most common cause of atrial tachycardia with block is digitalis toxicity.

TABLE 4-2. COMPARISON OF SUPRAVENTRICULAR TACHYCARDIAS

	Atrial Fibrillation	Atrial Flutter	Atrial Tachycardia
Atrial rate (bpm)	>400	240–350	100–240
Atrial rhythm	Irregular	Regular	Regular
AV block	Variable	2:1, 4:1, 3:1, or variable	2:1, 4:1, 3:1, or variable
Ventricular rate (bpm)	Variable	150, 75, 100, or variable	Variable

AV = atrioventricular; bpm = beats per minute.

47. **What is the significance of capture and fusion beats on ECG in differentiating between VT and SVT with aberrancy?**
Capture beats, fusion beats, and AV dissociation are virtually pathognomonic of VT (Table 4-3). A capture beat is a normally conducted sinus beat interrupting a wide-complex tachycardia. A fusion beat has a QRS morphology intermediate between a normally conducted narrow beat and a wide-complex ventricular beat. The clinical hallmark of AV dissociation is the presence of intermittent cannon waves in the jugular neck veins.

TABLE 4-3. DISTINGUISHING FEATURES OF WIDE-COMPLEX VENTRICULAR TACHYCARDIA AND SUPRAVENTRICULAR TACHYCARDIA

	VT	SVT
History of MI	+	−
Ventricular aneurysm	+	−
Fusion beats	+	−
Capture beats	+	−
Complete AV dissociation	+	−
Similar QRS when in sinus rhythm	−	+

TABLE 4-3. DISTINGUISHING FEATURES OF WIDE-COMPLEX VENTRICULAR TACHYCARDIA AND SUPRAVENTRICULAR TACHYCARDIA— *(continued)*

	VT	SVT
RBBB + QRS > 0.14 sec	+	−
LBBB + QRS > 0.16 sec	+	−
Positive concordance in V_1–V_6	+	−
LBBB + right QRS axis	+	−
Intermittent cannon waves	+	−

+ = present; − = absent; AV = atrioventricular; LBBB = left bundle branch block; MI = myocardial infarction; RBBB = right bundle branch block; SVT = supraventricular tachycardia; VT = ventricular tachycardia.

48. **What are the types of AV block?**
    - **First-degree:** Prolongation of the PR interval due to a conduction delay at the AV node.
    - **Second-degree:** Presence of dropped beats in which a P wave is not followed by a QRS complex (no ventricular depolarization and, therefore, no ventricular contraction). There are three types of second-degree AV block:
        - **Type I:** (Wenckebach phenomenon): PR interval lengthens with each successive beat until a beat is dropped and the cycle repeats itself.
        - **Type II:** PR intervals are prolonged but do not gradually lengthen until a beat is suddenly dropped. The dropped beat may occur regularly, with a fixed number (X) of beats for each dropped beat (called an "X·1 block"). Type II is much less common than type I and is commonly associated with bundle branch blocks.
        - **2:1 AV block:** Every other P wave is followed by a QRS alternating with P wave NOT followed by any QRS complex.
    - **Third-degree** (complete heart block): Separate pacemaker control of the atria and ventricles. The ECG shows widening of the QRS complex and a ventricular rate of 35–50 bpm.

49. **What ECG changes are seen first in hyperkalemia?**
    Tall, peaked, symmetrical T waves with a narrow base (so-called tented T wave) that usually are present in leads II, III, V_2, V_3, and V_4. As hyperkalemia progresses, the following may occur:
    - Shortened QT
    - Widened QRS interval
    - Depressed ST segment
    - Flattened P wave
    - Prolonged PR interval

    Eventually, the P waves disappear and the QRS complexes assume a configuration similar to a sine wave, eventually degenerating into VF. Widening of the QRS complex can assume a configuration consistent with atypical RBBB or LBBB, making the recognition of hyperkalemia more difficult. Unlike typical RBBB, hyperkalemia often causes prolongation of the entire QRS complex.

50. **Summarize the sequence of ECG changes in experimental hyperkalemia.**
    See Table 4-4.

TABLE 4-4. ELECTROCARDIOGRAM CHANGES IN EXPERIMENTAL HYPERKALEMIA	
Serum K$^+$ (mEq/L)	ECG Finding
>5.7	Tall, symmetrical T waves
>7.0	Reduced P wave amplitude
>7.0	Prolongation of PR interval
>8.4	Disappearance of P waves
9–11	Widening of QRS interval
>12	Ventricular fibrillation

ECG = electrocardiogram.

51. **What ECG signs suggest hypercalcemia? Are similar changes seen in other conditions?**
Shortened QT interval (particularly the interval between the beginning of the QRS complex and the peak of the T wave) and an abrupt slope to the peak of the T wave. Digitalis toxicity also causes shortened QT interval.

52. **Patients maintained on digitalis commonly exhibit some changes on ECG referred to as the "digitalis effect." What are these changes?**
Sagging of the ST segment and flattening and inversion of the T waves typically occurring in the inferolateral ECG leads that occurs when administered in therapeutic doses. Digitalis can cause a variety of other ECG abnormalities depending on the serum digoxin level.

53. **How do the ECG changes of "digitalis effect" compare with the ECG changes in myocardial ischemia?**
Typically, horizontal or down-sloping ST-segment depression, sharp-angled ST-T junctions, and U wave inversion are present in patients with subendocardial ischemia (coronary insufficiency). Less commonly, tall T waves may be a subtle ECG sign of myocardial ischemia.

54. **Where does the venous a-wave appear in the cardiac cycle and what specific component of the cardiac cycle does it correspond to?**
During the course of the cardiac cycle, the electrical events (corresponding to various ECG components of the PQRST complex) initiate and, therefore, precede the mechanical (pressure) events, and in turn, mechanical events are followed by auscultatory events (normal and extra heart sounds). Shortly after the ECG "P wave," the atria contract to produce the A wave, which may at times be visible by careful inspection of the jugular pressure waveform. In patients with longstanding systemic HTN, this atrial contraction may be "stronger" and a larger contributor to the total filling of the ventricle and as a result, a loud extra sound called "atrial gallop" or "S_4 sound" may be audible by cardiac auscultation in patients with HTN.

55. **Where does an S_3 occur in relation to the QRS complex?**
The QRS complex initiates ventricular systole, followed shortly by LV contraction and the rapid buildup of LV pressure. Almost immediately, LV pressure exceeds LA pressure to close the mitral valve and produces S_1. When LV pressure exceeds aortic pressure, the aortic valve opens, and when aortic pressure is once again greater than LV pressure, the aortic valve closes to produce S_2 and terminate ventricular ejection. The decreasing LV pressure drops below LA pressure to open the mitral valve, and a period of rapid ventricular filling commences. During this time, an S_3 may be heard (Fig. 4-3).

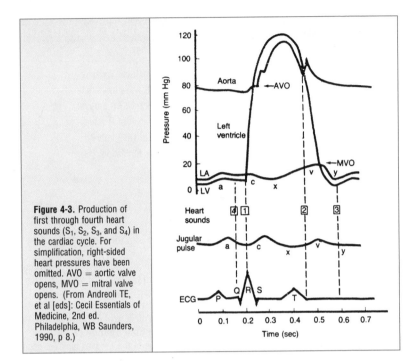

Figure 4-3. Production of first through fourth heart sounds (S₁, S₂, S₃, and S₄) in the cardiac cycle. For simplification, right-sided heart pressures have been omitted. AVO = aortic valve opens, MVO = mitral valve opens. (From Andreoli TE, et al [eds]: Cecil Essentials of Medicine, 2nd ed. Philadelphia, WB Saunders, 1990, p 8.)

DIAGNOSIS

56. **What are the cardiac and noncardiac causes of chest pain and their characteristics?**
See Tables 4-5 and 4-6.

57. **Is exercise treadmill ECG testing (ETT) helpful in confirming the diagnosis of exertional angina?**
Yes. Exercise testing is the most common provocative test used by clinicians to confirm the clinical diagnosis of exertional angina pectoris. An exercise ECG test is considered positive for CAD if it shows at least a 1-mm horizontal or downsloping ST segment depression during exercise. Myocardial ischemia is induced in these patients by an increase in myocardial O_2 demand, primarily due to the increase in heart rate with exercise.

58. **How does Bayes' theorem help determine the value of ETT in the detection of CAD?**
By allowing prediction of the presence or absence of CAD in a patient based on the prevalence of CAD in the population and the sensitivity and specificity of the diagnostic test. Bayes' theorem is the calculation that allows one to predict the posttest probability of a diagnosis based on the likely probability expected prior to performance of the diagnostic test. In general, the ability of noninvasive stress tests (treadmill ETT, treadmill thallium myocardial scintigraphy, treadmill or dobutamine echocardiography, or bicycle exercise radionuclide ventriculography) to predict the presence or absence of CAD in patients with a very low or very high pretest probability of CAD is poor. With either a high or a low pretest probability (based on clinical history), noninvasive testing does not help the clinician decide whether or

TABLE 4-5. CARDIOVASCULAR CAUSES OF CHEST PAIN

Condition	Location	Quality	Duration	Aggravating/Relieving Factors	Associated Signs and Symptoms
Angina	Retrosternal region; radiates to or occasionally isolated to neck, jaw, epigastrium, shoulder, or arms (left common)	Pressure, burning, squeezing, heaviness, indigestion	<2–10 min	Precipitated by exercise, cold weather, or emotional stress; relieved by rest or nitroglycerin; atypical (Prinzmetal's) angina may be unrelated to activity, often early morning	S₃ or murmur of papillary muscle dysfunction during pain
Rest or crescendo angina	Same as angina	Same as angina but may be more severe	Usually < 20 min	Same as angina, with decreasing tolerance for exertion or at rest	Similar to stable angina, but may be pronounced; transient heart failure can occur
Myocardial infarction	Substernal and may radiate like angina	Heaviness, pressure, burning, constriction	>30 min but variable	Unrelieved by rest or nitroglycerin	Shortness of breath, sweating, weakness, nausea, vomiting
Pericarditis	Usually begins over sternum or toward cardiac apex and may radiate to neck or left shoulder; often more localized than the pain of myocardial infarction	Sharp, stabbing, knifelike	Lasts many hours to days; may wax and wane	Aggravated by deep breathing, rotating chest, or supine position; relieved by sitting up and leaning forward.	Pericardial friction rub

(continued)

TABLE 4-5. CARDIOVASCULAR CAUSES OF CHEST PAIN—*(continued)*

Condition	Location	Quality	Duration	Aggravating/Relieving Factors	Associated Signs and Symptoms
Aortic dissection	Anterior chest; may radiate to back abdominal	Excruciating, tearing, knifelike	Sudden onset, unrelenting	Usually occurs in setting of hypertension or predisposition, such as Marfan syndrome	Murmur of aortic insufficiency, pulse or blood pressure asymmetry; neurologic deficit
Pulmonary embolism (chest pain often not present)	Substernal or over area of pulmonary infarction	Pleuritic (with pulmonary infarction) or like angina	Sudden onset; minute to < 1 hr	May be aggravated by breathing	Dyspnea, tachypnea, tachycardia, hypotension, signs of acute right ventricular failure, and pulmonary hypertension with large emboli; rales, pleural rub, hemoptysis with pulmonary infarction
Pulmonary hypertension	Substernal	Pressure, oppressive	Similar to angina	Aggravated by effort	Pain usually associated with dyspnea; signs of pulmonary hypertension

S_3 = third heart sound.
From Goldman L: Approach to the patient with possible cardiovascular disease. In Goldman L, Ausiello D (eds): Cecil Medicine, 23rd ed. Philadelphia, WB Saunders, 2007.

TABLE 4-6. NONCARDIAC CAUSES OF CHEST PAIN

Condition	Location	Quality	Duration	Aggravating/Relieving Factors	Associated Signs and Symptoms
Pneumonitis and pleurisy	Localized over involved area	Pleuritic, localized	Brief or prolonged	Painful breathing	Dyspnea, cough, fever, dull to percussion, bronchial breath sounds, rales, occasional pleural rub
Spontaneous pneumothorax	Unilateral	Sharp, well-localized	Sudden onset, lasts many hours	Painful breathing	Dyspnea, hyperresonance, and decreased breath and voice sounds over involved lung
Musculoskeletal disorders	Variable	Aching	Short or long duration	Aggravated by movement, history of muscle exertion or injury	Tender to pressure or movement
Herpes zoster	Dermatomal in distribution	Burning, itching	Prolonged	None	Vesicular rash appears in area of discomfort
Esophageal reflux	Substernal, epigastric	Burning, visceral discomfort	10–60 min	Aggravated by large meal, postprandial recumbency; relief with antacid	Water brash
Peptic ulcer	Epigastric, substernal	Visceral burning, aching	Prolonged	Relief with food, antacid	
Gallbladder disease	Epigastric, right upper quadrant	Visceral	Prolonged	May be unprovoked or follow meals	Right upper quadrant tenderness may be present
Anxiety	Often localized over precordium	Variable; location often moves from place to place	Varies; often fleeting	Situational	Sighing respirations, often chest wall tenderness

From Goldman L: Approach to the patient with possible cardiovascular disease. In Goldman L, Ausiello D (eds): Cecil Medicine, 23rd ed. Philadelphia, WB Saunders, 2007.

not to perform a definitive diagnostic test, such as coronary arteriography. Conversely, patients with an intermediate pretest probability of CAD (30–70%) are good candidates for noninvasive stress testing (Table 4-7). In the patient with typical exertional angina pectoris and two or more coronary risk factors (associated with $\geq$ 80% pretest probability of CAD), a negative ETT and thallium myocardial scintigram predict $<$ 30% probability of CAD. However, a positive treadmill thallium test in the same patient predicts a 90% probability of CAD. In such patients, coronary angiography is recommended in the latter case (positive treadmill thallium test) but not in the former.

TABLE 4-7. PROBABILITY OF CORONARY ARTERY DISEASE

Pretest Probability (%)	After Treadmill ECG (%)		After Treadmill Thallium (%)
80	Positive test: 95	→	Positive test: 99
		→	Negative test: 85
	Negative test: 60	→	Positive test: 90
		→	Negative test: 30

ECG = electrocardiogram.

59. **What are the medical contraindications to ETT?**

Acute or pending MI
Acute coronary syndrome (ACS)
Acute myocarditis or pericarditis
Left main CAD
Severe aortic stenosis
Uncontrolled HTN
Uncontrolled cardiac arrhythmias
Second- or third-degree AV block
Acute noncardiac illness

60. **A 31-year-old man complains of a sudden onset of sharp left chest pain, increased by deep inspiration and coughing. Physical findings, chest x-ray, and ECG are normal. What is your differential diagnosis?**
   - Acute pleuritis (coxsackievirus A, B)
   - Acute pericarditis (coxsackievirus B)
   - Pneumonia (viral, bacterial)
   - Pulmonary embolus or infarction
   - Pneumothorax

   In this patient, the most likely clinical diagnosis causing pleuritic chest pain in the presence of a normal physical, chest x-ray, and ECG findings is **acute viral pleuritis** or **pericarditis.**

61. **A 56-year-old man presents to the emergency department with acute onset of squeezing and diffuse, anterior chest pain associated with diaphoresis and dyspnea. What is your differential diagnosis?**
   - Acute MI
   - Angina pectoris
   - Acute pericarditis
   - Acute pulmonary embolus

- Acute aortic dissection
- Pneumothorax

62. **Which tests will help confirm your clinical suspicions?**
12-lead ECG, cardiac enzymes, and chest x-ray. Among these diagnoses, the first three are most common and should be carefully considered in the diagnostic work-up of this patient. A **12-lead ECG** is performed to look for ST segment elevations (evidence of acute myocardial injury due to infarction or pericarditis), ST segment depressions (evidence of subendocardial ischemia), or T wave changes. Determination of **serial cardiac enzymes** (troponin I or T or creatine kinase and MB CM isoenzyme) over the first 24–48 hours of hospitalization will help to confirm a diagnosis of acute MI. The absence of any ECG changes of acute MI or ischemia in a patient with severe anterior chest pain radiating to the back should suggest the clinical diagnosis of acute aortic dissection. Finally, a **chest x-ray** is helpful in the work-up of patients with acute chest pain to look for evidence of pneumothorax, cardiac enlargement suggestive of cardiac failure, or wedge-shaped pulmonary consolidation suggestive of acute pulmonary embolus.

63. **An 89-year-old woman was found unconscious in her backyard. She "woke up" a few minutes after arrival at the emergency department. Physical, neurologic, ECG, laboratory, and chest x-ray findings are all normal. She feels fine and demands to be released. Would you admit her to the hospital?**
Yes. Syncope, defined as a transient loss or impairment of consciousness, can be due to a wide variety of etiologies, both cardiovascular and noncardiovascular. Patients most likely to have cardiovascular syncope are older and may or may not have a prior history of documented cardiac disease (manifested by angina pectoris, MI, or resuscitated sudden cardiac death). Patients at high risk for cardiovascular syncope (similar to this elderly patient) should be hospitalized because they have a worse prognosis and may have potentially life-threatening complications of their underlying cardiovascular disease (CVD).

64. **List the common cardiovascular causes of syncope.**
- **Tachyarrhythmias:** VT or SVT (AF, atrial flutter, or paroxysmal SVT).
- **Bradyarrhythmias:** second- or third-degree AV block, AF with a slow ventricular response rate, or sinus bradycardia due to sick sinus syndrome.
- **LV outflow obstruction:** due to fixed lesions (valvular, subvalvular, or supravalvular aortic stenosis) or dynamic obstruction such as HCM. Characteristically, these patients present with syncope during or immediately after exercise.
- **LV inflow obstruction:** due to severe mitral stenosis or a large LA myxoma.
- **Primary pulmonary HTN.**

HYPERTENSION

See also Chapter 2, General Medicine and Ambulatory Care, and Chapter 18, Geriatrics.

65. **How do you classify or stage HTN severity?**
HTN is now classified into two stages:
- **Stage 1:** BP range 140–150/90–99
- **Stage 2:** BP range $\geq$160/$\geq$100

66. **How does the initial HTN stage predict treatment response?**
Patients with stage 2 HTN are rarely controlled to a goal BP of < 140/90 mmHg on a single BP-lowering drug. The Antihypertensive and Lipid-Lowering Treatment to Prevent Heart Attack Trial (ALLHAT) as well as several other trials have shown that at least two or more drugs are needed in two thirds of hypertensive patients and one third require three antihypertensives to achieve target BP.

ALLHAT Officers and Coordinators for the ALLHAT Collaborative Research Group: Major outcomes in high-risk hypertensive patients randomized to angiotensin-converting enzyme inhibitor or calcium channel blocker vs. diuretic: The Antihypertensive and Lipid-Lowering Treatment to Prevent Heart Attack Trial (ALLHAT), *JAMA* 288:2981–2997, 2002.

67. **Explain the significance of the ALLHAT clinical trial.**
The ALLHAT trial is the largest multicenter, double-blind, controlled clinical trial designed to evaluate the effects of four different classes of antihypertensive drugs (thiazide diuretics, angiotensin-converting enzyme [ACE] inhibitors, alpha blockers, and calcium blockers) on fatal and non-fatal CAD as well as on other cardiovascular endpoints such as stroke, angina, heart failure, and peripheral vascular disease risk. The study findings showed no superiority of the ACE inhibitor lisinopril, the dihydropyridine calcium blocker amlodipine, or the alpha blocker doxazosin over the diuretic chlorthalidone in preventing fatal or nonfatal CAD. However, one or more cardiovascular complications were less frequent with a thiazide diuretic than with any other antihypertensive drug.

ALLHAT Officers and Coordinators for the ALLHAT Collaborative Research Group: Major outcomes in high-risk hypertensive patients randomized to angiotensin-converting enzyme inhibitor or calcium channel blocker vs. diuretic: The Antihypertensive and Lipid-Lowering Treatment to Prevent Heart Attack Trial (ALLHAT), *JAMA* 288:2981–2997, 2002.

68. **Summarize the main results and clinical implications of the ALLHAT trial.**
- CAD risk was similar in all four treatment groups receiving a thiazide diurertic, an ACE inhibitor, a dihydropyridine calcium blocker, or an alpha blocker.
- Overall BP control was significantly better and systolic BP was 2 mmHg lower in diuretic-treated patients than in ACE inhibitor–treated patients. This difference was even higher (~4 mmHg) in African Americans.
- No overall difference in BP control or BP levels (0.7 mmHg lower systolic BP in diuretic-treated patients) between diuretic- and calcium blocker–treated patients.
- Between 10% and 15% higher risk of stroke and CAD morbid and fatal events in ACE inhibitor–treated compared with diuretic-treated patients. African Americans had a 40% higher stroke risk and a 19% higher CV risk compared with those treated with a diuretic; this was associated with a 4-mm higher systolic BP among African American patients.

ALLHAT Officers and Coordinators for the ALLHAT Collaborative Research Group: Major outcomes in high-risk hypertensive patients randomized to angiotensin-converting enzyme inhibitor or calcium channel blocker vs. diuretic: The Antihypertensive and Lipid-Lowering Treatment to Prevent Heart Attack Trial (ALLHAT), *JAMA* 288:2981–2997, 2002.

69. **What are the two key take-home messages from ALLHAT?**
- Control of HTN frequently requires multiple antihypertensive drugs used in combination. The recent Seventh Report of the Joint National Committee on Prevention, Detection, Evaluation, and Treatment of High Blood Pressure (JNC 7) report recommends initiation of two antihypertensive drugs whenever BP > 160/100 mmHg (now called "stage 2 HTN").
- More effective reduction of systolic BP in a high-risk older hypertensive patient results in more effective cardiovascular prevention.

Cushman WC, Ford CE, Cutler JA, et al: For the ALLHAT Collaborative Research Group: Success and predictors of blood pressure control in diverse North American settings: The Antihypertensive and Lipid-Lowering to Prevent Heart Attack Trial (ALLHAT), *J Clin Hypertens* 4:393–404, 2002.

70. **How effective are diuretics?**
Very effective. Thiazide diuretics appear to be unsurpassed in preventing cardiovascular complications of HTN and are, therefore, recommended by the JNC 7 report of the Joint National Committee for the Prevention, Detection, Diagnosis and Treatment of High Blood Pressure as preferred initial antihypertensive drug therapy in uncomplicated hypertension.

Seventh Report of the Joint National Committee on Prevention: Detection, Evaluation, and Treatment of High Blood Pressure: The JNC 7 report, *JAMA* 289:2560–2572, 2003. Available at www.nhlbi.nih.gov/guidelines/hypertension.

71. **Does antihypertensive therapy in older patients affect the risk of MI and angina?**
The Systolic Hypertension in the Elderly Program (SHEP) demonstrated that a thiazide-based antihypertensive regimen (chlorthalidone, 12.5–25 mg/day, alone or combined with atenolol, 25–50 mg/day) reduces stroke risk by 36% and nonfatal MI plus coronary death by 27% in older (>60 yr) patients with isolated systolic HTN (systolic BP > 160 mmHg/diastolic BP < 90 mmHg). Major cardiovascular events were reduced by 32%. As a result, overall all-cause mortality was 13% lower. Similar studies in younger hypertensive patients have shown a smaller beneficial effect or no effect of antihypertensive drug therapy on CAD events.

SHEP Cooperative Research Group: Prevention of stroke by anti-hypertensive drug treatment in older persons with isolated systolic hypertension. Final results of the Systolic Hypertension in the Elderly Program (SHEP), *JAMA* 265:3255–3264, 1991.

72. **Are calcium blockers as effective as diuretics in isolated systolic HTN in older patients?**
Yes. A multicenter clinical trial, the Systolic Hypertension in Europe (Syst-Eur) Trial, showed the same reduction in cardiac and stroke events in older (>60 yr) patients with systolic HTN (systolic BP > 160 mmHg) and normal or mildly elevated diastolic BP (<95 mmHg) with a long-acting dihydropyridine calcium blocker, alone or in combination with an ACE inhibitor. However, it has *not* yet been shown whether a dihydropyridine calcium blocker or a thiazide diuretic is *more* potent in reducing cardiovascular complications of HTN.

Staessen JA, Fagard R, Thijs L, et al: Randomised double-blind comparison of placebo and active treatment for older patients with isolated systolic hypertension. The Systolic Hypertension in Europe (Syst-Eur) Trial Investigators, *Lancet* 350:757–764, 1997.

73. **Which antihypertensive drug classes are currently recommended as first-line drugs in the treatment of HTN in patients at high risk for CAD?**
- Thiazide diuretics
- Beta blockers
- Calcium blockers
- ACE inhibitors

All of these drugs have been demonstrated to reduce the incidence of stroke and CAD in high-risk patients such as those with older age, dyslipidemia, or tobacco abuse history.

ALLHAT Officers and Coordinators for the ALLHAT Collaborative Research Group: Major outcomes in high-risk hypertensive patients randomized to angiotensin-converting enzyme inhibitor or calcium channel blocker versus diuretic: The Antihypertensive and Lipid-Lowering Treatment to Prevent Heart Attack Trial (ALLHAT), *JAMA* 288:2981–2997, 2002.

Seventh Report of the Joint National Committee on Prevention: Detection, Evaluation, and Treatment of High Blood Pressure: The JNC 7 report, *JAMA* 289:2560–2572, 2003. Available at www.nhlbi.nih.gov/guidelines/hypertension/.

Staessen JA, Fagard R, Thijs L, et al: for the Systolic Hypertension–Europe (Syst-Eur) Trial Investigators: Morbidity and mortality in the placebo-controlled European Trial on Isolated Systolic Hypertension in the Elderly, *Lancet* 350:757–764, 1997.

Yusuf S, Sleight P, Pogue J, et al: Effects of an angiotensin-converting-enzyme inhibitor, ramipril, on cardiovascular events in high-risk patients. The Heart Outcomes Prevention Evaluation Study Investigators, *N Engl J Med* 342:145–153, 2000.

74. **Although diuretics are the preferred agent for initial HTN treatment, for which patients should beta blockers be considered first?**
Those with a past history of a MI, compensated heart failure, or CAD. Contraindications to beta blockers must be carefully weighed against their potential therapeutic benefits. For example, a beta blocker should be avoided in a patient admitted to the hospital with acutely decompensated heart failure but may be started at lower doses then gradually increased in patients with well-compensated and stable heart failure. Withdrawal of beta blockers—particularly in patients with CAD—should be done gradually to avoid rebound increase in anginal symptoms upon their discontinuation.

75. **Is an angiotensin receptor blocker (ARB) equally effective as an ACE inhibitor in preventing cardiovascular complications of hypertension?**
Yes. Until recently, the evidence supporting the importance of ARB as an effective and safe BP-lowering drug class was quite limited. Recently, large prospective, randomized clinical trials have shown that an ARB is at least as effective as a beta blocker and as effective as an ACE inhibitor in preventing major cardiovascular complications. The largest clinical trials that support these conclusions are the Losartan Intervention For Endpoint reduction in Hypertension (LIFE) and ONgoing Telmisartan Alone and in combination with Ramipril Global Endpoint Trial (ONTARGET) clinical trials.

The ONTARGET Investigators: Telmisartan, ramipril or both in patients at high risk for vascular events, *N Engl J Med* 358:1547–1559, 2008.

76. **A 45-year-old hypertensive woman has been treated with amlodipine, a calcium channel blocker, for chronic stable angina pectoris and HTN. She complains of ankle edema that worsened after her dose was recently increased. Are diuretics indicated?**
No. Ankle edema is a common side effect of dihydropyridine calcium channel blockers, occurring in 7–20% of patients treated. Edema is a dose-dependent side effect and readily responds to lowering of the calcium channel blocker dose. Another novel strategy to minimize the occurrence of ankle edema combines calcium channel blockade with ACE inhibition. This combination is more effective than monotherapy with either drug in lowering BP and is associated with lower prevalence of any dose-related side effects, including ankle edema.

CORONARY ARTERY DISEASE AND ANGINA SYNDROMES

77. **Define "angina."**
The symptom complex that occurs during myocardial ischemia. Angina is typically described as a pressure or bandlike sensation in the middle of the chest that is precipitated by exertion and relieved by rest. Angina may also present with left arm or jaw pain and fatigue. Symptoms in women may be atypical and include dyspnea and palpitations.

78. **What is Prinzmetal's or variant angina?**
Described by Myron Prinzmetal in 1955, this disorder is associated with sudden localized spasm of a coronary artery that usually occurs near an atherosclerotic plaque. Typical ischemic ST changes (elevation) occur during the spasm.

79. **Is treadmill ETT helpful in confirming the diagnosis of variant angina?**
No. In patients with variant angina, myocardial ischemia is primarily due to a decrease in O_2 supply rather than to an increase in O_2 demand. Exercise testing is thus of limited diagnostic value in these patients and may show ST segment elevation, ST segment depression, or no change in ST segments during exercise.

80. **Do nitrates differ in efficacy when used in the management of variant angina compared with classic effort angina?**
No. Patients with both forms of angina respond promptly to nitrates.

81. **Do beta blockers differ in efficacy and safety when used in the management of variant angina compared with classic effort angina?**
Yes. Although the response of patients with effort angina to beta blockers is uniformly good, the response of patients with vasospastic or Prinzmetal's angina is variable. In some patients with vasospastic angina, the duration of episodes of angina pectoris may be prolonged during therapy with propranolol, a noncardioselective beta blocker. In others, especially those with associated fixed atherosclerotic lesions, beta blockers may reduce the frequency of anginal episodes. Noncardioselective beta blockers may, in some patients with vasospastic angina, leave a receptor-mediated coronary arterial vasoconstriction unopposed and thereby worsen anginal symptoms.

82. **Do calcium blockers differ in efficacy and safety when used in the management of variant angina compared with classic effort angina?**
No. In contrast to beta blockers, calcium blockers are quite effective in reducing the frequency and duration of episodes of vasospastic angina. Along with nitrates, calcium blockers are the mainstay of treatment of vasospastic angina because of their proven efficacy and safety.

83. **A 78-year-old asthmatic man has stable exertional angina of 3 years' duration. His past medical history reveals intermittent claudication after walking 50 yards. What is your approach to medical management of his anginal symptoms?**
This elderly man has three medical problems: asthma, intermittent claudication, and chronic stable angina. Of the available antianginal drugs, beta blockers are contraindicated because of the presence of asthma. Cardioselective beta blockers, such as metoprolol or atenolol, may be used cautiously in low doses in asthma, but noncardioselective beta blockers are not safe in this patient. However, the presence of peripheral vascular disease, manifested by intermittent claudication, also is a contraindication for the use of any beta blocker. Calcium channel blockers or nitrates are thus the antianginal drugs of choice in this patient.

84. **What is the HDL hypothesis?**
The observation that elevated high-density lipoprotein (HDL) cholesterol levels reduce the risk of coronary heart disease. Historically, the first hint of the validity of this "HDL hypothesis" was the finding of the Helsinki Heart Study that a 10% increase in HDL cholesterol levels induced by gemfibrozil accounted for the 15% larger reduction in CAD mortality compared with the first Lipid Research Clinic Coronary Primary Prevention Trial (LRC-CPPT) that used cholestyramine, a bile acid sequestrant resin. Both cholestyramine and gemfibrozil reduce low-density lipoprotein (LDL) cholesterol modestly by 10% but only gemfibrozil raises HDL cholesterol levels by as much as approximately 10%. More recent clinical trials have further supported an independent role of HDL in mediating coronary heart disease risk.

Frick MH, Elo O, Haapa K, et al: Helsinki Heart Study: Primary prevention trial with gemfibrozil in middle-aged men with dyslipidemia. Safety of treatment, changes in risk factors, and incidence of coronary heart disease, *N Engl J Med* 371:1237–1245, 1987.

ACUTE CORONARY SYNDROME

85. **Define "acute coronary syndrome (ACS)."**
    A clinical syndrome characterized by *chest pain suggestive of cardiac ischemia* that is further classified by ECG and cardiac biomarker findings as:
    - UA
      - ECG: may or may not show ST segment depression, transient ST segment elevation, or new T wave inversion.
      - Cardiac biomarkers: not elevated (no evidence of cardiac injury).
    - Non-ST elevation myocardial infarction (NSTEMI)
      - ECG: may or may not show ST segment depression, transient ST segment elevation, or new T wave inversion.
      - Cardiac biomarkers: elevated.
    - ST elevation myocardial infarction (STEMI)
      - ECG: ST segment elevation or depression.
      - Cardiac biomarkers: elevated.

86. **How common is ACS?**
    Very common. ACS is a common potentially life-threatening medical condition. In 2003, it accounted for over 750,000 hospital admissions in the United States.

87. **Is aspirin effective in the treatment of UA?**
    Yes. Unequivocal evidence from two clinical trials, the Veterans Administration (VA) and Canadian Cooperative Trials, indicates that aspirin reduces subsequent MI and mortality in UA patients. Both mortality and MI are reduced by approximately 50% in aspirin-treated patients. Aspirin should be administered immediately when UA is suspected. There is less evidence to suggest a beneficial effect of aspirin in chronic stable angina pectoris.

    Cairns JA, Gent M, Singer J, et al: Aspirin, sulfinpyrazone, or both in unstable angina: Results of a Canadian multicenter trial, *N Engl J Med* 313:1369–1375, 1985.

    Lewis HD, Davis JW, Archibald DG, et al: Protective effects of aspirin against acute myocardial infarction and death in men with unstable angina: Results of a Veterans Administration Cooperative Study, *N Engl J Med* 309:396–403, 1983.

88. **Is clopidogrel recommended in patients admitted with UA or NSTEMI already treated with aspirin?**
    Yes. The American Heart Association/American College of Cardiology (AHA/ACC) guidelines recommend clopidogrel in patients admitted with ACS with no ST segment elevation in addition to aspirin therapy. This recommendation is based on the Clopidogrel in Unstable Angina to Prevent Recurrent Events (CURE) trial, which showed a significant reduction in recurrent cardiac events with the addition of clopidogrel to standard therapy including aspirin, beta blockers, and statins.

    Anderson JL, Adams CD, Antman EM, et al: ACC/AHA 2007 Guidelines for the Management of Patients With Unstable Angina/Non–ST-Elevation Myocardial Infarction. A Report of the American College of Cardiology/American Heart Association Task Force on Practice Guidelines (Writing Committee to Revise the 2002 Guidelines for the Management of Patients With Unstable Angina/Non–ST-Elevation Myocardial Infarction) developed in collaboration with the American College of Emergency Physicians, the Society for Cardiovascular Angiography and Interventions, and the Society of Thoracic Surgeons endorsed by the American Association of Cardiovascular and Pulmonary Rehabilitation and the Society for Academic Emergency Medicine, *J Am Coll Cardiol* 50:1–157, 2007.

The Clopidogrel in Unstable Angina to Prevent Recurrent Events Trial Investigators: Effects of clopidogrel in addition to aspirin in patients with acute coronary syndrome without ST segment elevation, *N Engl J Med* 345:494–502, 2001.

89. **Is clopidogrel equally effective in all patients?**
No. Recent studies showed that approximately 3% of the population are poor metabolizers of clopidrogel and, therefore, the drug is less effective. The incidence among the Chinese population may be as high as 14%. Patients who take proton pump inhibitors (PPIs) and clopidrogel also have an increased risk of rehospitalization after MI or coronary stent placement, suggesting PPIs affect efficacy.

Mega JL, Close SL, Wiviott SD, et al: Cytochrome P-450 polymorphisms and response to clopidogrel, *N Engl J Med* 360:354–362, 2009.

Simon T, Verstuyft C, Mary-Krause M, et al: Genetic determinants of response to clopidogrel and cardiovascular events, *N Engl J Med* 360:363–375, 2009.

Stocki KM, Le L, Zahkaryan A, et al: Risk of rehospitalization for patients using clopidogrel with a proton pump inhibitor, *Arch Intern Med* 170:704–710, 2010.

90. **Based on clinical assessments, which patients with ACS are at highest risk for death or recurrent MI?**
Those with:
- Age $\geq$ 65 years
- Presence of at least three risk factors for CAD
- Prior coronary stenosis $\geq$ 50%
- ST segment deviation on ECG at presentation
- History of at least two anginal events in prior 24 hours
- Use of aspirin in prior 7 days
- Elevated serum cardiac markers

The scoring system listed (Thrombosis in Myocardial Infarction [TIMI] trial) counts one point for the presence of each characteristic and can be easily obtained at the bedside on initial evaluation of any patient with acute chest pain in the emergency department. In validation studies of the TIMI risk scoring variables, cardiovascular event rates increased significantly as the TIMI risk score increased (Table 4-8).

Antman EM, Cohen M, Bernik PJLM, et al: The TIMI risk score for unstable angina/non–ST elevation MI: A method for prognostication and therapeutic decision making, *JAMA* 284:835–842, 2000.

TABLE 4-8. CARDIOVASCULAR EVENT RATES BY THROMBOSIS IN MYOCARDIAL INFARCTION SCORE

TIMI Score	Event Rate Increase (%)
0–1	4.7
2	8.3
3	13.2
4	19.9
5	26.2
6–7	40.9

TIMI = Thrombosis in Myocardial Infarction (trial).

91. **Which patients with UA should undergo cardiac catheterization?**
    Those with:
    - UA refractory to medical management
    - Prior revascularization, including percutaneous coronary intervention (balloon angioplasty or coronary stent placement or both), or coronary artery bypass surgery
    - Depressed LV function (left ventricular ejection fraction [LVEF] < 50%)
    - Life-threatening "malignant" ventricular arrhythmias
    - Persistent or recurrent angina/ischemia
    - Inducible myocardial ischemia (provoked by exercise, dobutamine, adenosine, or dipyridamole) at a low exercise level

92. **Describe the pathophysiologic mechanisms of NSTEMI and STEMI.**
    In NSTEMI, the coronary artery is intermittently or incompletely occluded or both by platelet-rich "white" thrombus that is recently formed from platelet aggregation at the site of a damaged inner surface of a coronary artery. The trigger for this platelet aggregation is usually rupture of an atherosclerotic plaque in an artery with < 50% stenosis and causes acute subendocardial ischemia. Subendocardial ischemia may present with ST segment depression or T wave changes on ECG that are transient or dynamic in nature. This white thrombus is in sharp contrast to the mature red blood cell and fibrin-rich "red" or "mature" thrombus, which is the hallmark pathologic finding in patients with STEMI. Unlike the platelet-rich "white" thrombus, a mature "red" thrombus results in a complete or persistent coronary artery occlusion or both resulting in severe transmural ischemia characterized by acute ST segment elevation on ECG.

93. **Are the treatments different for NSTEMI and STEMI?**
    Yes. For patients with STEMI, thrombolytic or "clot-busting" drugs such as alteplase, tenecteplase, and reteplase are also indicated either as primary treatment or prior to percutaneous coronary intervention (PCI) such as balloon angioplasty with or without coronary stent placement. PCI should be attempted if available within the appropriate time frame. For NSTEMI, patients can be initially treated with potent platelet aggregation inhibitors such as aspirin in addition to more potent platelet aggregation inhibitors such as glycoprotein (GP) IIb/IIIa inhibitors (such as eptifibatide) or a platelet P2Y12 receptor blocker such as clopidogrel or both. Beta blockers are also indicated for NSTEMI patients. For some, calcium channel blockers, ARBs, and potassium and magnesium replacement should be considered. PCI will also play a role for many patients with NSTEMI.

94. **What are the contraindications to thrombolytic therapy in patients with STEMI?**
    - Bleeding disorders
    - Severe uncontrolled HTN (BP > 180/120 mmHg)
    - Recent history of thromboembolic cerebrovascular accident (within 2 mo)
    - Any prior history of a hemorrhagic cerebrovascular accident
    - Prolonged cardiopulmonary resuscitation (>10 min)
    - Active bleeding from a peptic ulcer or other noncompressible source
    - Known brain metastasis or cerebrovascular arteriovenous malformation (AVM) or aneurysm

    Kushner FG, Hand M, Smith SC Jr, et al: 2009 focused updates: ACC/AHA Guidelines for the Management of Patients With ST-Elevation Myocardial Infarction (Updating the 2004 Guideline and 2007 Focused Update) and ACC/AHA/SCAI Guidelines on Percutaneous Coronary Intervention (Updating the 2005 Guideline and 2007 Focused Update). A report of the American College of Cardiology Foundation/American Heart Association Task Force on Practice Guidelines, *Circulation* 20:2271–2306, 2009.

95. **Does early administration of thrombolytic therapy after STEMI decrease mortality?**

Yes. Thrombolysis is the most effective life-saving pharmacologic therapy in acute MI, saving approximately 40 lives for every 1000 treated patients and reducing 30-day and 1-year mortality by about 25%. In the GISSI (Gruppo Italiano per lo Studio della Sopravivenza nell' Infarto Miocardio) trial published in 1986, 11,806 patients with acute MI presenting within 12 hours of symptom onset were randomly assigned to receive intravenous (IV) streptokinase or placebo. The hospital mortality was significantly reduced in patients treated with streptokinase within the first 6 hours. Most important, there was a remarkable 50% reduction in hospital mortality in patients treated within 1 hour of symptom onset. Subsequent clinical trials of various thrombolytic drugs—including streptokinase (SK), alteplase (t-PA), reteplase (r-PA), and the most recent U.S. Food and Drug Administration (FDA)–approved thrombolytic, tenecteplase (TNK–t-PA)—confirmed the consistent improvement in survival with thrombolytic therapy in patients with acute ST elevation MI.

   GISSI Trial: Effect of time to treatment on reduction in hospital mortality observed in streptokinase-treated patients, *Lancet* 1:397–401, 1986.

96. **Which drug is more effective in achieving successful reperfusion of a thrombosed coronary artery: SK, t-PA, r-PA, or TNK–t-PA?**

t-PA. In the TIMI trial, t-PA resulted in approximately twice as many successful reperfusions (due to clot lysis) as SK. In the Global Utilization of Streptokinase and Tissue Plasminogen Activator for Occluded Coronary Arteries (GUSTO) trial, t-PA was more effective than SK in opening coronary arteries and preventing death in the first 30 days after acute MI. In the Reteplase (r-PA) Angiographic Phase II International Dose-finding Study (RAPID) I and RAPID II trials, approximately 60% of r-PA–treated patients experienced complete reperfusion at 90 minutes compared with about 50–55% of patients treated with t-PA. In the large-scale GUSTO III trial, however, despite the higher TIMI flow grade 3 in patients treated with r-PA, survival was similar in patients who received t-PA or r-PA. Angiographic trials of TNK–t-PA showed similar coronary angiographic success compared with t-PA, and the Assessment of the Safety and Efficacy of a New Thrombolytic (ASSENT-2) trial confirmed the equivalent efficacy of both agents in improving survival. Recent mortality trials of TNK–t-PA showed no survival benefit over t-PA. In summary, t-PA is clearly angiographically superior to SK in opening arteries and saving lives, whereas the newer r-PA and TNK-t-PA thrombolytics are not clearly superior to t-PA in overall efficacy, but are more convenient to administer as a bolus (single bolus for TNK–t-PA and double boluses, 30 min apart, for t-PA).

   GUSTO Angiographic Investigators: The effects of tissue plasminogen activator, streptokinase, or both on coronary-artery patency, ventricular function and survival after acute myocardial infarction, *N Engl J Med* 329:1615–1622, 1993.

97. **What are the third-generation thrombolytic drugs?**
   - Recombinant tissue plasminogen activator (r-PA): reteplase
   - TNK tissue plasminogen activator (TNK–t-PA): Tenecteplase
   - Novel plasminogen activator (n-PA): lanoteplase

   Third-generation thrombolytics (better called "fibrinolytics" because they basically degrade fibrin) are mutants of wild-type tissue plasminogen activator. Only r-PA and TNK–t-PA are currently FDA-approved and commercially available; n-PA was found to cause an unacceptably high risk of intracranial hemorrhage and is not approved by the FDA for general use in the United States.

98. **Explain the advantages of the third-generation thrombolytics.**

These drugs lack the finger moiety of wild-type t-PA that makes the drug less "sticky" to the fibrin on the surface of the clot and potentiates the clot-dissolving effect of r-PA and n-PA. The ability of the drug to "stick" to the outer clot surface is called "fibrin affinity." The main advantages of third-generation thrombolytic drugs are:

- **Efficacy:** Greater clot lytic effect.
- **Convenience:** Longer half-life makes these drugs "bolus-able" thrombolytics. Both r-PA and TNK–t-PA have longer half-lives than t-PA and can be given as bolus injections; r-PA is administered as a double bolus (10 units IV q30min) and TNK–t-PA is administered as a single 5-second IV bolus.
- **Fibrin specificity:** TNK–t-PA is 80-fold more fibrin-specific than t-PA.
- **Resistance to plasminogen activator inhibitor 1 (PAI-1),** making it more resistant to breakdown by naturally occurring inhibitors of plasminogen activator. This is the case for TNK–t-PA.

99. **How successful is the combination of thrombolysis and GP IIb/IIIa inhibitors for patients with acute coronary occlusion?**
    The combination of thrombolysis and GP IIb/IIIa inhibition is not routinely recommended. Three clinical trials have evaluated the angiographic results of thrombolytics in combination with an inhibitor of the platelet glycoprotein GP IIb/IIIa receptor: the TIMI 14, Strategies for Patency Enhancement in the Emergency Department (SPEED), GUSTO, and the INtegrelin and low dose ThRombolysis in Acute Myocardial Infarction (INTRO-AMI) trials. All three specifically evaluated angiographic outcome at 60 and 90 minutes after thrombolytics when combined with a platelet glycoprotein GP IIb/IIIa receptor. The TIMI 14 and GUSTO SPEED trials revealed that the proportion of patients who completely reperfuse (as evidenced by a TIMI flow grade 3) is significantly higher with the combination of half-dose t-PA or r-PA with the platelet glycoprotein GP IIb/IIIa receptor inhibitor abciximab (Reopro). The INTRO-AMI trial confirmed these results using the platelet glycoprotein GP IIb/IIIa receptor inhibitor eptifibatide (Integrelin) and showed a similar increase in rate and extent of thrombolysis at 90 minutes after thrombolysis is initiated. However, despite these promising angiographic results, none of the mortality trials showed any survival advantages for the combination of lysis + GP IIb/IIIa inhibitors.

Antman EM, Giugliano RP, Gibson CM, et al, for the TIMI 14 Investigators: Abciximab facilitates the rate and extent of thrombolysis: Results of the Thrombolysis in Myocardial Infarction (TIMI) 14 trial, *Circulation* 99:2720–2732, 1999.

Trial of abciximab with and without low-dose reteplase for acute myocardial infarction: Strategies for Patency Enhancement in the Emergency Department (SPEED) Group, *Circulation* 101:2788–2794, 2000.

KEY POINTS: PLATELET AGGREGATION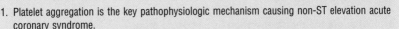

1. Platelet aggregation is the key pathophysiologic mechanism causing non-ST elevation acute coronary syndrome.

2. Strategies specifically targeting the inhibition of platelet aggregation, such as aspirin, low-molecular-weight or unfractionated heparin, and clopidogrel, are routinely recommended.

3. The use of more potent platelet aggregation inhibitors (the glycoprotein IIB/IIIA inhibitors such as tirofiban, eptifibatide, or abciximab) are reserved for patients with acute coronary syndromes at substantially high risk for major cardiovascular complications because of greater bleeding risk.

4. Patients may have genetic characteristics that make clopidogrel less effective.

5. Clopidogrel may have less efficacy in patients taking proton pump inhibitors.

100. **Is a PCI such as primary angioplasty using a balloon-tipped catheter as effective as pharmacologic reperfusion therapy with a thrombolytic drug in patients with STEMI?**

Yes. The Primary Angioplasty in Myocardial Infarction (PAMI) trial is the first published clinical trial designed specifically to compare balloon angioplasty with thrombolysis as the primary reperfusion therapy in patients with acute ST elevation MI. Survival rates (at 30 days and at 2 yr) after primary angioplasty were similar to those with thrombolysis in acute MI, but angioplasty conferred greater freedom from recurrent ischemia, reinfarction, and need for readmission to the hospital. Another important advantage of balloon angioplasty over thrombolytic drug therapy is reduced risk of intracranial hemorrhage, a dreadful complication of thrombolysis, particularly in elderly patients. Several subsequent trials using more modern and effective revascularization techniques such as coronary stenting have consistently demonstrated a clinical survival advantage of primary coronary intervention (coronary balloon angioplasty ± stent placement) over thrombolysis as well as less risk of intracranial hemorrhage. In clinical practice and included in the most current recommendations of the ACC, mechanical coronary reperfusion with primary stenting is recommended as a preferred reperfusion strategy in ST elevation MI patients over thrombolytic therapy in clinical settings in which percutaneous coronary intervention is feasible.

Nunn CM, O'Neill WW, Rothbaum D, et al: Long-term outcome after primary angioplasty: Report from the Primary Angioplasty in Myocardial Infarction (PAMI-I) trial, *J Am Coll Cardiol* 33:640–646, 1999.

Kushner FG, Hand M, Smith SC Jr, et al: 2009 Focused Updates: ACC/AHA Guidelines for the Management of Patients With ST-Elevation Myocardial Infarction (updating the 2004 Guideline and 2007 Focused Update) and ACC/AHA/SCAI Guidelines on Percutaneous Coronary Intervention (updating the 2005 Guideline and 2007 Focused Update): A report of the American College of Cardiology Foundation/American Heart Association Task Force on Practice Guidelines, *Circulation* 54:2205–2241, 2009.

101. **How common is restenosis after balloon angioplasty and bare metal noncoated coronary stent placement?**

About 40–45% of patients undergoing balloon angioplasty and about 25–35% of patients undergoing bare metal non-coated coronary stent placement develop restenosis.

KEY POINTS: PERCUTANEOUS CORONARY INTERVENTION ✓

1. Restenosis is the most common complication of percutaneous coronary balloon angioplasty (PCA).

2. The incidence of restenosis is significantly reduced with PCA and bare metal coronary artery stents.

3. The incidence is even more reduced with PCA and sirolimus or paclitaxel-coated drug-eluting coronary artery stents.

4. However, coated drug-eluting stents are more prone to thrombosis than bare metal stents and require a longer duration of treatment with the platelet inhibitor clopidogrel.

5. Restenosis is most common in the first 6 mo after balloon angioplasty or stent placement and presents with recurrent angina; stent thrombosis can occur up to several years after a coronary stent placement and presents with an acute myocardial infarction.

102. **Are drug-eluting coronary stents more or less likely to be complicated by restenosis compared with bare metal stents?**
Less likely. Two types of drug-eluting stents, sirolimus- and paclitaxel-eluting stents, have been extensively investigated in patients with CAD. These two coated stents have been developed specifically to inhibit proliferation of vascular smooth muscle cells, the primary mechanism for restenosis over the first 6 months after stent placement. Both drug-eluting coronary stents have now been demonstrated in large randomized clinical trials to cause significantly less restenosis than the so-called bare metal stents. Overall, restenosis occurs in 2–6% of patients receiving a drug-eluting coronary stent compared with about 25–35% with bare metal stents. Coated stents are also associated with substantially decreased need for readmission with recurrent angina and repeat coronary interventions.

Colombo A, Drzewiecki J, Banning A, et al: for the TAXUS II Study Group: Randomized study to assess the effectiveness of slow- and moderate-release polymer-based paclitaxel-eluting stents for coronary artery lesions, *Circulation* 108:788–794, 2003.

Moses JW, Leon MB, Popma JJ, et al: for the SIRUS investigators: Sirolimus-eluting stents versus standard stents in patients with stenosis in a native coronary artery, *N Engl J Med* 349:1315–1323, 2003.

Schofer J, Schluer M, Gershlick AH, et al: for the E-SIRIUS Investigators: Sirolimus-eluting stents for treatment of patients with long atherosclerotic lesions in small coronary arteries: Double-blind, randomized controlled trial (E-SIRIUS), *Lancet* 362:1093–1099, 2003.

103. **Why should IV ACE inhibitors be avoided in the first 24 hours after acute MI?**
Because they may cause a potentially harmful acute decrease in BP with a resultant reduction in coronary blood flow, as demonstrated in the CONSENSUS-II (Cooperative New Scandinavian Enalapril Survival Study II) trial.

Swedberg K, Held P, Kjekshus J, et al: Effects of the early administration of enalapril on mortality in patients with acute myocardial infarction: Results of the Cooperative New Scandinavian Enalapril Survival Study II (CONSENSUS-II), *N Engl J Med* 327:678–684, 1992.

104. **Should oral nitrates be administered routinely to all patients with uncomplicated MI?**
No. IV, transdermal, or oral nitrates or a combination have traditionally been used routinely in all patients admitted with suspected acute MI. However, despite the encouraging results of early small clinical studies, two large multicenter clinical trials, International Study of Infarct Survival (ISIS)-4 and GISSI-3, consisting of about 78,000 patients, showed no significant benefit of early oral nitrates on survival, infarct size, or ventricular function. Nitrate administration should be limited to patients with well-established indications for nitrates, such as postinfarction angina, ischemia or CHF.

Gruppo Italiano per lo Studio della Sopravivenza nell' Infarto Miocardio (GISSI-3): Effects of lisinopril and transdermal glyceryltrinitrate singly and together on 6-week mortality and ventricular function after acute myocardial infarction, *Lancet* 343:1115–1122, 1994.

ISIS-4: A randomized factorial trial assessing early oral captopril, oral mononitrate, and intravenous magnesium sulphate in 58,050 patients with suspected acute myocardial infarction, *Lancet* 345:669–685, 1995.

Morris JL, Zaman AG, Smyllie JH, Cowan JC: Nitrates in myocardial infarction: Influence on infarct size, reperfusion, and ventricular remodeling, *Br Heart J* 73:310–319, 1995.

105. **Do ACE inhibitors improve survival in patients recovering from acute MI?**
Yes. Long-term oral ACE inhibitors started 3–16 days after acute MI and maintained for about 3 years reduce mortality by about 19% in patients with asymptomatic LV systolic dysfunction (LVEF < 40%), as demonstrated in the Survival and Ventricular Enlargement (SAVE) Trial. Subsequent trials (ISIS-4 and GISSI-3) specifically showed that even a short

6-week course of an ACE inhibitor started within 24 hours of infarct onset decreases 6-week mortality by 7–12%, corresponding to 5 deaths prevented for every 1000 treated patients.

Pfeffer MA, Braunwald E, Moye LA, et al: on behalf of the SAVE Investigators: Effect of captopril on mortality and morbidity in patients with left ventricular dysfunction after myocardial infarction. Results of the Survival and Ventricular Enlargement Trial, *N Engl J Med* 327:669–677, 1992.

ISIS-4: A randomized factorial trial assessing early oral captopril, oral mononitrate, and intravenous magnesium sulphate in 58,050 patients with suspected acute myocardial infarction, *Lancet* 345:669–685, 1995.

Gruppo Italiano per lo Studio della Sopravivenza nell' Infarto Miocardio (GISSI-3): Effects of lisinopril and transdermal glyceryltrinitrate singly and together on 6-week mortality and ventricular function after acute myocardial infarction, *Lancet* 343:1115–1122, 1994.

106. **What is the most common cause of death in the first 48 hours after an acute MI?**
VF. Other causes of death include cardiac rupture, pump failure due to massive infarction, acute mechanical complication such as ventricular septal rupture or acute mitral regurgitation, and cardiogenic shock.

107. **Cardiac rupture is almost always a fatal complication of acute MI. List the three risk factors for its development.**
Female sex, hypertension, and first MI.

108. **List the clinical features of cardiac rupture.**
- Occurs more often in LV than in RV in a 7:1 ratio.
- Seen in anterior or lateral wall MI.
- Usually occurs with large MI.
- Usually occurs within 3–6 days after MI.
- Rarely occurs with LV hypertrophy or good collateral vessels.

109. **What complication of acute inferior wall MI typically presents with hypotension, elevated neck veins, clear lungs, and a normal cardiac silhouette on chest x-ray?**
RV MI. The diagnosis can be confirmed by demonstrating at least 1-mm ST elevation in right-sided chest leads V_3R or V_4R. Further confirmation of RV MI can be derived from noninvasive assessment of RV systolic function using radionuclide techniques or, more commonly, bedside two-dimensional echocardiography. A **right-sided ECG** should be done in **every** patient presenting to an emergency department with an acute inferior wall MI. Studies have shown that inferior MI patients with RV infarction are sicker, are more likely to die, and have an increased incidence of major cardiac complications of their inferior MI. Thus, these patients should be readily identified at initial clinical presentation and aggressively treated. Clinical management consists of volume expansion in combination with IV dopamine. In these patients, diuretics or preload-reducing drugs such as nitrates worsen the low cardiac output state and hypotension and should be avoided.

110. **What is the differential diagnosis of a new systolic murmur and acute pulmonary edema appearing 3 days after an acute anterior wall MI?**
Acute MR due to papillary muscle rupture and interventricular septal rupture. Both are potentially fatal complications and are most common 3–6 days after infarction. Rupture of the posteromedial papillary muscle, associated with inferior wall MI, is more common than rupture of the anterolateral papillary muscle. Unlike rupture of the interventricular septum, which occurs with large infarcts, papillary muscle rupture occurs with a small infarction in approximately 50% of cases.

111. **How do you differentiate between acute MR and ventricular septal rupture?**
     With two-dimensional and Doppler echocardiography (which can be done at the bedside), which will demonstrate the presence and severity of MR and localize the site of a ventricular septal defect (VSD). Further confirmation of the presence of a left-to-right shunt across a VSD can be obtained by a step-up in blood oxygen saturation from the RA to the pulmonary artery, documented by blood sampling using a Swan-Ganz catheter.

112. **What is the most likely cause of a persistent ST segment elevation several weeks after recovery from a large transmural anterolateral wall MI?**
     LV aneurysm. Persistent ST segment elevation is not an uncommon complication of a large anterolateral, transmural MI and may represent dyskinesis of the thinned-out, infarcted myocardium. However, persistent ST segment elevations should suggest the presence of an **LV aneurysm**, and noninvasive confirmation of this diagnosis by two-dimensional echocardiography or radionuclide ventriculography should be sought.

113. **Which MIs are most commonly complicated by LV aneurysms?**
     Acute transmural MI, developing in 12–15% of survivors. Aneurysms range from 1–8 cm in diameter and are four times more common at the apex and anterior wall than in the inferoposterior wall. Patients with larger infarcts are more likely to develop LV aneurysms, and the mortality is about six times higher in patients with an LV aneurysm than in those with comparable global LV function. Death is often sudden, suggesting an increased risk of sustained VT and VF in these patients.

114. **What is Dressler's syndrome?**
     Post-MI chest pain *not* due to coronary insufficiency. The syndrome was first described in 1854 and its exact etiology remains unclear. Dressler's syndrome occurs in 3–4% of MI patients 2–10 weeks after the event and is characterized by inflammation of the pericardium and surrounding tissues. Corticosteroids and nonsteroidal anti-inflammatory drugs (NSAIDs) are effective treatments.

115. **Summarize the current guidelines for use of an ACE inhibitor, an ARB, and an aldosterone antagonist in patients recovering from a STEMI.**
     The current guidelines for the management of patients with STEMI recommend the routine use of an ACE inhibitor in patients with no contraindications for an ACE inhibitor. An ARB is recommended for those intolerant of an ACE inhibitor who have heart failure or LV dysfunction defined as an LVEF $< 40\%$. Aldosterone antagonists are recommended in patients who recovered from an ST elevation MI without substantial renal dysfunction (defined as creatinine < 2.5 mg% in men and < 2.0 in women) or hyperkalemia who already are receiving an ACE inhibitor, have LVEF $< 40\%$, and have symptomatic heart failure or diabetes mellitus.

     Kushner FG, Hand M, Smith SC Jr, et al: 2009 focused updates: ACC/AHA Guidelines for the Management of Patients With ST-Elevation Myocardial Infarction (Updating the 2004 Guideline and 2007 Focused Update) and ACC/AHA/SCAI Guidelines on Percutaneous Coronary Intervention (Updating the 2005 Guideline and 2007 Focused Update). A report of the American College of Cardiology Foundation/ American Heart Association Task Force on Practice Guidelines, *Circulation* 120:2271–2306, 2009.

116. **Which lipid-lowering drug was shown in a prospective placebo-controlled clinical trial to reduce cardiovascular mortality in MI survivors with "average" blood cholesterol levels?**
     Pravastatin, a potent 3-hydroxy-3-methylglutaryl coenzyme A (HMG-CoA) reductase inhibitor, was evaluated in MI patients in the Cholesterol and Recurrent Events (CARE) Trial. In this

double-blind trial, 3583 men and 576 women who had survived a recent MI and had plasma total cholesterol levels below 240 mg/dL and LDL levels of 115–174 mg/dL received pravastatin (40 mg/day) or placebo for 5 years. The primary endpoint was a fatal coronary event or a nonfatal MI. The frequency of the primary endpoint was 10.2% in the pravastatin group and 13.2% in the placebo group (24% reduction in risk). Subgroup analysis revealed that most of the benefit occurred in patients with baseline serum LDL cholesterol levels > 125 mg/dL. In practical terms, patients with LDL cholesterol > 125 mg/dL and prior MI should receive an HMG-CoA reductase inhibitor for at least 5 years. More recently, the Pravastatin or Atorvastatin Evaluation and Infection Therapy (PROVE-IT) trial has demonstrated the superiority of a more potent statin, atorvastatin over pravastatin in preventing cardiovascular complications of a myocardial infarction. Based on the PROVE-IT and other recent statin clinical trials, the goal of lipid lowering in patients with ACS has been changed from < 100 mg% to a more optimal—yet still "optional"—goal LDL of < 70 mg%.

Cannon CP, Braunwald E, McCabe CH, et al: for the Pravastatin or Atorvastatin Evaluation and Infection Therapy—Thrombolysis in Myocardial Infarction: Intensive versus moderate lipid lowering with statins after acute coronary syndromes, *N Engl J Med* 350:1495–1504, 2004.

Sacks FM, Pfeffer MA, Moye LA, et al: for the Cholesterol and Recurrent Events Trial Investigators: The effect of pravastatin on coronary events after myocardial infarction in patients with average cholesterol levels, *N Engl J Med* 335:1001–1009, 1996.

117. **Do statins help prevent MI and stroke in patients with CAD (or other vascular disease) or diabetes mellitus or both, regardless of the LDL cholesterol level?**
Yes. The Heart Protection Study investigated the effect of simvastatin (40 mg/day) on fatal or nonfatal coronary heart disease events in about 20,000 patients, aged 40–79 years, with vascular disease and/or diabetes mellitus and a mildly elevated LDL cholesterol level of approximately 130 mg/dL. This trial showed the same overall 24% reduction in cardiovascular mortality and 30–35% reduction in coronary heart disease events and stroke in the 3800 patients with a baseline LDL cholesterol of < 100 mg/dL as in patients with higher LDL cholesterol levels (100–130 or > 130 mg/dL). These results indicate that patients aged 40–79 years with known vascular disease and/or diabetes mellitus should receive statin therapy, regardless of the LDL cholesterol level. A recent study of atorvastatin (10 mg/day) in diabetics 40–79 years reported similar results. As a result, the American Diabetes Association has recommended statin therapy in all diabetics 40 years or older regardless of LDL unless total cholesterol < 135 mg/dL.

Colhoun HM, Betteridge DJH, Durrington PN, et al: Primary prevention of cardiovascular disease with atorvastatin in type 2 diabetes in the Collaborative Atorvastatin Diabetes Study (CARDS): multicentre randomised placebo-controlled trial, *Lancet* 364:686–696, 2004.

Heart Protection Study Investigators: MRC/BHF Heart Protection Study of cholesterol lowering with simvastatin in 20,536 high-risk individuals: A randomised placebo-controlled trial, *Lancet* 360:7–22, 2002.

118. **Beta blockers are effective in the treatment of stable exertional angina pectoris. Should you recommend routine administration of oral beta blockers in MI survivors who are angina-free?**
Yes. Several large-scale, multicenter clinical trials conducted in the United States and abroad have shown a consistent reduction in total and cardiovascular mortality in survivors of acute transmural MI treated with oral beta blockers for 1–3 years. The largest published U.S. trial is the Beta-Blocker Heart Attack Trial, which randomized 3837 MI survivors to either propranolol (180 or 240 mg/day) or placebo. At 3 years of follow-up,

a 26% reduction in mortality was found in patients treated with propranolol compared with placebo-treated patients. Thus, regardless of the presence or absence of angina, oral beta blockers such as propranolol (180–240 mg), timolol (10 mg twice a day), or metoprolol (100 mg twice a day) should be routinely started 5–21 days post-MI and continued for at least 7 years.

Beta-Blocker Heart Attack Trial Research Group: A randomized trial of propranolol in patients with acute myocardial infarction: 1. Mortality results, *JAMA* 247:1707–1714, 1982.

119. **A 67-year-old man has stayed in bed for the past 3 days with flulike symptoms. A 12-lead ECG reveals new Q waves in leads V_1–V_6 and ST segment elevation of 3 mm in leads V_2–V_5, I, and aVL. What do you suspect in this patient?**
Anterolateral MI. This patient has ECG changes indicative of the recent evolution of an extensive anterolateral MI evidenced by: (1) 3-mm ST segment elevations in anterolateral leads V_2–V_5, I, and aVL; and (2) new Q waves in all anterolateral chest leads. The most likely clinical diagnosis is an acute, extensive anterolateral MI that occurred 3–4 days ago, when he first complained of flulike symptoms.

120. **Is plasma creatine kinase (CK) likely to be high in this patient?**
No. The laboratory confirmation of this clinical diagnosis is routinely done by measuring serum CK containing M and B subunits (CKMB) and CK levels at 6-hour intervals for 24–48 hours. Serum CKMB and CK levels are elevated starting at 4–8 hours after symptom onset, reach a peak at 18–24 hours, and normalize within 3–4 days. Thus, serum CKMB and CK levels in this patient are likely to be normal.

121. **What other laboratory tests are helpful in establishing the diagnosis of MI?**
Cardiac troponins T and I, which are newer, more specific enzymatic markers of MI that remain elevated up to 10–14 days after an MI. Troponins T and I are now routinely obtained in patients with chest pain syndromes and are of particular value in diagnosing MI in patients presenting late (>12–24 hr) after MI symptom onset as well as in risk-stratifying patients presenting with ACSs.

122. **A 48-year-old man presents with acute severe epigastric pain, anorexia, nausea, vomiting, and diaphoresis. Which myocardial wall is likely affected? Explain the rationale for such an unusual clinical presentation.**
Inferior wall. Patients with an **acute inferior wall MI** sometimes present with epigastric pain associated with gastrointestinal (GI) symptoms. Less commonly, they present with hiccupping, which may at times be intractable. These unique clinical manifestations are thought to be related to increased vagal tone and irritation of the diaphragm by the adjacent infarcted inferior wall.

CONGESTIVE HEART FAILURE

See also Chapter 2, General Medicine and Ambulatory Care.

123. **Name the types of cardiomyopathies.**
See Table 4-9.

TABLE 4-9. CHARACTERISTICS OF CARDIOMYOPATHIES

Characteristics	Cardiomyopathy		
	Hypertrophic	Dilated	Restrictive
Causes	Genetic Secondary to pressure overload (e.g., hypertension, aortic stenosis)	Myocarditis Chronic Genetic Arrhythmogenic right ventricular dysplasia	Infiltrative or storage diseases Endomyocardial (e.g., Löffler's, carcinoid)
Ejection fraction (normal > 55%)	>60%	<30%	25–50%
Left ventricular diastolic dimension (normal < 55 mm)	Often decreased	≥60 mm	<60 mm
Left ventricular wall thickness	Increased	Decreased	Normal or increased
Atrial size	Increased	Increased	Increased; may be massive
Valvular regurgitation	Mitral regurgitation	Mitral first during decompensation; tricuspid regurgitation in late stages	Frequent mitral and tricuspid regurgitation, rarely severe
Common first symptoms*	Exertional intolerance; may have chest pain	Exertional intolerance	Exertional intolerance, fluid retention
Congestive symptoms*	Primary exertional dyspnea	Left before right, except right prominent in young adults	Right often exceeds left
Risk for arrhythmia	Ventricular tachyarrhythmias, atrial fibrillation	Ventricular tachyarrhythmias; atrial fibrillation; conduction block in Chagas' disease, giant cell myocarditis, and some families	Atrial fibrillation; ventricular tachyarrhythmias uncommon except in sarcoidosis; conduction block in arcoidosis and amyloidosis

*Left-sided symptoms of pulmonary congestion: dyspnea on exertion, orthopnea, paroxysmal nocturnal dyspnea. Right-sided symptoms of systemic venous congestion: discomfort on bending, hepatic and abdominal distention, peripheral edema.

124. **List common signs and symptoms of CHF in order of decreasing specificity.**

RIGHT HEART FAILURE

Jugular vein distention
Hepatomegaly
Pleural effusion
Decreased albumin
Abdominal discomfort
Anorexia
Proteinuria
Increased prothrombin time
Peripheral edema
Increased aspartate
    aminotransferase (AST), bilirubin

LEFT HEART FAILURE

Chest x-ray with redistribution of
    perfusion or interstitial edema
S_3
Cardiomegaly
Pulmonary rales
Paroxysmal nocturnal dyspnea,
    orthopnea
Dyspnea on exertion

125. **What is the differential diagnosis of the etiology of CHF symptoms?**

ISOLATED RIGHT HEART FAILURE

Pulmonary embolus
Tricuspid stenosis
Tricuspid regurgitation
RA tumor
Cardiac tamponade
Constrictive pericarditis
Pulmonic insufficiency
RV infarction
Intrinsic lung disease
Ebstein's anomaly
High cardiac output states
    (e.g., anemia,
    systemic fistulae,
    beriberi, Paget's
    disease, carcinoid,
    thyrotoxicosis)

LEFT OR BIVENTRICULAR FAILURE

Aortic stenosis
Aortic insufficiency
Mitral stenosis
MR
Most cardiomyopathies
Acute MI
Myxoma
Hypertensive heart disease
Myocarditis
Supraventricular arrhythmias
LV aneurysm
Cardiac shunts
High cardiac output states

126. **What factors can precipitate an exacerbation of formerly well-controlled chronic CHF?**

Increased consumption of salt	Renal failure	Elevated BP
Fluid overload	Pregnancy	High environmental temperature
Pulmonary emboli	Paget's disease	Cardiac ischemia or MI
Fever, infection	Poor compliance with medications	Thyrotoxicosis
Anemia	Arrhythmias	

When patients with well-controlled, chronic CHF experience a sudden exacerbation, a search for the precipitating factors must be done.

127. **A 68-year-old man with HTN presents with a 2-week history of progressive exertional dyspnea, orthopnea, and paroxysmal nocturnal dyspnea. What is the differential diagnosis of CHF in hypertensive patients?**
    - CAD
    - Heart failure with normal ejection fraction (diastolic dysfunction) associated with HTN
    - Dilated cardiomyopathy (idiopathic or alcoholic)

- Valvular heart disease (MR, aortic stenosis, aortic insufficiency)
- Restrictive heart disease (amyloidosis)
- HCM

128. **What are the less common causes of GI symptoms in patients with CHF?**
Passive hepatic congestion or ascites. Differentiation of the various causes of nausea and vomiting in such patients, on clinical grounds alone, can be difficult.

129. **Which drugs are available at present for the treatment of CHF?**
- **Venous vasodilators:** nitrates to relieve pulmonary congestive symptoms
- **Arteriolar dilators:** ACE inhibitors or ARBs to reduce afterload, improve cardiac performance, and reduce progressive ventricular dilatation or "remodeling"
- **Inotropic drugs:** digoxin to reduce ventricular response to concomitant AF or improve cardiac performance
- **Diuretics:** loop diuretics to relieve congestive signs and symptoms of left- and right-sided CHF

130. **Which drug classes have been proved to decrease mortality in patients with CHF?**
- **ACE inhibitor:** enalapril
- **ARBs:** valsartan and candesartan
- **Beta blockers:** metoprolol succinate, carvedilol, bisoprolol, and nebivolol

These medications have been shown in a number of major clinical trials to reduce cardiovascular mortality in patients with systolic New York Heart Association (NYHA) functional classes II–IV and are now considered the standard treatment in patients with CHF. Generally, ARBs are recommended in patients who are intolerant of ACE inhibitors (particularly due to cough).

Consensus Trial Study Group: Effects of enalapril on mortality in severe congestive heart failure: Results of the Cooperative North Scandinavian Enalapril Survival Study (CONSENSUS), *N Engl J Med* 316:1429–1435, 1987.

Studies on Left Ventricular Dysfunction (SOLVE) Trial, *N Engl J Med* 325:293–302, 1991.

Cohn JN, Tognomi G: A randomized trial of the angiotensin-receptor blocker valsartan in chronic heart failure, *N Engl J Med* 345:1667–1675, 2001.

Foody JM, Farrell MH, Krumholz HM: Beta-blocker therapy in heart failure: Scientific review, *JAMA* 287:883–889, 2002.

Hunt SA, Abraham WT, Chin MH, et al: 2009 focused update incorporated into the ACC/AHA 2005 Guidelines for the Diagnosis and Management of Heart Failure in Adults: A report of the American College of Cardiology Foundation/American Heart Association Task Force on Practice Guidelines: Developed in collaboration with the International Society for Heart and Lung Transplantation, *Circulation* 119:e391–e479, 2009.

131. **What classes of antihypertensive drugs are recommended in a patient with CHF?**
- ACE inhibitors (captopril, enalapril, lisinopril, ramipril, or monopril).
- ARBs (losartan, irbesartan, valsartan, candesartan or telmisartan) if ACE inhibitors are not well tolerated or contraindicated.
- Vasodilators (hydralazine) if ACE inhibitors or ARBs if not tolerated. In African Americans with CHF, a combination of hydralazine plus isosorbide dinitrate is recommended in addition to an ACE inhibitor to prevent cardiovascular complications of CHF.
- Diuretics (furosemide). Loop diuretics are recommended in patients with CHF and clinical evidence of overt decompensated CHF with volume overload and should be titrated to minimize congestive symptoms without unduly reducing intravascular volume and worsening renal function.

132. **Which drugs should be usually avoided in patients with acutely decompensated CHF?**
    - Calcium channel blockers of the nondihydropyridine class (verapamil, diltiazem)
    - Beta blockers (e.g., propranolol, metoprolol, atenolol)
      These drugs have negative inotropic effects and should generally be avoided, particularly in patients with acutely decompensated CHF.

133. **How is acute pulmonary edema managed?**
    - IV diuresis
    - IV, cutaneous, or oral preload-reducing drug therapy
    - IV digitalization (in patients with acute pulmonary edema particularly with associated AF)
    - Oxygen therapy (depending on results of arterial oxygen saturation)
    - Bed rest and salt restriction
    - Afterload-reducing drugs

134. **Describe the effect of IV diuresis in heart failure patients**
    A loop diuretic, such as furosemide given as 20–60 mg IV push, lowers venous tone and thus lowers pulmonary wedge pressure even before inducing effective diuresis.

135. **Which drugs are useful for reducing preload?**
    Nitrates by acting as effective venodilators. In single oral doses of 40–60 mg (to be repeated three to four times daily), they are effective in lowering pulmonary capillary wedge pressure and, thus, improving congestive symptoms of heart failure: dyspnea, orthopnea, paroxysmal nocturnal dyspnea, and nocturnal cough.

136. **Describe the effects of afterload-reducing drugs.**
    Afterload-reducing drugs are effective in alleviating the signs and symptoms of CHF. ACE inhibitors such as captopril, enalapril, or lisinopril are effective afterload- and preload-reducing drugs and can be administered orally in patients with overt CHF. Unlike other drugs that effectively improve the symptoms of heart failure (such as diuretics and digoxin), ACE inhibitors (and ARBs in ACE inhibitor–intolerant patients) have been proved—in a large number of randomized, placebo-controlled clinical trials—to reduce cardiovascular mortality in patients with heart failure and depressed LV systolic function.

137. **Are all calcium channel blockers contraindicated in patients with heart failure?**
    No. Calcium channel blockers are not all created equal. Dihydropyridine calcium channel blockers such as amlodipine and felodipine have no clinically significant negative inotropic effects, have been evaluated in large, prospective, placebo-controlled clinical trials in patients with heart failure, and can be used safely in patients with impaired systolic function and/or CHF if there is an additional clinical indication for a calcium blocker, such as HTN or angina pectoris.

138. **Do beta blockers ever have a role in patients with heart failure?**
    Yes. Although beta blockers are generally contraindicated in patients with acute or decompensated heart failure or both, a large number of prospective, randomized clinical trials with beta blockers such as carvedilol, metoprolol and bucindolol at low and gradually titrated doses support a beneficial long-term effect in patients of NYHA functional classes II and III (mild-to-moderate symptomatic heart failure). Even low-dose beta blocker initiation in patients with heart failure should be done cautiously because a significant proportion as high as 30–40% of these patients may experience symptomatic hypotension and/or worsening heart failure symptoms in the first 4 weeks of beta blocker initiation.

139. **Why are digoxin, diuretics, and nitrates still used to treat CHF?**
Because they decrease the number of hospitalizations for acute CHF exacerbations and reduce mortality in patients with CHF.

140. **What is the mechanism of action of digitalis?**
Inhibition of Na^+-K^+-ATPase activity (the sodium pump) that blocks the transport of sodium and potassium across cell membranes, leading to an intracellular increase in sodium and decrease in potassium. The increase in intracellular sodium in turn leads to an exchange for calcium. The increased intracellular calcium, the contractile element of muscle, leads to increased contractility (positive inotropic effect). The antiarrhythmic effects of cardiac glycosides are probably not due to any direct effect of the drugs. Rather, they are mediated by an increase in vagal tone in the atria and AV junction.

141. **A 78-year-old man with a longstanding history of CHF and chronic AF presents with increasing generalized weakness, anorexia, nausea, and vomiting for the last few days. He has been receiving increasing digoxin doses up to 0.5 mg/day to slow the ventricular response to his AF and furosemide 120 mg twice a day to relieve his pulmonary congestive symptoms. What clinical diagnosis should you suspect in this patient?**
Digitalis toxicity. Any patient receiving digitalis who presents with GI symptoms, such as anorexia, nausea, or vomiting, should be suspected of having digitalis toxicity. The nausea and vomiting are thought to be mediated by stimulation of the area postrema in the medulla oblongata of the brainstem rather than by any direct effects of digitalis on the GI mucosa. These GI manifestations may occur in patients receiving excessive oral or IV doses of digitalis for the management of heart failure or rapid AF or both. Another diagnosis to consider in an elderly man receiving digoxin and with known peripheral vascular disease presenting with worsening GI symptoms is acute mesenteric ischemia, which is precipitated or worsened by digoxin's mesenteric vasoconstrictor effect. Early clinical suspicion and diagnosis followed by prompt and effective treatment of acute mesenteric ischemia are critically important to improve the clinical outcome. Acute mesenteric ischemia is a life-threatening vascular emergency associated with a 60–80% mortality and is almost uniformly fatal if unsuspected and not effectively and promptly treated.

Oldenbure QA, Lau LL, Rosenberg TJ, et al: Acute mesenteric ischemia: A clinical review, *Arch Intern Med* 164:1054–1062, 2004.

142. **List other manifestations of digitalis toxicity.**
   - **Neurologic symptoms:** headache, neuralgia, confusion, delirium, seizures
   - **Visual symptoms:** scotomata, halos, altered color perception
   - **Cardiac toxicity:** ventricular or junctional tachyarrhythmias, AV block
   - **Miscellaneous:** gynecomastia, skin rash

143. **What factors contribute to digitalis toxicity?**
   - Hypokalemia
   - Hypercalcemia
   - Hypomagnesemia
   - Renal insufficiency (digoxin)
   - Hepatic insufficiency (digitoxin)
   - Drugs (quinidine, verapamil, amiodarone, others)

144. **What arrhythmias are frequently found as complications of digitalis toxicity?**
   - PAT with AV block
   - Junctional tachycardia with or without AV block
   - First-degree or Mobitz I second-degree AV block

Any arrhythmia can be a manifestation of digitalis intoxication. The coexistence of increased automaticity or ectopic pacemakers with impaired AV conduction is also highly suggestive of digitalis intoxication. Cardiac manifestations are by far the most life-threatening complications of digitalis intoxication.

145. **What laboratory test helps confirm the diagnosis of digitalis toxicity?**
   Digoxin level. However, even serum digoxin levels in the "therapeutic range" may be toxic in elderly patients and patients with hypokalemia, hypercalcemia, acid-base disorders, or thyroid disorders.

146. **Which patients with CHF should be considered for implantable cardioverter-defibrillator (ICD) placement to prevent sudden cardiac death? For cardiac resynchronization therapy (CRT)?**
   Those with an LVEF < 35% and NYHA class II or III symptoms of ACC/AHA state B or C. Patient with either ischemic or nonischemic cardiomyopathy should be evaluated for ICD. CRT may be needed for patients with NYHA III or IV symptoms and ventricular dyssynchrony (intraventricular conduction delays or LBBB).

   McAliser FA, Ezekowitz J, Hooton N, et al: Cardiac resynchronization therapy for patients with left ventricular systolic dysfunction: A systematic review, *JAMA* 297:2502–2514, 2007.

147. **How is the B-type natriuretic peptide (BNP) used in the evaluation of CHF?**
   The BNP is elevated in patients with CHF and is most useful clinically in evaluating patients with acute symptoms of possible heart failure. CHF unlikely in a patient in the acute setting with BNP < 100 pg/mL. The test is currently under investigation for management of chronic CHF.

   Maisel AS, Krishnaswamy P, Nowak RM, et al: Rapid measurement of B-type natriuretic peptide in the emergency diagnosis of heart failure, *N Engl J Med* 347:161–167, 2002.

ARRHYTHMIAS, CONDUCTION DISTURBANCES, AND PACEMAKERS

148. **What arrhythmia is most commonly found in clinical practice?**
   AF.

149. **Why is the diagnosis of AF important?**
   AF is the *most common* clinically significant cardiac arrhythmia encountered in clinical practice and is a strong risk factor for embolic stroke. AF is common among middle-aged and older patients, and embolic stroke can be prevented by effective oral anticoagulation with warfarin.

150. **How is AF treated?**
   In most patients with AF with fast heart rates, effective rate control can be achieved by the use of AV nodal blocking drugs such as a beta blocker, a heart rate lowering nondihydropyridine calcium channel blocker (such as diltiazem or verapramil), digoxin, or amiodarone. Some patients are candidates for rhythm control with conversion to normal sinus rhythm with medications or direct-current cardioversion. Ablation therapy is also now used for patients with AF who may benefit from rhythm control. All patients with AF should be assessed for long-term anticoagulation with warfarin or dabigatran to prevent embolic stroke.

   Wilber DJ, Pappone C, Neuzil P, et al: Comparison of antiarrhythmic drug therapy and radiofrequency catheter ablation in patients with paroxysmal atrial fibrillation: A randomized controlled trial, *JAMA* 303:333–340, 2010.

151. **Is anticoagulation recommended before elective cardioversion of a patient with AF?**
Yes. A 4-week course of adequate anticoagulation decreases the risk of thromboembolic events during and shortly after cardioversion planned in a patient with chronic sustained AF. The risks and benefits of cardioversion and anticoagulation, however, must be weighed very carefully prior to elective cardioversion. The most important consideration is the urgency of cardioversion. Patients with AF presenting with markedly elevated ventricular response rate complicated by systemic hypotension and/or significant systemic hypoperfusion or signs of "hemodynamic instability" should undergo emergency cardioversion without the need for preceding anticoagulation. In patients with a recent onset of newly developed AF, a transesophageal echocardiogram (TEE) is recommended, and if no clots are detected in the left atrial appendage, cardioversion can be performed preferably within the next 24 hours without the need for a precardioversion anticoagulation period.

152. **Is anticoagulation similarly required in a patient with AF with a fast ventricular rate of 230 bpm and systolic BP of 70 mmHg?**
No. With clinical evidence of hemodynamic compromise (such as CHF, hypotension or systemic hypoperfusion, acute anginal symptoms, or acute MI), urgent cardioversion should be administered immediately, regardless of LA or LV size, systolic LV function, or prior anticoagulation. Thus, in a patient with AF complicated by a fast ventricular response rate of 230 bpm and severe hypotension with a systolic BP of 70 mmHg, emergency cardioversion absolutely should not be delayed until anticoagulation has been initiated or has successfully achieved desirable anticoagulation targets.

153. **What is the ECG triad of Wolff-Parkinson-White (WPW) syndrome?**
   - Short PR interval (<0.12 sec)
   - Wide QRS complex (>0.12 sec)
   - Delta wave or slurred upstroke of QRS complex (Fig. 4-4)

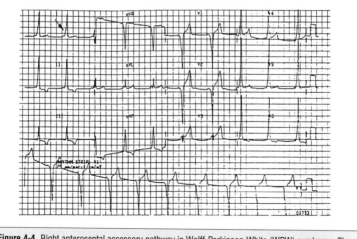

Figure 4-4. Right anteroseptal accessory pathway in Wolff-Parkinson-White (WPW) syndrome. The 12-lead ECG characteristically exhibits a normal to inferior axis. The delta wave is negative in V1 and V2; upright in leads I, II, aVL (augmented voltage for left arm), and aVF (augmented voltage for the foot); isoelectric in lead III; and negative in aVR (augmented voltage for the right arm). The *arrow* indicates delta wave (lead I). (From Braunwald E [ed]: Heart Disease: A Textbook of Cardiovascular Medicine, 3rd ed. Philadelphia, WB Saunders, 1988, p 686.)

154. **Discuss the mechanism underlying sudden cardiac death in patients with WPW syndrome.**
AF with antegrade conduction along the accessory pathway. This tachycardia presents a serious risk because of its propensity to degenerate into VF due to very rapid conduction over the accessory pathway. Patients with accessory pathways and short refractory periods (<200 msec) are at highest risk for this antegrade conduction AF and, therefore, sudden cardiac death.

155. **Are patients with intermittent preexcitation during sinus rhythm at risk for sudden cardiac death?**
No. Intermittent preexcitation during sinus rhythm and loss of conduction along the accessory pathway during exercise or during administration of ajmaline or procainamide suggest that the refractory period of the accessory pathway is long (>250 msec). These patients are not at risk of developing very rapid ventricular rates when AF or atrial flutter occurs and are, therefore, not at risk for sudden cardiac death.

156. **What is the holiday heart syndrome?**
Supraventricular arrhythmias following an acute alcoholic binge, sometimes associated with holiday parties or long weekends. These arrhythmias are often transient and do not require long-term antiarrhythmic drug therapy. The most common arrhythmias are AF and atrial flutter. Digitalis and beta blockers produce an effective and rapid therapeutic response. Supportive care is also essential to prevent alcohol withdrawal symptoms in these patients.

157. **Describe the three-letter code used to indicate the essential functions of a cardiac pacemaker.**
   - **First letter:** chamber(s) paced (A = atrial, V = ventricle, D = dual chamber)
   - **Second letter:** chamber(s) sensed (A = atrial, V = ventricle, D = dual chamber)
   - **Third letter:** mode of response to sensed event (O = no response, I = inhibition, T = triggering, and D = dual response)

158. **What are the two most commonly used pacemakers today?**
   - **VVI:** A pacemaker that can pace and sense the RV (VV) and has an inhibited mode of response (I).
   - **DDD:** The so-called dual-chamber AV sequential pacemaker can pace and sense either RV or RA (DD) and has both inhibited and triggered modes of response (D).

159. **What do the different modes of response indicate?**
   - **I = inhibited:** Pacemakers with an inhibited mode of response do not pace when a spontaneous depolarization (atrial or ventricular) is sensed by the pacemaker. Following a fixed interval, if no spontaneous depolarization is sensed, pacing occurs. The inhibited mode of response is most commonly used.
   - **T = triggered:** These pacemakers pace shortly after a spontaneous depolarization is sensed. After a fixed interval, pacing will occur if no spontaneous depolarization is sensed.
   - **D = dual-response:** The pacemakers have both inhibited and triggered modes of response.

160. **Who generally receives dual-chamber pacemakers (DDD)?**
Patients who are not good candidates for ventricular-demand pacemakers. DDD pacemakers are more expensive, are more difficult to implant, and require greater expertise from the clinician in charge of the patient's follow-up compared with ventricular-demand pacemakers (VVI). Examples of patients who benefit from DDD pacemakers include those with older age, CHF, or LV hypertrophy and physically active young adults who would not tolerate fixed-rate ventricular pacing.

161. **Who is not a good candidate for dual-chamber pacemakers?**
Patients who have a history of recurrent SVT are not good candidates for any pacing modality that involves atrial sensing, such as dual-chamber pacemakers. They are better served by a simpler VVI pacemaker.

162. **Describe the manifestations and pathophysiology of pacemaker syndrome.**
Dizziness, palpitations, a pounding sensation in the chest or neck, or dyspnea associated with ventricular pacing in patients who had symptomatic bradyarrhythmias. The underlying mechanism is the loss of the normal AV synchrony during ventricular pacing.

163. **How is pacemaker syndrome managed?**
By changing from ventricular to dual-chamber or AV sequential pacing. An improvement in cardiac output has been documented in various studies when the pacing modality was changed. Patients with LV hypertrophy or LV failure or older patients who have a large atrial contribution to LV filling are most prone to develop pacemaker syndrome and may be better candidates for AV sequential pacing using a DDD pacemaker.

AORTIC DISEASES

164. **What are the causes of acute, severe AR?**
- Infective endocarditis
- Dissecting aneurysm
- Rupture or prolapse of aortic leaflet(s)
- Traumatic rupture
- Spontaneous rupture of myxomatous valve
- Spontaneous rupture of leaflet fenestrations
- Sudden sagging of a "normal" leaflet
- Faulty incision of a stenotic aortic valve postoperatively

   Morganroth J, Perloff JK, Zeldis SN, et al: Acute severe aortic regurgitation: Pathophysiology, clinical recognition, and management, *Ann Intern Med* 87:223–232, 1977.

165. **Why is a wide pulse pressure, typically present in chronic severe AR, frequently absent in patients with acute AR?**
Because of the much higher left ventricular end-diastolic pressure (LVEDP) in the acute form. The acute development of a severe aortic valvular leak causes a much higher LVEDP in the normal-sized LV of patients with acute AR. Patients with chronic AR commonly have a dilated LV with increased compliance capable of accommodating large blood volumes without a significant rise of LVEDP.

166. **Explain the effects of the rapid elevation of LVEDP in acute AR.**
A much shorter and softer diastolic rumble results from the rapid elevation of LVEDP in acute AR and its rapid equilibration with aortic pressure. Another auscultatory manifestation of the rapid rise of LVEDP is premature mitral valve closure that is also considered a reliable echocardiographic sign of acute AR.

167. **Summarize the hemodynamic features of AR.**
See Table 4-10.

168. **What are the hemodynamic signs of chronic AR?**
- Dilated LV due to longstanding volume overload
- Large stroke volume
- Wide pulse pressure causing the peripheral arterial auscultatory signs

TABLE 4-10. HEMODYNAMIC FEATURES OF SEVERE AORTIC REGURGITATION

	Acute	Chronic
LV compliance	Not ↑	↑
Regurgitant volume	↑	↑
LV end-diastolic pressure	Markedly ↑	May be normal
LV ejection velocity	Not significantly ↑	Markedly ↑
Aortic systolic pressure	Not ↑	↑
Aortic diastolic pressure	→ to ↑	Markedly ↓
Systemic arterial pulse pressure	Slightly to moderately ↑	Markedly ↑
Ejection fraction	Not ↑	↑
Effective stroke volume	↓	↔
Effective cardiac output	↓	↔
Heart rate	↑	↔
Peripheral vascular resistance	↑	Not ↑

↔ = unchanged, ↑ = increased, ↓ = decreased; LV = left ventricular.
Data from Morganroth J, Perloff JK, Zeldis SN, et al: Acute severe aortic regurgitation: Pathophysiology, clinical recognition, and management, Ann Intern Med 87:223–232, 1977.

INFECTIONS

See also Chapter 12, Infectious Diseases.

169. **What are the indications for surgical intervention in infectious endocarditis?**
   ■ Severe or progressive heart failure due to valvular regurgitation
   ■ Perivalvular abscess
   ■ Fungal endocarditis
   ■ Persistent bacteremia despite appropriate antibiotic therapy
   ■ Vegetations > 10 mm
   ■ More than one systemic embolic event despite appropriate therapy

   Bonow RO, Carabello BA, Chatterjee K, et al: ACC/AHA 2006 guidelines for the management of patients with valvular heart disease. A report of the American College of Cardiology/American Heart Association Task Force on Practice Guidelines (Writing Committee to Revise the 1998 Guidelines for the Management of Patients with Valvular Heart Disease), *J Am Coll Cardiol* 48:e1–e142, 2006.

170. **What does the new onset of conduction system abnormalities in the setting of endocarditis imply?**
   Perivalvular or myocardial abscesses or both. Surgical drainage and valve replacement are usually necessary.

171. **Explain the pathophysiology of the so-called immunologic manifestations of subacute bacterial endocarditis (SBE).**
   Immunologic manifestations of infective endocarditis are believed to be mediated by the deposition of immune complexes within extracardiac structures, such as the retina, joints, fingertips, pericardium, skin, and kidney, rather than direct bacterial invasion. Interestingly, these immunologic manifestations of endocarditis are reported almost exclusively in patients with a prolonged course of SBE.

172. **List examples of the immunologic manifestations of SBE.**
    - **Roth spots:** cytoid bodies in the retina
    - **Osler nodes:** tender nodular lesions in the terminal phalanges
    - **Janeway lesions:** painless macular lesions on palms and soles
    - **Petechiae and purpuric lesions**
    - **Proliferative glomerulonephritis**

173. **What are the most common causes of acute pericarditis in the outpatient setting?**
    Idiopathic, although many of these cases are probably due to viral infections or autoimmune reactions.

174. **What are the most common causes of acute pericarditis in the inpatient setting?**
    - **T**rauma
    - **U**remia
    - **M**yocardial infarction (acute and post)
    - **M**edications (e.g., hydralazine and procainamide)
    - **O**ther infections (bacterial, fungal, tuberculous)
    - **R**heumatoid arthritis and other autoimmune disorders
    - **R**adiation
    This can be easily remembered with the mnemonic TUM(M)OR(R), which also serves as a reminder that metastatic cancer is a frequent cause of pericarditis and pericardial effusion in hospitalized patients.

175. **What is the major cardiac finding in Lyme disease?**
    AV conduction abnormalities, such as first-degree AV block, second-degree AV block, complete heart block, fascicular block, or bundle branch block. Complete heart block is often associated with syncope because of concomitant depression of ventricular escape rhythms. Temporary pacing is indicated (the AV block usually resolves), as is antibiotic treatment with high-dose IV penicillin or oral tetracycline. A mild myopericarditis may also occur. Cardiac findings are seen in about 1 in 10 patients.

CONGENITAL HEART DISEASE

176. **Which congenital heart disease (CHD) lesions most often present in adulthood?**
    - Bicuspid aortic valve
    - ASD, which accounts for about 30% of all CHD in adults
    Congenital cyanotic cardiac lesions rarely present in adulthood.

177. **List the types and frequencies of ASDs.**
    - Ostium secundum: 70%
    - Ostium primum: 15%
    - Sinus venosus: 15%

178. **What is the difference between ostium secundum ASD and ostium primum ASD?**
    Ostium secundum ASD occurs near the fossa ovalis in the atrial septum and ostium primum ASD occurs in the inferior portion of the septum.

179. *Coeur en sabot* ("boot-shaped heart") is a term coined in 1888 by a French scientist in his first report of a congenital cardiac disease. In which CHD is this heart configuration found?

Tetralogy of Fallot, a term first coined by E. L. Fallot that described the typical configuration of the cardiac silhouette on chest x-ray in affected patients. The four components of this malformation are:
- VSD
- Obstruction to RV outflow
- Overriding of the aorta
- RV hypertrophy

180. Summarize the radiographic findings in tetralogy of Fallot.

RV hypertrophy, which results in a fairly classic boot-shaped (or wooden shoe–shaped) configuration of the cardiac silhouette, with prominence of the RV and a concavity in the region of the underdeveloped RV outflow tract and main pulmonary artery.

181. Which cardiac disease most commonly presents in adulthood with RBBB, first-degree AV block, and left axis deviation on ECG?

Ostium primum ASD. Because of hypoplastic changes in the left anterior fascicle, patients with ostium primum ASD have left axis QRS deviation. Thus, the combination of RBBB and left axis QRS deviation is a fairly distinctive feature of ostium primum ASD, and it is often accompanied by first-degree AV block.

182. What are the most common sites of aortic coarctation?

In descending order of frequency:
- Postductal (adult-type coarctation)
- Localized juxtaductal coarctation
- Preductal (infantile-type coarctation)
- Ascending thoracic aorta
- Distal descending thoracic aorta
- Abdominal aorta

183. Which congenital cardiac lesions are associated with coarctation of the aorta?
- Bicuspid aortic valve
- Patent ductus arteriosus
- VSD
- Berry aneurysms of circle of Willis

184. What is the "figure 3" sign?

A finding on chest x-ray described as a characteristic "3" sign resulting from post-stenotic dilatation of the descending aorta and the dilated left subclavian artery. A barium swallow may reveal a reverse "3" sign. Along with rib notching, the presence of the "3" sign is almost pathognomic for **aortic coarctation.**

OTHER CARDIAC SYNDROMES

185. Identify the types of shock and their causes.

See Table 4-11.

186. How common are cardiac manifestations of ankylosing spondylitis?

3–10%, depending on the duration of the disease.

TABLE 4–11. CLASSIFICATION, MECHANISM, AND ETIOLOGY OF SHOCK

Hypovolemic		Cardiogenic		Extracardiac Obstructive		Distributive	
Mechanism	Etiology	Mechanism	Etiology	Mechanism	Etiology	Mechanism	Etiology
Hemorrhage	Trauma, gastrointestinal, retroperitoneal	Myopathic	Myocardial infarction (left ventricle, right ventricle) Myocardial contusion (trauma) Myocarditis Cardiomyopathy Postischemic myocardial stunning Septic myocardial depression Pharmacologic (anthracycline, calcium-channel blockers)	Impaired diastolic filling	Vena cava obstruction (tumor) Tension pneumothorax Mechanical ventilation Asthma Constriction pericarditis Cardiac tamponade	Septic	Bacterial Viral Fungal Viral Rickettsial
Fluid depletion (nonhemorrhaghic)	Dehydration Vomiting Diarrhea Polyuria	Mechanical	Valvular failure (stenotic or regurgitant) Hypertrophic cardiomyopathy Ventricular septal defect	Impaired systolic contraction	Pulmonary embolism Acute pulmonary hypertension Aortic dissection	Toxic shock syndrome	

(continued)

TABLE 4-11. CLASSIFICATION. MECHANISM. AND ETIOLOGY OF SHOCK—*(continued)*

Hypovolemic		Cardiogenic		Extracardiac Obstructive		Distributive	
Mechanism	Etiology	Mechanism	Etiology	Mechanism	Etiology	Mechanism	Etiology
Interstitial fluid redistribution	Thermal injury Trauma Anaphylaxis	Arrhythmic	Bradycardia Tachycardia			Anaphylactic Anaphylactoid	
Increased vascular capacitance (venodilation)	Sepsis Anaplylaxis Toxins/ drugs					Neurogenic Endocrinologic	Spinal shock Adrenal crisis Thyroid storm
						Toxic	Nitroprusside Bretylium

From Parrillo JE: Approach to the patient with shock. In Goldman L, Ausiello D (eds): Cecil Medicine, 23rd ed. Philadelphia, WB Saunders, 2007.

187. **What valvular dysfunction is commonly encountered in ankylosing spondylitis?**
Dilatation of the aortic valve ring and the sinuses of Valsalva as well as inflammatory changes in the aortic valve ring. The resultant clinical hallmark is aortic root dilatation and aortic regurgitation, often rapidly progressive and ultimately requiring aortic valve replacement. Echocardiography is the diagnostic technique of choice in the evaluation and follow-up of these patients.

188. **What is Marfan syndrome?**
A generalized disorder of connective tissue that is inherited as an autosomal dominant trait. Cardiac abnormalities occur in over 60% of patients and are almost always responsible for early death when present.

189. **What is the most common cardiac lesion in Marfan syndrome?**
Dilatation of the aortic ring, sinuses of Valsalva, and ascending aorta that leads to progressive AR. Acute aortic complication may occur and the risk of dissection is markedly increased during pregnancy.

190. **Describe another common valvular dysfunction in Marfan syndrome.**
MR due to a redundant myxomatous mitral valve (called "floppy" prolapsed mitral valve). In contrast to adults, children with Marfan syndrome are much more likely to have severe isolated MR than aortic root or aortic valve disease.

191. **To what does the term "Marfan syndrome–forme fruste" refer?**
MVP in the absence of other systemic manifestations of Marfan syndrome because of the similar pathologic appearance of the myxomatous mitral valve in both disorders. Isolated MVP is more common than Marfan syndrome.

192. **Which of the cardiac chambers is most frequently involved in an atrial myxoma?**
   - **LA:** 86%
   - **RA:** 10%
   - **LV:** 2%
   - **RV:** 2%
   - **Multiple locations:** 10%

193. **What surgical technique is used to prevent recurrence of myxoma?**
Wide resection of the fossa ovalis area of the interatrial septum. The most common site of origin of atrial myxomas is the fossa ovalis.

194. **What is the most common cause of chronic MR in the United States?**
MVP, which has replaced rheumatic heart disease (the most common cause of chronic MR in the 1950s and 1960s).

195. **How is MR treated medically? Surgically?**
Medically:
   - Afterload reduction (to maximize "forward" cardiac output)
   - Salt restriction
   - Diuretics (with symptoms of CHF)
   - Digitalis (with AF)
Surgically:
   - Mitral valve repair or valvuloplasty (particularly for patients with MVP or rheumatic heart disease)

■ Mitral valve replacement
Surgical mitral valve repair or replacement should be performed in patients refractory to medical management before they enter the severely symptomatic stage, or in asymptomatic patients before they develop irreversible ventricular dysfunction as evidenced by LVEF < 40% or progressive ventricular dilatation.

DRUG THERAPY

196. **In primary prevention trials aimed at reducing cardiovascular mortality with cholesterol-lowering statin drugs, which drugs have been shown to lower the risk of death from cardiac causes?**
■ Pravastatin
■ Lovastatin
■ Atorvastin
■ Rosuvastatin

Three primary coronary prevention trials—the West of Scotland Coronary Prevention Study (WOSCOPS), the AFCAPS/TexCAPS, and the Anglo-Scandinavian Cardiac Outcome Trial (ASCOT)—have demonstrated that pravastatin, lovastatin, and atorvastatin reduce coronary and cardiovascular fatal and nonfatal events in patients with baseline LDL cholesterol levels ranging from 130–190 mg/dL. These three clinical trials provide compelling evidence that reduction of LDL cholesterol to ≤ 100 mg/dL is effective in preventing heart disease and stroke in patients with no known vascular disease. More recently, the JUPITER trial showed efficacy in reducing major CVD in patients without hyperlipidemia but with elevated CRP (C-reactive protein). The FDA approved rosuvastatin for primary prevention of CVD in these patients.

Downs JR, Clearfield M, Weis S, et al: Primary prevention of acute coronary events with lovastatin in men and women with average cholesterol levels: Results of AFCAPS/TexCAPS. Air Force/Texas Coronary Atherosclerosis Prevention Study, *JAMA* 279:1615–1622, 1998.

Sever PS, Dahlof B, Poulter NR, et al: for the ASCOT Investigators: Prevention of coronary and stroke events with atorvastatin in hypertensive patients who have average or lower-than-average cholesterol concentrations, in the Anglo-Scandinavian Cardiac Outcomes Trial–Lipid Lowering Arm (ASCOT-LLA): A multicentre randomised controlled trial, *Lancet* 361:1149–1158, 2003.

Ridker PM, Danielson E, Fonseca FAH, et al: Rosuvastatin to prevent vascular events in men and women with elevated C-reactive protein, *N Engl J Med* 359:2195–2207, 2008.

197. **Which classes of lipid-lowering drugs are most effective in reducing LDL fraction and in reducing cardiovascular complications in patients with known CAD?**
A variety of lipid-lowering drug classes reduce total and LDL cholesterol levels. These lipid-lowering drug classes include:
■ **Bile acid resin sequestrants** (cholestyramine and colestipol): Reduce LDL cholesterol by approximately 10%. The Lipid Research Clinic Coronary Prevention Trial (LRC-CPPT) demonstrated a 20% reduction in CAD events but no change in total mortality during a 10-year treatment with cholestyramine in patients with no previous known CAD.
■ **Niacin and nicotinic acid:** Reduce LDL cholesterol by 15–25% and has been shown to reduce cardiovascular complications in clinical prospective trials.
■ **Fibrates** (gemfibrozil and fenofibrate): Reduce LDL cholesterol by approximately 10%. Gemfibrozil has been shown to reduce cardiovascular complications in patients without and patients with previous known CAD. A recent prospective placebo-controlled, randomized clinical trial of fenofibrate failed to show an overall reduction in fatal and nonfatal CAD complications in diabetic patients.
■ **Statins:** Achieve reductions of LDL of up to 60% unsurpassed by any other lipid-lowering class. Recent statin trials have suggested a clinical benefit related to both the reduction in

LDL cholesterol and the reduction in CRP, suggesting a non–LDL-dependent mechanism possibly mediated by the anti-inflammatory and/or endothelial protective benefits of statins.

Lipid Research Clinics Program: The Lipid Research Clinics Coronary Primary Prevention Trial results: Reduction in incidence of coronary heart disease, *JAMA* 251:351, 1984.

Frick MH, Elo O, Happa K, Heinonen OP: Helsinki Heart Study: Primary prevention trial with dyslipidemia, *N Engl J Med* 317:1237–1245, 1987.

Rubins HB, Robins SJ, Collins D, et al: Gemfibrozil for the secondary prevention of coronary heart disease in men with low levels of high-density lipoprotein cholesterol. Veterans Affairs High-Density Lipoprotein Cholesterol Intervention Trial Study Group, *N Engl J Med* 341:410–418, 1999.

Grundy S, Cleeman CN, Brewer HB, et al: Implications of recent clinical trials for the National Cholesterol Education Program Panel III Guidelines, *J Am Coll Cardiol* 44:720–732, 2004.

Sever P, Dahlof B, Poulter NR, et al: Prevention of coronary and stroke events with atorvastatin in hypertensive patients who have average or lower-than-average cholesterol concentrations, in the Anglo-Scandinavian Cardiac Outcomes Trial—Lipid Lowering Arm (ASCOT-LLA): A multicentre randomised controlled trial, *Lancet* 361:1149–1158, 2003.

198. **Are statins recommended in diabetic patients and have they been proved to prevent cardiovascular complications in such patients?**
Yes. Two leading recent randomized, placebo-controlled clinical trials have provided important insight into the role of statins in diabetics: the Heart Protection Study (HPS) of simvastatin and the Collaborative Atorvastatin Diabetes Study (CARDS) of atorvastatin. The HPS consisted of 5963 diabetic patients (33% of which had prior CAD) randomized to simvastatin 40 mg/day versus placebo and prospectively followed up for 4.8 years for the primary composite study outcome of MI or coronary death. LDL cholesterol levels were reduced from 125 to 85 mg%. Primary outcome was significantly reduced by 27% and stroke risk was reduced by 24% ($P <$ .0001, both comparisons). An important observation in this trial was that diabetics with no CAD or other vascular disease at baseline had a 33% reduction in coronary heart disease independently of baseline LDL cholesterol levels.

CARDS was the first prospective, randomized, placebo-controlled clinical trial of a statin, namely atorvastatin, in a population composed solely of adult-onset diabetic patients with NO known vascular disease. This CARDS trial randomized 2838 diabetics with at least one other cardiovascular risk factor to atorvastatin 10 mg or placebo. This trial was prematurely terminated 2 years early, after a median follow-up of 3.9 years because of the large statin benefit. It was noted that LDL cholesterol levels were reduced from 118 to 82 mg%. The primary study outcome (major coronary events, revascularization, UA, resuscitated cardiac arrest, and stroke) was reduced by 37% ($P = $ .001) and stroke risk was reduced by 48%.

The more recent Action to Control Cardiovascular Risk in Diabetes (ACCORD) trial, though, did not find that intensive treatment of cholesterol with fenobibrate in addition to simvastatin reduced combined occurrence of MI, strokes, or cardiovascular death in patients with diabetes.

ACCORD Study Group, Ginsberg HN, Elam MB, et al: Effect of combination lipid lowering therapy in type 2 diabetes mellitus, *N Engl J Med* 362:1563–1574, 2010.

Colhoun HM, Betteridge DJ, Durrington PN, et al: on behalf of the CARDS Investigators: Primary prevention of cardiovascular disease with atorvastatin in type 2 diabetes in the Collaborative Atorvastatin Diabetes Study (CARDS): Multicentre randomized placebo-controlled trial, *Lancet* 364:685–696, 2004.

Collins R, Armitage J, Parish S, et al: on behalf of the Heart Protection Study Collaborative Group: MRC/BHF Heart Protection Study of cholesterol-lowering with simvastatin in 5963 people with diabetes: A randomized placebo-controlled trial, *Lancet* 361:2005–2016, 2003.

199. **What does "cardioselectivity" of a beta blocking drug mean? Summarize the clinical implications of this pharmacologic property.**
That the drug predominantly blocks the beta$_1$ adrenergic receptors, which are mostly present in the heart. Cardioselective beta blockers, in low doses, have minimal blocking effects on

beta$_2$ receptors, the predominant beta receptors in the lungs. However, cardioselectivity is only relative; when drugs are administered in large doses, cardioselectivity is markedly diminished. Despite these limitations, cardioselective beta blockers are much safer than non-cardioselective beta blockers in patients with obstructive lung disease. There are three commercially available cardioselective beta blockers: atenolol, metoprolol, and acebutolol.

200. **What is the importance of intrinsic sympathomimetic activity (ISA) as it applies to beta blockers?**
ISA refers to the partial beta adrenergic agonist properties of some beta blockers. When sympathetic activity is low (at rest), these beta blockers produce low-grade beta stimulation. However, under conditions of stress (exercise), beta blockers with ISA behave essentially as conventional beta blockers without ISA. The clinical significance of ISA is not clearly established.

201. **Which beta blockers possess ISA?**
Pindolol and acebutolol. All other beta blockers currently available have no significant ISA. Beta blockers with ISA are rarely used today and are, in fact, contraindicated in patients recovering from a recent MI because they are not proved to be "cardioprotective," that is, effective in reducing the risk of a recurrent MI, cardiovascular mortality, or sudden cardiac death.

WEBSITES

1. American College of Cardiology: www:acc.org

2. American Heart Association: www.americanheart.org

BIBLIOGRAPHY

1. Fauci AS, Kasper DL, Hauser SL, et al, *Harrison's Principles of Internal Medicine*, ed 17, New York, 2008, McGraw-Hill.
2. Libby P, Bonow R, Mann DL, Zipes D: *Braunwald's Heart Disease: A Textbook of Cardiovascular Medicine*, ed 8, Philadelphia, 2007, WB Saunders.
3. Wagner GS: *Marriott's Practical Electrocardiography*, ed 11, Philadelphia, 2008, Lippincott Williams & Wilkins.

VASCULAR MEDICINE

Timothy R.S. Harward, M.D.

> *... Dr. DeBakey suspected that he was not having a heart attack ... but ... that the inner lining of the [thoracic aorta] had torn, known as a dissecting aortic aneurysm. ... [A]s a younger man, he devised the operation to repair such torn aortas, a condition virtually always fatal.*
> *The New York Times,* December 25, 2006.

GENERAL EVALUATION

1. **Describe the evaluation of a patient for arterial diseases.**
   - History. Ask the patient:
     - Do your symptoms get better or worse with activity?
     - Do you have a history of diabetes?
       - High blood pressure (BP)?
       - Heart disease, angina, or heart attack?
       - High cholesterol?
     - Does anyone in your family have a history of blood vessel aneurysms?
       - Strokes?
       - Surgeries on blood vessel in the neck, arm, or leg?
       - Amputation of a leg or arm?
   - Physical examination:
     - Examine all bilateral pulses including carotid, brachial, radial, femoral, popliteal, dorsalis pedis, and posterior tibial.
     - Listen for bruits at carotid pulse and any other pulse with abnormal palpation.
     - Examine for pulsatile masses at the abdomen, groin, and popliteal areas.
     - Listen for bruits in all quadrants of the abdomen.

2. **What tests can be used to evaluate blood flow if pulses are not palpable?**
   - Noninvasive vascular laboratory evaluation
     - BP measurements in upper arm, thigh, and lower leg to determine ankle-brachial index (ABI) and differences between BP on left and right sides
     - Doppler waveform analysis that evaluates velocity of blood flow
     - Ultrasound imaging that visualizes the arterial anatomy, morphology of any lesions seen, and hemodynamics of the blood flow
   - Computed tomography (CT) scan or magnetic resonance (MR) angiography that allows visualization of vascular anatomy through contrast injection into the venous system
   For initial evaluation of nonpalpable pulses, the noninvasive evaluation is preferable because of lower cost, less risk, and provision of both anatomic and hemodynamic data.

3. **How are noninvasive vascular laboratory tests interpreted?**
   By comparing BP measurements at different locations, analyzing waveforms representing the blood flow, and viewing ultrasound. All pressure measurements are compared with the arm BP. By dividing the ankle BP by the highest arm BP measurement, one can calculate an ABI. Values > 0.9 are considered normal, values < 0.4 are consistent with severe ischemia,

whereas values of 0.5–0.8 are consistent with complaints of claudication. These measurements are difficult to interpret in the diabetic patient because the arteries become very stiff secondary to calcification in the artery wall. Fortunately, toe pressures are still accurate in this setting for determining overall ischemia but do not help locate the site of obstruction. The addition of Doppler waveform analysis markedly increases the accuracy in determining the level of disease. A triphasic waveform is normal, whereas a monophasic waveform is consistent with a severe upstream obstruction. Finally, ultrasound helps detect aneurysms and delineate stenoses from occlusions. Overall, these criteria are 92–95% accurate in detecting the location and severity of arterial disease.

4. **When are noninvasive vascular laboratory tests indicated?**
When a clinician considers a peripheral arterial disease (PAD) diagnosis. In some cases, nothing other than the noninvasive study is needed to diagnose the problem and to plan treatment. In addition, the noninvasive study provides a baseline objective examination that can be repeated at no risk to the patient should the clinical situation change. In addition, the information learned will help steer future testing and intervention. After intervention, noninvasive vascular laboratory evaluation is used to follow the progress or regression of the intervention because the disease process has not been cured, only temporarily arrested.

ANEURYSM DISEASE

5. **What is an aneurysm?**
A dilatation of all three layers of the arterial wall measuring at least 50% larger than the expected normal diameter. When the dilatation is < 50% of the expected normal diameter, the artery is described as "ectatic."

6. **What are the most common sites for aneurysms?**
- **Infrarenal aorta:** 65%
- **Isolated thoracic aorta:** 16%
- **Infrarenal aorta with extension into the common iliac artery:** 13%
- **Peripheral aneurysms:** <3%

7. **Among *peripheral* arteries, which are the most frequent site for aneurysms?**
- Popliteal (70% of peripheral arterial aneurysms)
- Common femoral
- Carotid (rare)
- Mesenteric (rare)

8. **How does one detect an aneurysm?**
By a detailed physical examination with palpation of the aortic, femoral, and popliteal arteries. When an aneurysm is present, the pulsation feels broad and prominent. When a patient is obese, abdominal aortic and iliac artery aneurysms may not be palpable and are detected when an ultrasound or CT scan is performed for other reasons such as low back pain or gallbladder disease. When an aneurysm is suspected, CT or ultrasound confirms its presence. After an aneurysm is diagnosed, CT is used to follow the growth of a small abdominal aneurysm that is not yet large enough to warrant repair. For peripheral artery aneurysms, follow-up is done using ultrasound.

9. **What are the risks of an abdominal aortic aneurysm (AAA) or thoracic aneurysm?**
Rupture leading to death. The larger the diameter of the aneurysm, the greater the risk of rupture.

10. **How does the size of the AAA correlate with risk of rupture?**
Exponentially with increasing maximal diameter. A 3.0- to 4.4-cm-diameter aneurysm has a 2%/yr risk of rupture, whereas a 4.5- to 5.9-cm-diameter aneurysm has a 10%/yr risk of rupture. If the patient's aneurysm ruptures outside of the hospital setting, overall mortality is approximately 80–90%. Of these patients, 50% die at the scene of the rupture, 50% who make it to the hospital die in the operating room, and 50% of those who survive the operation die of other comorbid conditions prior to hospital discharge.

Brewster DC, Cronenwett JL, Hallett JW Jr, et al: Guidelines for the treatment of abdominal aortic aneurysms. Report of a subcommittee of the Joint Council of the American Association for Vascular Surgery and Society for Vascular Surgery, *J Vasc Surg* 37:1106–1117, 2003.

Thomas PR, Stewart RD: Abdominal aortic aneurysm, *Br J Surg* 75:733–736, 1988.

11. **What are the recommended methods of treating aortic aneurysms?**
Open surgical replacement or endovascular repair. Traditional therapy is open surgical replacement of the aneurysmal segment with an artificial conduit. Hospital stay is 5–7 days, whereas 30-day mortality is 1–5% depending on comorbidities. More recently, endovascular repair has become increasingly used. Under a light general anesthetic, this method utilizes a catheter delivery system to place a covered stent graft inside the aneurysm. Hospital stay is 1 day and operative mortality is < 1%; however, 30-day mortality is the same as for the open repair. More recent studies have found, though, that endovascular repair is associated with more late complications, higher late mortality, and higher cost that open surgical repair.

The United Kingdom EVAR Trial Investigators: Endovascular versus open repair of abdominal aortic aneurysm, *N Engl J Med* 362:1863–1871, 2010.

12. **Are there reasons why all patients do not undergo endovascular repair?**
Yes. The aortic or aneurysm anatomy precludes the proper placement of the stent graft by endovascular repair in 20–30% of patients.

13. **Which vasculitides are associated with thoracic aortic disease?**
   - Giant cell arteritis
   - Takayasu's arteritis
   - Behçet's disease

14. **What genetic disorders are most often associated with increased risk of thoracic aortic disease?**
   - Marfan syndrome (connective tissue disorder)
   - Loeys-Dietz syndrome (characterized by arterial aneurysms, hypertelorism, and cleft palate)
   - Turner's syndrome (characterized by genotype 45,X)
   - Ehlers-Danlos, type IV (characterized by easy bruising, thick skin, characteristic facial features, and rupture of arteries, uterus, and intestines)

Hiratzka LF, Bakris GL, Beckman JA, et al: 2010 ACCF/AHA/AATS/ACR/ASA/SCA/SCAI/SIR/STS/SVM guidelines for the diagnosis and management of patients with thoracic aortic disease, *J Am Coll Cardiol* 55: e27–e129, 2010.

15. **Should these patients with genetic disorders be followed regularly?**
Yes. Aortic imaging should be done at the time the genetic syndrome is identified and periodically as indicated for follow-up.

16. **What are the characteristics of the pain associated with acute thoracic aortic dissection (AoD)?**
   - Abrupt onset.
   - Severe intensity.
   - Sharp or stabbing in nature.

- Usually in the chest but also occurs in the back and abdomen depending on origin and progression of the dissection.
- May be asymptomatic with presenting symptoms of syncope, stroke, or congestive heart failure.

17. **What are the physical examination findings?**
    - Hypotension, hypertension, or normotension
    - Pulse deficits
    - Neurologic deficits
    - Symptoms of cardiac tamponade
    - Aortic insufficiency murmur

18. **How is a thoracic AoD diagnosed?**
    By thoracic CT scan, MR, or transesophageal echocardiogram (TEE).

19. **What are the two commonly used classification systems for thoracic AoD and their descriptions?**
    - DeBakey (Fig. 5-1)
        - Type I: Begins in the ascending aorta (proximal to the brachiocephalic artery) and propagates distally to at least the aortic arch. The descending aorta may also be involved.
        - Type II: Begins in and remains confined to the ascending aorta.
        - Type III: Begins in the descending aorta and propagates distally.
        - Type IIIa: Limited to descending thoracic aorta.
        - Type IIIb: Extends below the diaphragm.
    - Stanford
        - Type A: Involves the ascending aorta without regard to site of initial dissection.
        - Type B: All other dissections that do not involve the ascending aorta.

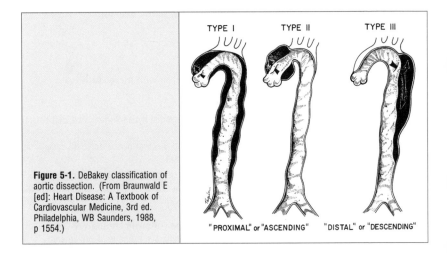

Figure 5-1. DeBakey classification of aortic dissection. (From Braunwald E [ed]: Heart Disease: A Textbook of Cardiovascular Medicine, 3rd ed. Philadelphia, WB Saunders, 1988, p 1554.)

20. **Which dissections should be considered for surgical repair?**
    Type I and type II for the DeBakey classification and type A for Stanford.

21. **Which dissections should be considered for medical treatment?**
    Type III (DeBakey) and type B (Stanford).

22. **Describe the medical management of thoracic AoD.**
    - Heart rate control with intravenous (IV) beta blockade to achieve a heart rate of < 60 beats per minute (bpm), if no contraindications to beta blockers. Non-dihydropyridine calcium channel blockers can be used for patients unable to receive beta blockers.
    - IV vasodilators (i.e., angiotensin-converting enzyme [ACE] inhibitors) if systolic BP remains > 120 mmHg after adequate beta blockade.
    - Pain control with IV opiates.

KEY POINTS: THORACIC AORTIC DISSECTION ✓

1. Patients with thoracic aortic dissection may have symptoms suggestive of myocardial ischemia.

2. Aortic dissection should be considered in all patients presenting with chest and upper back pain.

3. Improvement in pain does not rule out a thoracic aortic dissection.

4. Relatives of patients with thoracic aortic disease are at increased risk and should have appropriate screening.

23. **Who should be screened for thoracic aortic disease?**
    - Patients with identified genetic syndromes that have an increased risk
    - First-degree relative of patients with diagnosed thoracic aortic aneurysm or dissection
    - Patients with a bicuspid aortic valve
    - First-degree relatives of patients with bicuspid aortic valve

    Hiratzka LF, Bakris GL, Beckman JA, et al: 2010 ACCF/AHA/AATS/ACR/ASA/SCA/SCAI/SIR/STS/SVM guidelines for the diagnosis and management of patients with thoracic aortic disease, *J Am Coll Cardiol* 55: e27–e129, 2010.

24. **Do peripheral arterial aneurysms frequently rupture?**
    No. Only about 2% of peripheral arterial aneurysms rupture; however, peripheral arterial aneurysms can lead to distal embolization of intraluminal clot. Embolization can occur insidiously without symptoms until significant obstruction of smaller arteries is present. At this point, the upstream popliteal artery aneurysm thromboses, producing severe ischemic rest pain. In addition, peripheral aneurysm can enlarge sufficiently to compress the accompanying adjacent vein and/or nerve producing distal swelling and/or a burning discomfort as typically seen in patients with venous disease.

25. **When should peripheral arterial aneurysms be repaired?**
    When the aneurysm becomes > 2 cm in diameter or contains intraluminal clot. If a peripheral aneurysm clots and the patient develops rest pain, 20–30% will require an amputation.

26. **What is the treatment for peripheral arterial aneurysms?**
    Treatment methods differ based on the artery involved. Common femoral artery aneurysms are resected and replaced with a new prosthetic graft. Popliteal artery aneurysms are left in place but excluded from the circulation by ligating the artery above and below the aneurysm and constructing a bypass graft.

27. **What other arteries can become aneurysmal? How are they treated?**
Carotid, renal, superior mesenteric, splenic, and subclavian arteries. Carotid artery aneurysms are very rare but should be resected and repaired when found. Splenic artery aneurysms are more common and can rupture during pregnancy due to hormonal and hyperdynamic changes in blood flow and BP. Splenic artery rupture can be fatal to both mother and fetus and require resection. The renal artery aneurysm is treated much as the splenic artery aneurysm. Superior mesenteric artery (SMA) aneurysms are frequently mycotic or associated with infection and require removal and repair. Subclavian artery aneurysms may be associated with thoracic outlet syndrome. Symptoms of finger tip ulcers can occur from microemboli. Subclavian artery aneurysms are not true aneurysms but post-stenotic arterial dilatation generated by disturbed blood flow.

PERIPHERAL ARTERIAL OCCLUSIVE DISEASE

28. **What is the clinical spectrum of chronic PAD?**
- Asymptomatic
- Intermittent claudication
- Rest pain
- Nonhealing ulcers
- Gangrene

29. **What is intermittent claudication?**
A cramping pain or discomfort associated with activity that is relieved by rest, yet returns with resumption of activity. Claudication should not be confused with nocturnal cramps that have no association with PAD. The location of claudication discomfort suggests the level of the arterial obstruction. The disease is usually one level proximal to the discomfort. For example, calf claudication is associated with thigh level arterial obstruction.

30. **What is neurogenic claudication?**
Calf discomfort with activity that is both reproducible and relieved by rest and occurs in a patient with normal arterial circulation but with lumbar spine stenosis. The calf discomfort does not go away with just stopping activity. To make the discomfort dissipate, the patient must relieve pressure on the spine by either sitting or lying down. Noninvasive vascular laboratory testing is normal. Imaging evaluation of the lumbar spine shows lumbar spinal stenosis, often from protrusion of an intravertebral disc. This process often requires surgical decompression to relieve nerve compression.

31. **Describe the significance of rest pain, nonhealing ulcers, and gangrene.**
Ischemic rest pain, nonhealing ulcers, and gangrene develop with worsening of PAD and occur when the level of tissue perfusion is unable to maintain normal tissue viability, usually at approximately 40% of normal blood flow. Nonhealing ulcers and gangrene also suggest limb-threatening ischemia.

32. **What are the causes of claudication and tissue loss in the upper extremity?**
- Focal stenosis or total occlusion of the left subclavian artery due to atherosclerotic plaque
- Thoracic outlet syndrome
- Chronic trauma
- Giant cell arteritis (in women > 50–60 years old)

33. **What causes claudication, rest pain, and tissue loss in the lower extremity?**
- Atherosclerotic occlusive disease
- Popliteal artery entrapment due to an unusual anatomic location
- Adventitial cystic disease due to a mucin-secreting cell rest in the arterial wall

34. **Are there any medical therapies to help treat PAD?**
Yes. Risk modification can slow the progression of atherosclerotic arterial disease. Foremost is cessation of smoking. Smoking increases the incidence of PAD 16-fold.

Control of hypertension and diabetes mellitus also decreases progression of PAD. The ratio of total cholesterol to high-density lipoprotein (HDL) cholesterol is a strong predictor of developing PAD. Dietary modification to lower fat intake in combination with exercise improves this ratio. Statin medications help modify serum cholesterol levels. In addition, statins seem to have a protective effect unrelated to cholesterol control. This effect may be due to stabilization of the atherosclerotic plaque. Finally, pentoxifylline and cilostazol are medications used to increase pain-free walking distance in patients with claudication. Unfortunately, pentoxifylline does not work any better than placebo, but recent studies suggest that cilostazol may improve walking distance up to 200%. Antiplatelet therapy with aspirin is also helpful, particularly for the secondary prevention of cardiac and cerebrovascular disease, which are frequently concurrent (and sometimes without symptoms) in these patients.

Hirsch AT, Haskal ZJ, Hertzer NR, et al: ACC/AHA 2005 Practice Guidelines for the management of patients with peripheral arterial disease (lower extremity, renal, mesenteric, and abdominal aortic): A collaborative report from the American Association for Vascular Surgery/Society for Vascular Surgery, Society for Cardiovascular Angiography and Interventions, Society for Vascular Medicine and Biology, Society of Interventional Radiology, and the ACC/AHA Task Force on Practice Guidelines (Writing Committee to Develop Guidelines for the Management of Patients With Peripheral Arterial Disease): endorsed by the American Association of Cardiovascular and Pulmonary Rehabilitation; National Heart, Lung, and Blood Institute; Society for Vascular Nursing; TransAtlantic Inter-Society Consensus; and Vascular Disease Foundation, *Circulation* 113:e463–e654, 2006.

Sobel M, Verhaeghe R: Antithrombotic therapy for peripheral artery occlusive disease, *Chest* 133:1–38, 2008.

35. **Should patients with PAD receive anticoagulants?**
Generally no for patients with intermittent claudication. Anticoagulation is indicated for the initial treatment of acute arterial emboli or thrombosis.

36. **What are the surgical interventions used to improve arterial blood flow?**
Endarterectomy or bypass. Endarterectomy is done by removing the atherosclerotic plaque. This technique works well for short, focal lesions, but longer segments of disease are prone to early recurrent stenoses produced by development of both scar tissue and recurrent atherosclerotic plaque. Bypass is accomplished using a new conduit to redirect blood around an area of extensive arterial disease. This is best done using the patient's saphenous vein for the smaller arteries of the leg, whereas artificial conduits can be used for the larger arteries of the abdomen/pelvis. To ensure success of these techniques, one must originate the bypass in an area free of disease. The distal target artery needs to also be free of obstruction and have good runoff into the distal circulation.

37. **What are the endovascular procedures used to improve arterial blood flow?**
These newer percutaneous techniques focus on recanalizing the arterial lumen using balloon dilatation to fracture the atherosclerotic plaque away from the arterial wall followed by insertion of a stent to reexpand the arterial lumen. This technique was initially only utilized to treat short focal stenoses or occlusion (<5–10 cm in length). As stenting technology has evolved, longer and more complex segments of disease are being treated.

38. **What aspects of an open surgical intervention for treatment of PAD convey the greatest risk?**
General anesthesia and infection from a skin incision. In addition, both of these maneuvers (anesthesia and incision) stress the patient and increase the risk of myocardial infarction (MI), stroke, and death secondary to underlying comorbidities that are common in this patient

population; therefore, surgical intervention is reserved for patients with incapacitating symptoms (short-distance claudication < 100 yd and/or signs and symptoms of limb-threatening ischemia [rest pain, nonhealing ulcers, gangrene]). Appropriate patient selection and preoperative preparation produce perioperative mortality rates < 2% for inflow procedures such as aortic bypass, renal artery endarterectomy, and mesenteric artery bypasses, whereas outflow procedures to improve blood flow into the lower leg and foot have 30-day mortality rates of 4–5%.

39. **Are percutaneous endovascular procedures less risky than open surgical procedures?**
    Yes. The endovascular procedure is performed with a light sedation and requires only local anesthetic at the skin puncture site. Major risks consist of allergic reactions to the iodine contrast used to visualize arteries, potential renal failure created by the toxic effects of the iodine contrast in the renal tubules, and local arterial trauma secondary to the initial puncture and wire insertion where a dissection plane is created that leads to arterial thrombosis and embolization of the atherosclerotic plaque downstream during the balloon and stenting portion of the procedure.

40. **How do results of open surgical procedures compare with percutaneous endovascular interventions?**
    Short-term results in appropriately selected patients are excellent for both procedures. With endarterectomy or bypass, the 30-day patency rates > 95%, whereas 30-day patency rates for the majority of endovascular recanalization procedures > 80%; however, these endovascular results vary depending on the location, length, and severity of the disease treated. Shorter, more focal disease responds much better than longer, more diffuse disease. Long-term results for both surgical and endovascular procedures are excellent for aortoiliac PAD. Five-year patency rates for both techniques > 90%; therefore, balloon angioplasty and stenting have become the standard of care for this disease. For outflow artery PAD, surgical bypass is much better. If an adequate saphenous vein is used, 5-year patency rates are 70–80%. Unfortunately, even with the use of stenting, many arterial segments treated with endovascular repair develop recurrent disease within 6–12 months. Some reports suggest > 50% recurrence rates, but this topic is still under close study. The question of using drug-eluting coronary artery stents has been considered. In summary, the surgical bypass works better long-term but carries higher upfront risk whereas endovascular recanalization procedures are less risky but, at the present time, do not produce equivalent long-term results.

41. **Do medical therapies alter the outcome of surgical or endovascular procedures?**
    Yes. Smoking cessation dramatically improves maintenance of patency of both procedures. The use of statin drugs has been shown to improve patency of surgical bypass grafting and is being evaluated with endovascular recanalization procedures. At present, patient who have stents placed are started on clopidogrel, an antiplatelet adhesion medication. This decreases the incidence of stent thrombosis until the struts of the stent are covered. In addition, the use of aspirin or warfarin or both has been shown to improve long-term patency of leg bypass grafts, especially in patients requiring a second or third redo procedure; however, this advantage must be weighed against the risk of bleeding in an elderly population.

CAROTID DISEASE

42. **What causes carotid disease?**
    Atherosclerotic plaque in the proximal common carotid artery at the aortic arch (8%) or at the bifurcation extending into the internal carotid artery (ICA) (92%).

43. **How does carotid disease present clinically?**
When symptomatic, with a transient ischemia attack (TIA) (80%) or a stroke (20%) as the initial symptom. These are known as "hemispheric signs and symptoms," usually secondary to cholesterol or platelet or both and thrombus emboli breaking off of a friable atherosclerotic plaque.

44. **What are the symptoms of a TIA due to small emboli?**
   - Unilateral blindness in the eye ipsilateral to the carotid disease
   - Arm numbness or weakness or both contralateral to the carotid plaque
   - Leg numbness or weakness or both contralateral to the carotid plaque (may occur in association with arm symptoms)
   - Speech difficulties such as aphasia if the left side is involved or dysphasia if the right side is involved
   Events may last only seconds or hours and neuroimaging will not show any sign of ischemia.

45. **What is the initial evaluation for a patient presenting with a TIA?**
   - BP measurement and monitoring.
   - Head CT scan to evaluate for intracerebral bleed.
   - Duplex scanning (high-resolution ultrasound and Doppler) of the carotid arteries. This test allows one to diagnose the offending plaque without risk to the patient and is > 94% accurate.
   - Patients with TIAs require urgent evaluation and treatment to prevent complications of stroke.
   See also Chapter 17, Neurology.

   Luengo-Fernandez R, Gray AM, Rothwell PM: Effect of urgent treatment of transient ischaemic attack and minor stroke on disability and hospital costs (EXPRESS study): A prospective population-based sequential comparison, *Lancet* 8:235–243, 2009.

46. **What is the natural history of symptomatic carotid disease if not treated?**
An increased risk of stroke. The NASCET (North American Symptomatic Carotid Endarterectomy Trial) study provided this data. Phase I evaluated symptomatic patients with ≥ 70% stenosis and demonstrated a 12.5% stroke/yr with only medical therapy. Phase II evaluated symptomatic patients with 50–69% stenoses. This group of patients still presented with an unacceptable stroke rate of approximately 5%/yr. The natural history was shown to be dramatically altered by surgical intervention.

   North American Symptomatic Carotid Endarterectomy Trial: Methods, patient characteristics, and progress, *Stroke* 22:711–720, 1991.

47. **What is the treatment for patients with symptomatic carotid disease?**
If the duplex scan identifies a stenosis ≥ 50%, carotid endarterectomy is indicated. If the stenosis is < 50%, the patient should be treated with antiplatelet medications and followed closely with serial duplex scans. The only exception is when there is a significant ulcer in the atherosclerotic plaque. This situation is also an indication for surgical repair. However, if the patient is high risk for surgery (i.e., severe heart disease, prior neck irradiation or radical neck surgery, or is undergoing a repeat operation), the patient should be considered for a carotid artery balloon angioplasty and stenting.

48. **How should patients with asymptomatic carotid artery disease be treated?**
With regular follow-up with carotid duplex scanning. If the percentage of stenosis becomes > 60–70%, the surgeon can perform a carotid endarterectomy with a stroke rate < 3%, and the patient's life expectancy is at least 3 years, then prophylactic carotid endarterectomy should be performed. Antiplatelet therapy with aspirin and use of statin medications for cholesterol control is also important. These patients may also have asymptomatic coronary artery disease.

49. **What are the risks of carotid endarterectomy?**
Mainly perioperative stroke. This is usually due to intraoperative embolization but can be due to postoperative thrombosis usually caused by an operative technical defect. More common but less dramatic are cranial nerve injuries than can occur in approximately 10%. Most common of these is marginal mandibular nerve bruising that produces numbness around the ipsilateral mouth associated with droopiness. Other risks include bleeding and infection, both of which are moderately uncommon.

50. **Where does carotid angioplasty and stenting fit into the treatment of this disease?**
At this time, angioplasty is approved only for high-risk patients. The technique is still considered experimental for all other situations, and current trial results continue to be analyzed. The risk for periprocedure stroke from angioplasty and stenting is still higher than that for endarterectomy and its cost is more than twice that of surgical intervention. Still, for high-risk patients, the benefit outweighs the risk and cost.

> Brott TG, Hobson RW II, Howard G, et al: Stenting versus endarterectomy for treatment of carotid-artery stenosis. *N Engl J Med* 360:11–23, 2010.

51. **What are nonhemispheric TIAs?**
TIAs with signs and symptoms of drop attacks, dysarthria, ataxia, blurred vision secondary to bilateral eye involvement, dizziness, and occasionally, headaches. These events are due to ischemia in the posterior circulation distribution that includes the cerebellum and brainstem. They are usually due to vertebral artery pathology but can be due to generalized global ischemia when both ICAs are > 90% stenotic. In the latter situation, carotid endarterectomy will resolve these TIAs, especially if the posterior communicating artery off the circle of Willis is patent.

52. **What are crescendo TIA and stroke-in-evolution?**
Crescendo TIAs occur when the patient experiences several transient neurologic events within 24 hours, and a stroke-in-evolution is an acute neurologic deficit of mild-to-moderate degree that is progressive. Both entities can be associated with a severe carotid artery stenosis due to a friable, unstable atherosclerotic plaque. Emergent carotid endarterectomy or carotid balloon angioplasty and stenting are indicated for both these syndromes for qualifying patients.

53. **When is repair of an occluded carotid artery associated with a stroke indicated?**
Never. Complete occlusion should be treated with anticoagulation alone. Surgical procedures that attempt to reopen the artery are associated with possible progression of the stroke and an accompanying perioperative mortality of > 20%.

VENOUS DISEASE

54. **What is Virchow's triad?**
   - Stasis of flow
   - Hypercoaguable state
   - Vein wall injury

   The presence of these conditions increases the risk of deep venous thrombosis (DVT). Surgical procedures under general anesthesia, prolonged inactivity in patients suffering a neurologic event (e.g., strokes, brain surgery), severe diffuse trauma, orthopedic pelvic/knee surgery, and pelvic procedures all augment this situation and increase the risk for DVT development.

55. What are the physical findings of DVT?
Physical findings may be present in as few as 50% of patients with acute DVT. If present, unilateral leg swelling, warmth, pitting edema, or engorged superficial veins may be seen. Physical examination should not be relied upon to confirm or refute the suspected diagnosis.

56. How is DVT diagnosed?
The physical findings of DVT are nonspecific with an overall accuracy of 50%. This inaccuracy led to the development of noninvasive methods for detecting thrombosis. The examination includes both Doppler analysis of venous flow dynamics and ultrasonic imaging of the lower extremity veins. Intraluminal thrombus is detected when the vein is noncompressible and hemodynamic flow analysis shows a delay in flow with distal tissue compression due to upstream obstruction by clot.

57. What are the complications of DVT?
Pulmonary emboli, which are associated with a high mortality. Untreated DVT can also lead to chronic venous insufficiency with resultant swelling and predisposition to leg ulcerations.

58. What is the standard therapy for DVT?
Immediate anticoagulation with heparin and warfarin. Heparin should always accompany warfarin (Coumadin) administration initially to prevent warfarin skin necrosis. The heparin may be given by subcutaneous injections for 4–5 days while Coumadin takes effect and increases the International Normalized Ratio (INR). Anticoagulation is maintained for 3–6 months to allow for autolysis and recanalization of the thrombus, then discontinued. After 3–6 months, the risk of the Coumadin causing bleeding outweighs the risk of recurrent clot or pulmonary embolus. Currently, other oral anticoagulants are under investigation for prevention and treatment of DVT.

59. What is post-phlebitic syndrome?
Venous hypertension created by destruction of intraluminal valves during an initial thrombotic event with associated symptoms.

60. What are the symptoms of post-phlebetic syndrome?
- Lower extremity swelling: 95%
- Rust-colored skin discoloration (called "venous stasis dermatitis"): 50%
- Ulcerations located in the "gaiter zone" of the lower calf and ankle region: 5%

61. Describe a venous insufficiency ulcer.
An ulcer usually located on the medial leg with surrounding pigmentation of hemosiderin. The involved leg is usually swollen.

62. When does post-phlebitic syndrome occur?
Usually insidiously 5–10 years after the initial DVT.

63. How is post-phlebitic syndrome treated?
With external compression stockings to decrease soft tissue venous hypertension and to control lower extremity edema. Unfortunately, this treatment is for life. Valves cannot be repaired or replaced. Ulcerations may need débridement and attentive wound care in addition to compression.

64. What is May-Thurner syndrome?
A proximal left common iliac vein narrowing or occlusion caused by an anatomic abnormality. Normally, the left common iliac vein passes under the right common iliac artery as it joins the contralateral right common iliac vein to form the inferior vena cava (IVC). Constant pulsation of the artery causes fibrosis of the underlying left common iliac vein, producing severe narrowing or total occlusion. When occlusion occurs, the entire left iliac venous system

usually thromboses, and these patients are usually diagnosed as having an iliofemoral DVT. Treatment with thrombolysis can dissolve the clot and uncover the underlying pathology. If a wire can cross the narrowing, the area is treated with balloon angioplasty and stent placement. In addition, these patients still require anticoagulation.

65. **What is venous claudication?**
Pain with walking after short distances in which the patient has normal arterial circulation but a chronic, severe venous obstruction in either the iliac or the femoral veins or both. In addition, there are also few draining collaterals around the chronic obstruction.

66. **What is an IVC filter?**
A metallic device inserted into the flow stream of the IVC below the renal veins. It allows blood to pass through its interstices while having the ability to trap blood clots passing up from the pelvis/lower extremities and preventing pulmonary emboli. Original filters were permanent, but recent changes have produced a filter than can be removed 2–4 weeks after placement.

67. **What are the indications for placement of an IVC filter?**
Absolute indications are development of DVT in patients with contraindications to anticoagulation; recurrent pulmonary embolization despite proper anticoagulation; complications of anticoagulation forcing discontinuation of anticoagulant therapy; and chronic pulmonary embolism associated with pulmonary hypertension and cor pulmonale. Relative indications include free-floating clot in the iliofemoral region.

68. **What is Takayasu's arteritis?**
A chronic, large vessel vasculitis. The etiology of Takayasu's arteritis is unknown. Women are affected in nearly 90% of cases and are usually aged between 10 and 40 years.

69. **What arteries are involved?**
   - Aortic arch and brachiocephalic vessels (type I)
   - Thoracoabdominal aorta and renal arteries (type II)
   Type III Takayasu's arteritis has features of type I and type II involvement. Patients with Takayasu's arteritis may also have accelerated atherosclerosis of other blood vessels such as the carotid arteries.

70. **Describe the clinical prodrome associated with Takayasu's arteritis.**
Initially, these patients have systemic symptoms such as fever, fatigue, anorexia, weight loss, and arthralgias. Later in the disease, classic symptoms of arterial occlusive disease develop such as lack of palpable pulses, cool extremities, and upper or lower extremity claudication.

71. **Do these patients need revascularization procedures?**
Not always. Usually treatment with glucocorticoids or agents such as methotrexate and azothioprine may help abate the progression, although it remains a chronic disease. Revascularization procedures (either open repair or angioplasty with stent placement) are indicated in the presence of significant occlusion, but may have increased risks of restenosis. Aortic valve surgery is sometimes needed to repair aortic regurgitation.

LYMPHEDEMA

72. **What is the difference between primary and secondary lymphedema?**
Primary disease occurs when the lymphatic system is insufficient from birth (Milroy's disease) or puberty (lymphedema praecox), and secondary disease is from destruction of lymphatic channels due to trauma (usually surgical), radiation therapy, tumor invasion, and recurrent infections (bacteria and parasites).

73. **How does lymphedema present?**
Usually with unilateral, extensive swelling, worse at the distal end of the involved limb where one typically finds digit involvement. Late findings are verrucous skin changes. In severe cases caused by tropical filiaria infection, elephantiasis develops.

74. **Are there any specific diagnostic tests to perform to verify lymphedema?**
Yes. Lymphoscintigraphy with radiolabeled colloid is often used to verify lymphedema. In this test, the colloid is injected into the subcutaneous tissue. Normally, the colloid will move up into the abdomen within hours, but with lymphatic obstruction, the colloid never ascends but becomes trapped in the interstitial space of the lower limb.

75. **What is the treatment for lymphedema?**
Reduction of swelling with pneumatic compression pumps and stockings. Adjuvant therapies include weight control, exercise, and massage. Antibiotics are given whenever there are recurrent episodes of cellulitis. Lymphatic bypass procedures and reduction procedures are mentioned only to condemn them due to poor results.

WEBSITE

1. www.vascularweb.org

BIBLIOGRAPHY

1. Cronenwett JL, Johnston W, eds. *Rutherford's Vascular Surgery*, ed 7, Philadelphia, 2009, Elsevier.
2. Moore WD: *Vascular and Endovascular Surgery: A Comprehensive Review*, ed 7, Philadelphia, 2005, WB Saunders.

CHAPTER 6

PULMONARY MEDICINE

Adriano R. Tonelli, M.D., and Eloise M. Harman, M.D.

The orderly spoke of my father as a little man, but he was not, not until his black lung made its final assault. In a space of a few short weeks, he had shrunk, literally collapsing around his lungs as they became the entire focus of his being.

Homer Hickam, *October Sky*

ANATOMY

1. **Describe the main airway structure.**
   - **Trachea:** C-shaped cartilage with dorsal smooth muscle
   - **Main bronchi:** semicircular cartilage
   - **Bronchi:** irregularly shaped cartilage plates
   - **Bronchioles:** no cartilage support, surrounded by muscular layer

2. **What is the difference between conducting and respiratory airway zones?**
   - **Conducting airway:** Air gets filtered, humidified, and heated; extends from the trachea to the terminal bronchioles.
   - **Respiratory airway:** Site of gas exchange; includes the respiratory bronchioles, alveolar ducts, and sacs.

     The portion of lung supplied by a primary respiratory bronchiole is the *acinus*.

3. **What are the components of the alveolar-capillary surface?**
   Surfactant, alveolar epithelium (type 1 and type 2 alveolar cells, the latter producing surfactant), interstitium, and endothelium.

4. **Describe the respiratory muscles.**
   - **Diaphragm:** innervated by C3–5, and in supine position, provides more work than other muscles
   - **Inspiratory accessory:** external intercostals, scalene, and sternocleidomastoid muscles
   - **Expiratory accessory:** internal intercostals and abdominal muscles

PHYSIOLOGY AND PATHOPHYSIOLOGY

5. **What part of the brain generates spontaneous breathing?**
   The medulla, which integrates information from higher brain centers and reflexes from arterial, central chemoreceptors, lung, airways, and other components of the respiratory system.

6. **What size particles can reach the small airways?**
   Particles 2–5 μm in size. Particles > 10 μm are stopped in the upper airways. Particles 5–10 μm in size impact on the carina or main bronchi.

7. **What is the difference between lung volumes and capacities and how are they measured?**
   - **Lung volumes:** amount of air at specific points in the respiratory cycle
   - **Lung capacities:** the summation of volumes (Fig. 6-1)

   In general, lung volumes and capacities are measured by either helium equilibration or body plethysmography. Both methodologies allow the calculation of functional residual capacity (FRC). The rest of the volumes and capacities are then calculated using spirometric values. Helium equilibration may underestimate the FRC in patients with severe airflow limitation (trapped gas may not communicate with the airways).

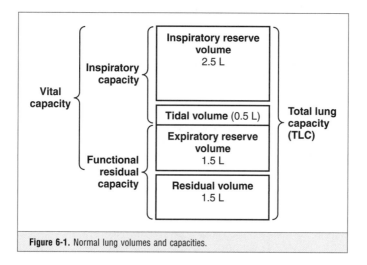

Figure 6-1. Normal lung volumes and capacities.

8. **What is the main determinant of airway resistance?**
   The radius of the medium-sized bronchi. The airway smooth muscle is mainly controlled by the autonomic nervous system including:
   - **Parasympathetic:** responsible for bronchoconstriction and mucus secretion
   - **Sympathetic (beta$_2$):** responsible for bronchodilatation and inhibition of glandular secretion

9. **What is lung compliance?**
   The change in lung volume generated by a change in pressure. Compliance is the inverse of elasticity. In a compliant lung, a small change in pressure will generate a large change in volume.

10. **Give examples of respiratory diseases associated with high and low compliance.**
    - **High compliance:** emphysema
    - **Low compliance:** interstitial lung diseases (ILDs), acute respiratory distress syndrome (ARDS), chest wall stiffness

11. **What is the difference between minute and alveolar ventilation?**
    - **Minute ventilation:** tidal volume × respiratory rate
    - **Alveolar ventilation:** (tidal volume − dead-space volume) × respiratory rate

    Dead space is the air that remains in the conducting airways and does not participate in gas exchange (1 mL/lb).

12. **How is the alveolar pressure of oxygen (PAO_2) calculated?**

$$PAO_2 = PIO_2 - PaCO_2/RQ$$

$$PIO_2 = FIO_2(P_{ATM} - PH_2O)$$

where FIO_2 = fraction of inspired oxygen; $PaCO_2$ = arterial partial pressure of carbon dioxide; P_{ATM} = atmospheric pressure; PH_2O = water vapor pressure; PIO_2 = partial pressure of inspired oxygen; RQ = respiratory quotient.

13. **What are the two extremes of the ventilation/perfusion ($\dot{V}/\dot{Q}$) relationship?**
Alveolar dead space (ventilation without perfusion) and right-to-left shunt (perfusion without ventilation). Ventilation and perfusion must match for optimal gas exchange.

14. **How is O_2 transported in the blood?**
Mainly through combination with hemoglobin, but a small amount of oxygen is dissolved in the blood. The dissolved portion contributes to the arterial partial pressure of oxygen (PaO_2).

15. **Why is the oxygen-hemoglobin dissociation curve important?**
The oxygen-hemoglobin curve is the relation between percent saturation hemoglobin (SO_2) and PaO_2 and explains how blood carries and releases O_2. An important measure is P50, defined as the PaO_2 at which the hemoglobin is 50% saturated. An increase in P50 indicates a shift to the right of the standard curve, or decreased affinity of the hemoglobin for oxygen (Fig. 6-2).

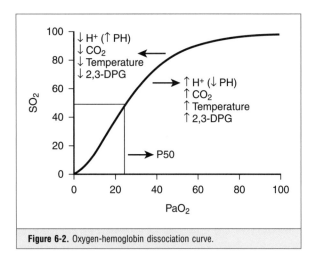

Figure 6-2. Oxygen-hemoglobin dissociation curve.

16. **What is the relationship between PaO_2 and aging?**
With aging, effective alveoli are decreased with a resultant decline in PaO_2. The expected PaO_2 can be calculated by the formula:

$$PaO_2 \text{ at sea level} = 100.1 - 0.32 \times \text{age (in yr)}$$

17. **Describe the mechanisms of arterial hypoxemia and give examples.**
 - **Low inspired O_2:** high altitude, air flight, and hypoxia inhalation test ($FIO_2 = 15\%$)
 - **Hypoventilation:** central nervous system (CNS) depressant drugs, cerebrovascular accident (CVA), and head injury

- **Diffusion impairment:** ILD, emphysema, pulmonary embolism (PE), pulmonary hypertension, and lung resection
- **V̇/Q̇ mismatch:** chronic obstructive pulmonary disease (COPD), atelectasis, ARDS, and pulmonary edema
- **Right-to-left-shunt:** Eisenmenger's syndrome and pulmonary arteriovenous malformation

18. **What is the value of measuring $PAO_2 - PaO_2$?**
The alveolar-arterial difference in partial pressure of O_2 is measured by the formula:

$$[FIO_2(P_{ATM}-PH_2O) - PaCO_2/RQ] - PaO_2$$

This equation allows the calculation of the shuntlike component in the lungs (due to shunting, diffusion, and V̇/Q̇ abnormalities). The normal value when breathing room air at sea level < 10–15. Generalized alveolar hypoventilation without V̇/Q̇ abnormalities will have normal $PAO_2 - PaO_2$.

19. **What is the best way of estimating the severity of hypoxemia in patients receiving supplemental O_2?**
By calculating the PaO_2/FIO_2 ratio. Ratios < 300 and 200 are considered moderate and severe hypoxemia, respectively.

SIGNS AND SYMPTOMS

20. **What physical examination maneuvers can help distinguish among pneumonia, atelectasis, pleural effusion, and pneumothorax?**
See Table 6-1.

TABLE 6-1. PHYSICAL EXAMINATION MANEUVERS AND FINDINGS OF COMMON PULMONARY DISORDERS

	Disorder			
Maneuver	Pneumonia	Atelectasis	Pleural Effusion	Pneumothorax
Inspection	↓ Chest wall movement	↓ Chest wall movement	↓ Chest wall movement	↓ Chest wall movement
Percussion	Dull	Dull	Dull	↑ Resonance
Fremitus	↑	↓	↓	↓
Auscultation	Crackles, bronchial breath sounds, whispered pectoriloquy, and egophony	↓ Breath sounds	↓ Breath sounds	↓ Breath sounds

21. **What are the most common causes of dyspnea?**
- **Respiratory:** COPD, asthma, and ILD
- **Cardiac:** congestive heart failure (CHF) and coronary artery disease (CAD)
- **Other:** metabolic acidosis, anemia, deconditioning, and anxiety

22. **What is the difference between orthopnea and platypnea?**
    - **Orthopnea:** Dyspnea increases on *recumbency* as found in CHF, COPD, and respiratory muscle weakness.
    - **Platypnea:** Dyspnea increases in the *upright* position as found in right-to-left shunts, $\dot{V}/\dot{Q}$ mismatch, hepatopulmonary syndrome, and PE.

23. **What is the definition of chronic cough?**
    A cough that has been present > 8 weeks.

24. **What are the most common causes of chronic cough?**
    - Gastroesophageal reflux disease (GERD)
    - Rhinitis or sinusitis
    - Asthma
    - Chronic bronchitis primarily related to cigarette smoking
    - Angiotensin-converting enzyme (ACE) inhibitor use
    - Bronchiectasis
    - Bronchogenic carcinoma
    - Interstitial lung disease
    - Upper airway cough syndrome (UACS; previously named "postnasal drip syndrome")
    - Nonasthmatic eosinophilic bronchitis (NAEB)
    - Hair or cerumen tickling the tympanic membrane ("ear-cough")
    - Aspirated foreign bodies
    - Chronic aspiration
    - Psychogenic cough

25. **How is a chronic cough evaluated?**
    Initial evaluation including history, physical examination, and chest x-ray may reveal a likely etiology such as ACE inhibitor use or smoking. Discontinuing the offending agent can improve the cough. Other etiologies identified initially include asthma, UACS, and GERD. These disorders can be empirically treated and cough symptoms reevaluated. Asthma can be further evaluated with spirometry, demonstrating bronchodilator reversibility. NAEB can be confirmed by the finding of sputum eosinophilia. If none of these more common etiologies are found, additional testing may include 24-hour esophageal pH monitoring (GERD), swallow evaluation (aspiration), sinus x-rays (sinusitis), high-resolution computed tomography scan (HRCT; lung lesions), bronchoscopy (endobronchial lesions and aspirated foreign bodies), and evaluation for environmental exposures.

    Irwin RS, Baumann MH, Bolser DC, et al: Diagnosis and management of cough. Executive Summary: ACCP Evidence-Based Clinical Practice Guidelines, *Chest* 129:1S–23S, 2006.

26. **What are the most common causes of wheezing?**
    Asthma, COPD, CHF, and UACS. The wheezing of UACS originates from the extrathoracic airway (most likely vocal cords). Wheezing lacks sensitivity and specificity for the diagnosis of asthma. Asthma can present without wheeze, and wheezing can be seen in other conditions that mimic asthma.

27. **What is massive hemoptysis and pseudohemoptysis?**
    Massive hemoptysis is the expectoration of $\geq$ 600 mL of blood within 24–48 hours. The most common causes of massive hemoptysis are bronchiectasis (as in cystic fibrosis [CF]), bronchogenic carcinoma, arteriovenous malformations, aortobronchial fistulas, PE with infarction, aspergilloma, invasive aspergillosis, cavitary lung disease (as in tuberculosis), necrotizing pneumonia, and diffuse alveolar hemorrhage. **Pseudohemoptysis** is the expectoration of blood coming from a source other than the respiratory tract, including the posterior pharynx or gastrointestinal (GI) tract.

28. **How is massive hemoptysis managed?**
Initially, the uninvolved lung must be protected from aspiration of blood because blood can flood the airway and cause asphyxia and death. Maneuvers that keep the bleeding lung dependent can help. In some cases, selective bronchial intubation with use of endobronchial balloons to occlude the bleeding bronchus is needed. Tamponade of tracheoarterial fistulas in patients with tracheostomies can sometimes be achieved by overinflation of the cuff of an endotracheal tube and applying forward pressure to the tube to compress the innominate artery. Definitive management of massive hemoptysis includes angiographic bronchial artery embolization or surgical resection.

THORACIC IMAGING

29. **What are the common diseases of the tracheobronchial tree?**
    - **Tracheal stenosis:** narrowing of the trachea
    - **Tracheobronchomalacia:** weakness of airway walls with excessive expiratory collapse
    - **Tracheobronchopathia osteochondroplastica:** calcified nodules on anterolateral walls of the trachea
    - **Amyloidosis:** concentric or nodular thickening of the trachea
    - **Relapsing polychondritis:** thickening of the anterolateral tracheal wall (occurs in approximately half of these patients)
    - **Wegener's granulomatosis:** usually lung nodules with or without cavitation, but rarely circumferential tracheal thickening
    - **Tracheobronchomegaly:** diffuse dilatation (>3 cm) of the trachea and main bronchi

30. **What are the radiographic findings in the posteroanterior chest x-ray of different lobar atelectasis?**
See Figure 6-3.

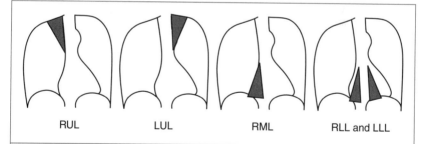

RUL   LUL   RML   RLL and LLL

Figure 6-3. Diagram showing atelectases of different lung lobes. **Right upper lobe (RUL) atelectasis** results in the elevation of the right hilum and minor fissure. **Left upper lobe (LUL) atelectasis** obliterates the left heart border. The **right middle lobe (RML) collapse** obscures the right heart border. **Right lower lobe (RLL) collapse** exposes the major fissure and the RLL pulmonary artery is obscured. **Left lower lobe (LLL) collapse** shifts the hilum downward with opacification behind the heart (sail sign) and obscuration of the left hemidiaphragm.

31. **What diseases can be found in the different regions of the mediastinum?**
See Table 6-2.

TABLE 6-2. LOCATIONS AND TYPES OF MEDIASTINAL MASSES

Mediastinal Location*		
Anterior	**Middle**	**Posterior**
Thymomas	Lymphomas	Neurogenic neoplasms
Lymphomas	Metastases	Esophageal lesions
Germ cell tumors	Sarcoidosis	Extramedullary hematopoiesis
Thyroid goiter or tumors	Mediastinal cysts	Descending aortic aneurysm
Morgagni hernia	Vascular lesions	Bochdalek hernia
Germ cell tumors		
Thyroid goiter or tumors		
Morgagni hernia		

*__Anterior mediastinum:__ from the sternum to the anterior aspect of the heart and great vessels; __middle mediastinum:__ between anterior and posterior compartments; __posterior mediastinum:__ from the posterior heart border and trachea to the posterior aspect of the vertebral bodies.

32. **What are the most common lesions found on chest x-ray in the right cardiophrenic angle?**
Prominent fat, lipoma, pericardial cyst, and Morgagni hernia. Most lesions in this area are benign.

33. **How is a solitary pulmonary nodule (SPN) defined and what are the characteristics of a benign lesion?**
A well-circumscribed single lung lesion that measures < 3 cm in diameter. Most common etiologies of SPN include granulomata, intrapulmonary lymph nodes, benign and malignant tumors, and vascular malformations. Characteristics of benign nodules include stability over time, presence of fat, and calcifications characterized as central, laminated, or popcorn-like.

34. **What are the most common HRCT patterns and the associated diseases?**
See Table 6-3.

35. **What are tree-in-bud opacities and in what conditions may they be seen?**
Dilated terminal bronchioles with impacted mucus that are often seen in atypical mycobacterial infections and aspiration but may also be seen in bacterial or viral infections, collagen vascular disease, fungal infections, collagen diseases, CF, or toxic inhalations. This abnormality is best seen on HRCT and is typical of bronchiectasis.

36. **What is PET scanning and how is it useful for assessment of pulmonary nodules?**
Positron-emission tomography (PET) scanning uses a D-glucose analogue labeled with ^{18}F to image the tissues. Metabolically active lesions will have increased uptake of this molecule. The degree of uptake is measured using a standardized uptake ratio (SUV). Typically, lung cancers will have an SUV > 2.5, and lesions with increased metabolism are highly likely to be malignant. False-positive results are found in infectious and inflammatory lesions, including sarcoidosis and atypical mycobacterial infections. False-negative results may be observed in bronchioloalveolar carcinoma, well-differentiated malignancies, or carcinoid.

TABLE 6-3. PATTERNS OF PULMONARY DISEASE ON HIGH-RESOLUTION COMPUTED TOMOGRAPHY SCAN

Pattern	Disorders	Anatomy
Linear	Pulmonary edema, lymphangitic spread	Due to thickening of interlobular septa (Kerley's lines)
Reticular	Pulmonary fibrosis, idiopathic pulmonary fibrosis, asbestosis, and collagen vascular disease	May appear as honeycombing
Nodular		Multiple nodules < 1 cm
Perilymphatic	Sarcoidosis, pneumoconiosis, lymphangitic carcinomatosis	Peribronchovascular interstitium and interlobular septa
Centrilobar	Hypersensitivity pneumonitis, infections	Center of pulmonary lobule
Randomly located	Metastatic disease, chronic histoplasmosis	
Ground-glass opacities	Pulmonary edema, *Pneumocystis jiroveci* pneumonia, hemorrhage, alveolar proteinosis	Hazy opacity that does not obscure pulmonary vessels
Cystic	Lymphangioleiomyomatosis, Langerhans' cell histiocytosis	Thin walled cysts < 1 cm in diameter

CHRONIC OBSTRUCTIVE PULMONARY DISEASE

37. **Define "COPD."**
A preventable and treatable disease state characterized by chronic airflow limitation that is not fully reversible and is usually progressive. The airflow limitation is usually associated with an inflammatory response of the lung to exposure to noxious substances or gases. COPD traditionally comprises chronic bronchitis and emphysema. **Chronic bronchitis** is characterized by productive cough for at least 3 consecutive months in 2 consecutive years. **Emphysema** is an abnormal enlargement of the air spaces distal to the terminal bronchioles with destruction of their walls.

   Rabe KF, Hurd S, Anzueto A, et al: Global strategy for the diagnosis, management, and prevention of chronic obstructive pulmonary disease: GOLD Executive Summary, *Am J Respir Crit Care Med* 176:532–555, 2007.

38. **What is the main risk factor for COPD?**
Cigarette smoking. Longstanding asthma may eventually result in COPD. Other risk factors include alpha$_1$-antitrypsin deficiency (AATD) and exposure to particulate matter.

39. **What is the prevalence of COPD?**
In the United States, >16 million people have COPD that frequently leads to hospitalization, increased mortality, and rising health costs. The prevalence and burden of COPD are projected to increase.

40. What are the comorbidities frequently encountered in COPD patients?
Weight loss, nutritional abnormalities, and skeletal muscle dysfunction. COPD patients also have an increased risk of CAD, osteoporosis, respiratory infection, lung cancer, diabetes, depression, sleep disorders, glaucoma, and anemia.

41. What are the Global Initiative for Chronic Obstructive Lung Disease (GOLD) guidelines stages for classifying COPD severity of based on postbronchodilator FEV$_1$ (forced expiratory volume in 1 second)?
- **Stage I** (mild): FEV$_1$/FVC (forced vital capacity) < 0.7 and FEV$_1$ ≥ 80% of predicted
- **Stage II** (moderate): FEV$_1$/FVC < 0.7 and FEV$_1$ 50–80% of predicted
- **Stage III** (severe): FEV$_1$/FVC < 0.7 and FEV$_1$ 30–50% of predicted
- **Stage IV** (very severe): FEV$_1$/FVC < 0.7 and FEV$_1$ < 30% of predicted, or FEV$_1$ < 50% of predicted with chronic respiratory failure (defined as PaO$_2$ < 60 mmHg with or without PaCO$_2$ > 50 mmHg while breathing room air at sea level).

The use of a fixed FEV$_1$/FVC ratio may result in inappropriate diagnosis of stage I COPD in the elderly.

Rabe KF, Hurd S, Anzueto A, et al: Global strategy for the diagnosis, management, and prevention of chronic obstructive pulmonary disease: GOLD Executive Summary, *Am J Respir Crit Care Med* 176:532–555, 2007.

42. What characteristics help differentiate between asthma and COPD?
See Table 6-4. However, patients with COPD can have features of asthma and vice versa. Patients with asthma may develop fixed airflow limitation. Subjects with COPD can have a mixed inflammatory pattern with increased eosinophils.

TABLE 6-4.	CHARACTERISTICS USEFUL TO DISTINGUISH BETWEEN ASTHMA AND CHRONIC OBSTRUCTIVE PULMONARY DISEASE	
Characteristic	**Asthma**	**COPD**
Airflow limitation	Largely reversible	Largely irreversible
Airway inflammation	CD4+ T lymphocytes and eosinophils	CD8+ T lymphocytes, macrophages and neutrophils
Onset	Early in life	Midlife
Symptoms	Vary from day to day and are worse at night or early morning	Slowly progressive
Risk factors	Family history of asthma	History of tobacco abuse

COPD = chronic obstructive pulmonary disease.

43. What are the risk factors for the development of COPD?
- Tobacco smoke
- Occupational dusts
- Indoor air pollution (biomass cooking and heating)
- Outdoor air pollution
- Genetic inheritance (AATD)

- Impaired lung growth and development (reduced maximal attained lung function)
- Age and gender (women may be more susceptible)
- Oxidative stress
- Low socioeconomic status
- Recurrent infections

44. **What features are associated with a poorer prognosis in COPD?**
- Decreased FEV_1
- Cigarette smoking
- Low body mass index (BMI ≤ 21)
- Human immunodeficiency virus (HIV) infection
- Decreased exercise tolerance and peak O_2 consumption
- High airway bacterial load and C-reactive protein (CRP)
- Advanced age
- Need for supplemental O_2
- Elevated BODE index

45. **What is the BODE index?**
An index used to calculate the 4-year survival of patients with COPD based on:
- **B**MI
- Airway **o**bstruction (FEV_1)
- Degree of **d**yspnea (based on Medical Research Council dyspnea score)
- **E**xercise capacity (6-min walk distance)

The 4-year survival decreases as the number of points increases (e.g., the 4-yr survival is only 18% when the score is 7–10 points).

Celli BR, Cote CG, Marin JM, et al: The body-mass index, airflow obstruction, dyspnea and exercise capacity index in chronic obstructive pulmonary disease, *N Engl J Med* 350:1005–1012, 2004.

46. **What are the steps for managing COPD according to the GOLD guidelines?**
- Assess and monitor disease:
  - Consider COPD in any patient with dyspnea, chronic cough, or sputum production or a history of exposure to risk factors for COPD.
  - Confirm the diagnosis with spirometry.
  - Consider arterial blood gas (ABG) analysis in patients with $FEV_1 < 50\%$ of predicted or clinical signs suggestive of respiratory or right heart failure.
  - Consider hereditary emphysema (AATD) in Caucasian patients who develop COPD at age < 50 years or have a strong family history for COPD.
  - Actively identify comorbidities.
- Reduce risk factor: Counsel about smoking cessation.
- Manage stable COPD: Use pharmacotherapy to decrease symptoms and complications.
- Manage exacerbations: Prescribe inhaled bronchodilators, oral steroids, and antibiotics for infections. If hospitalized, consider using noninvasive mechanical ventilation (MV), which reduces need for endotracheal intubations, length of hospital stay, and mortality.

47. **What is the basic treatment for COPD?**
Bronchodilators such as beta$_2$ agonists or anticholinergics or both in short-acting and long-acting forms with addition of:
- Inhaled steroids in patients with symptomatic COPD, repeated exacerbations, and $FEV_1 < 50\%$ of predicted
- Long-term administration of O_2 (>15 hr/day) in patients with chronic hypoxemic respiratory failure, characterized by a $PaO_2 < 55$
- Seasonal influenza vaccine annually

- Pneumococcal vaccine
- Pulmonary rehabilitation
- Consideration of alpha$_1$ augmentation therapy in AATD patients
- Consideration of lung volume reduction surgery (LVRS) in patients with upper lobe emphysema and low exercise capacity
- Consideration of lung transplantation for patients who fail other therapies

48. **What bacterial pathogens are most commonly involved in COPD exacerbations?**
    - *Streptococcus pneumoniae*
    - *Haemophilus influenzae*
    - *Moraxella catarrhalis*

    If the patient does not respond within 3–7 days of appropriate empirical antibiotic therapy for these organisms, consider sputum culture.

49. **What are the antibiotic treatments for COPD exacerbation?**
    - **Mild exacerbation:** oral beta-lactams (ampicillin, amoxicillin), tetracycline, or trimethoprim/sulfamethoxazole (TMP-SMX)
    - **Moderate exacerbation:** oral or intravenous (IV) beta-lactam/beta-lactamase inhibitor, IV second- and third-generation cephalosporins
    - **Severe exacerbations:** oral or IV fluoroquinolones or IV beta-lactam with *Pseudomonas aeruginosa* activity

50. **What are the indications for hospital admission in COPD exacerbation?**
    - Marked increase in symptoms
    - Severe underlying COPD
    - Failure of initial management as outpatient or in emergency department (ED)
    - Significant comorbidities
    - Older age
    - Insufficient home support

51. **What signs and symptoms of COPD suggest that intensive care unit (ICU) admission is indicated?**
    - Severe dyspnea poorly responsive to initial therapy
    - Change in mental status
    - Worsening hypoxemia (<40 mmHg), severe hypercapnia (>60 mmHg), or severe acidosis (pH < 7.25), or combination of all three
    - Need for MV
    - Need for vasopressors

52. **When is a hospitalized patient with COPD exacerbation ready for discharge?**
    When inhaled beta$_2$ agonists are used less than every 4 hours, and the patients is able to walk across the room, eat, and sleep without significant dyspnea. In addition, the patient should have stable blood gases or oxygen saturation for 24 hours and be able to maintain ventilation without the assistance of bilevel positive airway pressure (BPAP). The patient or caregiver or both also need to understand and accept the plan of care and follow-up arrangements.

ASTHMA

53. **Define "asthma."**
    As a complex disorder characterized by variable and recurring symptoms, airflow obstruction, bronchial hyperresponsiveness, and underlying inflammation. This disease appears to be due to a combination of genetic and environmental factors (e.g., airborne allergens, viral

infections, tobacco smoke, air pollution, and diet) as well as a dominant T helper 2 (Th2)–type cytokine response of the innate immunity.

Expert Panel Report 3 (EPR-3): Guidelines for the Diagnosis and Management of Asthma—Summary Report 2007, *J Allergy Clin Immunol* 120:S94–S138, 2007.

54. **How is the diagnosis of asthma established?**
By the identification of recurrent symptoms of airflow obstruction or airway hyperresponsiveness, the demonstration that the airflow obstruction is at least partially reversible on spirometry after administration of bronchodilator, and the exclusion of other diagnoses. Reversibility on pulmonary function testing is defined as 12% or 200 mL improvement in FEV_1 after bronchodilator. Asthma symptoms include cough that is typically worse at night, wheezing, dyspnea, and chest tightness. In general, the symptoms occur or worsen during exercise, viral infection, inhalation of allergens or irritants, change in weather, stress, and menstrual cycles. The finding of a negative bronchoprovocation challenge with methacholine practically excludes asthma.

55. **What other conditions can be confused with asthma?**
   - Vocal cord dysfunction (VCD)
   - Allergic rhinitis and sinusitis
   - COPD
   - CHF
   - PE
   - Mechanical airway obstruction
   - Cough secondary to ACE inhibitors use

KEY POINTS: VOCAL CORD DYSFUNCTION ✓

1. Symptoms are similar to asthma, including wheezing and stridor that may or may not be in response to irritants.

2. Can occur in patients who also have asthma and exercise-induced asthma.

3. Diagnosis is made by flow volume loops that show inspiratory cut-off.

4. Treatment includes speech therapy and behavior modification, NOT corticosteroids.

56. **What steps are followed for asthma management?**
   - Assess and monitor disease through the evaluation of:
     - Severity and control of asthma.
     - Response to treatment.
   - Educate patient to:
     - Develop asthma action plan.
     - Understand the difference between long-term control and quick-relief medications.
     - Use medications correctly.
     - Avoid environmental exposures.
     - Self-monitor disease.
     - Control environmental factors and comorbid conditions
   - Use medications based on asthma severity with frequent adjustment based on control.

Expert Panel Report 3 (EPR-3): Guidelines for the diagnosis and management of asthma—Summary Report 2007, *J Allergy Clin Immunol* 120:S94–S138, 2007.

57. How is asthma classified according to sign and symptom severity?
See Table 6-5.

TABLE 6-5. ASTHMA CLASSIFICATION BASED ON SIGN AND SYMPTOM SEVERITY

Signs and Symptoms	Intermittent	Persistent*		
		Mild	Moderate	Severe
Symptoms	$\leq$2 days/wk	>2 days/wk	Daily	Throughout the day
Nighttime awakenings	$\leq$2 nights/mo	3-4 nights/mo	>1 night/wk	Almost every night
SABA use	$\leq$2 days/wk	>2 days/wk	Daily	Several times a day
Interference with normal activity	None	Minor limitation	Some limitation	Severely limited
Lung function	Normal FEV_1 between exacerbations	FEV_1 80%	FEV_1 60–80% FEV_1/FVC reduced < 5%	FEV_1 < 60% FEV_1/FVC reduced > 5%
Need for systemic steroids	0–1/yr	$\geq$2/yr	$\geq$2/yr	$\geq$2/yr

FEV_1 = forced expiratory volume in 1 second; FVC = forced vital capacity; SABA = short-acting beta$_2$ agonist.
*The level of severity is determined by assessing impairment (previous 2–4 wk) and risk. Assign severity to the most severe category in which any feature occurs.
Adapted from Expert Panel Report 3 (EPR-3): Guidelines for the Diagnosis and Management of Asthma-Summary Report 2007. J Allergy Clin Immunol 120:S94–S138, 2007.

58. What comorbid conditions can complicate asthma management?
- GERD (even in the absence of suggestive GERD symptoms)
- Rhinitis or sinusitis (interrelationship between upper and lower airway)
- Obesity (weight loss may improve asthma control)
- Stress and depression
- Obstructive sleep apnea (OSA)
- Allergic bronchopulmonary aspergillosis (ABPA)

KEY POINTS: DIAGNOSTIC FEATURES FOR ALLERGIC BRONCHOPULMONARY ASPERGILLOSIS ✓

1. Eosinophilia.

2. Elevated serum immunoglobulin E (IgE) levels against *Aspergillus fumigates.*

3. Positive skin test for aspergillus.

59. **What medications are used for long-term control and quick relief of asthma?**
See Table 6-6.

TABLE 6-6. ASTHMA MEDICATIONS USED FOR LONG-TERM CONTROL AND IMMEDIATE SYMPTOM RELIEF	
Long-term Control	**Immediate Symptom Relief**
■ Inhaled corticosteroids (most effective) ■ LABAs (not to be used as monotherapy) ■ Leukotriene modifiers (adjunctive therapy) ■ Omalizumab (anti-IgE) (in patients with elevated IgE, documented allergy, and persistent asthma despite inhaled corticosteroids and LABA) ■ Methylxanthines (theophylline)	■ SABAs ■ Ipratropium bromide ■ Systemic corticosteroids (short course)
IgE = immunoglobulin E; LABAs = long-acting beta$_2$ agonist; SABAs = short-acting beta$_2$ agonists.	

60. **Describe the stepwise approach for asthma management in adults.**
See Table 6-7.

TABLE 6-7. STEPWISE APPROACH FOR ASTHMA MANAGEMENT IN ADULTS*	
Step	**Preferred Medication**
1	SABA as needed for intermittent asthma
2	Low-dose ICS[†]
3	Low-dose ICS + LABA or medium-dose ICS[†]
4	Medium-dose ICS + LABA[†]
5	High-dose ICS + LABA[‡]
6	High-dose ICS + LABA + oral corticosteroid[‡]

ICS = inhaled corticosteroid; LABA = long-acting beta$_2$ agonist; SABA = short-acting beta$_2$ agonist.
*Step up if poor control and step down if good control for ≥ 3 mo.
[†]Consider subcutaneous allergen immunotherapy in patients with allergic asthma.
[‡]Consider omalizumab for patients with allergies.
Adapted from Expert Panel Report 3 (EPR-3): Guidelines for the Diagnosis and Management of Asthma-Summary Report 2007. J Allergy Clin Immunol 120:S94–S138, 2007.

61. **What symptoms and objective clinical findings help determine whether a patient with an acute asthma exacerbation can receive treatment as an outpatient or in the hospital?**
The decision to admit a patient to the hospital incorporates the evaluation of signs and symptoms, pulse oximetry (SpO$_2$), and lung function measurements.
■ **Mild exacerbations:** dyspnea with activity and peak expiratory flow (PEF) ≥ 70% of personal best can be treated at home

- **Moderate exacerbations:** dyspnea with usual activity and PEF 40–69% of personal best require office or ED visit
- **Severe exacerbations:** dyspnea at rest and PEF < 40% of personal best require ED visit and likely hospitalization
- **Life-threatening exacerbation:** inability to speak, perspiration, and PEF < 25% of personal best require hospitalization, possibly ICU

In general, patients who have a good response after treatment in the ED as demonstrated by a sustained response after 60 minutes, no respiratory distress, normal physical examination, and PEF $\geq$ 70% can be discharged home. Those with poor response to ED treatment who exhibit severe symptoms, confusion, $PaCO_2 \geq 42$ mmHg or PEF < 40% generally need ICU admission.

62. **Which patients are at high risk of asthma-related death?**
Those with:
- Previous severe exacerbations
- Two or more hospitalizations or more than three ED visits in the past year
- More than two short-acting beta$_2$ agonist (SABA) canister uses per month
- Difficulty perceiving the severity of exacerbations
- Low socioeconomic status
- Illicit drug use
- Major psychosocial problems or psychiatric disease
- Presence of comorbidities

63. **What is exercise-induced asthma?**
Asthma symptoms (cough, dyspnea, chest tightness, or wheezing) that occur during exercise or immediately after exercise. A 15% decrease in FEV_1 after exercise (defined as 5-min intervals of exercise for 20–30 min) will establish the diagnosis.

64. **How is exercise-induced asthma managed?**
Usually with pretreatment with inhaled beta$_2$ agonists before exercise. (SABA may last for 2–3 hr whereas long-acting beta$_2$ agonists [LABAs] may protect for up to 12 hr.) If the symptoms are frequent or severe, initiate or step up long-term control medications. A warm-up period before exercise and the use of a mask or scarf over the mouth for patients with cold- and exercise-induced asthma may attenuate this condition. Leukotriene modifiers may also block exercise induced bronchospasm but are less effective than beta agonists.

65. **How is asthma managed during pregnancy?**
Usually with SABA (albuterol) and inhaled corticosteroids (budesonide) because more safety data during pregnancy are available for these medications. Asthma control during pregnancy is important for the well-being of the mother and the baby. Uncontrolled asthma increases perinatal mortality, preterm birth, low-birth-weight infants, and preeclampsia. Classically, asthma during pregnancy improves in one third of the patients and worsens in another third.

COMMUNITY-ACQUIRED PNEUMONIA

See also Chapter 12, Infectious Diseases.

66. **How is the diagnosis of community-acquired pneumonia (CAP) made?**
By the presence of suggestive clinical features and a demonstrable infiltrate by an imaging technique, with or without supporting microbiologic data. Patients should be evaluated for an etiologic diagnosis with pretreatment blood cultures, urinary antigens for *Legionella pneumophilia* and *S. pneumoniae*, and expectorated sputum culture when there is suspicion that these results may alter the empirical management or if there are concerns for unusual pathogens or antibiotic resistance.

67. **List the risk factors for CAP associated with specific pathogens.**
See Table 6-8.

TABLE 6-8.	RISK FACTORS FOR PNEUMONIA ASSOCIATED WITH SPECIFIC PATHOGENS
Risk Factor	**Pathogen(s)**
Alcoholism	*Streptococcus pneumoniae*, oral anaerobes, *Klebsiella pneumonia*
Aspiration	Gram-negative enteric pathogens, oral anaerobes
Exposure to bat/bird droppings	*Histoplasma capsulatum*
Exposure to birds	*Chlamydophila psittaci*
Exposure to rabbits	*Francisella tularensis*
Hotel/cruise ship stay	*Legionella* spp.
Travel to southwestern United States	*Coccidioides* spp., *Hantavirus*
Injection drug use	*Staphylococcus aureus*, anaerobes, *Mycobacterium tuberculosis*
Bioterrorism	*Bacillus anthracis*, *Yersinia pestis*, *Francisella tularensis*

From Mandell LA, Wunderink RG, Anzueto A, et al: Infectious Diseases Society of America/American Thoracic Society consensus guidelines on the management of community-acquired pneumonia in adults. Clin Infect Dis 44:S27–S72, 2007.

68. **What is a CURB-65 score?**
A prognostic index that helps to identify which patients require hospital admission for CAP. The score uses five variables and assigns one point for the presence of each variable. The variables are:
- **C**onfusion: defined as disorientation to person, place, and time
- **U**rea (blood urea nitrogen [BUN]): >20 mg/dL
- **R**espiratory rate: >30 breaths/min
- **B**lood pressure: systolic < 90 mmHg or diastolic < 60 mmHg
- Age >**65** years

   Patients with a score of 2 generally require hospital admission and patients with scores 3 and above should be considered for ICU admission. Other prognostic models include the Pneumonia Severity Index (PSI) that includes 20 different variables, which limits its practicality. All models should be supplemented by consideration of other factors such as the ability to take oral medications and have adequate outpatient support.

   Fine MJ, Auble TE, Yealy DM, et al: A prediction rule to identify low-risk patients with community-acquired pneumonia, *N Engl J Med* 336:243–250, 1997.

   Lim WS, van der Ferden MM, Laing R, et al: Defining community acquired pneumonia severity on presentation to hospital: an international derivation and validation study, *Thorax* 58:377–382, 2003.

69. **When do patients with CAP require ICU admission?**
When they need MV or vasopressors. ICU care is usually also required if patients meet at least three of the following criteria:

- Respiratory rate $\geq$ 30 breaths/min
- $PaO_2/FIO_2 \leq 250$
- Multilobar infiltrates
- Confusion
- BUN $\geq$ 20 mg/dL
- White blood cell (WBC) count 4000 cells/mm^3
- Platelets < 100,000 cells/mm^3
- Hypothermia (<36°C)
- Hypotension requiring aggressive fluid resuscitation

Mandell LA, Wunderink RG, Anzueto A, et al: Infectious Diseases Society of America/American Thoracic Society consensus guidelines on the management of community-acquired pneumonia in adults, *Clin Infect Dis* 44:S27–S72, 2007.

70. **What are the recommended empirical antibiotics for CAP?**
See Table 6-9.

TABLE 6-9. RECOMMENDED EMPIRICAL ANTIBIOTIC TREATMENT FOR PNEUMONIA

Outpatient	Inpatient (NON-ICU)	Inpatient (ICU)
Healthy and no antibiotics in previous 3 mo: ■ Macrolide ■ Doxycycline Comorbidities*: ■ Respiratory fluoroquinolone[†] ■ Beta-lactam + macrolide	■ Respiratory fluoroquinolone ■ Beta-lactam + macrolide	■ Beta-lactam[‡] + macrolide or respiratory fluoroquinolone ■ Respiratory fluoroquinolone + aztreonam

ICU = intensive care unit; MRSA = methicillin-resistant *Staphylococcus aureus*.
- If pseudomonas is a consideration, use (piperacillin-tazobactam, cefepime, imipenem, or meropenem) + ciprofloxacin or levofloxacin (750 mg) or aminoglycoside.
- If community-acquired MRSA is a consideration, add vancomycin or linezolid.
- For patients requiring admission, the first dose of antibiotic should be given within 4 hr of admission to the emergency department.
*Comorbidities include: heart, lung, liver, or renal disease, diabetes, alcoholism, malignancy, asplenia, immunosuppressing conditions, or use of immunosuppresing drugs.
[†]Respiratory fluoroquinolones include moxifloxacin, gemifloxacin, or levofloxacin.
[‡]Cefotaxime, ceftriaxone, or ampicillin-sulbactam.
Adapted from Mandell LA, Wunderink RG, Anzueto A, et al: Infectious Diseases Society of America/ American Thoracic Society consensus guidelines on the management of community-acquired pneumonia in adults. Clin Infect Dis 44:S27–S72, 2007.

71. **When can antibiotics be switched from IV to oral?**
When the following criteria are met:
- Temperature $\leq$ 37.8°C oral
- Heart rate $\leq$ 100 beats per minute (bpm)
- Respiratory rate $\leq$ 24 breaths/min

- Systolic blood pressure $\geq$ 90 mmHg
- SO_2 $\geq$90% on room air
- Able to maintain oral intake
- Mental status normal or approaching prehospital state

Mandell LA, Wunderink RG, Anzueto A, et al: Infectious Diseases Society of America/American Thoracic Society consensus guidelines on the management of community-acquired pneumonia in adults, *Clin Infect Dis* 44:S27–S72, 2007.

INTERSTITIAL LUNG DISEASES

72. **How are ILDs classified?**
- **Identified cause:** drugs and collagen vascular diseases
- **Granulomatous:** sarcoidosis
- **Other forms:** lymphangioleiomyomatosis (LAM) and Langerhans' cell histiocytosis (LCH)
- **Idiopathic**
  - Idiopathic pulmonary fibrosis (IPF)
  - Others
    - Desquamative interstitial pneumonia
    - Acute interstitial pneumonia
    - Nonspecific interstitial pneumonia (NSIP)
    - Respiratory bronchiolitis-associated ILD
    - Cryptogenic organizing pneumonia (COP)
    - Lymphocytic interstitial pneumonia (LIP)

American Thoracic Society, European Respiratory Society: American Thoracic Society/European Respiratory Society International Multidisciplinary Consensus Classification of the Idiopathic Interstitial Pneumonias, *Am J Respir Crit Care Med* 165:277–304, 2002.

Bradley B, Branley HM, Egan JJ, et al: Interstitial lung disease guideline: The British Thoracic Society in collaboration with the Thoracic Society of Australia and New Zealand and the Irish Thoracic Society, *Thorax* 63:v1–v58, 2008.

73. **What is the initial evaluation of ILD?**
History and physical examination, chest radiography, and lung function testing, looking for specific etiologies such as collagen vascular disease, environmental exposures, or drugs. If an etiology is not found from the initial evaluation, HRCT is helpful, followed by transbronchial or surgical lung biopsy, if needed.

74. **What is IPF?**
A distinct type of chronic fibrosing interstitial pneumonia of unknown etiology, limited to the lung. An interstitial pneumonia pattern is usually present on biopsy. On occasion, the diagnosis of ILD can be made without lung biopsy if the clinical setting and radiographic findings are consistent with IPF. In general, patients with IPF have no other known cause of ILD and are > 50 years old with insidious onset of unexplained dyspnea or cough or both that evolves over > 3 months. Examination finds bibasilar inspiratory crackles. HRCT shows predominantly bibasilar reticular abnormalities with minimal ground-glass opacities, associated with honeycombing, traction bronchiectasis, and volume loss. On pulmonary function tests, the total lung capacity (TLC) is reduced with decreased diffusing capacity for carbon monoxide (DLCO).

75. **What is the prognosis of IPF?**
Generally poor with a median length of survival from the time of diagnosis of 2.5–3.5 years. A decline in oxygen saturation during 6-minute walk test and a DLCO < 40% indicate advanced disease. During the course of the disease, patients can have episodes of rapid decline that may represent accelerated disease. A drop in the FVC $\geq$ 10% or in DLCO $\geq$ 15% in the first 6–12 months indicates a poorer prognosis.

76. **What is the treatment of IPF?**
No pharmacologic treatment improves survival or modifies the clinical course of disease. The current management includes oxygen supplementation, antireflux therapy, pulmonary rehabilitation, participation in clinical trials evaluating new therapies, and lung transplantation. Some specialists consider oral steroids, azathioprine and *N*-acetylcysteine for patients with mild-to-moderate disease who do not qualify for a clinical trial.

77. **What ILD(s) are associated with tobacco smoking?**
- IPF
- Desquamative interstitial pneumonitis
- Respiratory bronchiolitis-associated ILD
- LCH
Smokers are less likely to have hypersensitivity pneumonitis (HP) or sarcoidosis.

78. **What is HP?**
A lung disorder caused by repeated exposure to a sensitizing agent (organic and inorganic particles) and classified as acute, subacute, and chronic. The acute form is characterized by respiratory symptoms that occur in a few hours after a heavy exposure. The other forms occur with ongoing lower-level exposure. Patients with the chronic type have diffuse pulmonary fibrosis that may resemble IPF or NSIP. The features of acute and subacute HP on chest computed tomography (CT) scan include diffuse pulmonary nodules, ground-glass opacities, and mosaic attenuation. Treatment includes avoidance of the causative antigen and corticosteroids in severe or progressive disease.

79. **Which connective tissue diseases (CTDs) are most commonly associated with ILD?**
- Rheumatoid arthritis (RA)
- Systemic sclerosis (SSc)
- Polymyositis/dermatomyositis

SARCOIDOSIS

80. **What is sarcoidosis?**
A granulomatous disease with systemic involvement whose cause is unknown. Affected groups include young and middle-aged adults, women, and African Americans. Sarcoidosis is postulated to occur in genetically susceptible individuals exposed to certain unknown environmental agents.

Dempsey OJ, Paterson EW, Kerr KM, et al: Sarcoidosis, *BMJ* 339:b3206, 2009.

81. **Which organs are affected by sarcoidosis?**
In general, the disease can affect any organ, although the most commonly involved organs are:
- **Lungs** (>90%): hilar adenopathy, ILD, and nodules
- **Skin** (24%): erythema nodosum, maculopapular lesions, and lupus pernio
- **Liver** (18%): elevated liver enzymes, hepatosplenomegaly, intrahepatic cholestasis
- **Eyes** (12%): uveitis, conjunctival nodules, and lacrimal gland enlargement
- **Kidney** (5%): renal calculi, nephrocalcinosis, and interstitial nephritis
Nonspecific constitutional symptoms such as fever, fatigue, malaise, and weight loss are observed in up to one third of the patients. The disease can be asymptomatic in up to half of the patients. Mode of presentation and severity of disease are influenced by race and gender.

82. **What are the five radiographic stages of thoracic involvement?**
    - **Stage 0:** no visible thoracic finding
    - **Stage 1:** bilateral hilar adenopathy
    - **Stage 2:** bilateral hilar adenopathy + parenchymal infiltrates
    - **Stage 3:** parenchymal infiltrates
    - **Stage 4:** advanced fibrosis

    Stage 1 usually improves spontaneously or stabilizes. Spontaneous remission occurs less often as the disease stage progresses.

83. **What is Löfgren's syndrome?**
    A presentation of sarcoidosis with specific features that is usually seen in women. Lofgren's syndrome has an excellent prognosis, and patients usually recover spontaneously.

84. **Which are the features of Löfgren's syndrome?**
    - Erythema nodosum
    - Arthralgia
    - Malaise
    - Bilateral hilar adenopathy

85. **How is sarcoidosis diagnosed?**
    When patients present with Löfgren's syndrome, a clinical diagnosis of sarcoidosis is appropriate. In the remaining patients without this classic presentation, a tissue diagnosis is required. Most commonly, the diagnosis is made by bronchial or transbronchial biopsy, mediastinal lymph node biopsy, biopsy of skin lesions, or less commonly, conjunctival or lacrimal gland biopsy.

86. **Are noncaseating granulomas pathognomonic of sarcoidosis?**
    No. The characteristic lesion of sarcoidosis is a discrete, noncaseating epithelioid cell granuloma. However, noncaseating granulomas can be encountered in other diseases such as fungal and mycobacterial infections, foreign bodies, berylliosis, and common variable immunodeficiency. Any biopsy tissues obtained are routinely stained to exclude mycobacterial or fungal infections. In sarcoidosis, granulomas either resolve or lead to fibrotic changes.

87. **What is the utility of measuring ACE serum levels in sarcoidosis?**
    Limited. ACE levels have low sensitivity and specificity and are not helpful for monitoring patients for disease progression. Pulmonary function tests and chest CT scans monitor disease progression more effectively.

88. **What is the differential diagnosis of sarcoidosis?**

Tuberculosis	*Pneumocystis jiroveci*	Drug reaction
Atypical mycobacteria	infection	(interferon alpha)
Cryptococcosis	Brucellosis	Granulomatous lesions
Aspergillosis	Toxoplasmosis	of unknown
Coccidioidomycosis	Cat-scratch disease	significance (GLUS)
Blastomycosis	Lymphomas	

89. **Which pneumoconiosis resembles sarcoidosis?**
    Chronic beryllium lung disease. Berylliosis develops after a usual latent period of years following a low-level exposure to beryllium. The treatment is removal from further exposure to beryllium and steroids. Other hard metal–induced lung diseases due to aluminum and cobalt exposure are also characterized by the presence of sarcoid-like granulomas.

90. **What is the prognosis of sarcoidosis?**
    Generally good. Many patients are asymptomatic and spontaneous resolution occurs in up to two thirds of them. Risk factors for poor prognosis include age $\geq$ 40 years at onset of symptoms, African American race, lupus pernio, chronic uveitis, chronic hypercalcemia, nephrocalcinosis, progressive pulmonary sarcoidosis, neurosarcoidosis, myocardial compromise, and the presence of cystic bony lesions.

91. **What is the treatment of sarcoidosis?**
    Oral steroids, although treatment is usually not indicated in patients who are asymptomatic or in those with mild pulmonary function abnormalities. Steroid therapy is started in patients with progressive radiographic findings or moderate symptoms; hypercalcemia; and neurologic, cardiac, or ocular involvement. Treatment duration is 6–24 months. Other medications used in patients who cannot tolerate steroids or have progressive disease on steroid therapy include hydroxychloroquine, methotrexate, azathioprine, methotrexate, and tumor necrosis factor inhibitors (e.g., infliximab).

    Joint Statement of the American Thoracic Society (ATS), the European Respiratory Society (ERS) and the World Association of Sarcoidosis and Other Granulomatous Disorders (WASOG): Statement on sarcoidosis, *Am J Respir Crit Care Med* 160:736–755, 1999.

PULMONARY THROMBOEMBOLIC DISEASE

92. **What are the predisposing factors for the development of venous thromboembolism (VTE)?**
    - Age > 40
    - Prior VTE
    - Prolonged anesthesia (>30 min)
    - Prolonged immobilization
    - CHF
    - CVA
    - Cancer
    - Fracture of the pelvis, hip, or tibia
    - Hip or knee replacement
    - Pregnancy and postpartum period
    - Estrogen-containing medications
    - Tamoxifen
    - Obesity
    - Inflammatory bowel disease
    - Genetic or acquired thrombophilia including lupus anticoagulant, Factor V Leiden, anticardiolipin antibody syndrome, protein S or C deficiency, antithrombin III deficiency, prothrombin 20210A mutation

KEY POINTS: ANTICOAGULANT THERAPY FOR VENOUS THROMBOEMBOLISM ✓

1. The initial dose of warfarin for VTE should be between 5 and 10 mg for the first 1–2 days.

2. Use an initial warfarin dose of $\leq$ 5 mg for the elderly or patients who have CHF, liver disease, malnourishment, or recent major surgery or who are taking medications that can increase the sensitivity to warfarin.

3. Begin INR monitoring 2–3 days after the first warfarin dose.

CHF = congestive heart failure; INR = International Normalized Ratio; VTE = venous thromboembolism.

93. **Describe the initial evaluation of possible PE.**
Clinical grounds are insufficient for diagnosis and confirmation of PE. Clinical prediction tools, such as the Wells criteria, may be helpful in determining the clinical probability of PE and the need for further evaluation. In patients with a low or moderate clinical probability of PE, the D-dimer assay may be a useful screening tool. (D-dimers are cross-linked fibrin fragments that are released from thrombi soon after they are formed.) About 95% of patients with PE have an abnormal D-dimer, depending on the assay used. However, an elevated D-dimer level may be seen in many other conditions, such as malignancy or recent surgical procedures. In those patients with a low or moderate probability of PE, a D-dimer level < 500 ng/mL by quantitative enzyme-linked immunosorbent assay (ELISA) or semiquantitative latex agglutination is sufficient evidence to rule out PE. Helical (spiral) chest CT scan performed with contrast is often used to confirm the diagnosis of PE, but may miss small PEs. CT scan has the potential to identify other diagnoses that may explain the patient's symptoms. In patients with allergy to contrast or who have renal failure, a nuclear medicine $\dot{V}/\dot{Q}$ scan and compression ultrasonography of the lower extremity veins may be performed. The $\dot{V}/\dot{Q}$ scan is very sensitive but nonspecific.

94. **What is the Wells formula for predicting the clinical probability of PE?**
PE is unlikely with a score ≤ 4 and likely with a score of > 4. Points are assigned as follows:
- Clinical symptoms of deep venous thrombosis (DVT): 3
- Other diagnoses more likely than PE: 3
- Heart rate > 100 bpm: 1.5
- Immobilization ≥ 3 days: 1.5
- Surgery in previous 4 weeks: 1.5
- Previous DVT or PE: 1.5
- Hemoptysis: 1
- Malignancy: 1

vanBelle A, Buller HR, Huisman MV, et al: Effectiveness of managing suspected pulmonary embolism using an algorithm combining clinical probability, D-dimer testing, and computed tomography, *JAMA* 295:172–179, 2006.

95. **Summarize the chest x-ray findings associated with PE.**
Frequently chest x-rays in patients with PE are "normal," although subtle nonspecific abnormalities can be found. Examples of abnormal findings include differences in diameters of vessels that should be similar in size, abrupt cut-off of a vessel followed distally, increased radiolucency in some areas, regional oligemia (Westermark's sign), a peripheral wedge-shaped density over the diaphragm (Hampton's hump), or an enlarged right descending pulmonary artery (Palla's sign).

96. **What are the complications of pulmonary angiography?**
Death (<0.5%), cardiac perforation, arrhythmias, contrast reaction, renal insufficiency or failure secondary to dye, and bleeding. Pulmonary angiography is still the gold standard to demonstrate PE, but the procedure is not without risk and is usually reserved for unstable patients, when thrombolysis is considered, or when less invasive tests (guided by the clinical situation) are nondiagnostic. Overall, the risk of major complications is 4% and appears to be the highest in the most critically ill patients.

American Thoracic Society: The diagnostic approach to acute venous thromboembolism, *Am J Respir Crit Care Med* 160:1043–1066, 1999.

97. **What is the treatment of PE?**
IV unfractionated heparin (UH) or subcutaneous low-molecular-weight heparin (SC LMWH). Warfarin should be started simultaneously with any heparin, and both therapies continued for at least 4–5 days. Warfarin should be dosed to achieve an International

Normalized Ratio (INR) between 2 and 3. Heparin can be discontinued once the INR target is achieved for two consecutive measurements, 24 hours apart. Anticoagulation should be continued for at least 3 months, but longer treatment may be needed for patients with persistent risk factors. Patients at significantly high risk may require lifelong anticoagulation. Fondaparinux, is a more recent anticoagulant that is approved for the treatment of acute PE and DVT. Warfarin is also started simultaneously with fondaparinux and continued as described.

American Thoracic Society: The diagnostic approach to acute venous thromboembolism, *Am J Respir Crit Care Med* 160:1043–1066, 1999.

98. **When should thrombolytic therapy be considered?**
When patients have submassive or massive PE with associated hypotension, refractory hypoxemia, or right heart failure and do not have contraindications to thrombolytic therapy. The contraindications include a history of intracranial hemorrhage, brain tumor, recent intracranial surgery or trauma, and recent (<6 mo) or active internal bleeding. Patients with uncontrolled hypertension, thrombocytopenia, bleeding tendency, recent history of nonhemorrhagic stroke, and surgery within the previous 10 days also are considered at high risk of complications of thrombolytic therapy.

American Thoracic Society: The diagnostic approach to acute venous thromboembolism, *Am J Respir Crit Care Med* 160:1043–1066, 1999.

99. **What is the mortality rate for PE?**
PEs occur in over 600,000 people per year, resulting in over 100,000–200,000 deaths. Thirty percent of PEs are diagnosed antemortem.

100. **How common is pulmonary infarction?**
Approximately 1 in 10 PEs results in pulmonary infarction.

101. **What findings are associated with pulmonary infarction?**
Pleuritic chest pain, hemoptysis, and low-grade fever. Pulmonary infarction is classically described as a wedge-shaped infiltrate that abuts the pleura (Hampton's hump) and is often associated with a small pleural effusion that is usually exudative and hemorrhagic.

102. **List the causes of nonthrombotic PE.**
   - Fat embolism (following bone trauma or fracture)
   - Amniotic fluid embolism
   - Air embolism
   - Tumor emboli
   - Trophoblastic emboli

103. **What are the clinical manifestations of fat emoblism?**
Altered mental status, respiratory decompensation, anemia, thrombocytopenia, and petechiae that usually occur 12–36 hours after the inciting trauma.

PULMONARY HYPERTENSION

104. **Define "pulmonary hypertension (PH)."**
A mean pulmonary artery pressure (PAP) $\geq$ 25 mmHg. The normal resting PAP is 8–20 mmHg. The previous criterion of mean PAP $\geq$ 30 mmHg during exercise has been updated.

105. **How is PH classified?**
   - **Group 1, pulmonary arterial hypertension (PAH):** idiopathic, heritable (*BMPR2* mutations), drug- and toxin-induced (e.g., fenfluramine), and associated with CTD, HIV, portal hypertension, and CAD

- Group 2: Due to left heart disease
- Group 3: Due to lung diseases or hypoxia or both
- Group 4: Chronic thromboembolic
- Group 5: Unclear multifactorial mechanism: splenectomy, sarcoidosis, pulmonary LCH, thyroid disorders, and chronic renal failure on hemodialysis

106. **What is the gold standard for the diagnosis of PH?**
Right heart catheterization with the definition of mean PAP $\geq$ 25 mmHg. Doppler echocardiography can estimate the systolic PAP, though it has intrinsic and operator-related limitations. A tricuspid insufficiency jet > 2.8 m/sec that corresponds to an estimated systolic PAP of 36 mmHg is also considered PH.

107. **What factors predict poor prognosis in PH?**
Presence of New York Heart Association (NYHA) CHF functional class III or IV, brain natriuretic peptide (BNP) level $\geq$ 150 pg/mL, inability to walk more than 250 m in 6 minutes, low peak oxygen consumption, high right atrial pressure, low cardiac index, lack of response to acute vasodilator therapy, presence of pericardial effusion, right atrial and ventricular dilatation, and low tricuspid annular pansystolic excursion are some of the variables that predict worse outcome in PH.

108. **What is the treatment of PAH?**
In general, these patients should be treated by a physician with expertise in the condition. Supportive measures include oral anticoagulants, diuretics, oxygen, and digoxin. Pulmonary rehabilitation should be considered. An acute vasodilator response to inhalation of nitric oxide or administration of IV prostacyclin at the time of right heart catheterization supports the use of calcium channel blockers. In nonresponders, consider phosphodiesterase inhibitors type 5 (sildenafil or tadalafil), endothelin receptor antagonists (bosentan or ambrisentan), and prostacyclin analogues (epoprostenol, treprostinil, or iloprost), depending on the functional class, risk factors, and response to therapy.

109. **Which CTDs have an association with PH?**
SSc carries the highest risk of PH. The prevalence of PH in SSc is between 7 and 12% and its presence is associated with markedly poorer outcomes. The prevalence of PH is less common in systemic lupus erythematosus (SLE), mixed connective tissue disease (MCTD), Sjögren's syndrome, polymyositis, or RA.

110. **What percentage of patients with acute PE develops chronic thromboembolic pulmonary hypertension (CTEPH)?**
Up to 4% of patients. These patients may benefit from pulmonary thromboendarterectomy. This intervention is considered in centers with experience for patients with central obstruction of the pulmonary arteries who have abnormal hemodynamic findings and a small number of comorbidities.

PLEURAL DISEASES

111. **What is the difference between primary spontaneous pneumothorax (PSP) and secondary spontaneous pneumothorax (SSP)?**
PSP occurs in patients without apparent underlying lung disease (usually tall, thin subjects).
SSP occurs in patients with underlying lung disease. Other types of pneumothorax are:
- **Catamenial pneumothorax:** occurs in conjunction with menstruation
- **Traumatic pneumothorax:** classified as iatrogenic (central line placement) and noniatrogenic (blunt or penetrating chest injury)

Noppen M, De Keukelseir T: Pneumothorax, *Respiration* 76:7–15, 2008.

112. **What is the management of PSP?**
     - If the pneumothorax < 20% or < 3 cm (apex of the lung to cupula of the chest cavity) and the patient has few symptoms, the suggested approach is observation ± oxygen supplementation with appropriate follow-up.
     - If the pneumothorax > 20% or > 3 cm or the patient is symptomatic, air evacuation by aspiration or small catheter placement is needed.
     - If the pneumothorax occurred more than once, the recommended approach is recurrence prevention with thoracoscopy with talc insufflation or pleurodesis or chest tube drainage with chemical pleurodesis.

113. **Which are the diseases most commonly associated with SSP?**

Emphysema	IPF	Marfan syndrome
CF	Sarcoidosis	Lung cancer
P. jiroveci pneumonia	LCH	
Tuberculosis	LAM	

114. **What is the management of SSP?**
     SSP requires immediate evacuation of the air in the pleural space and recurrence prevention at the first episode. All patients should be hospitalized.

115. **What is the difference between transudative and exudative pleural effusions?**
     The differentiation between these two types of effusions is important because it helps narrow the diagnostic possibilities. **Transudative effusions** are usually due to an imbalance in the hydrostatic or oncotic pressures or both (e.g., CHF, hepatic hydrothorax, nephrotic syndrome, and atelectasis). **Exudative effusions** have a broader differential diagnosis and are generally caused by inflammation, infection, malignancy, and lymphatic abnormalities. According to **Light's criteria** the pleural fluid is an **exudate** if one of the following is present:
     - Pleural fluid protein-to-serum protein ratio > 0.5
     - Pleural fluid lactate dehydrogenase (LDH)–to-serum LDH > 0.6
     - Pleural fluid LDH > two thirds the upper limit of normal serum LDH
     Other criteria for exudative effusion include at least one of the following:
     - Pleural fluid cholesterol > 45 mg/dL
     - Pleural fluid protein > 2.9 g/dL
     - Pleural fluid LDH > 0.45 times the upper limit of normal LDH

116. **Describe the most relevant characteristic of the following exudative causes of pleural effusions.**
     See Table 6-10.

TABLE 6-10. DISORDERS ASSOCIATED WITH EXUDATIVE PLEURAL EFFUSIONS AND PLEURAL FLUID CHARACTERISTICS

Disorder	Pleural Fluid Characteristics
Complicated parapneumonic effusion	pH < 7.2, positive gram stain or culture.
Chylothorax	Triglycerides > 110 mg/dL, presence of chylomicrons.
Hemothorax	Hematocrit in fluid > 50% of blood.
Tuberculosis	Lymphocyte/neutrophil ratio > 0.75, adenosine deaminase > 50 IU/L, lysozyme > 15 mg/dL, <5% mesothelial cells, positive AFB or culture.

(continued)

TABLE 6-10.	DISORDERS ASSOCIATED WITH EXUDATIVE PLEURAL EFFUSIONS AND PLEURAL FLUID CHARACTERISTICS—(continued)
Disorder	**Pleural Fluid Characteristics**
Rheumatoid pleurisy	Glucose < 30 mg/dL, pH ~7, LDH > 1000 IU/L.
Malignancy (most commonly, lung and breast)	Positive cytology. Low glucose concentration in chronic effusion.
Esophageal rupture	pH ~6 and high salivary amylase.
Peritoneal dialysis	Protein of 0.5 g/dL, glucose of 300 mg/dL.
Pancreatitis	Pleural fluid/serum amylase of 3–6:1.

AFB = acid-fast bacilli; LDH = lactate dehydrogenase.
Adapted from Sahn SA: The value of pleural fluid analysis. Am J Med Sci 335:7–15, 2008.

117. **What are the diseases that can present with a predominantly lymphocytic exudate?**
   ■ Tuberculosis
   ■ Lymphoma
   ■ Sarcoidosis
   ■ Post–coronary artery bypass grafting (CABG) chylothorax
   ■ Yellow nail syndrome (triad of yellow nails, lymphedema, and pulmonary symptoms more commonly seen in women and associated with abnormal lymphatics).
   ■ Rheumatoid arthritis

118. **What are the diseases that can present with eosinophilic exudate (>10% eosinophils)?**

Hydropneumothorax	Drug-induced effusions	Fungal diseases
Hemothorax	Churg-Strauss	Parasitic diseases
Benign asbestos effusions	syndrome	

119. **What are the diseases that can present with pleural fluid acidosis (pH < 7.3)?**
   ■ Parapneumonic effusion or empyema
   ■ Esophageal rupture
   ■ RA
   ■ Malignancy

LUNG CANCER

See also Chapter 15, Oncology.

120. **How common is lung cancer?**
   Lung cancer is the second most common cancer after skin cancer, but is the leading cause of cancer death in both men and women. More men than women die from lung cancer, but the gap in mortality is steadily narrowing. Lung cancer occurrence is 45% higher among African American men than among white men. This neoplasia occurs more often in the poor

and less educated and has marked regional variation. Interestingly, in developed countries, the frequency of adenocarcinoma has increased while that of squamous carcinoma has decreased.

121. **What is the etiology of lung cancer?**
The risk of lung cancer is based on the interrelationship between the exposure to etiologic agents and individual susceptibility (genetic factors). In the United States, smoking is responsible for 90% of lung cancer. Compared with never smokers, smokers have an approximately 20-fold increase in lung cancer risk. The risk for lung cancer increases with the duration and number of cigarettes smoked per day. The risk of lung cancer decreases among those who quit smoking, but remains increased above that of nonsmokers for years after the quit date. Asbestos and cigarette smoking act synergistically to increase the risk of lung cancer. Cigar and pipe smoking are also established causes of lung cancer.

KEY POINTS: DIAGNOSTIC FEATURES OF ASBESTOSIS ✔

1. History of asbestos exposure.

2. Presence of latency period (20–30 yr) between exposure and symptoms.

3. Interstitial fibrosis on chest x-ray or CT scan.

4. Symptoms and signs of breathlessness, bibasilar inspiratory crackles, and clubbing.

5. Restrictive pattern on pulmonary function testing with reduced DLCO.

6. Exclusion of other pneumoconioses.

7. Presence of interstitial pneumonia pattern with asbestos bodies on biopsy (if needed).

CT = computed tomography; DLCO = diffusing capacity for carbon monoxide.

122. **Is there any benefit in screening patients at high risk for lung cancer?**
Early studies showed that screening with chest radiographs and sputum cytology did not decrease lung cancer mortality. More recent studies suggest that CT scanning is probably helpful. Early results from the National Lung Screening Trial (NLST) suggest a 20% reduction in lung cancer mortality in subjects screened with CT scans. The NLST compares the efficacy of chest x-ray and CT scan in early cancer detection. The data are currently undergoing further analysis.

Available at: www.cancer.gov/nlst/updates

123. **What are the clinical predictors for malignancy of SPNs?**
Independent predictors of malignancy includes older age, current or past smoking history, history of extrathoracic cancer > 5 years before nodule detection, larger nodule diameter, speculation, and upper lobe location.

124. **What is the management of an SPN?**
Initially, to review previous imaging tests to evaluate growth. If the nodule is growing, tissue diagnosis should be obtained unless contraindicated by the presence of severe comorbid conditions. If the nodule has been stable for at least 2 years, no additional diagnostic

evaluation is generally needed. An exception to the 2-year rule is bronchioloalveolar carcinoma, which may be slow growing and present as nodular ground-glass opacities. At the time a nodule is found, if it has a clear-cut benign pattern such as complete calcification, no additional evaluation is needed. PET scan is indicated in patients with low-to-moderate pretest probability and nodule(s) > 8–10 mm. If PET is positive or the patient has a high pretest probability (>60%) of cancer, then consider surgery.

125. **Which SPNs can be followed?**
Indeterminate nodules > 8–10 mm can be followed by CT scan if the clinical probability of cancer is very low (<5%) or low (<30%) and:
- PET scan is negative for malignancy,
- Needle biopsy is nondiagnostic and PET is negative, or
- Patient prefers a nonaggressive approach.
  Serial CT scans should be repeated at 3, 6, 12, and 24 months.

Alberts WM, American College of Chest Physicians: Diagnosis and management of lung cancer executive summary: ACCP evidence-based clinical practice guidelines (2nd ed). *Chest* 132:1S–422S, 2007.

126. **What is the difference between small cell carcinoma (SCLC) and non–small cell carcinoma (NSCLC) of the lung?**
- **SCLC:** High-grade, mitotically active, undifferentiated carcinomas that derive from neuroendocrine cells. SCLC usually presents as disseminated disease and is capable of secreting bioactive peptides.
- **NSCLC:** Some degree of cytoplasmic differentiation. Depending on the type, the carcinoma can have glandular features, cytoplasmatic mucin, and extracellular keratin.
  Adenocarcinoma and squamous cell and large cell carcinomas are classified as NSCLC.

127. **What is hypertrophic osteoarthropathy?**
A systemic disorder characterized by painful symmetrical arthropathy of the ankles, wrists, and knees with periosteal new bone formation in the distal long bones of the limbs, usually associated with clubbing.

128. **Which antibody is associated with paraneoplastic neurologic syndromes?**
Type 1 antineuronal nuclear antibodies (anti-Hu antibodies).

129. **Does the presence of paraneoplastic syndrome modify the treatment strategy?**
No. Patients with any of the paraneoplastic syndromes, and otherwise potentially treatable lung cancer, should not be excluded from potentially curative therapies.

CYSTIC FIBROSIS

130. **What are the clinical features of CF?**
- **Chronic sinopulmonary disease:** chronic productive cough, nasal polyps, digital clubbing, bronchiectasis, and colonization or infection with *Staphylococcus aureus*, mucoid and nonmucoid *P. aeruginosa*, *Stenotrophomonas maltophilia,* and *Burkholderia cepacia*
- **GI and nutritional abnormalities:** distal intestinal obstruction syndrome (DIOS), rectal prolapse, pancreatic insufficiency, chronic hepatic disease, and failure to thrive
- **Salt loss syndromes**
- **Obstructive azoospermia**

131. **How is the diagnosis of CF made?**
By analysis of sweat chloride by the quantitative pilocarpine iontophoresis sweat test. Sweat chloride levels are abnormally high (>60 mM) in > 90% of patients with CF. With recognition of the genetic basis of CF, analysis may also be done for the CF mutation (cystic fibrosis transmembrane conductance regulator [CFTR]). The most common mutation is ΔF508. Genetic analysis is usually done in patients suspected of having CF who have a normal or borderline sweat chloride test. The diagnosis of CF is usually made early in life, but the increasing awareness of the spectrum of disease has led to more frequent diagnosis of CF in adults. Patients diagnosed in adulthood usually have chronic respiratory symptoms, milder lung disease, fewer *Pseudomonas* infections, and more frequent pancreatic sufficiency than patients diagnosed during childhood.

132. **What is the treatment of CF?**
Airway clearance
- Antibiotic therapy for acute exacerbations and chronic antibiotic suppression (aerosolized tobramycin or colistin and oral azithromycin)
- Mucolytic agents (recombinant human DNase, hypertonic saline)
- Bronchodilators
- Anti-inflammatory agents (inhaled steroids and ibuprofen)
- Oxygen supplementation
- Pancreatic enzyme and vitamin supplements
- Control of hyperglycemia
- Nutritional support

   Yankaskas JR, Marshall BC, Sufian B, et al: Cystic fibrosis adult care: Consensus Conference report, *Chest* 125:1S–39S, 2004.

MECHANICAL VENTILATION

133. **What are the main modes of MV?**
Volume controlled (VC) or pressure controlled (PC) with assist control (AC) or synchronized intermittent mandatory ventilation (SIMV). In VC ventilation, the volume (based on patient height and ideal body weight) and flow rate or inspiratory time are set. In PC ventilation, the pressure above positive end-expiratory pressure (PEEP) and inspiratory time are set. In PCV, the volume delivered depends upon compliance and varies. Both VC and PC breaths may be delivered by AC or SIMV. In both modes, patients may trigger breaths. In AC, the patient receives a set number of ventilator breaths, and with self-initiated breaths, receives the same volume of pressure parameters set for ventilator controlled breaths. In SIMV, the patient receives a fixed number of ventilator breaths synchronized to their effort. If the patient breathes between ventilator breaths, some pressure support is provided which augments the spontaneous breath volume. The patient may also be allowed to breathe spontaneously with pressure support, often as a transition to weaning.

134. **What interventions on the respirator can increase oxygenation?**
An increase in inspiratory time and in the positive end-expiratory pressure (PEEP) or FIO_2.

135. **What ventilator changes can decrease hypercapnia?**
Those that increase MV by increasing the tidal volume or respiratory rate.

136. **Why are peak and plateau pressures important?**
These pressures are important to detect potential ventilator problems. When only the peak inspiratory pressure increases, consider bronchospasm and endotracheal tube narrowing by secretions or occlusion due to teeth clenching of the patient. When both peak and plateau pressures increase, consider parenchymal (pulmonary edema and pneumonia), pleural

(pneumothorax), chest wall (obesity), or abdominal (obesity and ascitis) abnormalities. High pressures can cause barotrauma such as pneumothorax and pneumomediastinum.

137. **In what setting does auto-PEEP occur?**
When there is incomplete exhalation (high respiratory rate or short exhalation time) as often occurs in the setting of COPD or asthma. Patients develop hyperinflation and increasing intrathoracic pressure that, when extreme, can lead to hypotension (reduced venous return and increased right ventricular afterload) and even cardiopulmonary arrest. Auto-PEEP can be treated by disconnecting the endotracheal tube from the ventilator and allowing passive exhalation. The ventilator should be adjusted to increase the expiratory time.

138. **What conditions should be met before discontinuation of a patient from MV?**
Patients should demonstrate some reversal of the cause of respiratory failure that led to intubation, adequate ventilatory endurance, and oxygenation (PaO_2/FIO_2 ratio $\geq$ 150–200) with PEEP $\leq$ 5 cmH$_2$O and FIO$_2$ 50%, pH $\geq$ 7.25, hemodynamic stability, appropriate cough strength, and mental status. The spontaneous breathing test (SBT) is used to assess lung mechanics and endurance.

139. **What are the indications of using noninvasive positive-pressure ventilation (NIPPV)?**
- Acute hypercapnic respiratory failure in COPD
- Cardiogenic pulmonary edema
- Pneumonia in immunocompromised hosts
- Postextubation respiratory distress due to upper airway obstruction
  Consider conventional MV if the NIPPV has not resulted in clear improvement of the condition in 2 hours.

140. **What are the main characteristics of ARDS?**
ARDS is characterized by acute onset (<7 days), hypoxemia (PaO_2/FIO_2 ratio < 200), diffuse bilateral pulmonary infiltrates, and absence of left heart failure (clinical assessment or wedge pressure < 18 mmHg). ARDS is caused by a multiplicity of conditions such as aspiration lung injury, pneumonia, inhalation injury, sepsis, and trauma, transfusion-related lung injury. Pneumonia and aspiration are the most common causes of direct lung injury. ARDS and sepsis are the most common cause of indirect lung injury ARDS. Mortality may be as high as 60%. In contrast to pulmonary edema, cardiomegaly, pleural effusion, and widening of the vascular pedicle are not prominent.

141. **What is the recommended strategy to ventilate patients with acute ARDS?**
The ARDSNet study showed that the application of low tidal volumes (6 mL/kg predicted body weight based on patient's height) reduced inflammation, lung injury, and duration of MV and improved survival.

The Acute Respiratory Distress Syndrome Network: Ventilation with lower tidal volumes as compared with traditional tidal volumes for acute lung injury and the acute respiratory distress syndrome, *N Engl J Med* 342:1301–1308, 2000.

MISCELLANEOUS

142. **What is the alveolar hemorrhage syndrome?**
The occurrence of bleeding into the alveolar spaces due to disorders that disrupt the alveolar-capillary basement membrane. Alveolar hemorrhage syndrome is diagnosed by progressive reddening of fluid aliquots on bronchoalveolar lavage (BAL) or presence of > 20% hemosiderin-laden macrophages on BAL.

143. **Which diseases are associated with alveolar hemorrhage syndrome?**
    - **Immunologic:** Goodpasture's syndrome, renal-pulmonary syndromes, glomerulonephritis, SLE, graft vs host disease
    - **Toxic:** crack cocaine, abciximab, penicillamine
    - **Traumatic**
    - **Increased vascular pressure:** mitral stenosis

144. **Which are the pulmonary complications of HIV infection?**
    See Table 6-11. Early in the course of disease, patients with HIV have respiratory disorders similar to those in the general population. As the disease progresses, opportunistic infections may occur. The CD4+ lymphocyte count is the most reliable marker for the risk of opportunistic infection.

TABLE 6-11. INFECTIOUS AGENTS IN PULMONARY COMPLICATIONS OF HUMAN IMMUNODEFICIENCY VIRUS INFECTION

Pulmonary Complication	Infectious Agent
Focal infiltrate	Bacteria, *Mycobacterium tuberculosis*, *Pneumocystis jiroveci*
Diffuse infiltrate	*P. jiroveci*, *M. tuberculosis*, Kaposi's sarcoma
Diffuse nodules	Kaposi's sarcoma, *M. tuberculosis*, fungi
Pneumothorax	*P. jiroveci*, *M. tuberculosis*
Pleural effusion	Bacteria, *M. tuberculosis*, Kaposi's sarcoma
Mediastinal adenopathy	*M. tuberculosis*, atypical mycobacteria, Kaposi's sarcoma
Cavities	*M. tuberculosis*, *P. jiroveci*, *Pseudomonas aeruginosa*

Adapted from Rosen MJ: Pulmonary complications of HIV infection. Respirology 13:181–190, 2008.

145. **What are the main characteristics of LAM?**
    LAM is a rare disease characterized by smooth muscle infiltration and cystic destruction of the lung due to mutations in tuberous sclerosis genes. LAM is found almost exclusively in women. Up to a third of the cases are associated with the tuberous sclerosis complex of seizures, brain tumors, and cognitive impairment. Clinically, LAM patients have progressive dyspnea, recurrent pneumothoraces, lymphadenopathy, chylothorax, and abdominal angiomyolipomas and lymphangiomyomas. There are no proven therapies for LAM.

    McCormack FX: Lymphangioleiomyomatosis: A clinical update, *Chest* 133:507–516, 2008.

146. **What are the main characteristics of pulmonary LCH?**
    Pulmonary LCH is a rare disorder of unknown etiology that predominantly affects young smokers, characterized by focal Langerhans' cell granulomas that infiltrate and destroy terminal bronchioles. Imaging studies show a combination of nodules (with or without cavitation) and thick- and thin-walled cysts. The diagnosis usually requires lung biopsy showing the characteristic granulomas. Treatment consists of smoking cessation, steroids, and cytotoxic agents. Many patients recover or remain stable after smoking cessation.

    Tazi A: Adult pulmonary Langerhans' cell histiocytosis, *Eur Respir J* 27:1272–1285, 2006.

147. **What is high-altitude pulmonary edema (HAPE)?**

A noncardiogenic form of pulmonary edema that usually occurs 2–3 days after rapid ascent to altitudes > 8500 feet. Hypoxic pulmonary vasoconstriction causes pulmonary hypertension with capillary stress fractures, release of inflammatory mediators, and decreased nitric oxide synthesis, leading to edema. HAPE can be prevented by a slow ascent, nifedipine, phosphodiesterase inhibitors (tadalafil, sidenafil), acetazolamide, and salmeterol. Treatment includes immediate descent to lower altitude, O_2, nifedipine, phosphodiesterase inhibitors, and dexamethasone.

148. **What determines if a patient with respiratory disease will need oxygen during air travel?**

- SpO_2 on room air > 95%: No oxygen.
- SpO_2 on room air < 92%: Oxygen supplementation.
- SpO_2 on room air between 92% and 95% with risk factors: Perform a hypoxic challenge. Oxygen will be needed if PaO_2 < 50 mmHg on FIO_2 of 15%.

The airplane cabin pressure is maintained at pressures that correspond to altitudes < 8000 feet. At this altitude, the PaO_2 is equivalent to an FIO_2 of 15.1%. Patients cannot carry their own oxygen tank on commercial flights but can use their own battery-powered O_2 concentrators. Patients already on oxygen can increase O_2 flow by 1–2 L.

149. **What is the difference between arterial gas embolism (AGE) and decompression sickness (DS) in divers?**

- **AGE:** Caused by air retention in the lungs that expands during ascent with rupture of alveoli and adjacent vessel. The air bubbles embolize and can reach the brain. Treatment includes 100% O_2 inhalation and hyperbaric oxygen recompression.
- **DS:** Caused by bubble formation on the tissues during rapid ascent because of inability of the nitrogen gas to leave the tissue in an orderly fashion. Patients have different symptoms such as skin itches, joint pain, paralysis, or unconsciousness. Treatment includes 100% O_2, aspirin, fluids, and hyperbaric oxygen recompression.

SLEEP

See also Chapter 2, General Medicine and Ambulatory Care, and Chapter 17, Neurology.

150. **What changes occur in the respiratory system during sleep?**

Decreased PaO_2 and increased $PaCO_2$ because the hypercapnic and hypoxic ventilator responses decrease when compared with responses during wakefulness The decreased responses become more prominent during rapid eye movement (REM). In addition, the upper airway dilator muscle tone decreases, favoring the development of upper airway obstruction in susceptible individuals.

151. **Define "apnea" and "hypopnea."**

- **Apnea:** Cessation or near cessation of air flow to < 20% of baseline for at least 10 seconds.
- **Hypopnea:** A 30% decrease in airflow for at least 10 seconds accompanied by at least a 4% decline in oxygen saturation. The apnea-hypopnea index (AHI) is the number of apneas plus hypopneas in 1 hour of sleep. This index defines the severity—mild (5–15), moderate (16–30), and severe (>30)—of sleep apnea.

152. **How are apneas classified?**

- **Obstructive:** Inspiratory effort is present.
- **Central:** Inspiratory effort is absent.
- **Mixed:** A central event is followed by an obstructive one.

153. **What are the risk factors for developing obstructive sleep apnea (OSA)?**

Male gender
Menopause
Older age
Obesity
Use of tobacco and
  alcohol
Hypothyroidism

Acromegaly
Neuromuscular
  disorders
Stroke
Increased neck
  circumference
Mandibular hypoplasia

Enlarged tonsils and
  adenoids
Medications (e.g.,
  muscle relaxants)

154. **What are the consequences of having OSA?**

Increased mortality
Insulin resistance
CAD
CHF

CVA
Cardiac arrhythmias
Hypertension
PH

Mood disorders
  (depression or
  anxiety or both)
Erectile dysfunction
GERD

155. **What is the treatment of OSA?**
   - **General measure:** sleep hygiene, appropriate positioning during sleep, safety counseling, weight loss, and avoidance of muscle relaxants and alcohol
   - **Positive airway pressure:** continuous positive airway pressure (CPAP), BiPAP, and autotitrating positive airway pressure (APAP)
   - **Oral devices:** mandibular repositioners and tongue-retainers
   - **Upper-airway surgery:** uvulopalatopharyngoglossoplasty, maxillomandibular advancement, and tracheostomy

156. **How is central sleep apnea (CSA) classified?**
   - **Hypercapnic:** decreased responsiveness to hypercapnias seen in neuromuscular disorders and use of opioids
   - **Nonhypercapnic:** increased response to hypercapnia as seen in idiopathic CSA, Cheyne-Stokes respiration, and high-altitude periodic breathing

157. **What is the treatment of CSA?**
   - Avoidance of respiratory depressants
   - Correction of underlying conditions such as heart failure
   - Positive airway pressure

158. **What are the main characteristics of narcolepsy?**
   Excessive sleepiness, cataplexy (episodes of muscle atonia/hypotonia precipitated by intense emotions), sleep paralysis, and sleep hallucinations (at sleep onset or on awakening). **Cataplexy is the only pathognomonic characteristic of narcolepsy.** Not all patients have all the components, and narcolepsy is usually diagnosed by history. Polysomnography followed by multiple sleep latency is required when cataplexy is absent. Treatment includes sleep hygiene and combination of modafinil or other stimulants, hypnotic agents, or sodium oxybate, and REM sleep-suppressants (selective serotonin reuptake inhibitors [SSRIs] and tricyclic antidepressants).

159. **What are parasomnias?**
   Physical or experiential phenomena that occur in association with both non–rapid eye movement (NREM) and REM sleep. NREM parasomnias are confusional arousals, sleep terrors (abrupt awakening with intense fear and autonomic discharge), and sleepwalking. REM parasomnias include nightmares and REM sleep behavioral disorder ("dream-enacting").

160. **What is restless leg syndrome (RLS)?**

An unpleasant sensation or urge to move in the legs that increases with inactivity and at night and improves transiently with movement. RLS may be associated with anemia, uremia, pregnancy, aging, Parkinson's disease, diabetes mellitus, alcohol intake, and certain medications. Polysomnography is rarely needed because the diagnosis is obtained by clinical history. Treatment includes iron if ferritin < 50 µg/L and dopaminergic agents such as pramipexole and ropinirole. Treatment is not indicated for asymptomatic periodic limb movement during sleep.

WEBSITES

1. American College of Chest Physicians: www.chestnet.org
2. National Heart, Lung, and Blood Institute: ww.nhlbi.nih.gov

BIBLIOGRAPHY

1. Berry RB, editor: *Sleep Medicine Pearls*, ed 2, Philadelphia, 2003, Mosby.

2. Strauss M, Aksenov I: *Diving Science*, Champaign, IL, 2004, Human Kinetics.

3. West JB, editor: *Pulmonary Pathophysiology: The Essentials*, ed 7, Philadelphia, 2008, Lippincott Williams & Wilkins.

CHAPTER 7

GASTROENTEROLOGY

Rhonda A. Cole, M.D., and Dang M. Nguyen, M.D.

GASTROINTESTINAL BLEEDING

1. **List the five ways in which gastrointestinal (GI) bleeding presents.**
   - **Hematemesis**: vomiting of blood that may appear bright red or similar to coffee-ground material
   - **Melena**: black, tarry, foul-smelling stool
   - **Hematochezia**: bright red blood per rectum, blood mixed with stool, bloody diarrhea, or clots
   - **Occult GI blood loss**: normal-appearing stool that is hemoccult-positive
   - **Symptoms only**: syncope, dyspnea, angina, palpitations, or shock

2. **Describe the initial care of the patient with acute GI bleeding.**
   In any patient with acute GI bleeding, the key word is *resuscitation!* The initial rapid evaluation assesses the patient's hemodynamic stability by measuring the blood pressure (including orthostatic readings if appropriate) and pulse. Venous access is obtained with a large-bore intravenous (IV) cannula, and normal saline infusion started immediately. The initial laboratory evaluation includes complete blood count (CBC), prothrombin time (PT), partial thromboplastin time (PTT), platelets, routine chemistry including liver function tests such as alanine aminotransferase (ALT, SGPT) and aspartate aminotransferase (AST, SGOT), and type and cross-match for blood transfusion.

3. **Describe the management of a hemodynamically unstable patient with GI bleeding.**
   - Immediate fluid infusion with normal saline
   - Blood transfusion (see Question 4)
   - Placement of a nasogastric (NG) tube to assess for evidence of an upper GI source and, if present, to document the rapidity of bleeding
   - Close monitoring of vital signs and urinary output in an intensive care unit (ICU) setting
   - Assessment of other underlying disease involving the cardiovascular, GI (especially liver), renal, pulmonary, and central nervous systems

4. **Cite a good rule of thumb for determining the use of blood transfusions.**
   Transfuse the blood as quickly as the patient loses or has lost blood. For example, if the patient presents with massive hematochezia and is hemodynamically compromised, packed red blood cells (RBCs) should be given immediately. Conversely, if the patient who presents with iron-deficiency anemia, hemoccult positive stools, and stable vital signs, blood transfusions may not be needed.

5. **How is the site of bleeding determined?**
   By inspecting the stool for melena or hematochezia and the NG tube aspirate for blood. The site of bleeding can frequently be determined from the patient's complaints. Upper GI bleeding often presents with hematemesis combined with melena. Hematochezia with a negative NG aspirate suggests a lower GI source. Note that NG tube aspirate can be negative

in up to 10% of patients with upper GI bleeding. When the patient is stable, upper and lower endoscopy can attempt to localize the bleeding source and perform any indicated endoscopy therapies.

6. **List the common causes of upper GI bleeding.**
   - Peptic ulcer disease (duodenal and gastric)
   - Esophageal or gastric varices in the cirrhotic patient
   - Mallory-Weiss tears (most commonly seen in alcoholic patients or patients with forceful vomiting)
   - Erosive gastritis as a result of nonsteroidal anti-inflammatory drugs (NSAIDs) or in intubated ICU patients (a newer term is "nonspecific mucosal abnormalities")
   - Esophagitis
   - Arteriovenous malformations (AVMs)
   - Tumors

7. **Is examination of the skin helpful in identifying the source of an upper GI bleed?**
   Yes. The skin examination suggests potential bleeding sources if certain stigmata are present (Table 7-1). Visible lymphadenopathy or abdominal masses may suggest an intra-abdominal tumor or malignancy as the bleeding source.

TABLE 7-1. SKIN FINDINGS IN CONDITIONS THAT CAUSE GI BLEEDING

Disease	Associated Skin Findings
Peutz-Jeghers	Pigmented macules on lips, palms, soles
Malignant melanoma	Melanoma
Hereditary hemorrhagic telangiectasias	Telangiectasias on lips, mouth, palms, soles (Osler-Weber-Rendu)
Blue rubber bleb nevus	Dark, blue soft nodules
Bullous pemphigoid	Oral and skin bullae
Neurofibromatosis	Café-au-lait spots, axillary freckles, neurofibromas
Cronkhite-Canada	Alopecia; hyperpigmentation of creases, hands, and face
Cirrhosis	Spider angiomata, Dupuytren's contracture
Neoplasm	Acanthosis nigricans
Kaposi's sarcoma	Cutaneous Kaposi's sarcoma
Ehlers-Danlos	Skin fragility, keloids, paper-thin scars
Pseudoxanthoma elasticum	Yellow "chicken fat" papules and plaques in flexural areas
Turner's	Webbing of neck, purpura, skin nodules

From Berger T, Silverman S: Oral and cutaneous manifestations of gastrointestinal disease. In Sleisenger MH, Fordtran JS (eds): Gastrointestinal Disease, 5th ed. Philadelphia, WB Saunders, 1994, pp 268–285.

8. **What are predictors of poor outcome in patients presenting with bleeding ulcers?**
   - Age > 60 years
   - Presence of fresh blood per NG tube or rectum

- Hemodynamic instability despite aggressive resuscitative measures
- Presence of four or more comorbid illnesses (e.g., cardiac disease, liver disease, diabetes, chronic obstructive pulmonary disease [COPD], sepsis, or renal failure)

9. **List the more common causes of lower GI bleeding.**
   - Hemorrhoids with rare presentation as massive bleeding requiring hospitalization
   - Diverticulosis with bleeding from either the right or the left colon
   - Angiodysplasia or vascular ectasias with bleeding from the cecum and ascending colon and increased frequency among patients aged > 60 years
   - Large bowel neoplasms that usually present with chronic occult bleeding but occasionally bleed acutely
   - Colitis

10. **What are the less common causes of lower GI bleeding?**
    Meckel's diverticulum, ischemic bowel disease, and solitary ulcers of the cecum and rectum.

11. **Does melena indicate a right-sided colonic source and hematochezia a left-sided source?**
    Not always. The stool color depends on colonic transit time. If the stool remains in contact with intestinal bacteria that degrade hemoglobin, the resulting stool is melanotic. Although right-sided lesions are usually associated with melena (dark, tarry stools) and left-sided lesions with hematochezia (the passage of bright red blood per rectum), the opposite can also be seen. Therefore, the evaluation of a patient with hematochezia must include examination of the proximal colon.

12. **What causes esophageal varices?**
    Any condition that elevates the pressure in the hepatic portal system leads to varices. The normal portal venous pressure is approximately 10 mmHg but increases to > 20 mmHg in portal hypertension. The causes of portal hypertension are classified as presinusoidal, sinusoidal, and postsinusoidal.

13. **List the presinusoidal cause of esophageal varices.**
    - Portal vein thrombosis
    - Splenic vein thrombosis
    - Primary biliary cirrhosis
    - Schistosomiasis

14. **What are the sinusoidal causes of esophageal varices?**
    Cirrhosis and idiopathic disease

15. **List the postsinusoidal causes of esophageal varices.**
    - Heart failure
    - Constrictive pericarditis
    - Hepatic vein thrombosis (Budd-Chiari syndrome)
    - Veno-occlusive disease

16. **What is the most common cause of esophageal varices in the Western world?**
    Alcohol-related cirrhosis

17. **What two factors determine whether esophageal varices will develop and whether they will bleed?**
    Portal pressure and variceal size. The portal to hepatic vein pressure gradient must be > 12 mmHg (normal $= 3–6$ mmHg) for varices to develop. Beyond this level, there is poor correlation between portal pressure and likelihood of bleeding. The best predictor of impending variceal

hemorrhage is size. When varices reach a large size (>5 mm in diameter), they are more likely to rupture and bleed. At any given pressure, the wall of a large varix is under greater tension than that of a small varix and must be thicker to withstand the pressure.

18. **List the classic features of Meckel's diverticulum.**
    - Occurs in 1–3% of the population
    - Usually found within 100 cm of the ileocecal valve
    - Causes 50% of lower GI bleeding in children
    - Rarely causes bleeding in patients > 40 years old
    - Has gastric mucosa present in approximately 40% of patients

19. **In the patient who has undergone multiple evaluations for the localization of recurrent occult GI bleeding such as upper GI endoscopies, colonoscopies, barium studies, and RBC scans without identification of a source, what test should be performed?**
    Enteroscopy with push enteroscopy, single or double balloon enteroscopy, or wireless capsule endoscopy. The source of bleeding is most likely from vascular ectasia (or angiodysplasias), usually hiding in the small intestine. Note that before a patient undergoes enteroscopy, the hemoglobin should be ≥ 10 g/dL to aid in detecting these tiny vessels.

LIVER DISEASE AND HEPATITIS

20. **What are the common blood tests used to assess liver function?**
    - **ALT, SGPT**: Relatively specific for liver injury
    - **AST, SGOT**: Less specific for liver injury because it is also found in skeletal muscles, cardiac muscles, and other organs
    - **Alkaline phosphatase**: Increased in cholestatic disease
    - **γ-glutamyltransferase (GGT)**: An enzyme of intrahepatic biliary canaliculi, more specific marker for cholestasis than alkaline phosphatase
    - **Bilirubin**: Conjugated versus unconjugated
    - **PT and albumin**: Markers of liver synthetic function

21. **Which type of viral hepatitis is a major health concern?**
    Hepatitis C virus (HCV). Currently, there are more than 170 million people infected with HCV worldwide, and 4 million people are infected with HCV in the United States. Over 50% of people who have served in the U.S. armed forces are positive for HCV, making the illness a priority for diagnosis and treatment in the federal health system. In addition to the known sources of risk and exposure, at least one third of all infected patients have no known exposures for this potentially debilitating illness.

22. **What complications are associated with HCV?**
    - Cirrhosis
    - Hepatocellular carcinoma (HCC)
    - Decompensated liver disease requiring liver transplantation

23. **What are the differences among hepatitis A, B, and C?**
    Hepatitis A, called "infectious hepatitis," is easily spread by the fecal/oral route. The hepatitis A virus (HAV) causes a short-lived, acute hepatitis that is not followed by chronic liver disease. Immunoglobulin G (IgG) antibodies to HAV remain positive for life. To determine whether the hepatitis is acute, one must look for IgM antibodies in the serum.

Hepatitis B, called "serum hepatitis," is contracted by contact with blood or other bodily secretions from an infected individual, usually through a break in the skin, sexual contact, perinatal transmission, use of a contaminated needle in IV drug users, or accidental needlestick in health-care workers. Transmission through blood transfusions is less common when blood donors are volunteers and are screened for hepatitis B surface antigen (HBsAg). Unlike HAV, the (HBV) may cause chronic disease and cirrhosis AND predisposes to HCC (hepatoma). A carrier state occurs when infected patients demonstrate persistent HBsAg without clinically evident disease and are able to transmit the disease.

Hepatitis C is the form of hepatitis most commonly contracted from blood transfusion. HCV infection is the most common viral cause of chronic liver disease and increases the patient's risk for developing hepatoma (HCC).

24. **Who should receive the HAV vaccine?**
    - All children 1 year of age (12–23 months old)
    - Travellers to endemic areas
    - Military personnel and others with occupational exposure
    - Users of illegal injectable and noninjectable drugs
    - People with high-risk sexual practices (e.g., men who have sex with men)
    - Children and adolescents in communities with routine HAV vaccination due to high incidence
    - Patients with clotting factor disorders
    - Patients with chronic liver disease
    - People who work with infected primates or in an HAV research laboratory

25. **Summarize the usual serologic response to naturally acquired HBV infection.** See Figure 7-1.

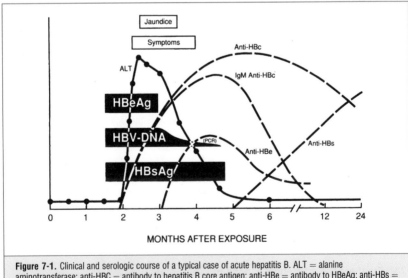

Figure 7-1. Clinical and serologic course of a typical case of acute hepatitis B. ALT = alanine aminotransferase; anti-HBC = antibody to hepatitis B core antigen; anti-HBe = antibody to HBeAg; anti-HBs = antibody to HbsAg; HBeAg = hepatitis Be antigen; HBsAg = hepatitis B surface antigen; HBV-DNA = hepatitis B virus DNA; PCR = polymerase chain reaction. (From Hoofnagle JH: Acute viral hepatitis. In Mandell GL, Bennett JE, Dolin R, et al [eds]: Principles and Practice of Infectious Diseases, 4th ed. New York, Churchill Livingstone, 1995, p 1143.)

26. **How should you treat a health-care worker with a recent (<48 hr) needlestick exposure to HBV?**
By administering hepatitis immunoglobulin, 0.06 mL/kg intramuscularly (IM), as soon as possible and within 7 days of exposure. If the health-care worker has not previously received the HBV vaccine, the vaccination program should be initiated with the usual three doses—the first dose within 14 days after exposure and again at 1 and 6 months.

27. **How is HCV transmitted? What are the possible courses of the disease?**
Blood transfusions, shared and/or contaminated needles among IV drug abusers, intranasal drugs, high-risk sexual behavior, tattoos, and vertical transmission from infected mothers to unborn children (accounts for 3–6%). Nearly 30% of persons infected with HCV have no known risk exposure. Detection of HCV-RNA by polymerase chain reaction is the definitive test for active HCV. Chronic infection developed in at least 55–85% of affected persons. Five to 20% of persons infected will develop cirrhosis over a period of 20–25 years, and they are at risk for the development of HCC.

28. **How can HCV transmission be prevented? How is HCV infection treated?**
Risk modification to minimize exposure is the only means of prevention. No vaccine is available for HCV. The standard treatment regimen for patients with HCV infection consists of pegylated interferon given weekly in combination with oral ribavirin for 24–48 months. Patients with genotype 2 or 3 have higher sustained virologic response rate of 80%, whereas patients with type 1 or 4 have lower sustained virologic response rates of about 50%.

29. **How is hepatitis D virus (HDV; delta virus) transmitted?**
HDV is a very small RNA virus that contains a defective genome and requires HBsAg to become pathogenic. Infection may occur under two circumstances:
- In conjunction with simultaneous infection with HBV in a previously unexposed patient (coinfection).
- In the chronic carrier of HBsAg (superinfection).
    HDV is diagnosed by detecting IgM antibody to HDV in acute serum or an increase in IgG antibody to HDV in convalescent serum.

30. **What is hepatitis E virus (HEV)?**
An enterically (fecal-oral) transmitted non-A, non-B hepatitis. HEV is endemic to Southeast and Central Asia, Africa, and Mexico and is responsible for large epidemics of acute hepatitis in these areas, but is rare in the United States. HEV may be transmitted from animal contact in areas where animal hosts are abundant, including pig farming areas in the United States. HEV illness is particularly severe in pregnant women with mortality rates from acute liver failure approaching 20%.

31. **What is hepatitis G virus (HGV)?**
An RNA virus transmitted primarily through blood and blood products, occurring frequently as a coinfection with HCV or other hepatitis viruses with which HGV shares common modes of transmission. Currently, no data support any role for HGV in chronic or serious liver disease.

32. **What conditions require hospitalization for a patient with acute viral hepatitis?**

Older age	Underlying chronic	PT >15 sec;
Underlying systemic	hepatitis of another	International
illnesses	etiology	Normalized Ratio
Encephalopathy	Volume depletion	(INR) > 1.4
Ascites	or inability to	Albumin < 3 mg/dL
Bilirubin > 15 mg/dL	hold down	Social problems that
Hypoglycemia	fluids	may result in loss
Pregnancy		to follow-up

33. **What blood tests predict fulminant hepatic failure?**
Worsening PT or bilirubin with improving transaminases.

34. **What three conditions result in very high transaminases (>1000)?**
   - Ischemia
   - Viral hepatitis
   - Drug-induced hepatitis

35. **What causes chronic liver disease?**
   - Viral HBV and HCV
   - Wilson's disease
   - Alcoholism
   - Drug-induced disease
   - Autoimmune hepatitis
   - Alpha$_1$ antitrypsin deficiency (AATD)
   - Hemochromatosis
   - Nonalcoholic fatty liver disease (NAFLD)

36. **Discuss the significant features of fulminant hepatic failure.**
Fulminant hepatic failure usually occurs in a previously healthy patient who develops acute and progressive liver failure. Early symptoms include malaise, anorexia, and low-grade fever with progression to signs and symptoms of liver failure (e.g., jaundice, encephalopathy). The mortality rate is approximately 80% if untreated. The most common cause of death in fulminant hepatic failure is either brain edema due to increased intracranial pressure or sepsis. The most definitive therapy is liver transplantation.

37. **List the common causes of fulminant hepatic failure.**
   - **Drugs**: acetaminophen (most common cause of acute liver failure in the United States), amiodarone, Ecstasy (illicit drug), isoniazid, ketoconazole, NSAIDs, rifampin, phenytoin, prophythiouracil, sulfonamides, tetracycline, tricyclic antidepressants, and troglitazone
   - **Indeterminate** (second most common cause of acute liver failure in the United States)
   - **Viral:** HAV, HBV, HCV, HDV, and HEV (HBV is the most common viral causes of fulminant hepatic failure)
   - **Herbal medications**: Jin bu huan, comfrey, germander
   - **Toxins**: *Amanita phalloides*, carbon tetrachloride, trichloroethylene
   - **Vascular**: Budd-Chiari syndrome, veno-occlusive disease, ischemia or hypoxia, portal vein thrombosis
   - **Miscellaneous**: malignant infiltration, Wilson's disease, acute fatty liver of pregnancy, Reye's syndrome, heatstroke, autoimmune hepatitis

38. **What is Budd-Chiari syndrome?**
Partial or complete obstruction of blood flow out of the liver, usually involving the hepatic veins. The patient characteristically presents with hepatomegaly, ascites, and abdominal pain. Underlying etiologies include myeloproliferative disorders (~50%), malignancy, infections of the liver, oral contraceptive pills, pregnancy, collagen vascular diseases, and hypercoagulable states.

39. **What is Wilson's disease?**
An autosomal recessive genetic disorder characterized by an accumulation of copper in the liver, basal ganglia, and cornea with resulting Kayser-Fleischer rings. The Wilson's gene is *ATP7B*, which is either absent or markedly diminished in Wilson's disease. The lack of the gene results in diminished synthesis of ceruloplasmin and/or defective transport of hepatocellular copper into bile for excretion. The diagnosis of Wilson's disease is suspected in patients with low serum ceruloplasmin, increased copper in the liver on biopsy, and increased urinary copper excretion.

40. **What is alpha₁ antitrypsin deficiency (AATD)?**
A relatively common autosomal recessive disease resulting from a defect in the gene for the q arm of chromosome 14. The disorder is characterized by hepatic disease including cirrhosis and HCC, pulmonary emphysema mainly involving the lung bases, panniculitis, vascular disease including arterial aneurysms and fibromuscular dysplasia, and glomerulonephritis. The actual degree of organ involvement depends on the phenotype of the patient.

41. **What is hereditary hemochromatosis (HH)?**
An autosomal recessive disorder resulting from the mutations in the *HFE* gene that lead to increased intestinal iron absorption. Patients with HH have increased iron deposition in their vital organs resulting in liver disease, skin pigmentation, diabetes mellitus, arthropathy, impotence, and cardiac enlargement with heart failure or conduction defects.

NUTRITION

42. **Name six common vitamins and trace minerals and the clinical manifestations of their respective deficiency states.**
   - **Thiamine**: beriberi, muscle weakness, tachycardia, heart failure
   - **Niacin**: pellagra, glossitis
   - **Vitamin A**: xerophthalmia, hyperkeratosis of skin
   - **Vitamin E**: cerebellar ataxia, areflexia
   - **Zinc**: hypogeusia, acrodermatitis
   - **Chromium**: glucose intolerance

43. **What disorders lead to major and minor folate deficiency?**
Major
   - Chronic alcoholism
   - Celiac sprue
   - Tropical sprue
   - Blind loop syndrome
   Minor
   - Crohn's disease
   - Following partial gastrectomy
   Because folate is mainly absorbed in the upper small intestine, malabsorption is worse in disorders that affect the upper gut; however, any intestinal disorder accompanied by a decrease in dietary folate intake or rapid transport may result in folate deficiency.

44. **An elderly man presents with profound peripheral neuropathy and a markedly low serum level of vitamin B_{12}. Physical examination reveals an abdominal scar consistent with previous laparotomy, but the patient does not remember what kind of surgery was done. What two operations may result in vitamin B_{12} deficiency? Why?**
Gastrectomy and terminal ileum resection. Vitamin B_{12} absorption starts in the stomach, where it binds to intrinsic factor and R proteins produced there. In the duodenum, the R proteins are hydrolyzed off the vitamin B_{12} in the presence of an alkaline environment, which then allows for further binding of vitamin B_{12} with intrinsic factor. Vitamin B_{12} cannot be absorbed unless it is bound to intrinsic factor. If the patient's stomach was completely or partially removed, he would have insufficient intrinsic factor.
   This patient may also have had Crohn's disease and undergone resection of a large portion (>100 cm) of terminal ileum, the site of absorption of the vitamin B_{12}–intrinsic factor complex.

45. **How are vitamin B_{12} deficiencies related to surgery treated?**
With IM vitamin B_{12} injections.

46. **What is the most common disorder of carbohydrate digestion in humans?**
Lactase deficiency. Lactase-deficient adults retain 10–30% of intestinal lactose activity and develop symptoms (diarrhea, bloating, and gas) only when they ingest sufficient lactose. Symptoms result from the colonic bacteria metabolizing lactose to methane, carbon dioxide, and short-chain fatty acids.

47. **After avoiding dairy products, the patient's GI symptoms have disappeared. Does this confirm the diagnosis of lactose deficiency?**
No. The diagnosis cannot be made simply by advising the patient to avoid dairy products for 2 weeks to determine whether the altered bowel habits revert to normal because many patients who respond to these manipulations are actually not lactase-deficient. The diagnostic test to be used is the lactose hydrogen breath test.

48. **Outline the fundamental principles of total parenteral nutrition (TPN).**
   - Maintain 25–35 kcal/kg/day.
   - Achieve an optimal calorie-to-nitrogen ratio approximately 160 cal/g N.
   - Provide 30 mL water/kg body weight/day.
   - Provide nonprotein calories through IV lipid emulsions that contribute to conservation of body protein.
   - Provide calories through both dextrose solution and lipid emulsions, with fat providing 20–30% of the total calories.

49. **What are the most common complications of TPN?**
Infections as well as venous thrombosis, nonthrombotic occlusion, and other mechanical complications during line placement. Catheter-related complications can be minimized by maintaining strict and reproducible technique as well as meticulous line care.

50. **What long-term complications may arise?**
   - Liver dysfunction. In prolonged TPN, especially when excessive carbohydrate calories are given, patients frequently develop liver tenderness and transaminase elevations. The increased liver values are thought to reflect hepatic steatosis. AST and ALT abnormalities usually return to normal when TPN is discontinued. If TPN is continued, one should decrease the dextrose infusion and increase the amount of fat calories provided.
   - Metabolic bone disease similar to osteomalacia and osteoporosis. The addition of acetate or phosphate may offset the urinary calcium losses and restore positive calcium balance in these patients.
   - Cholelithiasis and cholecystitis related to gallbladder stasis.

51. **Which vitamin deficiencies might develop in a patient maintained on long-term TPN (> 6 mo) containing only Na^+, K^+, Cl^- HCO_3^-, glucose, and amino acids?**
Magnesium, zinc, and water-soluble vitamins (with the exception of B_{12}). Over several months, vitamin K and copper deficiencies would develop. Over a period of years, deficiencies in the fat-soluble vitamins A and D as well as selenium, chromium, and vitamin B_{12} would result. This preparation is also deficient in essential fatty acids.

52. **What is body mass index (BMI)?**
A calculation determined by the weight in kilograms divided by the height in meters squared (kg/m^2). An online BMI calculator can be accessed at http://www.nhlbisupport.com/bmi/. BMI is the most widely used measure of obesity.

53. **Summarize the standards of weight and obesity according to BMI.**

BMI	CATEGORY
<18.5 kg/m^2	Underweight
18.5–24.9 kg/m^2	Normal
25.0–29.9 kg/m^2	Overweight
>30 kg/m^2	Obese
≥40 kg/m^2	Extreme obesity

54. **Define "obesity." What is its impact on American society?**
A chronic disease of excess body fat. More than 30% of all Americans are categorized as obese. Obesity is at epidemic proportions among school-age children. Fifty percent of all African American and Latino women are obese. Annually, 300,000 deaths are attributable to obesity. Obesity is second only to smoking as a leading cause of preventable death.

55. **What comorbid diseases are directly attributable to obesity?**

Type 2 diabetes mellitus
Hypertension
Pulmonary embolus
Thrombophlebitis
Low back pain
Lower extremity edema
Sleep apnea
Varicose veins
Pickwickian syndrome
Coronary artery disease
Deep venous thrombosis
Lymphedema
Osteoarthritis of hips knees, ankles, and feet
Herniated intravertebral disc
Asthma
Pseudotumor cerebri
Intertriginous dermatitis
Cancer (breast, uterine, and prostate)

56. **What GI disorders are associated with obesity?**
- **Esophagus**: Gastroesophageal reflux disease (GERD) symptoms, erosive esophagitis, Barrett's esophagitis, esophageal adenocarcinoma
- **Gallbladder**: stones and cancer
- **Pancreas**: cancer, worsened acute pancreatitis
- **Colon**: adenoma and cancer
- **Liver**: NAFLD, advanced HCV-related disease, cirrhosis, and HCC
- **Stomach**: nonspecific abdominal pain, bloating, diarrhea, cancer

CANCER

57. **When should screening for colorectal cancer (CRC) begin?**
At age 50 in asymptomatic people without increased risk of CRC.

58. **What are appropriate methods for colon cancer screening?**
- Fecal occult blood testing (FOBT) with high sensitivity or fecal immunochemical testing (FIT): annually.
- Flexible sigmoidoscopy with insertion to the splenic flexure: every 5 years.
- Double-contrast barium enema (DCBE): every 5 years.
- Computed tomographic colonography (CTC): every 5 years.
- Colonoscopy: every 10 years. Colonoscopy should be used to evaluate the patient with a positive FOBT, abnormal DCBE or CTC, or polyp on flexible sigmoidoscopy.

The U.S. Preventive Services Task Force currently recommends the following:

- Annual high-sensitivity FOBT
- Sigmoidoscopy every 5 years with high-sensitivity blood testing every 3 years
- Colonoscopy at 10-year intervals

The Task Force found insufficient evidence to recommend CTC, although the Joint Colorectal Cancer Screening Guideline by the American Cancer Society (ACS), the U.S. Multisociety Task Force (MSTF) on Colorectal Cancer, and the American College of Radiology (ACR) included CTC and fecal DNA testing as possible options.

U.S. Preventive Services Task Force: Screening for Colorectal Cancer: U.S. Preventive Services Task Force Statement, *Ann Intern Med* 149:627, 2008.

59. **List the risk factors for CRC.**
    - Colon cancer in a first-degree relative < 60 years old
    - Chronic ulcerative colitis with involvement beyond left colon
    - Familial adenomatous polyposis
    - Hereditary nonpolyposis colon cancer (HNPCC)
    - Personal history of uterine, endometrial, or breast cancer
    - Lynch's syndrome (HNPCC)
    - Personal history of CRC or adenomatous polyp > 1 cm
    - Cancer family syndrome
    - Advanced age > 80 years

60. **What is the significance of an adenomatous polyp?**
    Adenomatous polyps have malignant potential and are most often in the colon, giving rise to symptoms only when they become large. They are frequently detected incidentally on colonoscopic examination or barium enema. Nearly all colonic carcinomas arise from adenomatous polyps. About 75% of adenomatous polyps are tubular adenomas, 15% are tubulovillous adenomas, and the rest are villous adenomas.

61. **What factors increase the likelihood that a polyp is malignant?**
    Villous tumors are more likely to be malignant than tubular adenomatous polyps. Other factors that relate to malignant potential include tumor size > 1 cm, degree of cellular atypia, and number of polyps present.

62. **How are adenomatous polyps managed?**
    Through endoscopic polypectomy. Patients with polyps should undergo colonoscopy at routine intervals so that additional polyps may be removed before they progress to malignancy.

63. **Summarize the guidelines for repeat surveillance time intervals of patients after polypectomy.**
    - Hyperplastic polyps that should be considered "normal": 10 years.
    - One or two adenomatous polyps < 1 cm, and negative family history of CRC: 10 years.
    - Two adenomatous polyps or adenomatous polyp > 1 cm: 5 years.
    - Villous histology or high-grade dysplasia: 3 years.
    - Family history of CRC: 3 years.
    - Large, sessile, or numerous adenomatous polyps: 3–5 years, based on clinical judgment that should be individualized for each patient.
    - Dirty preparation: Variable based on clinical judgment with acknowledgment that patient had suboptimal examination and, therefore, lesions may have been missed.

- Piecemeal resection of > 2 cm sessile adenoma: 2–6 months to exclude dysplasia of the flat mucosa then subsequent follow-up based on clinical judgment.
- Negative follow-up for new polyps: Every 5 years.

64. **Summarize the guidelines for surveillance of patients after CRC resection.**
Colonoscopy should be performed in the perioperative period to clear the colon of any synchronous lesions. The next colonoscopy following clearing should be 3 years postoperatively *or* according to postpolypectomy surveillance guidelines if a polyp is detected in the perioperative colonoscopy. In the patient with a history of HNPCC, follow-up should be every 1–2 years. In patients with rectal cancer, a flexible sigmoidoscopy or rectal endoscopic ultrasound should be performed every 3–6 months for 2 years because rectal cancer has a greater tendency to recur locally.

65. **Name the most common malignant neoplasms of the small intestine.**
- Adenocarcinoma (45%)
- Carcinoid (34%)
- Leiomyosarcoma (18%)
- Lymphoma (3%)

66. **List, in order of frequency, the most common benign neoplasms of the small intestine.**
Leiomyoma > lipoma > adenoma > hemangioma.

67. **What is the most common primary cancer of the liver?**
HCC ranks fourth in the annual mortality cancer rate in the United States. HCC often coexists with cirrhosis, but it can also occur in noncirrhotic patients, including those with HBV infection.

68. **What are the risk factors for HCC?**
Major risk factors
- Chronic HBV and HCV
- Dietary exposure to aflatoxin B1
- Cirrhosis
Minor risk factors
- Cigarette smoking
- Oral contraceptives
- HH
- Wilson's disease
- AATD

69. **How is HCC diagnosed?**
According to the American Association for the Study of Liver Diseases (AASLD), the diagnosis of HCC is guided by the nodule size and characteristic features on imaging studies.
- For nodule < 1 cm: No initial diagnosis of HCC but surveillance with ultrasound every 3–6 months.
- For nodule from 1–2 cm in a cirrhotic liver: The diagnosis of HCC is made when the lesion has an appearance typical of HCC on two dynamic studies (computed tomography [CT] scan, contrast ultrasound, or magnetic resonance imaging [MRI] with contrast).
- For nodule > 2 cm: the diagnosis of HCC is made when there are typical features of HCC on one dynamic imaging technique or an alpha-fetoprotein (AFP) > 200 ng/mL.
- Biopsy is recommended for nodules > 1 cm when the diagnosis is not clear on dynamic imaging studies or AFP.

70. **What are the GI endocrine tumors and their associated findings and symptoms?**
    - **Gastrinoma (Zollinger-Ellison syndrome [ZES])**: Peptic ulcer disease, diarrhea, and gastric acid hypersecretion. Frequently associated with multiple endocrine neoplasia type I (MEN I).
    - **Insulinoma**: Hypoglycemia.
    - **VIPoma**: Watery diarrhea, hypokalemia, and achlorhydria known as "WDHA syndrome" or "Verner-Morrison syndrome."
    - **Glucagonoma**: Dermatitis, glucose intolerance, weight loss, and anemia.
    - **Somatostatinomas**: Abdominal pain, weight loss.

INFLAMMATORY BOWEL DISEASE

71. **How do Crohn's disease and ulcerative colitis differ?**
    See Table 7-2.

TABLE 7-2. DISTINGUISHING FEATURES OF CROHN'S DISEASE AND ULCERATIVE COLITIS

	Crohn's Disease	Ulcerative Colitis
Symptoms	Pain is more common; bleeding is uncommon	Diarrhea with a bloody-mucosal discharge, cramping
Location	Can affect GI tract from mouth to anus	Limited to colon
Pattern of colonic involvement	Skip lesions	Continuous involvement
Histology	Transmural inflammation, granulomas, focal ulceration	Mucosal inflammation, crypt abscesses, crypt distortion
Radiologic	Terminal ileal involvement, deep ulcerations, normal haustra between involved areas, strictures, fistulas	Rectum involved, shortened colon, absence of haustra (lead-pipe sign)
Complications	Obstruction, fistulas, abscesses, kidney stones, gallstones, vitamin B_{12} deficiency	Bleeding, toxic megacolon, colon cancer

GI = gastrointestinal.

72. **What are the pathologic gold standards for differentiating between Crohn's disease and ulcerative colitis?**
    The finding of a granuloma = Crohn's disease. The finding of crypt abscesses = ulcerative colitis. Again, these findings are documented in fewer than one third of patients, but when found, they are considered pathognomonic for these diseases.

73. **What are the extraintestinal manifestations of inflammatory bowel disease (IBD)?**
    - **Musculoskeletal**: Arthritis, ankylosing spondylitis, sacroileitis, osteoporosis
    - **Mucocutaneous**: erythema nodosum, pyoderma gangrenosum, aphthous ulcers

- **Ocular**: iritis, uveitis, episcleritis
- **Hepatobiliary**: fatty liver, gallstones, pericholangitis, sclerosing cholangitis, cholangiocarcinoma
- **Renal**: kidney stones
- **Miscellaneous**: venous thrombosis, weight loss, hypoalbuminemia, anemia, vitamin and electrolyte disturbances

ULCERS

74. **What are the two major functions of acid secretion in the stomach?**
   - Activation of the enzyme pepsin by converting pepsinogen to pepsin, initiating the first stages of protein digestion.
   - Antibacterial barrier that protects the stomach from colonization.

75. **List the factors that lead to recurrent ulcer after ulcer surgery.**
   - Untreated *Helicobacter pylori* infection
   - NSAID use
   - Incomplete vagotomy
   - Adjacent nonabsorbable suture that acts as an irritant
   - "Retained antrum" syndrome, in which antral tissue left behind at surgery produces a continued source of gastric production
   - Antral G-cell hyperplasia (uncommon)
   - ZES (gastrinoma)
   - Gastric cancer
   Other factors that may contribute to recurrent ulcers but have not necessarily been implicated as primary causes include smoking, enterogastric reflux (bile acid reflux), primary hyperparathyroidism, and gastric bezoar.

76. **List the most common causes of peptic ulcer disease in order of frequency.**
   - *H. pylori* infection (duodenal $>>$ gastric)
   - NSAIDs (gastric $>>$ duodenal)
   - Hyperacidity states (e.g., ZES)

77. **How common is *H. pylori* infection?**
   Approximately 1 in 10 persons worldwide are infected, and *H. pylori* infection is the most infectious disease worldwide. This microaerophilic spiral bacterium that inhabits the mucous layer of the stomach is associated with the development of peptic ulcer disease and occurs in $> 90\%$ of patients with duodenal ulcers. Although millions are infected, only about 10% develop peptic ulcer disease.

78. **Which diseases are strongly associated with *H. pylori* infection?**
   - Peptic ulcer disease (duodenal $>>$ gastric)
   - Chronic active gastritis
   - MALToma (mucosa-associated lymphoid tissue)
   - Gastric carcinoma

79. **How is *H. pylori* infection treated?**
   Over 60 treatment regimens for *H. pylori* have been used. Triple therapy (two antibiotics plus a proton pump inhibitor) is the most widely used regimen, resulting in eradication of *H. pylori* in approximately 80% of patients. At present, no regimen results in 100% cure. Knowledge of the antibiotic resistance patterns in the community assists in antibiotic selection. A typical oral treatment regimen with an eradication rate of 70-80% includes:

- Clarithromycin, 500 mg twice daily
- Amoxicillin, 1000 mg twice daily
- Proton pump inhibitor, maximum dose twice daily

80. **What are the diagnostic tests for *H. pylori*?**
Noninvasive tests (do not require sampling of the gastric mucosa):
- Serologic (IgG antibody, useful for initial diagnosis, but not useful to confirm cure after treatment)
- Urea breath tests (useful to confirm eradication)
- Stool antigen tests (e.g., the *H. pylori* stool antigen test, useful to confirm eradication)
Invasive tests (require sampling of the gastric mucosa):
- Histologic examination
- Special stains for *H. pylori* (Warthin-Starry silver stain, Giemsa stain and El-Zimaity stain)
- Culture
- Urease testing (e.g., Campylobacter-like organism test, hpfast, PyloriTek)

81. **What is the clinical triad of ZES?**
Gastric acid hypersecretion, severe ulcer disease of the upper GI tract, and a non–beta cell pancreatic tumor that secretes the hormone gastrin (gastrinoma).

82. **What are other diagnostic features of ZES?**
In addition to symptoms of peptic ulcer disease (abdominal pain, heartburn, GI bleeding, and weight loss), diarrhea is common and may be present for many years before diagnosis. ZES should be suspected in patients with a compatible clinical history and gastric acid hypersecretion or a personal/family history of MEN I.

83. **How is the diagnosis of ZES made?**
- Serum fasting gastrin concentration $>$ 1000 pg/mL
- Secretin stimulation test with an increase serum gastrin level of $\geq$ 200 pg/mL
- Localization studies: octreotide scan, endoscopic ultrasonography, CT of the abdomen.

PANCREATITIS

84. **What are the most common causes of acute pancreatitis in the United States?**
Choledocholithiasis, ethanol abuse, and idiopathic etiologies account for $>$ 90% of cases of acute pancreatitis in the United States. Most patients previously classified with idiopathic pancreatitis have subsequently been found to have diminutive gallstones (microlithiasis). In the private hospital setting, 50% of patients with acute pancreatitis have gallstones (gallstone pancreatitis). In public hospitals, up to 66% of first episodes are caused by excessive alcohol consumption.

85. **Which drugs have the strongest association with acute pancreatitis?**

Asparaginase	6-mercaptopurine	Pentamadine
Azathioprine	Dideoxyinosine	Vinca alkaloids

86. **List other drugs that may be associated with acute pancreatitis.**
- **Analgesics**: acetaminophen, piroxicam, NSAIDs, morphine
- **Diuretics**: furosemide, thiazides, metolazone
- **Antibiotics**: sulfonamides, tetracyclines, erythromycin, ceftriaxone
- **Anti-inflammatory agents**: salicylates, 5-aminosalicylic acid (5-ASA) products, sulfasalazine, corticosteroids, cyclosporine
- **Toxins**: ethanol, methanol

- **Hormones**: estrogens, oral contraceptive pills
- **Others**: octreotide, cimetidine, valproic acid, ergotamine, methyldopa, propofol, alpha interferons, zalcitabine, isotretinoin, ritonavir, ranitidine

87. **List Ranson's criteria for the prognosis in acute pancreatitis.**
    See Table 7-3.

TABLE 7-3. RANSON'S CRITERIA FOR PROGNOSIS IN ACUTE PANCREATITIS

On Admission	In Initial 48 Hours
Age > 55 yr	Hematocrit decrease of > 10%
WBC > 16,000/mm^3	BUN rise of > 5 mg/dL
Serum LDH > 350 IU/L	Serum calcium < 8 mg/dL
Blood glucose > 200 mg/dL	PaO$_2$ < 60 mmHg
SGOT/AST > 250 IU/L	Base deficit > 4 mEq/L
	Estimated fluid sequestration > 6 L

BUN = blood urea nitrogen; LDH = lactate dehydrogenase; PaO2 = arterial oxygen pressure; SGOT/AST = aspartate aminotransferase; WBC = white blood cell.
From Ranson JH: Etiologic and prognostic factors in human acute pancreatitis: A review. Am J Gastroenterol 77:633–638, 1982.

---

88. **How are Ranson's criteria used to make a prognosis?**
    By calculating the number of criteria present. When there are fewer than three positive signs, the patient has mild disease and an excellent prognosis. The mortality rate is 10–20% with three to five signs and > 50% with six or more signs.

89. **What conditions other than acute pancreatitis may cause an increase in serum amylase?**

    Macroamylasemia
    Renal failure
    Mesenteric infarction
    Parotitis
    Burns
    Cholecystitis
    Post–endoscopic retrograde cholangio-pancreatography

    Perforated peptic ulcer disease
    Ruptured ectopic pregnancy
    Diabetic ketoacidosis
    Peritonitis
    Tumors of pancreas, salivary glands, ovary, lung, prostate

    Pancreatitis complications (pseudocyst, abscess, ascites)

90. **What features of a pancreatic pseudocyst suggest that surgery or percutaneous drainage is indicated?**
    - Development of symptoms, including abdominal pain, nausea, emesis, obstruction (intestinal, biliary), and weight loss
    - Increasing size of pseudocyst
    - Onset of complications (infection)
    - Possible malignancy

91. **What may be a serious vascular complication of pancreatitis?**
    Splenic vein thrombosis, which is associated with pancreatic or peripancreatic inflammation and/or tumors. Splenic vein thrombosis classically results in gastric varices without accompanying esophageal varices. The definitive therapy is surgical splenectomy.

92. **What is chronic pancreatitis?**
    Irreversible damage to the pancreas resulting in inflammation, fibrosis, and destruction of exocrine and endocrine tissue.

93. **What are the causes of chronic pancreatitis?**
    - **Alcohol**: most common cause
    - **Genetic**: mutations in cationic trypsinogen gene (*PRSS*1 mutation), cystic fibrosis transmembrane conductance regulator gene (*CFTR*), and pancreatic secretory trypsin inhibitor gene (*SPINK*1)
    - **Metabolic**: hypercalcemia and hyperlipidemia
    - **Other**: autoimmune, tropical calcific pancreatitis, and pancreatic duct obstruction

VASCULAR DISEASE

94. **What is dysphagia lusoria?**
    Dysphagia causing vascular compression of the esophagus by an aberrant right subclavian artery. The right subclavian artery in dysphagia lusoria arises from the left side of the aortic arch and compresses the esophagus as it courses from the lower left to the upper right side posterior to the esophagus.

95. **What is intestinal angina?**
    Symptoms of pain after eating that occur when all three of the major intestinal arteries (celiac axis, superior mesenteric, and inferior mesenteric) (Fig. 7-2) to the bowel are obstructed by atherosclerosis. Patients with intestinal angina usually have the triad of crampy, epigastric discomfort (postprandial pain), nausea, and occasional diarrhea. The discomfort is similar to that of cardiac angina (substernal chest pressure with exercise), hence the term "intestinal

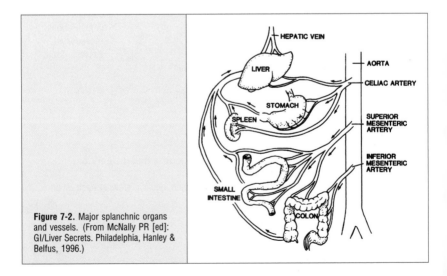

Figure 7-2. Major splanchnic organs and vessels. (From McNally PR [ed]: GI/Liver Secrets. Philadelphia, Hanley & Belfus, 1996.)

angina." Patients lose weight simply by avoiding meals secondary to a fear of recurrent symptoms.

96. **How is chronic mesenteric ischemia diagnosed and treated?**
By noninvasive evaluation using ultrasound and Doppler evaluation of the mesenteric arteries. If the noninvasive tests are suggestive of significant disease, a more invasive angiogram is performed to verify findings. Treatment for severe stenoses is balloon angioplasty and stenting of *both* the celiac axis and the superior mesenteric artery. If occlusions are noted, surgical bypass or endarterectomy is the more accepted therapy.

97. **Which two colonic segments are most commonly involved in ischemic colitis? Why?**
The splenic flexure, which lies between the inferior and the superior mesenteric arteries, and the rectosigmoid junction, which lies between the inferior mesenteric and the interior iliac arteries. Ischemic colitis most commonly occurs in the regions lying in the "watershed" areas between two adjacent arterial supplies.

98. **Describe the presentation of hepatic hemangioma.**
A benign blood vessel tumor that is most commonly found incidentally on imaging examinations of the liver. Hemangiomas are usually single, asymptomatic, and measure < 5 cm. The incidence is thought to range from 0.4–20%.

99. **Define "superior mesenteric artery syndrome."**
A narrowing of the aortomesenteric angle may lead to compression of the duodenum that may be caused by weight loss, immobilization, scleroderma, neuropathies that reduce duodenal peristalsis (e.g., diabetes), and use of narcotics. Because of its anatomic position anterior to the aorta and posterior to the superior mesenteric vessels, the third portion of the duodenum is prone to luminal compression by these vessels.

DIARRHEA

100. **What are the four pathophysiologic mechanisms of diarrhea?**
- **Osmotic**: Due to the presence of an osmotically active agent in the intestinal lumen that cannot be absorbed and, therefore, draws fluid in the intestinal lumen
- **Exudative**: Due to infection, food allergy, celiac sprue, IBD, collagenous colitis, and graft-versus-host disease
- **Secretory**: Due to mucosal stimulation of active chlorine ion secretion associated with *Escherichia coli*, *Vibrio cholerae*, hormone-producing tumors, bile acids, and long-chain fatty acids
- **Altered intestinal transit**

101. **What causes osmotic diarrhea?**
The ingestion of excessive amounts of a poorly absorbable but osmotically active solute. Substances such as mannitol or sorbitol (seen in patients chewing large quantities of sugar-free gum), magnesium sulfate (Epsom salt), and some magnesium-containing antacids can cause osmotic diarrhea. Carbohydrate malabsorption also may cause osmotic diarrhea through the action of unabsorbed sugars (lactulose). Clinically, osmotic diarrhea stops when the patient fasts (or stops ingesting the poorly absorbable solute).

102. **Explain the mechanism of secretory diarrhea.**
Secretory diarrhea involves a disruption of normal bowel function. Small intestinal epithelial cells normally secrete less than they absorb, ultimately leading to a net absorption of fluid and electrolytes. If this process is interrupted by a pathologic process that stimulates increased secretion or inhibits absorption, secretory diarrhea may occur.

103. **Which three diagnostic features can distinguish secretory from osmotic diarrhea?**
See Table 7-4.

TABLE 7-4. SECRETORY VERSUS OSMOTIC DIARRHEA		
	Secretory	**Osmotic**
Stool osmolar gap	<50 mOsm/kg	>50 mOsm/kg
Effect of fasting	None	Ceases
Presence of WBCs, RBCs, fat	None	May be present
RBCs = right blood cells; WBCs = white blood cells.		

104. **What organisms are responsible for bacillary dysentery?**
Shigella, Salmonella, Campylobacter, and enteroinvasive or enterohemorrhagic *E. coli*. The term "dysentery" refers to a diarrheal stool that contains inflammatory exudate (pus) and blood. "Bacillary dysentery" refers to infectious diarrhea caused by invasive pathogens.

105. **A 50-year-old woman complains of six to eight loose stools per day for 1 month. The cause is not immediately evident after a careful history and physical examination. What diagnostic tests should be performed at this stage?**
- **Blood tests**: CBC, serum chemistry profile, urinalysis
- **Stool studies**: Bacterial culture and sensitivity, Sudan stain for fat, Wright's stain, white blood cells (WBCs), occult blood testing, phenolphthalein test for the presence of laxative ingestion

106. **Discuss the role of proctosigmoidoscopy in the diagnosis of diarrhea.**
Proctosigmoidoscopy is a very important part of the examination in most patients with chronic and recurrent diarrhea. In patients aged ≥ 50 years, this should be expanded to a full colonoscopy to allow screening for polyps. Examination of the rectal mucosa may reveal pseudomembranes seen with antibiotic-associated diarrhea, discrete ulceration typical of amebiasis, or a diffusely inflamed granular mucosa seen in ulcerative colitis. Biopsy specimens can be obtained through the scope for histologic examination, and fresh stool samples can be collected for cultures.

107. **What is the most common cause of antibiotic-associated colitis?**
Clostridium difficile. Patients usually have a history of antibiotic use, especially clindamycin or one of the quinolone antibiotics, or recent hospitalization. The diagnosis is based on a history of recent antibiotic use, detection of *C. difficile* toxin A or B in stool sample, or a sigmoidoscopy revealing colonic pseudomembranous.

108. **What are the risk factors for *C. difficile* infection?**
   - Drugs: antibiotic, chemotherapy, or acid antisecretory medication
   - Comorbidity: older age, human immunodeficiency virus (HIV), or IBD
   - Use of an NG tube
   - GI procedures
   - Length of hospital stay

109. **What is traveler's diarrhea?**
   A common term given to the onset of diarrhea in patients who have traveled to other countries, usually in the Third World, where the enteric flora are different. Eighty percent of cases are caused by bacteria that can be transmitted via a fecal-oral route. Viruses account for 10% of cases, and parasites cause 2–3%. In the remainder of cases, the cause is unknown.

110. **How can traveler's diarrhea be prevented?**
   - Eat only foods that are recently cooked and served hot.
   - Avoid nonbottled water, ice, and cold beverages diluted with nonbottled liquids (e.g., fruit juices).
   - Drink only bottled, sealed, carbonated, or boiled beverages.
   - Avoid fresh, unpeeled fruits and vegetables that are washed in nonbottled water.

111. **What are most common organisms implicated in traveler's diarrhea?**

Enterotoxigenic *E. coli*	*Cryptosporidium* spp.	Norwalk virus
Shigella spp.	Enteroaggregative	*Giardia* spp.
Campylobacter jejuni	*E. coli*	*Cyclospora* spp.
Plesiomonas spp.	*Salmonella* spp.	
Rotavirus	*Aeromonas* spp.	

112. **What prophylactic regimens are recommended for traveler's diarrhea?**
   Nonantimicrobial agent
   - Bismuth subsalicylate (Pepto-Bismol), 2 tablets with every meal and at bedtime

   Antimicrobial agents
   - Rifaximin, 200 mg once or twice daily
   - Ciprofloxacin, 500 mg once daily (or one of the other fluoroquinolones)

   The U.S. Centers for Disease Control and Prevention (CDC) currently recommends antibiotic prophylaxis only for short-term travelers with high-risk conditions such as immunosuppression or those taking critical trips where acute diarrhea may significantly impede the trip's purpose.

113. **How does the time of onset of illness relate to the possible causes of food poisoning?**
   See Table 7-5.

TABLE 7-5. CAUSES OF FOOD POISONING

Onset	Symptoms and Signs	Agents
1 hr	Nausea, vomiting, abdominal cramps	Heavy metal poisoning (copper, zinc, tin, cadmium)
1 hr	Paresthesias	Scrombroid poisoning, shellfish poisoning, Chinese restaurant syndrome (MSG), niacin poisoning

(continued)

TABLE 7-5. CAUSES OF FOOD POISONING—*(continued)*

Onset	Symptoms and Signs	Agents
1–6 hr	Nausea and vomiting	Preformed toxins of *Staphylococcus aureus* and *Bacillus cereus*
2 hr	Delirium, parasympathetic hyperactivity, hallucinations, disulfiram reaction, or gastroenteritis	Toxic mushroom ingestion
8–16 hr	Abdominal cramps, diarrhea	In vivo production of enterotoxins by *Clostridium perfringens* and *B. cereus*
6–24 hr	Abdominal cramps, diarrhea, followed by hepatorenal failure	Toxic mushroom ingestion (*Amanita* spp.)
16–48 hr	Fever, abdominal cramps, diarrhea	*Salmonella, Shigella, Clostridium jejuni,* invasive *Escherichia coli, Yersinia enterocolitica, Vibrio parahemolyticus*
16–72 hr	Abdominal cramps, diarrhea	Norwalk agent and related viruses, enterotoxins produced by *Vibrio* spp., *E. coli*, and occasionally *Salmonella, Shigella*, and *C. jejuni*
18–36 hr	Nausea, vomiting, diarrhea, paralysis	Food-borne botulism
72–100 hr	Bloody diarrhea without fever	Enterotoxigenic *E. coli*, most frequently serotype 0157:H7
1–3 wk	Chronic diarrhea	Raw milk ingestion

MSG = monosodium glutamate.
From Mandell GL, Bennett JE, Dolin R, et al (eds): Principles and Practice of Infectious Diseases, 4th ed. New York, Churchill Livingstone, 1995.

NONHEPATITIS LIVER DISEASE

114. **Explain the Child-Pugh system for staging cirrhosis.**
See Table 7-6.

TABLE 7-6. CHILD-PUGH STAGING OF CIRRHOSIS

Parameter	Score 1	Score 2	Score 3
Albumin	>3.5	3.0–3.5	<3.0
Bilirubin	<2.0	2.0–3.0	>3.0
Prologation of PT	<4 sec	4–6 sec	>6 sec
Ascites	None	Moderate	Massive
Encephalopathy	None	Moderate	Severe
Child's score:	A = 5–6	B = 7–9	C = >9

115. **What is a model for end-stage diseases (MELD) score?**
A validated chronic liver disease severity scoring system that uses a patient's serum bilirubin, serum creatinine, and the INR for PT to predict survival. The MELD score is mainly used to allocate donor organs for liver transplantation. A MELD calculator can be found at www.unos.org/resources/MeldPeldCalculator.asp?index=98

116. **Summarize the clinical manifestations of liver disease and their pathogenetic basis.**
See Table 7-7.

TABLE 7-7. CLINICAL MANIFESTATIONS OF LIVER DISEASE

Sign/Symptom	Pathogenesis	Liver Disease
Constitutional		
Fatigue, anorexia, malaise, weight loss	Liver failure	Severe acute or chronic hepatitis Cirrhosis
Fever	Hepatic inflammation or infection	Liver abscess Alcoholic hepatitis Viral hepatitis
Fetor hepaticus	Abnormal methionine metabolism	Acute or chronic liver failure
Cutaneous		
Spider telangiectasias, palmar erythema	Altered estrogen and androgen metabolism	Cirrhosis
Jaundice	Diminished bilirubin excretion	Biliary obstruction Severe liver disease
Pruritus		Biliary obstruction
Xanthomas and xanthelasma	Increased serum lipids	Biliary obstruction/ cholestasis

(continued)

TABLE 7-7. CLINICAL MANIFESTATIONS OF LIVER DISEASE—*(continued)*

Sign/Symptom	Pathogenesis	Liver Disease
Endocrine		
Gynecomastia, testicular atrophy, diminished libido	Altered estrogen and androgen metabolism	Cirrhosis
Hypoglycemia	Decreased glycogen stores and gluconeogenesis	Liver failure
Gastrointestinal		
RUQ abdominal pain	Liver swelling, infection	Acute hepatitis
		Hepatocellular carcinoma
		Liver congestion (heart failure)
		Acute cholecystitis
		Liver abscess
Abdominal swelling	Ascites	Cirrhosis, portal hypertension
GI bleeding	Esophageal varices	Portal hypertension
Hematologic		
Decreased RBCs, WBCs, platelets	Hypersplenism	Cirrhosis, portal hypertension
Ecchymoses	Decreased synthesis of clotting factors	Liver failure
Neurologic		
Altered sleep pattern, subtle behavioral changes, somnolence confusion, ataxia, asterixis, obtundation	Hepatic encephalopathy	Liver failure, portosystemic shunting of blood

GI = gastrointestinal; RBCs = red blood cells; RUQ = right upper quadrant; WBCs = white blood cells. From Andreoli TE, et al (eds): Cecil Essentials of Medicine, 2nd ed. Philadelphia, WB Saunders, 1990, p 312.

117. **A patient with known cirrhosis of the liver presents with massive swelling of the abdomen. A fluid wave can be elicited on examination of the abdomen by striking one flank and feeling the transmitted wave on the opposite flank. What is the appropriate diagnostic procedure at this point?**
Abdominal paracentesis. After the diagnosis of new-onset ascites on physical examination, all patients should undergo abdominal paracentesis with ascitic fluid analysis. A small amount of fluid is aspirated from the midline of the abdomen between the umbilicus and the pubis with a small-gauge needle. The most important tests to order are the serum albumin value and ascitic fluid cell count and albumin.

118. **Explain the significance of the serum albumin value.**
To determine the serum–to–ascitic fluid albumin gradient. The serum albumin value should be measured within a few hours of the abdominal paracentesis to ensure accuracy. Ascitic fluid with a serum–to–ascitic fluid albumin gradient (S-A AG) > 1.1 g/dL is designated as high-gradient ascites. Fluids with values < 1.1 g/dL are designated as low-gradient ascites. The terms "high-albumin gradient" and "low-albumin gradient" should replace the terms "transudative" and "exudative" in the description of ascites.

119. **Which diseases are associated with high-gradient ascites?**

Portal hypertension (i.e., cirrhosis)	Nephrotic syndrome (occasionally)	Meigs' syndrome
Constrictive pericarditis	Congestive heart failure	Fulminant hepatic failure
Hypoalbuminemia	Inferior vena cava obstruction	Mixed ascites
Myxedema		

120. **Which diseases are associated with low-gradient ascites?**

Peritoneal neoplasms	Bowel obstruction or infarction	Nephrotic syndrome
Tuberculosis	Pancreatic ascites	Connective tissue diseases

121. **Explain the significance of the ascitic fluid cell count.**
A large number of RBCs in the fluid or grossly bloody ascites suggests neoplasm. An ascitic fluid WBC count of > 500/mL is strongly suggestive of a peritoneal infection or an inflammatory process.

122. **What other ascitic fluid tests should be considered in the diagnosis of ascites?**
Cytology; lactic dehydrogenase (LDH); specific tumor markers; glucose; and cultures for bacteria, mycobacteria, and fungi.

123. **List the benign primary hepatic lesions.**
- Cavernous hemangioma (most common benign tumor of the liver)
- Focal nodular hyperplasia (composed of nodules of benign hyperplastic hepatocytes)
- Hepatic adenoma (associated with the use of oral contraceptive steroids)
- Bile duct adenoma
- Bile duct hamartoma
- Biliary cyst
- Focal fat

124. **List the malignant primary hepatic lesions.**
- HCC (most common primary malignant tumor of the liver)
- Hepatoblastoma (most common malignant tumor of the liver in children)
- Intrahepatic cholangiocarcinoma (originates from small intrahepatic bile ducts)
- Angiosarcoma (most common malignant mesenchymal tumor of the liver)
- Biliary crystadenoma and/or carcinoma
- Sarcoma

125. **How is acetaminophen toxic to the liver?**
Through the accumulation of the toxic metabolite of acetaminophen, *N*-acetyl-p-benzoquinone. When the dosage of acetaminophen is excessive or the protective detoxifying pathway in the liver is overwhelmed the metabolite accumulates and leads to hepatocyte death. Acetaminophen is the second most common cause of death from poisoning in the United States.

126. **At what doses does acetaminophen become toxic to the liver?**
>7.5 g in nonalcoholic patients. A potentially lethal effect is seen with ingestion of > 140 mg/kg (10 g in a 70-kg man). Chronic alcoholics are at greater risk of acetaminophen injury due to alcohol induction of the cytochrome P450 system and attendant malnutrition and low levels of glutathione. Glutathione is an intracellular protectant naturally found in the hepatocyte.

127. **What are contraindications to liver transplantation?**
- Extrahepatic malignancy
- Acquired immunodeficiency syndrome (AIDS)
- Active/ongoing substance abuse
- Uncontrolled systemic infection
- Inability to comply with the posttransplant immunosuppression regimen
- Advanced cardiopulmonary disease

128. **What is the most prevalent liver disease in the United States?**
Nonalcoholic steatohepatitis (NASH), also known as "nonalcoholic fatty liver disease (NAFLD)." This disease is present in approximately 20% of the American population and perhaps as high as 30–80% of people who are obese. NAFLD is clinically silent except for abnormal liver tests and is most often discovered incidentally, but it can be progressive and result in end-stage liver disease. Imaging studies usually show steatosis of the liver.

ESOPHAGEAL DISEASE

129. **Describe the approach to treatment of GERD.**
See Table 7-8.

130. **What are the extraesophageal manifestations of GERD?**
- **Cardiac**: atypical chest pain, arrhythmias, ischemia, electrocardiogram (ECG) abnormalities.
- **Vocal cords**: laryngitis, granuloma, polyps, ulcers, neoplasm.
- **Respiratory**: adult-onset asthma, recurrent bronchitis, aspiration or chronic interstitial pneumonia, irreversible airway disease, pulmonary fibrosis, sleep apnea, chronic or recurrent cough.
- **Pharyngeal**: globus sensation (globus pharynges), pharyngitis, recurrent sore throat, hoarseness.
- **Oral**: burning mouth syndrome, dental erosions.
- **Other**: sudden infant death syndrome, otitis media.

131. **How is extraesophageal GERD treated?**
With proton pump inhibitors twice daily for a minimum of 3 months.

132. **What is Barrett's esophagus?**
A complication that develops in patients with longstanding reflux peptic esophagitis that represents a unique reparative process in which the original squamous epithelial cell lining of the esophagus is replaced by a metaplastic columnar-type epithelium. In most adults, this epithelium resembles intestinal mucosa, complete with goblet cells.

133. **Summarize the clinical significance of Barrett's esophagus.**
There is an increased risk (30- to 125-fold above the general population) of esophageal adenocarcinoma arising in Barrett's epithelium. The actual incidence is unknown, but the average is approximately 10%. Currently, adenocarcinoma of the junction, which primarily arises from Barrett's epithelium, is the fastest growing GI cancer among white men in the United States.

TABLE 7-8. TREATMENT OF GASTROESOPHAGEAL REFLUX DISEASE

Dietary and Lifestyle Changes

- Postural therapy: elevate head of bed 6–8 inches; avoid lying down after eating; remain upright at least 2 hr after eating (most important lifestyle change).
- Limit intake of foods and drink that reduce LES pressure: fatty foods, peppermint, acidic foods, onions, chocolate, caffeine, alcohol.
- Avoid medications that reduce LES pressure: theophylline, nitrates, tranquilizers, progesterone, calcium blockers, anticholinergic agents, beta adrenergic agonists.
- Stop smoking.
- Decrease the size of meals.
- Weight reduction if obese (BMI > 30).
- Avoid tight-fitting garments around abdomen.

Proton Pump Inhibitor

- Most potent single agent for treating severe reflux esophagitis (e.g., omeprazole, lansoprazole, rabeprazole, pantoprazole, and esomeprazole).
- Acts to increase the pH of gastric contents and heal erosive esophagitis.

Endoscopic Therapy

- To increase LES pressure.

Surgery (Endoscopic or Open)

- Aimed at restoring LES competence or preventing reflux.

BMI = body mass index; LES = lower esophageal sphincter.

---

134. **How is Barrett's esophagus managed?**
In a similar way as GERD. Acid suppression with proton pump inhibitors in high doses controls symptoms and heals esophageal damage. Although the inflammatory changes associated with Barrett's epithelium can be healed, once Barrett's epithelium has developed, the process cannot be reversed by any form of antireflux therapy.

135. **Is routine surveillance for esophageal cancer necessary in patients with Barrett's esophagus?**
Probably. The benefits of periodic endoscopic screening for dysplasia have not been shown, but endoscopic surveillance and four-quadrant biopsies of each 2-cm segment of the esophagus at 2-year intervals are advocated by most experts.

136. **Name the three types of esophageal dysphagia.**
   - **Transfer**: Pathologic alteration in the neuromotor mechanism of the oropharyngeal phase.
   - **Transit**: Abnormal peristalsis and lower esophageal sphincter (LES) function. Transit dysphagia is due to motor disorders in which the primary peristaltic pump of the esophagus fails.
   - **Obstructive**: Mechanical narrowing of the esophagus. Obstructive dysphagia may be due to intrinsic lesions blocking the esophagus (e.g., peptic strictures, esophageal webs, carcinoma) or to extrinsic lesions (e.g., mediastinal tumors) compressing the esophagus.

137. **Describe the typical history of a patient with transfer dysphagia.**
Difficulty in swallowing liquids, while solids pass normally. Transfer dysphagia is frequently seen in patients with stroke, myasthenia gravis, amyotrophic lateral sclerosis, or botulism.

138. **What is the typical history of a patient with transit dysphagia?**
Difficulty in swallowing both liquids and solids. Transit dysphagia is commonly seen in such entities as achalasia and scleroderma. Dysphagia that worsens on ingesting cold liquids and improves with warm liquids suggests a motor disorder of transit dysphagia.

139. **How does obstructive dysphagia typically present?**
Difficulty in swallowing solids that may progress to difficulty in swallowing liquids. Patients usually give a history of eating only soft foods, chewing foods longer, and avoiding steak, apples, and fresh bread. Solid-food dysphagia associated with a long history of heartburn and regurgitation suggests a peptic stricture. If the bolus can be dislodged by repeated swallowing or drinking water, a motor disorder is usually the cause.

140. **What is the initial diagnostic step for obstructive dysphagia after a thorough history and examination?**
An upper GI endoscopy is the standard for diagnosis and any therapeutic intervention.

141. **Define "achalasia."**
A disorder of unknown etiology with lack of peristalsis in the lower esophagus and failure of the LES to relax. Achalasia is the best-known motor disorder of the esophagus and usually occurs in patients aged 25–60 years, with an equal frequency between the sexes. Symptoms include dysphagia with solids, liquids, regurgitation of undigested foods, heartburn, and chest pain.

142. **How is achalasia diagnosed?**
By esophageal manometry, which yields the following characteristic findings:
- Loss of peristalsis (absolute requirement)
- Failure of the LES to relax
- Increased LES pressure

143. **Define "pseudoachalasia."**
Other esophageal conditions that mimic the clinical and x-ray findings of achalasia. The majority of causes are neoplasms that obstruct the LES either directly by tumor or as a paraneoplastic disorder. Common causes are amyloidosis, sarcoidosis, Chagas' disease, eosinophilic gastroenteritis, neurofibromatosis, idiopathic intestinal pseudo-obstruction, Anderson-Fabry disease, and MEN IIB.

144. **How is 24-hour pH monitoring endoscopy used to assess patients with suspected esophageal disease?**
Through correlation of symptoms with a temporal profile of acid reflux events and acid clearance. Specific variables measured include the number of reflux episodes in 24 hours, acid clearance times from the esophagus, and esophageal exposure to acid. These values can be determined while the patient is in the upright or recumbent position. pH monitoring is the gold standard for documenting or excluding GERD and determining whether atypical GERD symptoms are a result of acid reflux. Anyone who undergoes surgery for GERD must have a 24-hour pH probe and esophageal manometry.

145. **Summarize the role of esophageal manometry in the assessment of esophageal disease.**
To evaluate patients with noncardiac chest pain and a history suggestive of esophageal motor disorder, achalasia, or esophageal reflux disease.

146. **Why is endoscopy useful in assessing esophageal disorders?**
It provides a direct view of the esophageal mucosa and allows directed biopsy when necessary. Endoscopy and biopsy are necessary to make a definitive diagnosis of many esophageal diseases (e.g., malignancy). The benefits of endoscopy include the ability to perform therapeutic intervention such as biopsy, cytology, brushing, dilatations, and stent placement.

MALABSORPTION

147. **What causes Whipple's disease?**
Tropheryma whippelii, a bacterium. Whipple's disease is a systemic disease that may affect almost any organ system of the body, but in most cases, it involves the small intestine. Patients present with intestinal malabsorption, weight loss, diarrhea, abdominal pain, fever, anemia, lymphadenopathy, and arthralgias. Nervous system symptoms, pericarditis, or endocarditis may also be present.

148. **How is Whipple's disease diagnosed?**
By small intestinal biopsy that shows infiltration of involved tissues with large glycoprotein-containing macrophages that stain strongly positive with a periodic acid–Schiff stain. One can also see characteristic rod-shaped, gram-positive bacilli that are not acid-fast.

149. **How is Whipple's disease treated?**
With prolonged antibiotic therapy, usually oral double-strength trimethoprim/sulfamethoxazole given for a minimum of 1 year. Repeat intestinal biopsy should document the disappearance of the Whipple bacillus before therapy is discontinued. Relapses are common and are retreated for a minimum of 6–12 months. Patients allergic to sulfonamides should receive parenteral penicillin.

150. **In a small bowel biopsy, the mucosa shows flat villa with markedly hyperplastic crypts. What is the diagnosis?**
Celiac sprue, also called "gluten enteropathy." Celiac sprue is an allergic disease characterized by malabsorption of nutrients secondary to the damaged small intestinal mucosa. The responsible antigen is gluten, a water-insoluble protein found in cereal grains such as wheat, barley, oats, and rye. Withdrawal of gluten from the diet results in complete remission of both the clinical symptoms and the mucosal lesions. Although this disease is present worldwide, the distribution varies; the highest prevalence is in western Ireland.

151. **What is dermatitis herpetiformis?**
A pruritic skin condition that may be reversed with gluten restriction and is characterized by papulovesicular lesions in a symmetrical distribution on the elbows, knees, buttocks, face, scalp, neck, and trunk.

152. **How does dermatitis herpetiformis relate to celiac sprue?**
Patients with dermatitis herpetiformis usually have the spruelike mucosal lesion in the small bowel, although most patients with celiac sprue do not develop skin lesions of dermatitis herpetiformis. The two diseases appear to be distinct entities that respond to the same dietary restrictions. Unlike the intestinal disease, the skin lesions can be treated with the antibiotic dapsone, with a clinical response within 1–2 weeks.

153. **What is the blind-loop syndrome?**
A constellation of symptoms and laboratory abnormalities that include malabsorption of vitamin B_{12}, steatorrhea, hypoproteinemia, weight loss, and diarrhea attributed to overgrowth

of bacteria within the small intestine. Bacterial overgrowth is associated with a number of diseases and surgical abnormalities. The common link between these conditions is abnormal motility of a segment of small intestine, resulting in stasis. The aim of therapy is to reduce the bacterial overgrowth and consists of antibiotics and, when feasible, correction of the small intestinal abnormality that led to the condition.

KEY POINTS: GASTROENTEROLOGY ✓

1. Proton pump inhibitors should be given 15–30 min prior to a meal to be most effective.

2. CT scan with contrast is the most accurate radiographic test to diagnose pancreatitis.

3. Hepatocellular carcinoma is the fifth most common malignancy worldwide—accounting for > 1 million deaths/yr.

4. The mechanism for GERD is inappropriate, transient relaxation of the lower esophageal sphincter.

5. Irritable bowel syndrome is more common in men in areas outside the United States.

6. The two most common symptoms of GERD are heartburn (burning sensation that patients feel behind the breast bone area) and regurgitation (effortless passage of fluid into the back of the mouth or throat).

7. In patients presenting with lower GI bleeding no definite source is found in ~20% at the time of endoscopy.

8. Bariatric surgery is the most effective management of morbid/extreme obesity.

9. The U.S. incidence of GI cancers has declined overall except adenocarcinoma of the GE junction.

10. Nearly 25% of patients are inappropriately diagnosed with lactose intolerance based upon dietary symptoms.

CT = computed tomography; GE = gastroesophageal; GERD = gastroesophageal reflux disease; GI = gastrointestinal.

154. **Describe the process of normal fat absorption.**
Normal fat absorption requires all phases of digestion to be intact. The process begins with secretion of pancreatic lipase and colipase. These enzymes are activated intraluminally and require an optimal pH of 6–8. Both enzymes are necessary for triglyceride hydrolysis in the duodenum. The products of triglyceride hydrolysis (i.e., fatty acids and monoglycerides) then must be solubilized by bile salts to form micelles, which are subsequently absorbed by the small intestinal epithelium.

155. **What mechanisms may lead to fat malabsorption?**
   ■ Deficiencies of pancreatic enzyme secretion.
   ■ Presence of an acidic intraluminal environment
   ■ Interruption of the enterohepatic circulation or secretion of bile salts may impair micelle formation
   ■ Diseased intestinal epithelial cell leading to impairment of monoglyceride absorption and processing into chylomicrons for transport
   ■ Diseased intestinal lymphatics with impaired chylomicron transport

156. **Which diseases can affect fat absorption?**
    - Chronic pancreatitis
    - Cystic fibrosis
    - Pancreatic carcinoma
    - Postgastrectomy syndrome
    - Biliary tract obstruction
    - Terminal ileal resection or disease
    - Cholestatic liver disease
    - Intestinal epithelial disease (Whipple's disease, sprue, eosinophilic gastroenteritis)
    - Lymphatic disease (abetalipoproteinemia, intestinal lymphangiectasia, lymphoma, tuberculous adenitis)
    - Small bowel bacterial overgrowth (bile salts are deconjugated and inactivated by bacteria)
    - ZES (low intraluminal pH)

157. **What type of kidney stones are most often seen in a person with fat malabsorption?**
    Calcium oxalate stones. Fat malabsorption leads to excess free fatty acids in the intestine, which then bind to luminal calcium, decreasing the calcium available to bind and clear oxalate. The increased luminal oxalate is absorbed, resulting in hyperoxaluria, which leads to calcium oxalate stone formation in the kidney.

158. **Summarize the pathologic mechanism of small bowel bacteria overgrowth. How is it diagnosed?**
    Any abnormality of the small intestine that results in local stasis or recirculation of intestinal contents is likely to be associated with marked proliferation of intraluminal bacteria. The gold standard for diagnosing bacterial overgrowth is a culture of aspirate from the upper small bowel showing > 100,000 colony-forming units (CFU)/mL.

159. **What disorders are associated disorders with small bowel bacteria overgrowth?**
    - Hypochlorhydric or achlorhydric states that lead to gastric proliferation of bacteria particularly when in combination with motor or anatomic disturbances
    - Small intestinal stagnation associated with anatomic alterations following surgery, such as afferent loop syndrome after a Bilroth II procedure
    - Duodenal and jejunal diverticulosis, particularly as seen in scleroderma
    - Surgically created blind loops, such as end-to-side anastomoses
    - Chronic low-grade obstruction secondary to small intestinal strictures, adhesions, inflammation, or carcinoma
    - Motor disturbances of the small intestine (e.g., scleroderma, idiopathic pseudo-obstruction, diabetic neuropathy)
    - Abnormal communication between the proximal small intestine and the distal intestinal tract, as seen in gastrocolic or jejunocolic fistulas or resection of the ileocecal valve
    - Immunodeficiency syndromes (e.g., AIDS, primary immunodeficiency states, malnutrition)

160. **How does bacterial overgrowth of the small bowel result in fat malabsorption?**
    Through the excess production of enzymes that deconjugate intraluminal bile salts to free bile acids. Free bile acids are reabsorbed in the jejunem and are, therefore, unable to solubilize monoglycerides and free fatty acids into micelles for absorption by the intestinal epithelial cells. The result is impaired absorption of fat and fat-soluble vitamins.

161. **What constitutes a normal fecal fat concentration? What is steatorrhea?**
Normal concentration is 4–6 g/day, ranging to an upper limit of normal of approximately 7 g/day. The typical U.S. diet consists of 100–150 g of fat/day. Fat absorption is extremely efficient, and most of the ingested fat is absorbed with very little excretion into the stool. Patients with steatorrhea, or increased excretion of fecal fat, may have up to 10 times this amount in the stool.

162. **How is steatorrhea detected?**
Through a 72-hour stool sample collected while the patient is on a defined dietary fat intake of > 100 g/day. Chemical analysis of the stool collection measures the amount of fat present. This test is highly reliable but neither specific nor sensitive in determining the etiology of steatorrhea.

OBSTRUCTION

163. **Name the four most common causes of mechanical small bowel obstruction in adults.**
- Adhesions ($\sim$74%)
- Hernias (8%)
- Malignancies of the small bowel (8%)
- IBD with stricture formation

164. **Define "small bowel ileus."**
Distention due to intestinal muscle paralysis. Paralytic ileus is a relatively common disorder and occurs when neural, humoral, and metabolic factors combine to stimulate reflexes that inhibit intestinal motility.

165. **What seven entities may cause small bowel ileus?**
- Abdominal surgery
- Peritonitis
- Generalized sepsis
- Electrolyte imbalance (especially hypokalemia)
- Retroperitoneal hemorrhage
- Spinal fractures
- Pelvic fractures

166. **What role do drugs play in small bowel ileus?**
Drugs such as phenothiazines and narcotics inhibit small bowel motility and also may contribute to paralysis.

167. **How is small bowel ileus treated?**
With NG suction to relieve distention and IV fluids to replace fluid losses, followed by correction of the underlying disorder.

168. **What conditions may aggravate or be associated with colonic pseudo-obstruction?**
See Table 7-9.

169. **What are bezoars?**
Clusters of food or foreign matter that have undergone partial digestion in the stomach then failed to pass through the pylorus into the small bowel, forming a mass in the stomach. Substances typically composing bezoars include hair (trichobezoars) and, more commonly, plant matter (phytobezoars).

TABLE 7-9. CONDITIONS ASSOCIATED WITH COLONIC PSEUDO-OBSTRUCTION

1. Trauma (nonoperative) and surgery (gynecologic, orthopedic, urologic)
2. Inflammatory processes (pancreatitis, cholecystitis)
3. Infections
4. Malignancy
5. Radiation therapy
6. Drugs (narcotics, antidepressants, clonidine, anticholinergics)
7. Cardiovascular disease
8. Neurologic disease
9. Respiratory failure
10. Metabolic disease (diabetes, hypothyroidism, electrolyte imbalance, uremia)
11. Alcoholism

---

170. **How do patients with bezoars present?**
With abdominal mass, gastric outlet obstruction, attacks of nausea and vomiting, and peptic ulceration when bezoars become large. Factors important in the formation of bezoars include the amount of indigestible materials in the diet (pulpy, fibrous fruit or vegetables such as oranges), the quality of the chewing mechanism, and loss of pyloric function, which limits the size of food particles that may enter the duodenum.

BILIARY TRACT DISEASE

171. **Which U.S. ethnic groups have the highest prevalence of cholesterol gallstone formation?**
American Indians and Mexican Americans.

172. **List the types of gallstones.**
- **Cholesterol** (70–80% of all stones in Western countries): Risks are female gender, obesity, age > 40 years, and multiparity.
- **Pigmented** (20–30%).
- **Black calcium bilirubinate**: Risks are cirrhosis, chronic hemolytic syndromes.
- **Brown calcium salts**: Can form de novo in bile ducts; risks are infections of biliary system.

173. **What is Charcot's triad?**
Right upper quadrant pain, jaundice, and fever. Charcot's triad is present in approximately 50% of patients with bacterial cholangitis.

174. **What is Reynold's pentad?**
Charcot's triad (right upper quadrant pain, jaundice, and fever), plus hypotension and altered mental status.

175. **Which tests are used in the initial diagnostic evaluation of a patient with suspected obstructive jaundice?**
Clinical history, physical examination, and routine laboratory tests (serum total and unconjugated or indirect bilirubin, alkaline phosphatase, PT, ALT, AST, and albumin). The only special study that is routinely useful in the early evaluation of obstructive jaundice is an ultrasound of the gallbladder, bile ducts, and liver. Ultrasound is fairly specific for detecting gallstones and ductal dilatation (the latter signifying ductal obstruction). However, a

negative ultrasound does not prove the absence of stones or obstruction, because the sensitivity of ultrasound in detecting obstruction is only about 90%.

176. **What are the advantages of endoscopic ultrasound (EUS)?**
   - Noninvasive
   - Images the entire pancreaticobiliary system
   - Detects presence of tumors, stones, or strictures
   - Can be used with fine-needle aspiration for biopsy or tissue samples

177. **Discuss the role of CT in the evaluation of obstructive jaundice.**
   Abdominal CT is fairly sensitive for detecting ductal dilatation and can be useful in localizing the site of ductal obstruction. A CT scan is less able to detect stones of the gallbladder and common bile duct than ultrasound, but it is better able to image mass lesions and to evaluate the pancreas.

178. **Is magnetic retrograde cholangiopancreatography (MRCP) useful in the evaluation of obstructive jaundice?**
   Yes. MRCP is a useful diagnostic tool in the evaluation of jaundice. MRCP can reveal the size of the ducts and document presence of stones and other masses. In many centers, the MRCP has supplanted the diagnostic endoscopic retrograde pancreatography (ERCP) as a primary screening modality.

179. **Are liver scans helpful in the evaluation of jaundice?**
   No. Liver scan in the patient with extrahepatic ductal obstruction is not routinely useful. It may reveal evidence of cholestasis and cholangitis but will not help to determine the cause. A liver scan using technetium sulfur colloid is of very little value in the jaundiced patient.

180. **What causes air in the biliary system?**
   - Previous surgery or endoscopy procedures (most common)
   - Penetrating ulcers
   - Erosion of gallstone into the bowel lumen
   - Traumatic fistula
   - Neoplasms
   - Bowel obstruction

IRRITABLE BOWEL SYNDROME

181. **What is irritable bowel syndrome (IBS)?**
   A functional bowel disorder that is characterized by at least 3 months, which do not have to be consecutive, in the past 12 months of abdominal discomfort or pain that has two or three of the following Rome III criteria:
   - Relief with defecation; and/or
   - Onset associated with a change in frequency of stool; and/or
   - Onset associated with a change in form or appearance of stool

182. **What findings suggest organic disease instead of IBS?**

New onset of symptoms in an elderly patient	Weight loss	Diarrhea that awakens the patient
Pain that interferes with normal sleep patterns	Anemia	Fever
	Blood in the stools	Steatorrhea
	Pain on awakening from sleep	Physical examination abnormalities

183. **What is the differential diagnosis of IBS?**

Psychiatric disorders
(depression,
anxiety,
somatization)
Diabetes
Scleroderma

IBD
Chronic pancreatitis
Postgastrectomy
syndromes
Side effects of
medications

Hypothryoidism
Lactose malabsorption
Endocrine disorders
Celiac sprue
Infectious diarrhea

WEBSITES

1. The DAVE project: www.daveproject.org
2. GastroSource: www.gastrosource.com
3. Medscape Gastroenterology: www.medscape.com/gastroenterology
4. UpToDate: www.uptodate.com
5. WebMD: www.webmd.com

BIBLIOGRAPHY

1. Feczko PJ, Halpert RD, editors. *Case Review: Gastrointestinal Imaging*, St. Louis, 2000, Mosby.
2. Lichetenstein GR, Wu GD, editors. *The Requisites in Gastroenterology: Vol 2: Small and Large Intestines*, St. Louis, 2003, Mosby.
3. Reddy KR, Long WB, editors. *The Requisites in Gastroenterology: Vol 3: Hepatobiliary Tract and Pancreas*, St. Louis, 2003, Mosby.
4. Rustgi AK, editor: *The Requisites in Gastroenterology: Vol 1: Esophagus and Stomach*, St. Louis, 2003, Mosby.
5. Feldman M, Friedman LS, Brandt LJ, editors. *Gastrointestinal and Liver Disease: Pathophysiology, Diagnosis, and Management*, ed 8, Philadelphia, 2006, WB Saunders.
6. Tytgat GNJ, Classen M, Waye JD, et al: *Practice of Therapeutic Endoscopy*, ed 2, London, 2000, WB Saunders.
7. United Network for Organ Sharing: *MELD/PELD calculator*. Available at: www.unos.org/resources/MeldPeldCalculator.asp?index=98. Accessed December 14, 2008.

CHAPTER 8

NEPHROLOGY

Sharma S. Prabhakar, M.D., M.B.A., F.A.C.P., F.A.S.N.

> *Present facilities cannot care for [all those] being treated [on dialysis].... [A]n anonymous committee of laymen has been set up to narrow the selection [and] includes a bank president, a labor leader, a minister, two physicians, a housewife and a lawyer. It must choose who is to live and who is to die.*
>
> "Panel Holds Life-or-Death Vote in Allotting of Artificial Kidney"
> *The New York Times*, May 6, 1962

ASSESSMENT OF RENAL FUNCTION

1. **What is the glomerular filtration rate (GFR)?**
   The ultrafiltrate of plasma that exits the glomerular capillary tuft and enters Bowman's capsule to begin the journey along the tubule of the nephron. The GFR is the initial step in the formation of urine and is usually expressed in milliliters per minute.

2. **How is the GFR measured clinically?**
   Indirectly with a marker substance contained in glomerular filtrate, which is then excreted in the urine. The amount of this substance leaving the kidney (urinary mass excretion) must equal the amount of marker substance entering the kidney as glomerular filtrate. The marker substance must not be reabsorbed, secreted, or metabolized after entering the kidney tubule. The marker substance is chosen so that its concentration in the glomerular filtrate is equal to its concentration in the plasma (i.e., the substance is freely filterable across the glomerular capillary). Therefore, the amount of substance X entering the kidney equals the GFR multiplied by the plasma concentration of the substance (P_x). Likewise, the amount of the substance leaving the kidney in the urine equals the urinary concentration of the substance (U_x) multiplied by the urine flow in mL/min (V). Therefore, the formula for calculating GFR using our marker substance X becomes:

   $$GFR \times P_x = U_xV \; or \; GFR = U_xV/P_x$$

   A stable plasma concentration of the substance (steady-state situation) is required to make this equation useful.

3. **Why is creatinine used as a marker substance for GFR determinations in clinical settings?**
   Because creatinine is an endogenous substance, derived from the metabolism of creatine in skeletal muscle and fulfills almost all of the requirements for a marker substance: it is freely filterable, not metabolized, and not reabsorbed once filtered. A small amount of tubular secretion makes the creatinine clearance a slight overestimate of the GFR, but this overestimate becomes quantitatively important only at low levels of GFR. Creatinine is released from muscle at a constant rate, resulting in a stable plasma concentration. The creatinine clearance is commonly determined from a 24-hour collection of urine. This time period is used to average out the sometimes variable creatinine excretion that may occur from hour to hour. Creatinine is easily measured, making it a nearly ideal marker for GFR determination.

4. **Is any other substance used as a marker of GFR in laboratory settings?**
The polysaccharide **inulin** is often used in laboratory determinations of GFR. However, it requires constant intravenous infusion, making it somewhat impractical for routine clinical use in patients.

5. **Can the completeness of a 24-hour urine collection be judged?**
Yes, by knowing the estimated creatinine excretion value. Because total creatinine excretion in the steady state is dependent on muscle mass, day-to-day creatinine excretion remains fairly constant for an individual and is related to lean body weight. In general, men excrete 20–25 mg creatinine/kg body weight/day, whereas women excrete 15–20 mg/kg/day. Therefore, a 70-kg man excretes approximately 1400 mg creatinine/day. Creatinine excretion levels measured on a 24-hour urine collection that are substantially less than the estimated value suggest an incomplete collection.

6. **What is the relationship between the plasma creatinine concentration (P_{Cr}) and GFR?**
Because creatinine production and excretion remain constant and equal, the amount of creatinine entering and leaving the kidney (urinary creatinine [U_{Cr}]) remains constant. Thus:

$$\text{GFR} \times P_{Cr} = U_{Cr} \times V = \text{constant} \ or \ \text{GFR} = (1/P_{Cr}) \times \text{constant}$$

Creatinine excretion remains constant as GFR declines until the GFR reaches very low levels. Therefore, the GFR is a function of the reciprocal of the P_{Cr}.

7. **Does a given P_{Cr} reflect the same level of renal function in different patients?**
Not necessarily. Remember that creatinine production is directly proportional to muscle mass, and that the P_{Cr} is determined in part by creatinine production. Examination of the creatinine clearance (C_{Cr}) for an 80-kg man compared with that of a 40-kg woman, assuming both individuals have P_{Cr} of 1.0 mg/dL (0.01 mg/mL), shows the following:
For the 80-kg man, creatinine excretion should be:

$$80 \text{ kg} \times 20 \text{ mg/kg/day} = 1600 \text{ mg/day} = 1.11 \text{ mg/min}$$

$$\text{GFR} = (1.11 \text{ mg/min})/(0.01 \text{ mg/mL}) = 111 \text{ mL/min}$$

For the 40-kg woman, creatinine excretion should be:

$$40 \text{ kg} \times 15 \text{ mg/kg/day} = 600 \text{ mg/day} = 0.42 \text{ mg/min}$$

$$\text{GFR} = (0.42 \text{ mg/min})/(0.01 \text{ mg/mL}) = 42 \text{ mL/min}$$

This example demonstrates that the same P_{Cr} can represent markedly different GFRs in different individuals.

8. **What formulas are used to estimate GFR when a measured C_{Cr} is not immediately available?**
The following formula was first devised to provide a rough estimate of the GFR when a measured C_{Cr} is not immediately available:

$$C_{Cr(mL/min)} = \frac{(140 - age \ in \ years) \times lean \ body \ weight \ in \ kg}{(P_{Cr} \times 72)} \times (0.85 \text{ if female})$$

This is the Cockcroft-Gault formula, which gives C_{Cr} in milliliters per minute. These estimates are in the range of those determined previously and serve to illustrate the relative differences in the GFR calculated for two individuals with the same P_{Cr}. Recognizing this fact and using this formula to estimate GFR could prevent a serious error when selecting the dose of a drug that is excreted by the kidneys. The modification of diet in renal disease (MDRD) formula is now the most used method (and has replaced the use of Cockcroft-Gault formula in many instances) to estimate the GFR (eGFR) in the context of CKD:

$$eGFR = 170 \times SCr^{-1.154} \times age^{-0.203} \times [1.21 \text{ if black}]or[0.74 \text{ if female}] \times BUN^{-0.170}$$
$$\times \text{ albumin}^{+0.138}$$

where the serum creatinine (SCr) and blood urea nitrogen (BUN) concentrations are both in mg/dL. The albumin concentration is in g/dL. The GFR is expressed in mL/min/1.73 m^2. However, this formula underestimates the GFR in healthy people with GFR > 60 mL/min. The **Chronic Kidney Disease Epidemiology Collaboration (CKD-EPI) formula** was developed recently to circumvent this problem:

$$eGFR = 141 \times \min(Scr/k, 1)^a \times \max(Scr/k, 1)^{-1.209} \times 0.093^{age} \times (1.108 \text{ if female}) \text{ or}$$
$$\times (1.159 \text{ if black})$$

where k is 0.7 for females and 0.9 for males, a is −0.329 for females and −0.411 for males, min indicates the minimum of SCr/k or 1, and max indicates the maximum of SCr/k or 1. This formula is slowly replacing the MDRD formula to estimate C_{Cr}.

Levey AS, Stevens LA, Schmid CH, et al: A new equation to estimate glomerular filtration rate, *Ann Intern Med* 50:604–612, 2009.

9. **How does the BUN relate to the GFR?**
   BUN is excreted primarily by glomerular filtration and the plasma level tends to vary inversely with GFR. BUN, however, is a much less ideal marker of GFR than is creatinine. The production of urea is not constant and varies with protein intake, liver function, and catabolic rate. In addition, urea can be reabsorbed once filtered into the kidney, and this reabsorption increases in conditions with low urine flow, such as volume depletion. Volume depletion is one cause of a high (>15:1) BUN-to-creatinine ratio in plasma. Thus, creatinine is the better marker for GFR. The plasma level of BUN can be used along with the C_{Cr} to indicate the presence of certain states, such as volume depletion.

10. **What is the difference between urinary excretion and clearance?**
    Urinary **excretion** of a substance is simply the total amount of a substance excreted per unit of time, usually expressed in mg/min. **Clearance** expresses the efficiency with which the kidney removes a substance from the plasma. The volume of plasma that must be completely cleared of a substance per unit of time accounts for the amount of that substance appearing in the urine per unit of time. Clearance is expressed in volume per unit of time, usually mL/min.

11. **Give an example of clearance.**
    Substance (X) with a plasma concentration (P_x) of 1.0 mg/mL, urine concentration (U_x) of 10 mg/mL, and urine flow (V) of 1.0 mL/min has the following clearance:

    $$Cl_x = (U_x/P_x) \times V = (10 \text{ mg/mL} \times 1 \text{ mL/min})/1.0 \text{ mg/min} = 10 \text{ mL/min}$$

    The calculated clearance of 10 mL/min indicates that the amount of substance X appearing in the urine is the same as if 10 mL of plasma were completely cleared of the substance and excreted in the urine each minute. The urinary excretion of X is 10 mg/min, but this measurement does not indicate the efficiency with which the substance is removed from the plasma.

12. **How does measurement of urinary protein excretion help in the evaluation of renal disease?**
    Normal urinary protein excretion < 150 mg/day, with albumin constituting < 50% of this protein. Failure of the tubules to reabsorb the normally filtered small-molecular-weight (MW) proteins leads to **tubular proteinuria.** This occurs in diseases that affect tubular function, and the proteins are almost entirely of smaller MW rather than albumin. **Glomerular proteinuria** occurs when the normal glomerular barrier to the passage of plasma proteins is disrupted. This results in variable quantities of albumin and sometimes larger MW proteins

spilling into the urine. Quantitatively, tubular proteinuria is usually < 1 g/24 hr, and glomerular proteinuria is usually > 1 g/24 hr. When the proteinuria > 3.5 g/1.73 m^2 body surface area, it is said to be in the **nephrotic range.** Significant degrees of proteinuria (>150 mg/day) could indicate intrinsic renal disease. Quantification and characterization of the proteinuria are useful in detecting the presence of renal disease and also in determining involvement of the tubule, glomerulus, or both.

13. **What information can be gained from examining urine sediment?**
Urine sediment is normally almost cell free, is usually crystal free, and contains a very low concentration of protein ($<1+$ by dipstick). Examination of this sediment is an important part of the work-up of any patient with renal disease. The examination should be performed by the physician before diagnostic or therapeutic decisions are made. The information must be correlated with all other aspects of the patient's history, physical examination, and laboratory database. The examination can provide evidence of many conditions, including renal inflammation (cells, protein), infection (white blood cells [WBCs], bacteria), stone disease (crystals), and systemic diseases (e.g., bilirubin, myoglobin, and hemoglobin).

14. **Define "oliguria."**
A urine volume that is inadequate for the normal excretion of the body's metabolic waste products. Because the daily load of metabolic products amounts to approximately 600 mOsm and the maximal urine concentrating ability of the human kidney is about 1200 mOsm/kgH$_2$0, there is a minimal obligate urine volume of 500 mL/day for most people. Therefore, a 24-hour urine volume $<$ **500 mL/day** is said to represent oliguria. When associated with acute kidney injury (AKI), oliguria portends a poorer prognosis than does nonoliguric AKI.

15. **Define "anuria."**
A 24-hour urine volume < 100 mL. Anuria denotes a severe reduction in urine volume that is commonly associated with obstruction, renal cortical necrosis, or severe acute tubular necrosis (ATN). It is important to make the distinction between oliguria and anuria so that these diagnostic entities will be considered and appropriate therapy planned.

PROTEINURIA, NEPHROTIC SYNDROME, AND NEPHRITIC SYNDROME

16. **List the four general mechanisms by which abnormally increased urinary protein excretion (>150 mg/day) occurs.**
   - Glomerular
   - Tubular
   - Overflow
   - Secretory

17. **What causes glomerular proteinuria?**
Damage to the glomerular filtration barrier (in glomerulonephritis), leading to leakage of plasma proteins into the glomerular ultrafiltrate.

18. **Describe the mechanism behind tubular proteinuria.**
Suboptimal reabsorption of the normally filtered protein as a result of tubular disease. This recovery of the small amount of normally filtered protein (usually ~2 g/day) allows for the normal excretion of < 150 mg/day of protein.

19. **Explain overflow proteinuria.**
Proteinuria resulting from disease states that lead to excessive levels of plasma proteins (e.g., in multiple myeloma). The proteins are filtered and overload the reabsorptive capacity of the renal tubules.

20. **What is secretory proteinuria?**
Proteinuria that occurs because of the addition of protein to the urine after glomerular filtration. The protein may come from the renal tubules (e.g., Tamm-Horsfall protein from the ascending limb of the loop of Henle) or from the lower genitourinary (GU) tract.

21. **What conditions are associated with heavy proteinuria despite severely reduced GFR?**
Usually glomerular disease. In most glomerular diseases, proteinuria tends to decrease with diminishing GFR as the filtration of proteins also tends to decrease. However, in certain conditions, such as diabetic nephropathy, amyloidosis, focal glomerulosclerosis, and probably reflex nephropathy, proteinuria (often in the nephrotic range) persists despite severely diminished GFR.

22. **Define "nephrotic syndrome."**
A symptom complex resulting from various etiologies and characterized by heavy proteinuria (usually >3.5 g/day), generalized edema, and lipiduria with hyperlipidemia. Because all the other features are a consequence of marked proteinuria, some authorities restrict the definition of "nephrosis" to heavy proteinuria alone.

23. **What are the common causes of nephrotic syndrome in adults and children?**
In **adults,** the most common cause is diabetes nephropathy, which is a secondary cause of nephritic syndrome. Membranous nephropathy is the most common primary glomerulopathy in adults. In **children,** the most common cause of nephrotic syndrome is minimal change disease, also called "lipoid nephrosis" or "nil disease." Other causes of nephrotic syndrome include focal and segmental glomerulosclerosis and amyloidosis.

24. **When evaluating patients with nephrotic syndrome, which diseases must you rule out before considering the syndrome to be due to a primary renal disease?**
   - Drugs that may result in excessive urinary protein excretion (gold and penicillamine)
   - Systemic infections (hepatitis B and C, human immunodeficiency virus [HIV], malaria)
   - Neoplasia (lymphomas)
   - Multisystem collagen vascular diseases (systemic lupus erythematosus [SLE])
   - Diabetes mellitus (DM)
   - Heredofamilial diseases (Alport's syndrome)

25. **Why is it important to distinguish primary renal disease from these conditions?**
The distinction between these causes and primary renal disease is important for a number of reasons. Diagnostically, identification of some of these processes may help to identify the renal lesion without the need for a renal biopsy (as in DM). Treatment of such disorders may involve simple discontinuation of the offending agent (e.g., a drug). Management may need to be directed at a systemic disease (infection) rather than at the renal lesion itself.

26. **Name the common complications of the nephrotic syndrome.**
   - **Edema** and **anasarca**.
   - **Hypovolemia** with acute prerenal or parenchymal renal disease or both. In the nephrotic syndrome, decreased effective arterial blood volume can lead to various degrees of renal underperfusion, resulting in renal failure in severe cases.
   - **Protein malnutrition** due to massive protein losses in excess of dietary replacement.
   - **Hyperlipidemia,** which raises the risk of atherosclerotic cardiovascular disease.

- **Increased susceptibility to bacterial infection** often involving the lungs, meninges (meningitis), and peritoneum. Common organisms include Streptococcus (including *Streptococcus pneumoniae*), *Haemophilus influenzae*, and *Klebsiella* spp.
- **Proximal tubular dysfunction** leading to Fanconi's syndrome with urinary wasting of glucose, phosphate, amino acids, uric acid, potassium, and bicarbonate.
- **Hypercoagulable state** manifested by an increased incidence of venous thrombosis, particularly in the renal vein, which may be due to urinary loss of antithrombotic factors.

27. **Define "nephritic syndrome."**
A renal disorder resulting from diffuse glomerular inflammation characterized by the sudden onset of gross or microscopic hematuria, decreased GFR, oliguria, hypertension (HTN), and edema. Nephritic syndrome results from many different etiologies but is traditionally represented by postinfectious glomerulonephritis following infections with certain strains of group A beta-hemolytic streptococci.

28. **What are the various causes of an acute nephritic syndrome?**
   - **Postinfectious glomerulonephritis**: bacterial (pneumococci, *Klebsiella* spp., staphylococci, gram-negative rods, and meningococci), viral (varicella, infectious mononucleosis, mumps, measles, hepatitis B, and coxsackievirus), rickettsial (Rocky Mountain spotted fever, and typhus), and parasitic (e.g., *Falciparum* malaria, toxoplasmosis, and trichinosis)
   - **Idiopathic glomerular diseases**: membranoproliferative glomerulonephritis, mesangial proliferative glomerulonephritis, and immunoglobulin A (IgA) nephropathy
   - **Multisystem diseases**: SLE, Henoch-Schönlein purpura, essential mixed cryoglobulinemia, and infective endocarditis
   - **Miscellaneous**: Guillain-Barré syndrome and post-irradiation of renal tumors

29. **Are the syndromes of nephritis and nephrosis mutually exclusive?**
No. Some forms of glomerular diseases are characteristically nephrotic in their presentation whereas some aggressive forms of proliferative glomerulopathies present as nephritic syndrome. Some others manifest mixed features (Table 8-1).

TABLE 8-1. INTERRELATIONSHIP OF MORPHOLOGIC AND CLINICAL MANIFESTATIONS OF GLOMERULAR INJURY

	Nephrosis	Nephritis
Minimal change glomerulopathy	++++	
Membranous glomerulopathy	+++	
Focal glomerulosclerosis	++	+
Mesangioproliferative glomerulopathy	++	++
Membranoproliferative glomerulopathy	++	+++
Proliferative glomerulonephritis	+	+++
Acute diffuse proliferate glomerulonephritis	+	++++
Crescentic glomerulonephritis		++++

From Mandal AK, et al: Diagnosis and Management of Renal Disease and Hypertension. Philadelphia, Lea & Febiger, 1988, p 248.

30. **A 62-year-old man with nephrotic syndrome is found to have no systemic etiology. What is the differential diagnosis?**
As opposed to minimal lesion in children, minimal lesion on renal biopsy in an elderly patient warrants an extensive search to rule out underlying malignancy, especially lymphomas (both Hodgkin's and non-Hodgkin's) and other solid tumors (e.g., renal cell carcinoma). One third of elderly patients with membranous nephropathy have underlying malignancy (colon, stomach, or breast).

GLOMERULAR DISORDERS

31. **Define "primary glomerulopathy."**
A heterogeneous group of kidney diseases in which the glomeruli are predominantly involved. Extrarenal involvement, if present, is usually secondary to consequences of the glomerular insult. Most of these disorders are idiopathic. The cardinal manifestations of the primary glomerular disorders or glomerulopathy are proteinuria, hematuria, alterations in GFR, and salt retention leading to edema, HTN, and pulmonary congestion.

32. **What are the characteristics of the clinical syndromes that are manifested by the primary glomerulopathies?**
   - **Acute glomerulonephritis**: Acute onset of variable degrees of hematuria, proteinuria, decreased GFR, and fluid and salt retention that is usually associated with an infectious agent and tends to resolve spontaneously.
   - **Nephrotic syndrome**: Insidious onset characterized primarily by heavy proteinuria of usually > 3.5 g/day in an adult and usually associated with hypoalbuminemia, lipidemia, and anasarca.
   - **Chronic glomerulonephritis**: Insidious onset of vague symptoms with progressive renal insufficiency and a protracted downhill course of 5–10 years' duration. Varying degrees of proteinuria, hematuria, and HTN are present.
   - **Rapidly progressive glomerulonephritis (RPGN)**: Subacute onset of symptoms but with rapid progression to renal failure and no tendency toward spontaneous recovery. Patients are usually hypertensive, hematuric, and oliguric.
   - **Asymptomatic urinary abnormalities**: No clinical symptoms but microscopic hematuria and/or proteinuria (usually < 3 g/day).

33. **How does routine urinalysis help in the evaluation of a primary glomerular disease?**
In glomerular disease, the urinary sediment usually conforms to one of three different forms:

NEPHROTIC	NEPHRITIC	CHRONIC
Heavy proteinuria	Red cells	Less proteinuria and hematuria
Free fat droplets	Red cell casts	Broad, waxy casts
Oval fat bodies	Variable proteinuria	Pigmented granular casts
Fatty casts	Frequent white cell	
Variable hematuria	and granular cells	

Schreiner GE: The identification and clinical significance of casts, *Arch Intern Med* 99:356–369, 1957.

34. **Which strains of streptococci cause poststreptococcal glomerulonephritis (PSGN)?**
Only certain serotypes of group A (beta-hemolytic) streptococci are nephritogenic. Type 12 is the most common type, but types 1, 2, 3, 18, 25, 49, 55, 57, and 60 are also nephritogenic.

In contrast, all strains of streptococci can cause acute rheumatic fever, which is why the incidence of nephritis differs from that of rheumatic fever in outbreaks of streptococcal infection. The M-protein in streptococci is poorly linked to nephritogenicity. Recent evidence indicates that nephritogenicity is more closely related to endostreptosin, a cell membrane antigen. Other streptococcal cytoplasmic antigens and autologous antigens also have been implicated.

35. **What abnormalities are seen in patients with PSGN?**
The urinalysis in PSGN is characterized by a nephritic sediment, high specific gravity, and nonselective proteinuria. The proteinuria is < 3 g/day in > 75% of patients, although proteinuria in the nephrotic range is occasionally seen. Pyuria is often noted, indicating glomerulitis. Hematuria is almost always present in either gross (smoky urine) or microscopic form. Red blood cell (RBC) casts, if present, are very diagnostic. Dysmorphic erythrocytes are found in abundance. However, a benign urinary sediment does not rule out acute PSGN if clinical features are suggestive. In some cases, biopsy studies have confirmed PSGN.

36. **What is the prognosis in acute PSGN? What are the poor prognostic signs?**
In **children,** the immediate and late prognosis are quite favorable in both epidemic and sporadic cases. A diuresis occurs in 1 week, and SCr returns to normal in 3–4 weeks. The mortality in acute cases is < 1%, and chronic sequelae are uncommon. Microscopic hematuria may last 6 months, and proteinuria may persist for as long as 3 years in 15% of patients. In **adults,** the prognosis is good in epidemic forms but less predictable in sporadic cases.

37. **What are the poor prognostic signs in PSGN?**
In **adults,** severe impairment of renal function at the onset, persistent proteinuria, elderly age, and crescent formation on biopsy are poor prognostic factors. In **children,** the factors indicating a poor prognosis include persistent heavy proteinuria, extensive crescents or atypical humps in initial biopsy, and severe disease in the acute phase requiring hospitalization.

38. **What is RPGN?**
Histologically, RPGN is characterized by extensive glomerular crescent formation, in most cases involving over 75% of glomeruli. The cells of the crescents are thought to be derived from blood-borne monocytes.

39. **Is RPGN synonymous with crescentic nephritis?**
No. RPGN is strictly a clinical expression, whereas crescentic nephritis denotes the histologic picture in such patients. Several primary glomerulopathies demonstrate variable degrees of crescent formation, but they do not progress as rapidly as in RPGN.

40. **Define "fibrillary" and "immunotactoid glomerulonephritis (GN)."**
These are two related yet distinct glomerular diseases characterized by deposition of Congo red–negative fibrils and characterized by a variety of light microscopic features and progressive clinical course. **Fibrillary GN** is defined as Congo red-negative fibrils < 30 nm in diameter, whereas **immunotactoid GN** is defined by glomerular deposition of hollow stacked microtubules > 30 nm in diameter. Both entities are relatively uncommon, accounting for less than 1% of native renal biopsies. Recurrence of these diseases is common after transplantation.

Rosenstock JL, Markowitz GS, Valeri AM, et al: Fibrillary and immunotactoid glomerulonephritis: Distinct entities with different clinical and pathologic features, *Kidney Int* 63:1450–1461, 2003.

41. What are the renal manifestations of infective endocarditis?

Initially, microscopic or gross hematuria and proteinuria. Renal failure is usually mild or absent. The histologic examination in these cases reveals focal proliferative glomerulonephritis. Rarely, a rapidly progressive renal failure with extensive crescent formation is reported. Nephrotic syndrome is rare. Serum IgG and C3 levels are often decreased, and immunofluorescence often demonstrates IgG, IgM, and subendothelial and subepithelial deposits, suggesting an immune-complex etiology.

42. What are the current strategies for treatment of lupus nephritis?

Active treatment of HTN, especially with angiotensin-converting enzyme (ACE) inhibitors, delays the progression of all classes of lupus nephritis. In general, classes II and V lesions are amenable to therapy and are associated with better prognosis. A combination of cyclophosphamide (oral or intravenous [IV]) with oral low-dose steroids is effective in improving the prognosis of classes III and IV lupus nephritis. IV pulse cyclophosphamide has become popular in view of less gonadal and bladder toxicities. Azathioprine and mycophenolate mofetil are used as alternates to cyclophosphamide. Treatment is generally ineffective in class VI lesions.

Berden JHM: Lupus nephritis, *Kidney Int* 52:538–558, 1997.

43. What are the main causes of recurrent isolated glomerular hematuria?

- Berger's disease (IgA nephropathy)
- Thin basement nephropathy
- Idiopathic hypercalciuria

Berger's disease and thin basement nephropathy may require biopsy for confirmation.

44. What are the signs and symptoms of Berger's disease?

Recurrent episodes of painless hematuria, often gross, and presence of RBC casts in urine. HTN and proteinuria are often minimal or modest. Only 25% of the patients progress to end-stage renal disease (ESRD). Berger's disease is the most common primary glomerulopathy worldwide.

DIABETIC RENAL DISEASE

45. What is the incidence of renal involvement in DM?

Among type 1 diabetics, 40–60% develop chronic kidney disease (CKD) between 10 and 30 years after onset of DM. Although about one third of type 2 diabetics develop proteinuria, only 4% develop nephrotic syndrome and 6% develop ESRD. However, owing to the large number of type 2 diabetics, they constitute the majority of diabetics on dialysis. DM contributes up to 40% of all cases of ESRD in the United States.

46. What is the earliest evidence of renal involvement in DM?

An increase in GFR of 25–50% (hyperfiltration) and a slight enlargement of the kidney (hypertrophy) that persists for 5–10 years. At this stage, there may be a slight increase in albumin excretion rate (microalbuminuria), but the total protein excretion remains in the normal range. Studies indicate that patients with this "microalbuminuria" (>20 μg/min of albumin) are more likely to develop overt diabetic nephropathy than those who do not exhibit microalbuminuria. The clinical phase starts with the appearance of proteinuria (corresponding to > 300 mg/day) on urine dipstick.

47. **Why is diabetic nephropathy associated with large kidneys?**
Elevated levels of growth hormone, often seen with uncontrolled hyperglycemia, are incriminated in this renal hypertrophy; however, the exact etiology remains unknown. Renal size is increased early in the course of diabetic renal disease and involves hypertrophy and hyperplasia.

48. **What interventions are used for renal protection in diabetic nephropathy?**
Control of blood pressure, blood sugar levels, and dietary protein restriction has been shown to decrease proteinuria and retard the progression of renal failure. The hyperfiltration and hypertrophy seen early in the course of diabetic nephropathy can be corrected with insulin treatment. Strict glycemic control can reverse the elevated GFR and renal hypertrophy and also can decrease the spontaneous or exercise-induced microalbuminuria seen in the preclinical phase. Renin-angiotensin system inhibitors are also renoprotective.

49. **What are the goals of glucose and blood pressure control in diabetic patients?**
Maintenance of a blood glucose level within or close to the normal range while avoiding hypoglycemic attacks and maintaining a hemoglobin A_1c < 7%. However, once overt nephropathy begins and progressive renal insufficiency ensues, the benefit of tight glycemic control is still observed, although less pronounced than in the preclinical phase. HTN control significantly slows the progression of diabetic nephropathy. The blood pressure target level is < 130/80 mmHg for patients without proteinuria and < 125/75 mmHg for patients with significant proteinuria. ACE inhibitors have been shown to slow diabetic nephropathy progression, as do angiotensin receptor blockers (ARBs). The more recent Action to Control Cardiovascular Risk in Diabetes (ACCORD) and Action in Diabetes and Vascular Disease: Preterax and Diamicron Modified Release Controlled Evaluation (ADVANCE) trials, though, suggest that a lower hemoglobin A_1c may be associated with increased cardiovascular mortality, although these data continue to be analyzed carefully. At this time, most experts continue to recommend modification of all cardiovascular risk factors, including control of blood glucose and HTN.

Boyko EJ: ACCORD glycemia results continue to puzzle, *Diabetes Care* 33:1149–1150, 2010.

Diabetes Control and Complications Trial Research Group: The effect of intensive treatment of diabetes on the development and progression of long-term complications in insulin-dependent diabetes mellitus, *N Engl J Med* 329:977–986, 1993.

The Action to Control Cardiovascular Risk in Diabetes Study Group: Effects of intensive glucose lowering in type 2 diabetes, *N Engl J Med* 358:2545–2559, 2008.

The ADVANCE Collaborative Group: Intensive blood glucose control and vascular outcomes in patients with type 2 diabetes, *N Engl J Med* 358:2560–2572, 2008.

50. **How do inhibitors of the renin-angiotensin-aldosterone system (RAAS) slow the renal disease in diabetic nephropathy?**
Activation of RAAS occurs early in diabetic nephropathy and contributes to glomerular HTN by causing efferent arteriolar constriction. The resulting hyperfiltration leads to microalbuminuria, which predisposes to overt proteinuria. In addition, angiotensin II directly leads to oxidative stress. Other intracellular mediators result in functional and structural demise of the kidney in DM. By inhibiting angiotensin II production and action, the inhibitors of RAAS such as ACE inhibitors and ARBs slow down the progression of renal damage in diabetic nephropathy.

51. **What are the agents of choice to treat HTN in DM?**
ACE inhibitors should be the first-line agents in therapy for HTN in DM. Shortly after ACE inhibitors are started, SCr and potassium should be monitored to detect patients who develop hyperkalemia or an abrupt reduction in GFR. If no adverse effects are seen for at least 2 weeks, ACE inhibitors can be safely continued. ARBs can be used in place of ACE inhibitors when the latter are not tolerated. They are the preferred agents in DM in view of their renoprotective effects.

52. **Why are ACE inhibitors preferred in diabetic kidney disease?**
Because ACE inhibitors reduce intraglomerular HTN and thereby reduce proteinuria by decreasing the tone of efferent arterioles. Sufficient data now exist to support the use of ACE inhibitors, especially in diabetic patients with clinical or subclinical renal involvement, to retard the progression of diabetic nephropathy (in terms of both proteinuria as well as renal failure). A recent, large-scale, multicenter, prospective study concluded that captopril treatment was associated with a 50% reduction in the risk of death, dialysis, or transplantation in diabetics. This renal protective effect was independent of blood pressure control. Patients with insulin-dependent DM with microalbuminuria (30–300 mg/day in at least two out of three measurements) or overt albuminuria (>300 mg/day) should receive an ACE inhibitor even in the absence of HTN or renal failure.

Lewis EJ, Hunsicker LG, Bain RP, et al: The effect of angiotensin-converting enzyme inhibition on diabetic nephropathy, *N Engl J Med* 329:1456–1462, 1993.

53. **What other agents may be considered?**
ARBs such as losartan and valsartan are also effective and reno-protective. Direct renin inhibitors (aliskirin) can effectively control hypertension in the context of diabetes. Although effective in controlling blood pressure in renal failure, calcium channel blockers may not be as effective as ACE inhibitors in slowing the renal damage from DM. Nondihydropyridine calcium channel blockers (diltiazem and verapamil) have some renoprotective and antiproteinuric effects, whereas dihydropyridine calcium channel blockers (nifedipine and amlodipine) have no such benefits. Beta blockers may be effective, but their effects on the lipid profile and need for dose modification in renal failure and dialysis make them less desirable.

Parving HH, Smidt UM, Hommel E, et al: Effective antihypertensive treatment postpones renal insufficiency in diabetic nephropathy, *Am J Kidney Dis* 22:188–195, 1993.

54. **Do diabetics with renal failure tolerate dialysis as well as nondiabetics?**
No. Several years ago, it was thought that diabetics were not good candidates for dialytic therapy because about 80% of diabetics with ESRD who were placed on hemodialysis died in the first year. More recently, results have improved significantly. One recent report indicates a 1-year survival of 85% and a 3-year survival of 60% in diabetics on hemodialysis. However, even today, diabetics tend to do poorly compared with nondiabetics. Their 3-year survival is 20–30% less, and their mortality is 2.25 times higher than that of nondiabetics. Atherosclerotic cardiac disease is the most common cause of death, with infections a close second.

ACUTE KIDNEY INJURY

55. **What is AKI?**
A syndrome of many etiologies characterized by a sudden decrease in renal function leading to a compromise in the kidney's ability to regulate normal homeostasis. The kidney is unable to maintain the content and volume of the extracellular fluid or perform its routine endocrine functions. In most cases, AKI is a potentially reversible process. The clinical manifestations of AKI are generally more severe than those associated with chronic renal failure (CKD) because of the rapidity of development of symptoms. Unlike CKD, a cause for AKI can usually be identified and must be addressed to prevent further kidney or other organ damage. AKI is a potentially reversible disorder if the causative factor or factors are identified and corrected, and appropriate supportive care must be given to optimize the chances for recovery of renal function. The etiology of AKI is frequently multifactorial.

56. **What is the RIFLE classification of AKI?**
The Acute Dialysis Quality Initiative group proposed a stratified definition of AKI into five groups. This classification has been proposed to allow consistency across studies and to allow greater ability to compare clinical results (Table 8-2).

TABLE 8-2. RIFLE CLASSIFICATION

	GFR Criteria	Urine Output Criteria
Risk	SCr > 1.5 times baseline or GFR decrease > 25%	<0.5 mL/kg/hr × 6 hr
Injury	SCr > 2.0 times baseline or GFR decrease > 50%	<0.5 mL/kg/hr × 12 hr
Failure	SCr > 3.0 times baseline or GFR decrease > 75%; or SCr > 4.0 mg/dL	<0.5 mL/kg/hr × 24 hr
Loss	Persistent AKI = complete loss of renal function for > 4 wk	
ESRD	End-stage kidney failure > 3 mo	

AKI = acute kidney injury; ESRD = end-stage renal disease; GFR = glomerular filtration rate; RIFLE = risk, injury, failure, loss, ESRD; SCr = serum creatinine.
From Ricci Z, Cruz D, Ronco C: The RIFLE criteria and mortality in acute kidney injury: A systematic review. Kidney Int 73:538–546, 2008.

57. **How are the causes of AKI classified?**
As prerenal, renal, or postrenal.

58. **What is meant by prerenal failure?**
A decrease in renal function resulting from a decrease in renal perfusion. The decrease in renal perfusion leads to functional changes within the kidney, which in turn compromise the kidney's ability to perform its homeostatic functions. This disorder is potentially correctable by addressing the factors leading to renal hypoperfusion. In some cases, renal hypoperfusion can be severe and prolonged enough to result in structural damage and, hence, can lead to the "renal" category of AKI. Therefore, it is important that the prerenal syndrome be identified and corrected promptly.

59. **List the common prerenal causes of AKI in the United States.**
- True volume depletion, as seen with gastrointestinal (GI) losses (vomiting, diarrhea, and bleeding), renal losses (diuretics, osmotic diuresis [glucose], hypoaldosteronism, salt-wasting nephropathy, and diabetes insipidus), skin or respiratory losses (insensible losses, sweat, and burns), and third-space sequestration (intestinal obstruction, crush injury or skeletal fracture, and acute pancreatitis)
- Hypotension (shock)
- Edematous states (heart failure, hepatic cirrhosis, and nephrosis)
- Selective renal ischemia (hepatorenal syndrome, nonsteroidal anti-inflammatory drugs [NSAIDs], bilateral renal artery stenosis, and calcium channel blockers)

60. **List the typical findings in the urine of patients with prerenal azotemia.**
- Low urinary sodium concentration (<20 mEq/L)
- Low fractional excretion of sodium (<1.0%)
- Low free-water excretion (high urine osmolality > 500 and urine specific gravity > 1.015)

61. **What are the renal causes of AKI?**
- **Ischemia**: All causes of severe prerenal disease, particularly hypotension.
- **Nephrotoxins**: Drugs and exogenous toxins. Common examples include aminoglycoside antibiotics, radiocontrast media, cisplatin, and NSAIDs. Rare examples include cephalosporins, rifampin, amphotericin B, polymyxin B, methoxyflurane, acetaminophen

overdose, heavy metals (mercury, arsenic, and uranium), carbon tetrachloride, ethylenediamine tetraacetic acid, and tetracyclines. In addition, heme pigments may lead to rhabdomyolysis (myoglobinuria) and intravascular hemolysis (hemoglobinuria).

62. **Define "acute tubular necrosis (ATN)."**
A syndrome characterized by structural and functional damage of the renal tubules and a functional decrease of glomerular function. If the patient survives, ATN is self-limited, with most patients recovering renal function within 8 weeks. It is most commonly caused by ischemia, but there are a multitude of other causes.

63. **How can the use of urinary indices help to distinguish prerenal failure from ATN?**
Patients with prerenal azotemia have intact tubular function. The kidney, in this setting, is attempting to minimize solute and water excretion in an effort to preserve extracellular fluid volume, and this will be reflected in the urinary excretion of sodium and water. By contrast, the tubules of patients with ATN do not properly recover solutes and water that have been filtered into the kidney.

64. **What are the urinary indices of patients with ATN?**
The urinary indices of patients with ATN reveal the kidney's relative inability to reabsorb sodium (urinary Na > 40 mEq/L and fractional excretion of sodium [FE_{Na^+}]> 3.0%) and to reabsorb water (urine osmolality < 350 mOsm/L and urine specific gravity < 1.010). Remember that there is considerable crossover between renal and prerenal failure with regard to these indices, and hence, no value absolutely indicates one or the other diagnosis. The indices should be used along with other data (i.e., history and physical examination) to arrive at a clinical impression.

65. **How is the FE_{Na^+} calculated?**

$$FE_{Na^+} = (U_{Na^+} \times P_{Cr} \times 100)/(P_{Na^+} \times U_{Cr})$$

where U_{Na^+} and P_{Na^+} = urinary and plasma sodium concentrations (in mEq/L) and U_{Cr} and P_{Cr} = urinary and plasma creatinine in mg/dL.

66. **What is the relevance of FE_{Na^+} to the diagnosis of AKI?**
An FE_{Na^+} value < 1% favors prerenal states, whereas a value > 1% indicates intrarenal states or ATN. The test is more accurate than urinary Na measurement in this differentiation. An FE_{Na^+} < 1% is occasionally reported for various causes of AKI other than prerenal states. In addition, an intact sodium reabsorptive capacity is necessary for the use of this test. Thus, in conditions such as underlying chronic renal disease, hypoaldosteronism, diuretic therapy, or metabolic alkalosis with bicarbonaturia, the FE_{Na^+} will be inappropriately high despite the presence of volume depletion.

67. **What are the postrenal causes of AKI?**
   - Obstruction due to strictures
   - Stones
   - Malignancies
   - Prostatic enlargement

68. **What is renal-dose dopamine?**
A widespread practice to use a low-dose dopamine IV infusion in critically sick patients with oliguria to prevent or treat AKI. This practice is based on the belief that dopamine increases the urine output through direct tubular effects and may also help to increase the tubular delivery of diuretics and renal blood flow. However, in low doses, dopamine may cause

tachycardia and myocardial ischemia. In extreme cases, dopamine may also predispose to digital and bowel ischemia. Low-dose dopamine infusion is not without risk.

Chertow GM, Sayegh MH, Lazarus JM: Is dopamine administration associated with adverse or favorable outcomes in AKI? *Am J Med* 101:49–53, 1996.

69. **List the indications for dialysis in patients with AKI.**
    - Uncontrolled hyperkalemia
    - Acute pulmonary edema
    - Uremic pericarditis
    - Uremic encephalopathy (coma)
    - Bleeding diathesis due to uremia
    - Refractory metabolic acidosis (HCO_3^- 10 mEq/L)
    - Severe azotemia (BUN > 100 mg/dL, SCr > 10 mg/dL)

70. **What are CRRTs? What is their role in AKI?**
    Continuous renal replacement therapies, which are now increasingly used for treatment of AKI. These therapies are slow forms of dialytic treatments that are performed continuously. They are particularly beneficial in patients with hemodynamic instability that may preclude the use of conventional hemodialysis and are specifically advantageous when fluid removal is an important aspect of therapy.

71. **What is the mortality rate of AKI?**
    Approximately 40–60% despite the availability of dialysis. The mortality is worse in the subcategory of patients with a history of surgery or trauma. The prognosis is better in the absence of respiratory failure, bleeding, or infection and also in patients with nonoliguric ATN. AKI in the obstetric setting also has a better prognosis, with only a 10–20% mortality rate.

72. **In which situations do ACE inhibitors lead to AKI?**
    Bilateral renal artery stenosis and renal artery stenosis of a single kidney or transplant kidney. AKI under these conditions may be mediated by ACE inhibitor–induced poststenotic dilatation of efferent arterioles and consequent reduction of glomerular hydrostatic pressure. In normal persons, this effect is offset by dilatation of afferent sites and maintenance of GFR. There have been reports of reversible renal failure in patients with chronic essential HTN treated with ACE inhibitors. In patients with severe nephrosclerosis, GFR depends on angiotensin-induced efferent arteriolar constriction. In patients with decreased effective renal blood flow, as in congestive heart failure, cirrhosis, or nephrosis, systemic hypotension and effective arteriolar dilatation caused by ACE inhibitors result in AKI.

Toto RD, Mitchell HC, Lee HC, et al: Reversible renal insufficiency due to angiotensin-converting enzyme inhibitors in hypertensive nephrosclerosis, *Ann Intern Med* 115:513–519, 1991.

73. **Name the important risk factors for contrast-induced AKI.**

Azotemia (Cr > 1.5 mg/dL)	Dehydration	Contrast medium > 2 mL/kg
Albuminuria > 2+	Uric acid > 8.0 mg/dL	Multiple myeloma with renal insufficiency
HTN	Multiple radiologic studies	
Age > 60 years	Solitary kidney	

Berns AS: Nephrotoxicity of contrast media, *Kidney Int* 36:730–740, 1989.

KEY POINTS: NEPHROLOGY ✔

1. Maintenance of adequate hydration and minimizing the dose of contrast media, combined with the routine use of *N*-acetylcysteine, reduce the frequency of contrast-induced renal failure.

2. Despite the recent advances in dialysis and continuous filtration techniques, mortality remains high in AKI; hence, the need for early detection and intervention, because half of these patients regain normal renal function.

3. Renal replacement therapy in the form of hemodialysis, CAPD, or renal transplantation should be considered once creatinine clearance drops to 10 mL/min (15 mL/min in diabetics).

4. Diabetic patients with microalbuminuria or overt proteinuria should be treated with ACE inhibitors or ARBs even if BP is not elevated.

5. Reduction of proteinuria is critical in the management and prognosis of diabetic and nondiabetic glomerulopathies since proteinuria not only affects the progression of renal disease but is also an independent risk factor for cardiovascular complications.

ACE = angiotensin-converting enzyme; AKI = acute kidney injury; ARB = angiotensin receptor blockers; BP = blood pressure; CAPD = chronic ambulatory peritoneal dialysis.

CHRONIC RENAL FAILURE

74. **List the five stages of CKD.**
    - **Stage 1**: Kidney damage with normal renal reserve (GFR > 90 mL/min)
    - **Stage 2**: Mild renal insufficiency (GFR 60–89 mL/min)
    - **Stage 3**: Moderate renal failure (GFR 30–59 mL/min)
    - **Stage 4**: Severe renal failure or uremic syndrome (GFR 15–29 mL/min)
    - **Stage 5**: ESRD (GFR < 15 mL/min)

75. **Summarize the evolution of CKD through the five stages.**
    Patients with normal renal function have nephron mass in excess of that necessary to maintain a normal GFR. With progressive loss of renal mass, the **renal reserve** is initially lost, and subsequently, there is not a rise of BUN and creatinine or a disturbance of homeostasis. If the progression continues, mild **renal insufficiency** occurs, associated with mild elevation of BUN and creatinine and very mild symptoms, such as nocturia and easy fatigability. With further progression, moderate **renal failure** ensues. Abnormalities of renal excretory function become apparent, including disturbances in water, electrolyte, and acid-base metabolism. Continued worsening of renal function is followed by the stage of severe renal failure with **uremic syndrome,** which includes multiple dysfunction of major organ systems in addition to the abnormalities of excretory function described. Finally, **ESRD** appears, at which time renal replacement therapy (dialysis or transplantation) is required to sustain life.

76. **How do the remaining intact nephrons adapt in the diseased kidney?**
    When nephron mass is lost, the remaining intact (functioning) nephrons compensate to maintain the same excretory function performed by the normal kidney by increasing the GFR and excretion of salt and water. The increased excretory function is accomplished by reducing reabsorption of filtered salt and water, often resulting in polyuria and nocturia.

77. **What happens to the adaptation process in patients with chronic renal insufficiency?**

Patients with chronic renal insufficiency have a reduced ability to respond to changes in intake with appropriate changes in excretory function. The remaining functioning nephrons of persons with decreased GFR are chronically excreting a higher salt load and are, thus, much closer to their maximum salt-excreting ability. Hence, these patients are less able to adjust to an increased salt intake by increasing salt excretion. At the opposite extreme, the remaining nephrons of the patient with a decreased GFR are less able to reduce their high salt excretion to compensate for a reduction in salt intake. These patients are more at risk of becoming salt-depleted in response to salt restriction than are patients with normal renal function.

78. **Why is the renal potassium excretory ability usually well-maintained down to very low (10–15 mL/min) levels of GFR in patients with progressive CKD?**

As is the case for salt excretion, the remaining intact nephrons increase potassium excretion and the level of excretion per nephron is much higher than when there was a full contingent of nephrons, allowing for a total renal K^+ excretion that is nearly normal. In addition, there is evidence that the extrarenal K^+ excretion, especially by the colon, is increased in patients with CKD. By these mechanisms, patients with a significant decrease in GFR are unlikely to be hyperkalemic purely as a result of chronic renal insufficiency. In this clinical situation, if hyperkalemia is seen, consideration should be given to acute rather than chronic renal insufficiency, hormonal disorders (i.e., hyporeninemic hypoaldosteronism), or tubular disorders (i.e., obstructive uropathy).

79. **Name the common causes of CKD and the frequency of occurrence.**
   - **DM**: 42%
   - **HTN**: 31%
   - **Glomerulonephritis**: 10%
   - **Obstructive uropathy**: 2%
   - **Polycystic kidney disease and other interstitial diseases**: 3%
   - **Others**: 10%

   U.S. Renal Data Systems: 2008. Available at: www.usrds.org.

80. **Discuss the new developments in the treatment of anemia of CKD.**

The most important development is the use of recombinant human erythropoietin. Studies have documented the efficacy of this agent in improving the anemia and minimizing the need for blood transfusion. More important, the significance of correcting the iron deficiency in these patients by not only restoring the iron stores but also decreasing the requirements of the more expensive erythropoietin has been recognized.

   Eschbach JW, Abdulhadi MH, Browne JK, et al: Recombinant human erythropoietin in anemic patients with end stage renal disease, *Ann Intern Med* 111:992–1000, 1989.

81. **What are ESAs?**

Erythropoietin-stimulating agents. These agents are human recombinant erythropoietin preparations that have been approved for the use for treatment of anemia in CKD and ESRD. These include erythropoietin alpha and darbepoietin.

82. **Is it safe to normalize hemoglobin in CKD and dialysis patients?**

No. The target hemoglobin in CKD and dialysis subjects that need ESAs is usually 11–12 g/dL. The Correction of Hemoglobin Outcomes in Renal Insufficiency (CHOIR) study showed that such higher hemoglobin levels of 13–15 gm/dL are associated with increased cardiovascular morbidity and mortality.

   Singh AK, Szczech L, Barnhart H, et al: Correction of anemia with epoetin alfa in chronic kidney disease, *N Engl J Med* 355:2085–2098, 2006.

DIALYSIS

83. What are the indications for dialysis in a patient with CKD?
When conservative management fails to maintain the patient in reasonable comfort. Usually, dialysis is required when the GFR drops to 5–10 mL/min, but it is both unnecessary and risky to adhere to strict biochemical indications. Broadly speaking, the development of uremic encephalopathy, neuropathy, pericarditis, and bleeding diathesis is an indication to start dialysis immediately. Fluid overload, congestive heart failure, hyperkalemia, metabolic acidosis, and HTN uncontrolled by conservative measures are also indications for starting patients on dialysis therapy.

84. What are the contraindications for dialysis?
The presence of potentially reversible abnormalities is a major contraindication for dialysis. These include volume depletion, urinary tract infection (UTI), urinary obstruction, hypercatabolic state, uncontrolled HTN, hypercalcemia, nephrotoxic drugs, and low cardiac output state.

85. Which clinical manifestations of uremia (CKD) can be improved with dialysis? Which ones persist or worsen?

IMPROVE	PERSIST	DEVELOP OR WORSEN
Uremic encephalopathy	Renal osteodystrophy	Dialysis dementia
Seizures	Hypertriglyceridemia	Nephrogenic ascites
Pericarditis	Amenorrhea and infertility	Dialysis pericarditis
Fluid overload	Peripheral neuropathy	Dialysis bone disease
Electrolyte imbalances	Pruritus	Accelerated atherosclerosis
GI symptoms	Anemia	Carpal tunnel syndrome
Metabolic acidosis	Risk of hepatitis	(amyloid-related)

86. Which poisons and toxins are dialyzable?
- Alcohols: ethanol, methanol, ethylene glycol
- Salicylates
- Heavy metals: mercury, arsenic, and lead
- Halides

    In addition, hemoperfusion successfully removes barbiturates, sedatives (meprobamate, methaqualone, and glutethimide), acetaminophen, digoxin, procainamide, quinidine, and theophylline.

87. What is chronic ambulatory peritoneal dialysis (CAPD)?
A manual form of peritoneal dialysis, usually performed by the patient, in which 1–2 L of dialysate fluid are infused into the peritoneal space through a Tenckhoff catheter and then drained after a dwell time of 4–6 hr. The exchanges are repeated four to five times a day. CAPD is indicated in any patient with ESRD.

88. What are the indications and contraindications for CAPD?
CAPD is the treatment of choice for diabetics with severe peripheral vascular disease because hemodialysis is not a viable option for such patients. This method provides more independence and mobility, and it should be offered to all young patients leading active lives. The contraindications include blindness, severe disabling arthritis, presence of colostomy, poor patient motivation, and quadriplegia.

89. **What are the common mechanical complications of CAPD?**
    Pain, bleeding, leakage, inadequate drainage, intraperitoneal catheter loss, abdominal wall edema, scrotal edema, incisional hernia, other hernia, intestinal hematoma, and intestinal perforation.

90. **What are the common metabolic complications of CAPD?**
    Hyperglycemia, hyperosmolar nonketotic coma, postdialysis hypoglycemia, hyperkalemia, hypokalemia, hypernatremia, hyponatremia, metabolic alkalosis, protein depletion, hyperlipidemia, and obesity.

91. **List other potential complications of CAPD.**
    - **Infections and inflammation**: bacterial or fungal peritonitis, tunnel infection, exit-site infection, diverticulitis, sterile peritonitis, eosinophilic peritonitis, sclerosing peritonitis, and pancreatitis
    - **Cardiovascular**: acute pulmonary edema, fluid overload, hypotension, arrhythmia, cardiac arrest, and HTN
    - **Pulmonary**: basal atelectasis, aspiration pneumonia, hydrothorax, respiratory arrest, and decreased forced vital capacity (FVC)

92. **What are the causes of peritonitis in a patient on peritoneal dialysis?**
    - *Staphylococcus epidermidis* and *Staphylococcus aureus*: 70%
    - Gram-negative organisms: 20%
    - Fungi and mycobacterial: 5%

    The frequency of infection has decreased considerably since this dialysis method was first introduced, to about one episode every 18–24 patient-months. This decrease is mainly due to the addition of a Luer-Lok adapter between the catheter and the tubing and the institution of monthly tubing changes.

93. **What is dialysis-associated amyloidosis?**
    The accumulation and deposition of amyloid fibrils containing beta$_2$ microglobulin associated with long-term dialytic therapy. Amyloidosis is usually manifested after 5–7 years of chronic dialytic therapy and is seen in most patients after 10 years of dialysis. Clinical findings include asymptomatic lytic bone lesions, carpal tunnel syndrome (often bilateral), tenosynovitis, scapulohumeral periarthritis, and destructive arthropathy. No satisfactory preventive measures are available.

    Koch KM: Dialysis related amyloidosis, *Kidney Int* 41:1416–1429, 1992.

NEPHROLITHIASIS

94. **What three mechanisms are important in the development of nephrolithiasis?**
    - Precipitation of a substance from supersaturated solutions to form stones that is related to many factors, including solubility and concentration of the substance and urine characteristics (e.g., pH).
    - Reduced concentration of normal constituents of urine that inhibit stone formation including citrate, pyrophosphate, and magnesium.
    - Contribution of the protein matrix to the formation, growth, and/or aggregation of stones. This matrix derives in part from renal tubular epithelial cells and from the uroepithelium.

95. **What are the common constituents of urinary stones in the United States and their frequency?**
    - Calcium oxalate: 35%
    - Calcium apatite: 35%

- Magnesium ammonium phosphate (struvite): 18%
- Uric acid: 6%
- Cystine: 3%

96. **Summarize the conditions that favor the formation of each kind of stone.**
In general, an alkaline urine pH favors precipitation of inorganic stone such as calcium phosphate that undergoes rearrangement into hydroxyapatite. Alkaline urine pH and high concentrations of urinary ammonia lead to supersaturation of magnesium ammonium phosphate (struvite). This environment is created by the presence of urea-splitting bacteria (commonly *Proteus, Pseudomonas, Klebsiella,* and *Staphylococcus*), which contain the enzyme urease and convert urea to ammonia and CO_2. An acid pH favors precipitation of organic stone such as uric acid and cystine. Urine pH has little effect on calcium oxalate solubility and, therefore, little influence on formation of these stones.

97. **List common metabolic conditions that predispose to the formation of urinary stones.**
- **Idiopathic hypercalciuria** (50%): due to excessive GI calcium absorption of renal calcium leakage
- **Low urinary citrate excretion** (50%): contributes to stone formation in most states
- **Hyperuricosuria** (30%): occurs with and without gout and may contribute to calcium stone formation
- **Hyperoxaluria** (15%): due to various causes

98. **What are the less common causes of urinary stones?**
- Chronic UTI
- Primary hyperparathyroidism
- Cystinuria
- Distal renal tubular acidosis (RTA)
   Typically, more than one of these conditions are present in a stone-forming patient.

99. **What are the symptoms of urinary obstruction by a stone?**
Usually severe, colicky pain that radiates toward the lower abdomen and genital area. The ureteropelvic junction, the midureter as it crosses the iliac artery, and the ureterovesical junction are the common sites for urinary obstruction by stones. In women who have children, the pain is often described as more severe than the pain of labor. The increased pressure inside the collecting system decreases the net pressure for glomerular filtration, resulting in a decreased GFR. The resulting urinary stasis predisposes to infection.

100. **Do the consequences of urinary obstruction have permanent effects?**
No. The GFR corrects toward normal if the stone passes or is removed from the urinary tract within a few days. If the obstruction becomes chronic, permanent renal injury can ensue, with an irreversible reduction in GFR and chronic dilatation of the collection system. This dilated collecting system is less efficient in delivering urine to the bladder (because of compromised peristalsis), predisposing to urinary stasis and infection.

101. **How should you manage the patient with acute urinary obstruction due to a stone?**
Initially with supportive management with analgesics and oral fluids because most stones spontaneously pass in a few hours to days. Serum chemistries should be done to document the degree of renal dysfunction (if any) and an imaging procedure (e.g., IV pyelography, renal ultrasound [US]) to locate the stone and estimate its size in order to help determine the possible need for surgical intervention.

102. **What should you do once the acute phase of obstruction ends?**
Evaluate the patient for underlying conditions that led to the formation of the stone, which will lead to a protocol for long-term management. A reasonable percentage of patients recover stone material from their urine. However, laboratory analysis is usually not readily available, and the approach to further management is more often empirical than based on analysis of recovered stones.

103. **Describe the general approach to avoidance of recurrent stones.**
Maintenance of a dilute urine through high intake of hypotonic fluids. More specific management depends on the predisposing condition.

104. **What measures are appropriate for patients with absorptive or renal hypercalciuria?**
Absorptive hypercalciuria can be managed by reducing dietary calcium (type 2 only), reducing intestinal calcium absorption by using cellulose sodium phosphate (type 1), or a thiazide diuretic, which promotes renal calcium reabsorption. **Renal** hypercalciuria can also be treated with thiazides.

105. **How is primary hyperparathyroidism treated?**
With parathyroidectomy in selected patients. (See also Chapter 16, Endocrinology.)

106. **Summarize the management of uricosuric states.**
Uricosuric states result from the overproduction of uric acid and can be treated with allopurinol or with potassium citrate if patients have hyperuricosuria associated with calcium oxalate stones.

107. **Describe the treatment of patients with excessive intestinal oxalate absorption.**
With a low-oxalate diet and use of magnesium or calcium salts, which bind oxalate and inhibit its reabsorption.

108. **How is cystinuria treated?**
With conservative management and maintenance of a dilute or alkaline urine or with penicillamine, which increases the solubility of cysteine if the conservative measures are ineffective.

109. **How should you manage patients with struvite stones?**
Treat UTIs with antibiotics and use the urease inhibitor acetohydroxamic acid, if needed.

110. **What is lithotripsy?**
Litho (stone or calculus) *tripsy* (crushing) is a way of breaking up stones by use of shock waves or US and may serve as an alternative to operation or cystoscopy for the removal of stones in the kidney and urinary tract.

111. **What are the three forms now available for lithotripsy?**
- Extracorporeal shock-wave lithotripsy
- Percutaneous ultrasonic lithotripsy
- Endoscopic ultrasonic lithotripsy

URINARY TRACT OBSTRUCTION

112. **List the common causes of ureteric obstruction in adults.**
- Renal stones
- Prostatic, bladder, or pelvic malignancy

- Retroperitoneal lymphoma, metastasis, or fibrosis
- Accidental surgical ligation
- Blood clot
- Pregnancy
- Stricture

113. **How do unilateral and bilateral obstructions differ in their effects on the GFR?**
Unilateral obstruction does not necessarily lead to a clinically measurable decrease in GFR in patients with normal renal function, but bilateral obstruction quite often leads to a decreased GFR in patients with both normal and abnormal renal function.

114. **Describe in detail how unilateral obstruction affects the GFR.**
In patients with normal renal function, unilateral obstruction with complete obliteration of ipsilateral function forces recruitment of the nephron reserve of the unaffected, contralateral kidney, resulting in no changes or only small changes in total GFR. Relatively large reductions in functioning nephron mass ($\sim$40%) are necessary to elicit an appreciable rise in the P_{Cr} concentrations when baseline renal function is normal (P_{Cr} 0.8–1.2 mg/dL). The relatively small change in GFR in patients with normal baseline renal function who are subjected to unilateral obstruction probably will not be reflected by a rise in P_{Cr}. The response is different for patients with baseline renal insufficiency. Such patients have already lost their reserve nephron mass and are likely using compensatory mechanisms to maintain their GFR. Unilateral obstruction in such patients may result in a significant fall in GFR and is more likely to be associated with a rise in P_{Cr}.

115. **Describe the differences in clinical presentation between acute and chronic obstruction of the urinary tract.**
Partial or complete obstruction of the urinary tract compromises urine passage whether it is acute or chronic. Nevertheless, the urinary findings and clinical consequences differ depending on the duration of the obstruction. After release of an **acute (> 24 hr) obstruction**, there is commonly a decrease in excretion of sodium, potassium, and water. This results in excretion of a urine low in sodium and with increased osmolarity, a situation also seen with volume depletion. In contrast, release of **chronic obstruction** commonly results in increased excretion of sodium and water and decreased excretion of acid (with urinary loss of bicarbonate) and potassium. These abnormalities can lead to volume depletion, free-water deficit (reflected by hypernatremia), and hyperkalemic non–anion-gap metabolic acidosis.

116. **What abnormalities of tubular function can occur with chronic obstruction?**
Chronic obstruction affects primarily distal rather than proximal nephron functions, including reabsorption of sodium and water and secretion of acid and potassium. The decreased **water** reabsorption results from decreased responsiveness of the collecting tubule to antidiuretic hormone, yielding a form of nephrogenic diabetes insipidus. The **acid** secretory defect results in incomplete bicarbonate recovery from the urine and a non–anion-gap metabolic acidosis. The **potassium** secretory defect results in potassium retention and hyperkalemia. Therefore, obstructive nephropathy is a common cause of hyperkalemic, hyperchloremic, non-anion-gap metabolic acidosis. These abnormalities usually resolve after correction of the obstruction but may require weeks or months to do so. In addition to the decrease in GFR and the potential tubular abnormalities, the resulting urinary stasis can predispose to infection, renal stones, and papillary necrosis. The salt and water retention can lead to HTN.

117. **Which components of polyuria (postobstructive diuresis) are seen immediately after correction of chronic obstruction?**
The patient with obstruction and compromised renal function accumulates solute and water that are ordinarily excreted by the normally functioning kidney. Correction of the

obstruction results in appropriate excretion of the accumulated urea, NaCl, and water in an effort to return the volume and content of the extracellular fluid to normal. This polyuria is physiologic. However, a minority of such patients have a pathologic polyuria, resulting from poor salt and/or water reabsorption. These abnormalities commonly resolve within a few hours but may last for days. Usually, the polyuria is physiologic, but the patient must be observed. Pathologic polyuria may occur because of either salt or water loss (or both). Pathologic salt loss is reflected by continued excretion of a large amount of urinary sodium in the setting of volume depletion. Pathologic water loss is reflected by excretion of large volumes of dilute urine in spite of rising serum osmolality.

118. **Should the polyuria after correction of obstruction be treated?**
In pathologic polyuria, appropriate fluid replacement therapy should be instituted. If replacement is instituted during the physiologic polyuria, one will "chase" the patient's volume status so that polyuria continues as a result of the fluids that are administered.

119. **Explain "functional" obstruction of the urinary tract.**
Abnormalities that compromise the exit of urine from the kidney in the absence of anatomic obstruction of the outflow tract. Two examples are an atonic bladder and vesicoureteral reflux.

120. **What is an atonic bladder?**
A bladder that is unable to empty itself completely and hence contains urine, continuously yielding a higher than normal hydrostatic pressure. This high bladder pressure is transmitted via the ureters and may cause the abnormalities described earlier.

121. **What causes vesicoureteral reflux?**
Retrograde flow of urine into the ureter or kidney or both during voiding due to an incompetent vesicoureteral valve. The transmitted pressure is felt to contribute to the renal abnormalities. Both of these conditions also predispose to infection.

122. **How is the diagnosis of lower urinary tract obstruction (LTO) made?**
By history, clinical setting, and the laboratory findings. A palpable urinary bladder on examination is strong evidence for LTO or an atonic bladder. A postvoid residual urine of > 100 mL on Foley catheter insertion is supportive of LTO. Imaging studies help confirm the diagnosis.

123. **Which imaging studies are helpful in the diagnosis of LTO?**
   - Plain abdominal x-rays show distended bladder as well as large kidney.
   - Renal US can detect hydronephrosis. Abdominal computed tomography (CT) scan if further imaging is needed.
   - Retrograde pyelography (selective catheterization and insertion of contrast dye into both ureters via cystoscopy) may be necessary if LTO is suspected but not found by x-ray or US.
   - Radionuclide renal scans suggest LTO when there is prompt uptake of the dye with prolonged excretion.
   Intravenous pyelograms should be avoided owing to the risk of additional renal injury from the contrast dye.

124. **How does imaging help determine the prognosis of LTO?**
Development of hydronephrosis usually up to 48 hours; therefore, the absence of hydronephrosis does not rule out LTO. The chances of recovery of renal function in LTO can be predicted based on the extent and duration of parenchymal injury. The US studies will reflect this by the degree of cortical thinning and echogenicity of the renal parenchyma.

RENAL BONE DISEASE

125. **What is Bricker's "trade-off" hypothesis?**
The trade-off hypothesis propounded by Neil Bricker that is the basis for the secondary hyperparathyroidism seen in renal failure.

126. **Explain the trade-off hypothesis.**
Early in the course of renal failure, the kidney fails to excrete phosphorus, leading to a transient and often undetectable rise in serum phosphorus. This tends to lower the serum level of ionized calcium temporarily, leading to stimulation of parathyroid hormone (PTH) secretion. The increased levels of PTH reduce tubular reabsorption of phosphate, leading to phosphate excretion and thereby tending to normalize the serum calcium and phosphorus levels. However, this process occurs at the expense of an elevated PTH level. With further declines in renal function, the serum phosphorus tends to rise, and the whole cycle is repeated. With advancing renal failure, these changes tend to keep serum calcium and phosphorus levels below normal at the expense of increasing serum PTH levels. The serum level of PTH is increased in an attempt to normalize serum phosphate and calcium levels, but the "trade-off" is the bone disease caused by the elevated PTH levels (osteitis fibrosa cystica).

127. **List the three major bone histologic subtypes found in renal osteodystrophy.**
Osteitis fibrosa cystica, which is a result of high bone turnover (bone changes due to secondary hyperparathyroidism), **osteomalacia,** and occasionally, **osteosclerosis.** With better management of patients with ESRD, the long-term course of renal bone disease and its clinical features has changed, and newer entities have emerged. Adynamic or aplastic bone disease or low bone turnover has become a fairly common bone disease. Aluminum accumulation causes osteomalacia, which is one cause of adynamic bone disease. Decreased vitamin D, DM, and iron accumulation are other factors associated with adynamic bone disease.

128. **Why do patients with CKD and marked hypocalcemia often fail to manifest tetany?**
Because of the acidemia seen in CKD, ionized calcium is usually not reduced enough to cause tetany. Tetany is the result of decreased ionized calcium, which is decreased in the presence of alkemia. Tetany is usually only manifested in the presence of an alkaline pH. However, if the acidosis of CKD is excessively treated with alkalizing agents, tetany may become manifest.

129. **How do you manage secondary hyperparathyroidism in patients with CKD?**
By reducing the serum parathormone levels with vitamin D analogues. However, vitamin D therapy should not be attempted before the serum phosphorus level is normalized or the product of calcium and phosphorus is lowered to < 70. The most commonly used vitamin D preparation is calcitriol (1,25 dihydroxycholecalciferol) as either oral or IV form. More recently, other analogues of vitamin D such as 19-nor-cholecalciferol and 1-alpha calcidiol have been successfully used and may cause less hypercalcemia.

130. **Does bone disease improve with dialysis?**
No. Renal osteodystrophy does not always improve with dialytic therapy. Indeed, the symptoms may worsen or progress because a number of additional factors are introduced that either directly or indirectly influence the severity of renal bone disease, including the aluminum content of dialysate, heparin administration, and administration of large amounts of acetate.

Sherrard DJ, Hercz G, Pei Y, et al: The spectrum of bone disease in end stage renal failure—An evolving disorder, *Kidney Int* 43:436–442, 1993.

131. **Does renal transplantation improve bone disease?**
Yes. In patients who undergo renal transplantation, the uremic bone disease improves to a great extent. Increased osteoclastic and osteoblastic activities are noted within a few weeks after transplantation. However, in some patients, osteoporosis and the effects of secondary hyperparathyroidism may persist for as long as 1–2 years. In addition, steroid therapy may be responsible for osteoporosis and osteonecrosis that complicate the later phases of the posttransplant period. Another abnormality that may develop in the posttransplant phase is a renal phosphate leak, which, if severe, may contribute to osseous abnormalities.

RENAL TRANSPLANTATION

132. **Who is a potential candidate for renal transplantation?**
All patients with ESRD who need some form of renal replacement therapy should be considered for transplantation.

133. **What are the absolute contraindications to renal transplantation?**
- Reversible renal disease
- Active infection
- Recent malignant disease
- Active glomerulonephritis
- Presensitization to donor class I major transplantation antigens
- Acquired immunodeficiency syndrome (AIDS)

134. **List the relative contraindications to renal transplantation.**
- Fabry's disease (an inherited lysosomal storage disease)
- Oxalosis
- Advanced age
- Psychiatric problems
- Presence of anatomic urologic abnormality
- Iliofemoral occlusion
- Chronic active hepatitis

135. **What are the donor-selection criteria for living-related transplantation?**
Donors should have a normal physical examination, be younger than age 65 years and have the same ABO blood group as the recipient or type O. An angiogram is necessary to exclude the presence of multiple or abnormal renal arteries, because such abnormalities make the surgery prolonged and difficult. In general, the left kidney is preferred because of the longer renal vein. Some relative contraindications for kidney donation include severe HTN, DM, HIV positivity, active medical illness, urologic abnormalities, persistently abnormal urinalyses, and family history of nephritis, polycystic kidney disease, or other renal disease.

136. **What factors are considered important in evaluating suitability of a cadaver kidney?**
The donor should have been free of neoplastic or infectious disease, *preferably* be younger than 60 years, and have had good urine output and a normal SCr before death. Urinalyses should be normal, and urine cultures should be negative. The kidney should be transplanted as early after harvesting as possible. The graft function tends to be worse 24 hours after harvesting. The donor should be free of infection with hepatitis B virus and HIV.

137. **Give the current survival figures for renal transplant recipients in the United States.**
The 1-year patient survival rate for living-related renal transplantation is now around 95–100%, and for cadaveric transplantation, approximately 90%. With cyclosporine therapy, graft survivals are 90% and 80%, respectively, for living and cadaveric kidney transplants.

138. **What are the common immunosuppressive agents used in renal transplantation?**
   - **Induction therapy (perioperatively)**: corticosteroids (IV methylprednisolone at engraftment followed by oral prednisone tapered over the first 3 months) and possibly monoclonal antibodies such as baxilisimab or daclizumab that block interleukin-2 (IL-2) receptors
   - **Maintenance therapy (during the life of the kidney)**: oral corticosteroids, antimetabolites (mycophenolate mofetil), and calcineurin inhibitors (cyclosporine and tacrolimus)

139. **What is acute rejection and how is it treated?**
An acute deterioration in renal allograft function associated with specific pathologic changes in the graft. Acute rejection can occur at any time but most often occurs in the first 6 months after transplant. As a result of better immunosuppressive regimens, the incidence of acute rejection is declining and is currently < 20% in the first year in many transplant centers. Acute rejection could be acute cellular or acute humoral rejection. The treatment of acute cellular rejection usually includes high-dose IV corticosteroids, polyclonal antibodies such as antithymocyte globulins, or monoclonal antibodies such as OKT3 and rituximab. Acute humoral rejection can also be treated with plasmapheresis, steroids, and intravenous immunoglobulin (IVIG).

MISCELLANEOUS RENAL DISORDERS

140. **How is a patient with recurrent hematuria evaluated?**
Initially with renal imaging and urinary instrumentation to exclude urinary stones and other structural lesions such as tumors of the upper and lower urinary tract. The presence of dysmorphic erythrocytes or RBC casts helps to distinguish glomerular bleeding from lower tract bleeding. Glomerular bleeding accounts for recurrent hematuria in over a quarter of patients younger than age 40 years.

141. **What are the risk factors associated with aminoglycoside nephrotoxicity?**

Dose and duration of drug therapy	Preexisting renal or liver failure	Concurrent nephrotoxin administration
Recent aminoglycoside therapy	Older age Volume depletion	Potassium or magnesium depletion or both

Fumes D: Aminoglycoside nephrotoxicity, *Kidney Int* 33:900–911, 1988.

142. **How should antibiotic doses be adjusted in patients with renal failure?**
Several antibiotics need dosage modification in the presence of renal failure, notably aminoglycosides, most cephalosporins, many penicillins, most fluoroquinolones, and vancomycin. The adjustments can be made by maintaining the usual dose and varying the dosing interval, maintaining the dosing interval and varying the dose, or a combination of the two. The objective is to obtain a therapeutic drug concentration–time profile that is therapeutic and not toxic. For most commonly used antibiotics, dosing guidelines are established and readily accessible. No adjustment is needed for erythromycin, doxycycline,

rifampin, and oral vancomycin. Tetracyclines, nitrofurantoin, nalidixic acid, and bacitracin should be totally avoided in renal failure.

Brier ME, Aronoff GR, Burns JS, et al: *Drug Prescribing in Renal Failure*, ed 5, Philadelphia, 2007, American College of Physicians, pp 45–75.

143. **How do drugs interfere with assessment of renal function?**
Cimetidine, trimethoprim, and acetylsalicylic acid increase SCr by interfering with the tubular creatinine secretion, whereas methyldopa and cefoxitin interfere with creatinine assay, artificially elevating the SCr level. Tolbutamide, penicillins, cephalosporins, sulfonamides, and contrast media can cause a false-positive reaction for protein in the urine.

144. **Explain the interaction of digoxin with other drugs in renal failure.**
Concomitant use of **metoclopramide** with digoxin decreases the absorption of the digoxin owing to decreased gastric motility. The digoxin dose may have to be increased. Conversely, **quinidine** impairs renal excretion of digoxin, and hence, the digoxin dose may have to be decreased.

145. **How do antacids interact with other drugs in cases of renal failure?**
Antacids impair the gastric absorption of **beta blockers** and **ferrous sulfate.** These drugs should be given 1–2 hours apart.

146. **With what drug may Scholl's solution interact in patients with renal failure?**
Aluminun hydroxide. Scholl's solution contains sodium citrate, and citrate increases aluminum absorption so that aluminum toxicity may result. The combination has to be avoided.

147. **Explain the interaction between azathioprine and allopurinol.**
Azathioprine levels in the blood are elevated when used in conjunction with allopurinol owing to decreased xanthine oxidase metabolism of azathioprine. The azathioprine dose, therefore, has to be decreased and leukocyte counts followed.

148. **Which drugs alter cyclosporine levels in the plasma?**
Phenytoin, phenobarbital, and **rifampin** increase cyclosporine clearance by the liver, and higher doses may be needed. Conversely, **erythromycin, amphotericin B,** and **ketoconazole** decrease cyclosporine clearance by the liver; thus, the dose needs to be decreased.

149. **How does pregnancy affect healthy kidneys?**
Owing to increased blood volume and hyperdynamic circulation in pregnancy, renal hemodynamics are altered. Most important, clearances of urea, creatinine, and uric acid are increased, leading to a decrease in the serum concentrations of these compounds. Urine protein excretion rates are increased. There is some dilatation of the collecting system, including the ureters, partially due to the pressure from the gravid uterus but mainly due to the effect of progestational hormones on the muscular tone of the ureters. All of these changes revert to normalcy once the patient delivers.

150. **How does pregnancy affect diseased kidneys?**
Most renal diseases with proteinuria demonstrate increases in proteinuria during pregnancy. In diabetics with no renal disease, pregnancy does not adversely affect the renal function. However, there are no data about effects of pregnancy on renal function in patients with advanced diabetic nephropathy. Lupus nephritis is associated with an increased rate of spontaneous abortion and increased fetal loss. However, there is no evidence that pregnancy affects the long-term prognosis of lupus nephritis.

151. **What is a simple renal cyst?**
Simple cysts represent 60–70% of renal masses. They are common after age 50, most often asymptomatic, and usually detected as incidental findings in radiologic procedures done for other reasons.

152. **How is a simple renal cyst distinguished from a malignant cyst?**
On sonography, a simple cyst has smooth, sharply delineated margins, no echoes within the mass, and a strong posterior wall echo indicating good transmission through the cyst. These features generally exclude the possibility of malignancy. However, if there is any further suspicion, a CT scan should be done. CT findings consistent with a simple cyst include fluid that is homogeneous with a density of 0–20 Hounsfield units and no enhancement of the cyst fluid following the administration of radiocontrast media. Characteristics of renal cysts are summarized in Table 8-3.

153. **You are asked to examine a 53-year-old man admitted to the hospital with fever, chills, right flank pain, and dysuria. Two years ago when he was evaluated for newly detected HTN, he was noted to have polycystic kidney disease. Urinalysis showed 15–20 RBCs, plenty of WBCs, and 3+ bacteria. An abdominal US is unremarkable except for bilateral polycystic kidneys, showing one of the renal cysts in the right kidney filled with highly echogenic material. What should be done first?**
Start IV ciprofloxacin. One does not need to wait for urine culture results, but empirical therapy should be started. An antibiotic such as ampicillin would not penetrate the cyst wall (demonstrated on US as infected) and reach adequate concentration to clear the infection. Surgical drainage is needed only in cases resistant to IV antibiotics.

154. **What are the renal manifestations of HIV disease?**
The most common chronic renal disease from HIV infection is a type of focal glomerulosclerosis, the so-called HIV nephropathy. Typically, nephrotic proteinuria, large echogenic kidneys, minimal or modest HTN, and rapidly progressive renal failure characterize the disease. Dialysis is well tolerated; however, the mean survival is less than 1 year in patients with full-blown AIDS. Transplantation is contraindicated in HIV nephropathy. The other renal manifestations include hyponatremia, hyperkalemia (often secondary to adrenal disease or hyporenin hypoaldosteronism), hypouricemia, and AKI, often due to anti-HIV medications. (See also Chapter 13, AIDS and HIV Infection.)

155. **Describe the major differences between fibromuscular dysplasia (FMD) and atherosclerotic renal artery stenosis.**
See Table 8-4.

156. **How do you diagnose renovascular HTN?**
Onset of HTN before age 20 or after age 50 should suggest the possibility of renovascular HTN. Similarly, the development of a refractory phase in a previously stable hypertensive patient, the presence of spontaneous hypokalemia and the presence of an abdominal bruit are also suggestive.

157. **What laboratory tests are useful in screening for renovascular HTN?**
Imaging techniques have largely replaced these tests now in diagnosing renovascular HTN, but previously, **high plasma renin** profile was found in 80% of patients with renovascular HTN, Another previously used screening is the **captopril test.** The administration of oral captopril causes a reactive rise of renin that is greater in patients with renovascular as opposed to essential HTN. The overall sensitivity is 74% and specificity is 89%.

TABLE 8-3. CHARACTERISTICS OF RENAL CYSTIC DISORDERS

Feature	CYSTS	ADPKD	ARPKD	ACKD	MCD	MSK
Inheritance pattern	None	Autosomal dominant	Autosomal recessive	None	Often present, variable pattern	None
Incidence or prevalence	Common, increasing with age	1/200–1/1000	Rare	40% in patients on dialysis	Rare	Common
Age of onset	Adult	Usually adults	Neonates, children	Older adults	Adolescents, young adults	Adults
Presenting symptom	Incidental finding, hematuria	Pain, hematuria, infection, family screening	Abdominal mass, renal failure, failure to thrive	Hematuria	Polyuria, polydipsia, enuresis, renal failure, failure to thrive	Incidental, UTIs, hematuria, renal calculi
Hematuria	Occurs	Common	Occurs	Occurs	Rare	Common
Recurrent infections	Rare	Common	Occurs	No	Rare	Common
Renal calculi	No	Common	No	No	No	Common
Hypertension	Rare	Common	Common	Present from underlying disease	Rare	No
Diagnosis	Ultrasound	Ultrasound, gene linkage analysis	Ultrasound	CT scan	None reliable	Excretory urogram
Renal size	Normal	Normal to very large	Large initially	Small to normal, occ. large	Small	Normal

ACKD = acquired cystic kidney disease; ADPKD = autosomal dominant polycystic kidney disease; ARPKD = autosomal recessive polycystic kidney disease; MCD = medullary cystic disease; MSK = medullary sponge kidney; UTIs = urinary tract infections.
Adapted from Grantham JJ: Cystic diseases of kidney. In Goldman K, Bennett JC, et al (eds): Cecil Textbook of Medicine, 21st ed. Philadelphia, WB Saunders, 2000.

TABLE 8-4. FIBROMUSCULAR DYSPLASIA VERSUS ATHEROSCLEROTIC RENAL ARTERY STENOSIS

	FMD	ATHEROSCLEROSIS
Age at onset	<40 yr	>45 yr
Gender	80% female	Primarily male
Distribution of lesion	Distal main renal artery	Aortic orifice and proximal main renal artery and intrarenal branches
Progression	Uncommon	Common; may progress to complete occlusion

FMD = fibromuscular dysphasia.

158. **What imaging techniques are useful in screening for renovascular HTN?**
Duplex renal sonography, CT angiography or magnetic resonance (MR) angiography are the most useful screening tests for renal artery stenosis. The gold standard test for confirmation of renal artery stenosis is renal angiography.

Hirsch AT, Haskal ZJ, Hertzer NR, et al: ACC/AHA 2005 practice guidelines for the management of patients with peripheral arterial disease (lower extremity, renal, mesenteric, and abdominal aortic). *Circulation* 113:1474–1547, 2006.

159. **What are ANCAs?**
Antineutrophil cytoplasmic antibodies that are autoantibodies directed against intracellular antigens in neutrophils. ANCAs have two immunofluorescence patterns: cytoplasmic (c-ANCA) or perinuclear (p-ANCA) staining. c-ANCAs are directed toward proteinase-3, and p-ANCAs are specific for myeloperoxidase (MPO). (See also Chapter 10, Rheumatology.)

160. **How do ANCAs help in distinguishing glomerular disorders?**
ANCAs are often positive in pauci-immune vasculitidis. Approximately 85–90% patients with Wegener's granulomatosis are positive for c-ANCA, and 50–80% with microscopic polyarteritis are positive for p-ANCA. However, many other autoimmune disorders with small vessel vasculitis, such as SLE, rheumatoid arthritis, and Sjögren's syndrome, are also positive for p-ANCA. It is highly recommended to obtain tissue biopsy in ANCA-positive vasculitis before immunosuppressive therapy is begun.

Jeaneete JC, Falk RJ: Small vessel vasculitis, *N Engl J Med* 337:1512–1523, 1997.

161. **What causes AKI secondary to rhabdomyolysis?**
Frequently, ATN. Rhabdomyolysis occurs in various clinical conditions, including trauma, ischemic tissue damage after a drug overdose, alcoholism, seizures, and heat stroke (especially in untrained subjects or those with sickle cell trait). Hypokalemia and severe hypophosphatemia can also precipitate rhabdomyolysis. It is the most common cause of AKI in patients abusing illicit IV drugs.

162. **Summarize the signs and symptoms of AKI secondary to rhabdomyolysis.**
Typical patients have pigmented granular casts in urine sediment, a positive orthotolidine test in the urine supernatant (indicating the presence of heme), and markedly elevated plasma creatine kinase and other muscle enzymes, owing to their release from damaged muscle tissue. Other characteristics of AKI due to rhabdomyolysis include hyperphosphatemia,

hyperkalemia, and a disproportionate increase in P_{Cr} (all of these being due to release of cellular constituents). A high–anion-gap metabolic acidosis and severe hyperuricemia are also characteristic, and oliguria or anuria is common.

163. **What is the mechanism of renal failure in rhabdomyolysis?**
The mechanism of renal failure is not completely understood. Although myoglobin is not directly nephrotoxic, concurrent vasoconstriction or volume depletion decreases the renal perfusion and rate of urine flow in tubules, thereby promoting the precipitation of these pigment casts.

BIBLIOGRAPHY

1. Brenner EM, editor: *Brenner & Rector's The Kidney*, ed 8, Philadelphia, 2007, Saunders Elsevier.
2. Goldman L, Ausiello D, editors. *Cecil Textbook of Medicine*, ed 23, Philadelphia, 2007, Saunders.
3. Greenberg A: *Primer on Kidney Diseases—National Kidney Foundation*, ed 5, Philadelphia, 2009, Saunders Elsevier.
4. Rose BD, Post TW: *Clinical Physiology of Acid-Base and Electrolyte Disorders*, ed 5, New York, 2001, McGraw-Hill.
5. Schrier RW, editor: *Diseases of the Kidney*, ed 7, Philadelphia, 2007, Lippincott Williams & Wilkins.
6. Schrier RW, editor: *Renal and Electrolyte Disorders*, ed 7, Philadelphia, 2010, Lippincott Williams & Wilkins.
7. Singh A, editor: *Educational Review Manual in Nephrology*, ed 2, New York, 2008, CCGM.

CHAPTER 9

ACID–BASE AND ELECTROLYTES

Sharma S. Prabhakar, M.D., M.B.A., F.A.C.P., F.A.S.N.

In all things you shall find everywhere the Acid and the Alcaly.

Otto Tachenius (1670)
Hyppocrates Chymacus, Chapter 21

Hence if too much salt is used in food, the pulse hardens.

Huang Ti (The Yellow Emperor) (2697–2597 BC)
Nei Chung Su Wen, Bk. 3, Sect. 10, trans. by Ilza Veith,
in *The Yellow Emperor's Classic of Internal Medicine*

REGULATION OF SODIUM, WATER, AND VOLUME STATUS

1. **List the osmolality and electrolyte concentrations of serum and commonly used intravenous (IV) solutions.**
    See Table 9-1.

2. **How do you estimate a patient's serum osmolality?**
    A close estimate can be derived from measurements of the serum sodium concentration ($[Na^+]$), glucose, and blood urea nitrogen (BUN), using the following equation:

    $$\text{Osmolality} = 1.86 \times [Na^+] + \frac{\text{Glucose}}{18} + \frac{\text{BUN}}{2.8} + 9$$

3. **What percentage of the adult human body consists of water? What percentage of the water content is intracellular versus extracellular?**
    Approximately 60% of the adult man and 50% of the adult woman is water. About two thirds of this volume is intracellular, and one third is extracellular. About 20% of the extracellular fluid (ECF) volume is plasma water.

4. **What are the sources and daily amounts of water gain and loss?**
    The average adult male gains and loses 2600 mL of water each day. The gains occur from direct fluid ingestion (1400 mL/day), from the fluid content of ingested food (850 mL/day), and as a product of water produced by oxidation reactions (350 mL/day). Water losses occur through urine (1500 mL/day), perspiration (500 mL/day), respiration (400 mL/day), and feces (200 mL/day).

5. **List the factors necessary to allow the kidney to excrete free water.**
    - A filtrate must be formed to allow renal excretion of free water.
    - Glomerular filtrate must escape reabsorption in the proximal tubule to reach the diluting segment (ascending loop of Henle), where free water is created.
    - An adequately functioning diluting segment must be present.
    - The free water formed by the diluting segment must leave the nephron without being reabsorbed by the collecting tubule. This nephron segment is intrinsically impermeable to water but is made permeable by antidiuretic hormone (ADH).

TABLE 9-1.	OSMOLALITY AND ELECTROLYTE CONCENTRATIONS OF COMMONLY USED INTRAVENOUS SOLUTIONS			
Serum and Solutions	Osmolality (mOsm/kg)	Glucose (g/L)	Sodium (mEq/L)	Chloride (mEq/L)
Serum	285–295	65–110	135–145	97–110
5% D/W	252	50	0	0
10% D/W	505	100	0	0
50% D/W	2520	500	0	0
½ NS (0.45% NaCl)	154	0	77	77
NS (0.9% NaCl)	308	0	154	154
3% NS	1026	0	513	513
Ringer's lactate*	272	0	130	109

D/W = dextrose in water; NS = normal saline.
*Ringer's lactate also contains 28 mEq/L lactate, 4 mEq/L K^+, and 4.5 mEq/L Ca^{2+}.

6. **Summarize the relationship between glomerular filtration rate (GFR) and excretion of free water.**
   The lower the GFR, the lower the kidney's ability to respond rapidly to a free-water challenge with excretion of free water.

7. **What pathologic states can affect fluid reabsorption in the proximal tubule?**
   True volume depletion and states of decreased effective arterial blood volume, such as congestive heart failure, cirrhosis, and nephrotic syndrome. These states involve vigorous fluid reabsorption in the proximal tubule and are associated with a compromised ability to excrete free water.

8. **What pathologic states can affect functioning of the diluting segment?**
   Intrinsic disorders of function of the diluting segment are unusual. Endogenous prostaglandin E_2 and loop diuretics inhibit NaCl transport in this segment and can thereby limit formation of free water.

9. **Explain the meaning of serum sodium concentration with respect to sodium balance and water balance.**
   [Na^+], measured in mEq/L, reflects the concentration of this cation in ECF. Because its units are measured as mass per unit volume, [Na^+] indicates the relationship between Na^+ and water in the body. It is not indicative of total body Na^+ content but is more an indication of the water status (hydration) of the body. [Na^+] may be low, normal, or increased with any given perturbation of total body Na^+ content. Alterations of the [Na^+] reflect alterations in free-water balance. Therefore, a true low [Na^+] indicates a free-water excess compared with Na^+ content, and a high [Na^+] indicates a relative free-water deficit.

10. **Why is normal saline (with 154 mEq/L of Na^+) isotonic with plasma, which has a sodium of 145 mEq/L?**
    The plasma sodium is the concentration of sodium that reflects the concentration of sodium per liter of water in the plasma. Because the plasma has other solid components, the sodium concentration per liter of just water in the blood compartment is 154 mEq/L, and hence, the sodium concentration in normal saline.

11. **What is meant by a state of decreased effective arterial blood volume?**
    The extracellular space is dynamic, with an ongoing balance between its capacity and
    its actual volume. Both parameters are biologically monitored and normally coordinated
    to maintain optimal tissue perfusion. A state of decreased effective arterial blood
    volume occurs when a large capacity is combined with a smaller volume, as seen
    most commonly with congestive heart failure, cirrhosis, and nephrotic syndrome.
    Isotonic fluid losses, such as hemorrhage, cause a decrease in ECF volume with no
    change in $[Na^+]$. If, however, these losses are replaced with hypotonic fluids, dilutional
    hyponatremia results.

12. **Why does Na^+ have an effective distribution in total body water (TBW) despite
    being confined largely to the extracellular space?**
    Na^+ is the major determinant of serum osmolality, and changes in its concentration lead
    to water shifts between the extracellular and the intracellular compartments. This osmotic
    shift of water gives Na^+ an effective distribution greater than its chemical distribution and
    equivalent to that for TBW.

13. **What is the initial step in evaluating a patient with hyponatremia?**
    Determining the serum osmolality (both measured and calculated) (Fig. 9-1).

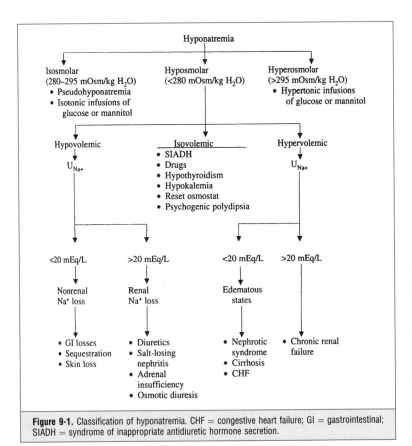

Figure 9-1. Classification of hyponatremia. CHF = congestive heart failure; GI = gastrointestinal;
SIADH = syndrome of inappropriate antidiuretic hormone secretion.

14. **What is hyperosmolar hyponatremia?**
Serum osmolarity > 295 mOsm/kg H_2O. It usually results from administration of hypertonic solutions of dextrose or mannitol.

15. **Define "isotonic hyponatremia."**
Serum osmolality of 280–295 mOsm/kg H_2O. It is seen with administration of isotonic solutions of dextrose and mannitol.

16. **What is hyposmolar hyponatremia?**
Serum osmolality < 280 mOsm/kg H_2O. It can be associated with low, normal, or increased volume status and is seen with diuretic administration, salt-losing renal conditions, syndrome of inappropriate antidiuretic hormone secretion (SIADH), chronic kidney disease (CKD), and a wide range of other causes.

17. **How can patients with hyposmolar hyponatremia be categorized according to history and physical findings?**
As hypovolemic, hypervolemic, or euvolemic.

18. **What findings suggest a hypovolemic state?**
A history of volume loss or decreased intake and orthostatic blood pressure changes on examination.

19. **How is the hypovolemia treated?**
By replacement of the lost volume to turn off the factors that limit the kidney's ability to excrete free water.

20. **How do you recognize the hypervolemic patient?**
By a history of a condition with decreased effective arterial blood volume and an examination showing edema.

21. **Describe the treatment of the hypervolemia.**
Therapeutic attention must be directed to the underlying disorder. If the hyponatremia is mild and asymptomatic, free-water restriction, in addition to specific treatment of the underlying disorder, is the suggested initial therapeutic approach. If the hyponatremia is severe and symptomatic, more aggressive treatment with hypertonic saline and furosemide may be required.

22. **Summarize the approach to euvolemic hyposmolar hyponatremia.**
In patients with hyposmolar hyponatremia and apparently normal volume status or euvolemia, a wide variety of pathologic processes must be considered in the diagnostic evaluation, including SIADH and drugs that can limit free-water excretion (e.g., chlorpropamide).

23. **Define "pseudohyponatremia."**
Pseudohyponatremia occurs when a quantitative $[Na^+]$ measurement is performed on a given volume of plasma that contains a greater-than-normal amount of water-excluding particles, such as lipid or protein. In this setting, plasma water (which contains the Na^+) composes a smaller fraction of the plasma volume, leading to a factitiously low serum $[Na^+]$ (when expressed in mEq/L). The $[Na^+]$ in plasma water is normal, and therefore, patients are asymptomatic. Attention should be directed to hyperlipidemia or hyperproteinemia.

24. **How is spurious hyponatremia different from pseudohyponatremia?**
Spurious hyponatremia results from hyperosmolality of the serum (i.e., from hyperglycemia), resulting in movement of intracellular water to the extracellular space and subsequent dilution

of the Na^+ in the ECF. These patients are not symptomatic from hyposmolality (unlike patients with true hyponatremia). If they are symptomatic at all, it is due to their hyperosmolar state. Attention should be directed to correcting the hyperosmolar state. It is important to distinguish these two categories of hyponatremia from true hyponatremia associated with hyposmolality because the diagnostic work-up and therapeutic management are different.

25. **How do you correct the [Na^+] for a given level of hyperglycemia?**
Hyperglycemia, one of the causes of spurious hyponatremia, causes a decrease in the measured [Na^+]. For each increase in serum glucose of 100 mg/dL up to 600 mg/dL (an increase of 500, or 5 × 100 mg/dL), the [Na^+] decreases by 8.0 mEq/L (5 × 1.6 mEq/L). However, recent studies suggested that the relationship is not linear, especially with plasma glucose levels of more than 400 mg/dL, and a factor of 2.4 mEq/L may be a more accurate correction factor.

26. **Define "essential hyponatremia."**
Hyponatremia in the absence of a water diuresis defect. One hypothesis is that the osmoreceptor cells in the hypothalamus are reset so that they maintain a lower plasma osmolality. This is seen in several conditions, such as congestive heart failure, cirrhosis, and pulmonary tuberculosis, and is diagnosed by demonstrating normal urinary Na^+ concentration and dilution in the face of hyponatremia. Generally, this entity does not require treatment, and is sometimes called "sick cell syndrome."

27. **What are the signs and symptoms of hyponatremia?**
The manifestations are mainly attributable to central nervous system (CNS) edema, which is usually not seen until the [Na^+] falls to $\leq$ 120 mEq/L. Symptoms range from mild lethargy to seizure, coma, and death. The signs and symptoms of hyponatremia are more a function of the rapidity of the drop in [Na^+] than the absolute level. In patients with chronic hyponatremia, there has been time for solute equilibration, resulting in less CNS edema and less severe manifestations. In acute hyponatremia, there is no time for equilibration, and so smaller changes in [Na^+] are accompanied by larger degrees of CNS edema and more severe manifestations.

28. **Why is hyponatremia often seen after transurethral resection of the prostate (TURP)?**
Because large volumes of solutions containing mannitol, glycerol, or sorbitol are used to irrigate the prostate. A variable fraction of these fluids is absorbed into the systemic circulation, producing hyponatremia.

29. **How do you manage hyponatremia in edematous states?**
Treatment depends on the underlying etiology, any symptoms, and the rapidity of the drop in [Na^+]. In general, patients with edematous states such as the nephrotic syndrome, who have ECF expansion, have some degree of hyponatremia if they are not water-restricted. Generally, this condition is asymptomatic and requires no treatment. Treatment is required only if the hyponatremia is severe (<125 mEq/L), and especially if there are symptoms such as lethargy, confusion, stupor, and coma.

30. **A 41-year-old black man is hospitalized with acute bacterial meningitis. His chemistry profile shows a BUN and creatinine of 11 and 1.2 mg/dL, respectively, but his [Na^+] is 127 mEq/L. What is the likely cause of his hyponatremia?**
SIADH. Hyponatremia in the setting of bacterial meningitis (or any pathologic CNS process) is usually due to SIADH. SIADH is a form of hyponatremia involving sustained or spiking levels of ADH that are inappropriate for the osmotic or volume stimuli that normally affect ADH secretion.

31. **List the essential points in the diagnosis of SIADH.**
- Presence of hypotonic hyponatremia
- Inappropriate antidiuresis (urine osmolality higher than expected for the degree of hyponatremia)
- Significant Na^+ excretion when the patient is normovolemic
- Normal renal, thyroid, and adrenal function
- Absence of other causes of hyponatremia, volume depletion, or edema

32. **Describe the work-up for the patient with suspected SIADH.**
Measurement of serum and urine Na^+ concentration and osmolality. In most cases, urinary osmolality exceeds plasma osmolality, often by > 100 mOsm/L. Urinary Na^+ excretion exceeds 20 mEq/L unless the patient is wasting, and it improves with fluid restriction. In most cases, restriction of fluids to 1000–1200 mL/day is all that is needed. Occasionally, patients with symptomatic and marked hyponatremia may require demeclocycline therapy and/or hypertonic saline.

33. **What is cerebral salt-wasting?**
A syndrome that mimics SIADH in all aspects including hypouricemia except that in cerebral salt-wasting, patients are volume-depleted. In SIADH, patients are euvolemic. Owing to impaired renal water excretion, this condition is associated with hyposmolar hyponatremia in patients with cerebral trauma or disease. The high urinary Na^+ despite hypovolemia reflects renal salt-wasting. The etiology of this salt-wasting is unknown, although increased secretion of cerebral natriuretic factors is one likely explanation. A circulating factor that impairs renal tubular Na^+ reabsorption is another likely possibility.

Al-Mufti H, Arieff AI: Cerebral salt wasting syndrome: Combined cerebral and distal tubular lesion, *Am J Med* 77:740–746, 1984.

34. **How do you estimate the free-water deficit in a patient with hypernatremia?**
It can be assumed that the patient has lost free water without salt, and thus the patient has reduced TBW but maintains the same total body Na^+ content. This change results in an increase in the $[Na^+]$ that is proportional to the decrease in TBW. In other words, the ratio of the initial $[Na^+]$ (which is assumed to be normal) to the current $[Na^+]$ (which is higher than normal) is equal to the ratio of the present TBW (which is less than normal) to the initial TBW (which is assumed to have been normal).

$$\text{Current TBW} \div \text{Initial TBW} = \text{Initial } [Na^+] \div \text{Current } [Na^+]$$

This relationship can be used to calculate the current TBW. Subtracting this value from the initial (normal) TBW yields the estimated free-water deficit. This calculated free-water deficit must be replaced with fluids.

35. **What are the manifestations of hypernatremia?**
Basically those of hyperosmolality and are similar to the symptoms manifested by other causes of hyperosmolality, such as hyperglycemia. These are produced mainly by fluid shifts from the CNS and increased CNS osmolality, resulting in "shrinking" of the brain. The symptoms range from lethargy to seizures, coma, and death. The severity of the symptoms depends on the severity of the hyperosmolality and the speed with which it develops.

36. **What are some common causes of hypernatremia?**
Diabetes insipidus, severe dehydration due to extrarenal fluid losses (e.g., burns, excessive sweating), and hypothalamic disorders (e.g., tumors, granulomas, cerebrovascular accidents) leading to defective thirst and vasopressin regulation.

37. **How do you correct hypernatremia?**
By replacement of the water. In mild cases, this can be accomplished by simply having the patient drink, or if IV fluids are used, dextrose in water can be given. If salt-containing fluids are deemed necessary, the equivalent free-water volume must be given. For example, if half-normal saline is used (1 L of which contains 500 mL of normal saline and 500 mL of free water), then twice the amount of the estimated free-water deficit is needed to correct the free-water deficit. This volume deficit should be replaced slowly. The first half is given over 24 hours. If the patient is hemodynamically unstable, with signs of severe ECF volume depletion, therapy with 0.9% normal saline is warranted before dextrose infusion is started.

POTASSIUM BALANCE

38. **How is potassium (K^+) distributed between the intracellular fluid (ICF) and the ECF compartments?**
A 70-kg man contains approximately 3500 mEq of K^+ ($\sim$50 mEq/kg body weight). The vast majority of this (98%) is in the ICF space. Therefore, the amount in the ECF compartment (the portion that we routinely measure) represents only a small percentage of the total body K^+.

39. **How is the large chemical gradient between intracellular and extracellular K^+ concentration maintained?**
The Na^+-K^+ adenosine triphosphate (ATPase) pump actively extrudes Na^+ from the cell and pumps K^+ into the cell. This pump is present in all cells of the body. In addition, the cell is electrically negative compared with the exterior, which serves to keep K^+ inside the cell.

40. **Because the extracellular K^+ concentration is relatively small compared with the intracellular concentration of K^+, why are some electrical processes (cardiac conduction, skeletal and smooth muscle contraction) sensitive to changes in the ECF K^+ concentration?**
Because the ratio of the ECF to the ICF K^+ concentration is more significant than the absolute level of either in determining the sensitivity of these electrical processes. Because the ECF concentration of K^+ is small compared with the ICF concentration, a small absolute change in ECF K^+ concentration results in a large change in the ECF-to-ICF K^+ ratio.

41. **What factors commonly influence the movement of K^+ between the intracellular and the extracellular compartments?**
    - **Acid-base changes:** Acidemia (increased concentration of H^+ in serum) leads to intracellular buffering of H^+, with subsequent extrusion of K^+ into the ECF, increasing the concentration of K^+ in this compartment. Similarly, alkalemia leads to hypokalemia.
    - **Hormones:** Insulin, epinephrine, growth hormone, and androgens all promote net movement of K^+ into cells.
    - **Cellular metabolism:** Synthesis of protein and glycogen is associated with intracellular K^+ binding.
    - **Extracellular concentration:** All other things being equal, K^+ tends to enter the cell when its extracellular concentration is high and vice versa.

42. **How is K^+ handled by the kidney?**
Through reabsorption in the proximal tubule, and there is net secretion or net resorption in the distal nephron, depending on the body's K^+ needs. Under most conditions, we are in K^+ excess, and the kidney must excrete K^+ to maintain whole body K^+ balance. K^+ restriction leads to renal K^+ conservation, but this process is neither as rapid nor as efficient as the process for Na^+.

43. **How does aldosterone influence K^+ metabolism?**
By promoting Na^+ resorption and K^+ secretion in the distal nephron, gut, and sweat glands. Aldosterone is the main regulatory hormone for K^+ metabolism. Quantitatively, its greatest effect is in the kidney. Its secretion is increased by an increasing K^+ concentration in the ECF and is decreased by low K^+ concentrations.

44. **How does hypoaldosteronism affect K^+ and Na^+ levels?**
Asymptomatic hyperkalemia is a common presentation of patients with mineralocorticoid deficiency. Na^+ deficiency and volume depletion are not seen unless there is concomitant glucocorticoid deficiency. Na^+ balance is maintained by other factors, such as angiotensin II and catecholamines, although the ability to conserve Na^+ maximally is generally lost. Thus, urine $Na^+ < 10$ mEq/L is unusual in primary hypoaldosteronism.

45. **How is hypoaldosteronism diagnosed?**
First by excluding drug-induced hyperkalemia (such as caused by angiotensin-converting enzyme [ACE] inhibitors, beta blockers, nonsteroidal anti-inflammatory drugs [NSAIDs], heparin, or K^+-sparing diuretics). The next step is to obtain morning samples of plasma for renin, aldosterone, and cortisol measurements. Administration of furosemide (20–40 mg) at 6 pm and 6 am before samples are drawn enhances the utility of the test by stimulating plasma renin activity in normal persons but not in those with hypoaldosteronism.

46. **What is meant by transtubular K^+ gradient (TTKG)?**
An indirect method of evaluating the effect of aldosterone on the kidney. The principle is to measure K^+ at the end of the cortical collecting tube, after all the distal K^+ secretion has taken place:

$$TTKG = \frac{U_{K^+}/(U_{osm}/P_{osm})}{P_{K^+}}$$

where P_{K^+} is plasma K^+ concentration. It is assumed that urine osmolality (U_{osm}) at the end of the cortical collecting tube is the same as that of plasma (P_{osm}) because the interstitium here is iso-osmotic. It is also assumed that no further K^+ secretion or resorption takes place. But, because ADH-mediated water permeability continues in the medullary collecting tubule, the K^+ concentration in this duct rises. This formula is applicable as long as the urine Na^+ concentration is 25 mEq/L, because Na^+ delivery should not be a limiting factor.

47. **What is the TTKG value in normal and hyperkalemic subjects?**
The TTKG in normal subjects is 8–10 on a normal diet. On a high K^+ diet, TTKG > 11 because of increased K^+ secretion. Thus, in a hyperkalemic subject, a TTKG < 5 mEq/L indicates impaired tubular K^+ secretion and is highly suggestive of hypoaldosteronism.

Ethier JH, Kamel KS, Magner PO, et al: The trans-tubular potassium gradient in patients with hypokalemia and hyperkalemia, *Am J Kidney Dis* 15:309–315, 1990.

48. **List conditions that can lead to increased renal K^+ excretion.**
   - Increased dietary K^+ intake
   - Increased aldosterone secretion (as in volume depletion)
   - Alkalosis
   - Increased flow rate in the distal tubule
   - Increased Na^+ delivery to the distal nephron
   - Decreased chloride concentration in tubular fluid in the distal nephron
   - Natriuretic agents

49. **How does increased sodium delivery promote renal excretion of K^+?**
Increased Na^+ delivery to the distal nephron promotes Na^+ resorption in exchange for K^+ secretion. The process is accelerated in the presence of aldosterone.

50. **Explain how decreased chloride concentration leads to an increased renal excretion of K^+.**
Decreased chloride concentration in tubular fluid in the distal nephron allows Na^+ to be resorbed with a less permeable ion (e.g., bicarbonate or sulfate) that increases the negativity of the tubular lumen in the distal nephron. The increased negativity of the tubular lumen promotes K^+ secretion.

51. **How do natriuretic agents increase renal excretion of K^+?**
Natriuretic agents, such as loop diuretics, thiazides, and acetazolamide, lead to increased Na^+ delivery to the distal nephron, volume depletion with increased aldosterone secretion, and subsequent increased renal K^+ excretion.

52. **In addition to the kidney, what is the other major route of K^+ loss?**
The gastrointestinal (GI) tract. Fluids in the lower GI tract, particularly those of the small bowel, are high in K^+. Therefore, diarrhea can result in significant losses of K^+. However, upper GI losses, such as vomiting or nasogastric suction, cause renal K^+ loss. This renal K^+ loss is multifactorial and includes the following:
- Alkalosis
- Volume depletion, which leads to increased aldosterone secretion
- Chloride depletion from the loss of HCl in gastric fluid, which leads to a high tubular concentration of HCO_3^-, a relatively nonresorbable anion

53. **What causes a spuriously elevated serum K^+ determination?**
- **Hemolysis,** with the release of intraerythrocytic K^+.
- **Pseudohyperkalemia,** seen in marked thrombocytosis or leukocytosis due to the disproportionately increased amounts of the normally released K^+ that occurs with clotting. This condition can be corrected by inhibiting clotting and measuring the plasma K^+ concentration.

54. **List the four common mechanisms by which hyperkalemia develops.**
- Inadequate excretion of K^+
- Excessive intake of K^+
- Shift of potassium from tissues
- Pseudohyperkalemia (due to thrombocytosis, leukocytosis, poor venipuncture technique, in vitro hemolysis)

   Singer GG, Brenner BM: Fluids and electrolytes. In Fauci A, Braunwald E, Kaspar DL, et al, editors: *Harrison's Principles of Internal Medicine*, ed 17, New York, 2008, McGraw-Hill.

55. **What factors lead to inadequate potassium excretion?**
- Renal disorders (acute renal failure, severe CKD, tubular disorders)
- Hypoaldosteronism
- Adrenal disorders
- Hyporeninemia (as with tubulointerstitial diseases, drugs such as NSAIDs, ACE inhibitors, and beta blockers)
- Diuretics that inhibit potassium secretion (spironoloactone, triamterene, amiloride)

56. **Is there a difference in the risk for hyperkalemia between ACE inhibitors and angiotensin receptor blockers (ARBs)?**
The risk of hyperkalemia caused by ARBs is similar to that of ACE inhibitors, although in many large-scale clinical studies, the frequency was found to be less with ARBs than with

ACE inhibitors. Although the exact reason is unclear, it may depend partly on the differential degree of inhibition of aldosterone with these two classes of agents.

57. **What factors lead to a shift of potassium from tissues?**
    - Tissue damage (muscle crush, hemolysis, and internal bleeding)
    - Drugs (succinylcholine, arginine, digitalis poisoning, and beta blockers)
    - Acidosis
    - Hyperosmolality
    - Insulin deficiency
    - Hyperkalemic periodic paralysis

58. **What is the first step in the diagnostic approach to patients with disturbances in serum K^+ concentration?**
    Determine whether the disturbance results from:
    - Abnormal K^+ intake or metabolism (excessive catabolism or anabolism)
    - Intra- and extracellular compartmental shifts
    - Disturbances in renal excretion or extrarenal loss

59. **What should you do next?**
    After the patient is placed in one of these three categories, it is possible to narrow the differential diagnosis, order appropriate diagnostic tests, and decide on the appropriate management. Disturbances of intake can be investigated by history and physical examination. The possibility of cellular shifts can be investigated by looking for any of the disturbances that result in compartmental movement of this cation. Determination of the urinary K^+ concentration can help in distinguishing renal from nonrenal causes. High urinary K^+ excretion in the setting of hypokalemia is compatible with a renal cause for K^+ deficiency. In contrast, an appropriately low urinary K^+ excretion in the setting of hypokalemia suggests extrarenal (possibly GI) losses.

60. **How does hypokalemia present clinically?**
    Usually with neuromuscular symptoms. When K^+ falls to 2.0–2.5 mEq/L, muscular weakness and lethargy are seen. With further decreases, the patient manifests paralysis with eventual respiratory muscle involvement and death. Hypokalemia also can cause rhabdomyolysis, myoglobinuria, and paralytic ileus. Prolonged hypokalemia can lead to renal tubular damage (called "hypokalemic nephropathy").

61. **How do you manage a patient with hypokalemia?**
    First with correction of the disturbance causing the abnormal K^+ concentration. If hypokalemia is associated with alkalosis, then the alkalosis should be corrected in addition to providing K^+ supplements. In general, patients with K^+ depletion should be given supplements slowly to replace the deficit. The oral route is preferred because of its safety as well as its efficacy. Some instances require more rapid repletion with IV supplements, but this should not exceed 20 mEq/hr. Cardiac monitoring should accompany infusions of > 10 mEq/hr.

62. **What are the manifestations of hyperkalemia besides electrocardiogram (ECG) changes?**
    The most important manifestation is the increased excitability of cardiac muscle. With severe elevations in K^+, a patient can suffer diastolic cardiac arrest. Skeletal muscle paralysis also can be seen. Again, the symptoms produced by hyperkalemia are dependent on the rapidity of the change. Patients with chronically elevated serum K levels can tolerate higher levels with fewer symptoms than patients with acute hyperkalemia. (See also Chapter 4, Cardiology.)

63. **How is chronic hyperkalemia generally managed?**

Treatment depends on the extent of the hyperkalemia and the clinical setting. Mild levels of hyperkalemia (5.0–5.5 mEq/L) associated with the hyporenin-hypoaldosterone syndrome are tolerated well and usually require no treatment. Higher levels not associated with ECG changes may require treatment with a synthetic mineralocorticoid.

64. **Describe the management of hyperkalemia as a medical emergency.**

- IV calcium must be administered to immediately counteract the effect of hyperkalemia on the conduction system.
- Calcium administration must be followed by maneuvers to shift K^+ into cells, thereby decreasing the ratio of extra- to intracellular K^+. This goal can be accomplished by administering glucose with insulin and/or bicarbonate to increase serum pH.
- Finally, a maneuver to remove K^+ from the body must be instituted, such as a cation-exchange resin (Kayexalate) and/or hemodialysis or peritoneal dialysis.

65. **A 61-year-old woman with end-stage renal disease missed her dialysis twice and presents to the emergency department with a serum K^+ of 6.4 mEq/L. How should you manage this patient?**

The severity of hyperkalemia is assessed by both the serum K^+ level and ECG changes. If the ECG shows only tall T waves and the serum $K^+ < 6.5$ mEq/L, the hyperkalemia is mild, whereas K^+ levels of 6.5–8.0 mEq/L are associated with more severe ECG changes, including absent P waves and wide QRS complexes. At higher K^+ levels, ventricular arrhythmias tend to appear, and the prognosis is grave unless proper treatment is given.

66. **If the ECG shows only tall T waves, which agents should you administer? Why?**

- **Hypertonic glucose infusion,** along with 10 units of insulin (e.g., 10 units of insulin with 200–500 mL of 10% glucose in 30 min followed by 1 L of the same in the next 4–6 hr).
- **Sodium bicarbonate,** 50–150 mEq given by IV (if the patient is not in fluid overload).

Both of these agents shift K^+ into cells and start acting within an hour. Total body K^+ can be decreased by using cation-exchange resins, such as sodium polysterone sulfonate; usually 20 g with 20 mL of 70% sorbitol solution is started every 4–6 hours.

67. **If the ECG shows the more severe changes, what should you do?**

Give 10% calcium gluconate (10–30 mL IV) with cardiac monitoring. Arrangements must be made to dialyze the patient as soon as possible to correct the hyperkalemia.

68. **A 71-year-old diabetic with a nonhealing foot ulcer is on tobramycin and piperacillin. This patient has a resistant hypokalemia. How do you approach this problem?**

Aminoglycosides and penicillins are both known to deplete serum K^+. The former do this by defective proximal tubular K^+ resorption and the latter by increased renal K^+ excretion induced by the poorly resorbable anion (penicillin). With aminoglycosides, magnesium-wasting is another complication. Hence, in addition to K^+ repletion, correction of hypomagnesemia is important, because hypokalemia is often resistant to correction unless the magnesium deficit is also corrected.

69. **A 67-year-old man with congestive heart failure treated with furosemide has a serum K^+ of 2.4 mEq/L. How would you correct his K^+ deficit?**

Hypokalemia is an important complication of diuretic therapy (except with K^+-sparing diuretics). It is important to monitor serum K^+ periodically in these patients, especially those with cardiac illnesses who are likely to be on digoxin because hypokalemia can exacerbate digitalis toxicity. The K^+ deficit requires replacement (except in patients who are on minimal doses of diuretics), particularly if serum $K^+ < 3$ mEq/L. The serum K^+ level is not an exact indicator of the total body deficit, but severe hypokalemia with serum $K^+ < 3$ mEq/L is usually associated with a deficit of approximately 300 mEq. KCl elixir or tablets are the treatment of choice. Enteric-coated K^+ supplements are known to cause gastric ulceration.

70. **What is the primary defect in Bartter's syndrome?**
Impaired NaCl reabsorption in the thick ascending loop of Henle or distal tubule. Recent genetic studies indicate the defect involves a mutation of Na^+-K^+-2Cl co-transporter or K^+ channel in the thick ascending limb of Henle. The diagnosis is often made by exclusion. Surreptitious use of diuretics and vomiting (urine Cl^- is often low!) can mimic most of the findings of this syndrome.

71. **Describe the treatment of Bartter's syndrome.**
A K^+-sparing diuretic (such as amiloride in doses of 10–40 mg) and NSAIDs to raise the plasma K^+ by reversing the physiologic abnormalities.

72. **A 55-year-old man with a history of congestive heart failure and chronic obstructive pulmonary disease (COPD) presents with extreme weakness and fatigue. His medications include digoxin 0.25 mg/day, furosemide 40 mg/day, and albuterol inhalations for his asthma. The patient reports a few days of exacerbation of COPD symptoms, forcing him to use the inhaler more frequently. What is the likely cause of his weakness?**
Severe hypokalemia resulting from overuse of beta agonists such as albuterol especially in the presence of potassium-losing diuretics, because both effects could be additive. The hypokalemic effects of inhaled beta agonists are often so potent that they are used to treat patients with hyperkalemia acutely.

ACID–BASE REGULATION

73. **What is the Henderson-Hasselbalch equation?**
An acid-base disorder is suspected on clinical grounds and confirmed by arterial blood gas (ABG) analysis of the pH, arterial carbon dioxide pressure ($PaCO_2$), or HCO_3^- concentration. The Henderson-Hasselbalch equation is used to test whether a given set of parameters is mutually compatible:

$$pH = pKa + \log \frac{(HCO_3^-)}{\alpha CO_2 \times paCO_2} = 6.1 + \log \frac{(HCO_3^-)}{0.03 \times paCO_2}$$

The value of pK_a, the negative log of the equilibrium constant K, and the CO_2 solubility coefficient (αCO_2) are constant at any given set of temperature and osmolality. In plasma, at $37°C$, the $pK_a = 6.1$ and the $\alpha CO_2 = 0.03$.

74. **Explain the significance of the Henderson-Hasselbalch equation.**
The Henderson-Hasselbalch equation shows that pH is dependent on the ratio of $[HCO_3^-]$ to $PaCO_2$ and not on the absolute individual values alone. A primary change in one of the values usually leads to a compensatory change in the other value. This serves to limit the degree of the resulting acidosis or alkalosis.

75. **The integrated action of which three organs is involved in acid-base homeostasis?**
Liver, lungs, and **kidneys.** The **liver** metabolizes proteins contained in the standard American diet such that net acid (protons) is produced. Hepatic metabolism of organic acids (lactate) can

consume acid, which is the equivalent of producing bicarbonate. Acid released into the ECF titrates HCO_3^- to H_2O and CO_2. The **lungs** excrete this CO_2 and the CO_2 produced from cellular metabolism. The **kidney** reclaims the filtered HCO_3^- and excretes the accumulated net acid.

76. **What is the fate of a load of nonvolatile acid administered to the body?**
    Initially, buffering by extracellular (40%) and intracellular (60%) buffers and eventual excretion by the kidneys. The buffers minimize the decrease in pH that otherwise would occur. The major ECF buffer is the HCO_3^- system, and most intracellular buffering is provided by histidine-containing proteins. The administered acid reduces ECF HCO_3^-, and new HCO_3^- is then regenerated by the kidney during the process of proton (acid) secretion.

77. **How does the kidney excrete acid to maintain the acid-base balance?**
    The kidney must **reclaim** the filtered HCO_3^- and **regenerate** the HCO_3^- lost by acid titration. This latter process is equivalent to acid excretion. Reclamation of HCO_3^- is quantitatively a more important process than regeneration (4500 mEq/day vs. 70 mEq/day). Nevertheless, without regeneration of new HCO_3^- (excretion of acid), the plasma HCO_3^- concentration could not be maintained, and net acid retention would result. Two principal urinary buffers allow net acid excretion (new HCO_3^- regeneration): dibasic phosphate and ammonia. By accepting a proton, they become monobasic phosphate and ammonium ions, respectively, and are excreted in the urine. The phosphate is measured as titratable acid, and the ammonium is measured directly. Urinary excretion of these two substances minus urinary HCO_3^- excretion constitutes net acid excretion.

78. **List the four primary acid-base disturbances.**
    - Metabolic acidosis
    - Metabolic alkalosis
    - Respiratory acidosis
    - Respiratory alkalosis

79. **Explain what is meant by "acidosis" and "alkalosis."**
    Acidosis refers to an imbalance in the steady-state acid-base balance that leads to a net increase in $[H^+]$. **Alkalosis** refers to an imbalance that leads to a net decrease in $[H^+]$. In the maintenance of normal acid-base balance, the addition of H^+ to the body fluids is balanced by their excretion, such that the H^+ concentration of the ECF remains relatively constant at 40 nM (40×10^{-9} M, or pH = 7.40).

80. **What is meant by "metabolic" and "respiratory" in referring to acid-base disturbances?**
    "Metabolic" and "respiratory" are terms used to describe how the imbalance occurred. Describing a disorder as **metabolic** infers that the imbalance leading to the change in H^+ occurred either because of addition of nonvolatile acid or base or because of a gain or loss of available buffer (HCO_3^-). HCO_3^- as a buffer reduces the concentration of free H^+ in solution. Referring to an acid-base disorder as **respiratory** infers that the net change in $[H^+]$ occurred secondary to a disturbance in ventilation that resulted in either a net increase or decrease in CO_2 gas in the ECF.

81. **Define "metabolic acidosis."**
    A net increase in $[H^+]$ as a result of a net gain in nonvolatile acid or from a net loss of HCO_3^- buffer.

82. **Define "respiratory acidosis."**
    A net increase in $[H^+]$ as a result of decreased ventilation, leading to CO_2 retention.

83. **Define "metabolic alkalosis."**
A net decrease in [H$^+$] as a result of gain of HCO$_3^-$ or loss of acid.

84. **Define "respiratory alkalosis."**
A net decrease in [H$^+$] because of increased ventilation leading to decreased CO$_2$.

85. **What important points should be kept in mind about these four disorders?**
These disorders refer to the imbalance that leads to the directional change in [H$^+$] and do not
denote what the final [H$^+$], PCO$_2$, and [HCO$_3^-$] will be. Two important facts should be kept in mind:
1. Compensatory changes occur in response to these disorders.
2. More than one acid-base disturbance may occur simultaneously; the final parameters
   measured depend not only on the algebraic sum of the different disorders but also on their
   respective compensatory responses.

86. **How are the four primary acid-base disorders diagnosed?**
See Table 9-2.

TABLE 9-2.	RELATIONSHIPS BETWEEN BICARBONATE AND ARTERIAL CARBON DIOXIDE PRESSURE IN SIMPLE ACID-BASE DISORDERS			
Condition	**pH**	**HCO$_3$**	**PaCO$_2$**	**Predicted Response**
Metabolic acidosis	↓	↓	↓	ΔPaCO$_2$ (↓) = 1–1.4 ΔHCO$_3^-$*
Metabolic alkalosis	↑	↑	↑	ΔPaCO$_2$ (↑) = 0.4–0.9 ΔHCO$_3^-$*
Respiratory acidosis	↓	↑	↑	Acute: ΔHCO$_3^-$ (↑) = 0.1 ΔPaCO$_2$
				Chronic: ΔHCO$_3^-$ (↑) = 0.25–0.55 PaCO$_2$
Respiratory alkalosis	↑	↓	↓	Acute: ΔHCO$_3^-$ (↓) = 0.2–0.25 ΔPaCO$_2$
				Chronic: ΔHCO$_3^-$ (↓) = 0.4–0.5 ΔPaCO$_2$

HCO$_3^-$ = bicarbonate; PaCO$_2$ = arterial carbon dioxide pressure.
*After at least 12–24 hr.
From Hamm L: Mixed acid-base disorders. In Kokko JP, Tannen KL (eds): Fluids and Electrolytes, 3rd
ed. Philadelphia, WB Saunders, 1996, p 487.

87. **What are secondary acid-base disturbances?**
Compensatory physiologic responses to the cardinal acid-base disturbances. The phrase
"secondary acid-base disturbance" is actually a misnomer. They usually alleviate the change
in H$^+$ concentration and, therefore, the pH change that otherwise would occur.

88. **What equation helps explain the compensatory physiologic responses to
acid-base disturbances?**
The mass-action equation, derived from the more familiar Henderson-Hasselbalch equation,
defines the relationship of H$^+$, HCO$_3^-$, and the PaCO$_2$:

$$[H^+] = \frac{PaCO_2}{(HCO_3^-)} \times 24$$

One can see that in the setting of metabolic acidosis, with a primary decrease in [HCO$_3^-$],
the [H$^+$] increases. It is also evident that the increase in [H$^+$] in this setting can be alleviated

by concomitantly decreasing the $PaCO_2$, which is exactly what occurs as a result of a **physiologic** increase in ventilation. This situation is properly described as metabolic acidosis with a directionally appropriate respiratory response. It is incorrect to describe the condition as primary metabolic acidosis with secondary respiratory alkalosis. To say that a patient has respiratory alkalosis is to say that a patient has **pathologic** hypoventilation, which is not the case in this situation. Tables and formulas can be used to calculate the expected respiratory response to a given degree of metabolic acidosis.

89. **What is a mixed acid-base disorder?**
If the decrease in $PaCO_2$ in response to the degree of metabolic acidosis is exactly what we would have predicted from the formulas, the patient is said to have one acid-base disorder: metabolic acidosis. In contrast, if the measured decrease in $PaCO_2$ is more than that predicted for the degree of metabolic acidosis, then the patient has an additional (not secondary) acid-base disorder: respiratory alkalosis in addition to metabolic acidosis. In other words, the patient has a mixed disorder, which is actually very common. If the measured $PaCO_2$ is higher than predicted, then the patient has an additional respiratory acidosis.

90. **What causes respiratory acidosis?**
Alveolar hypoventilation that leads to a drop in the pH. The alveolar hypoventilation leads to a rate of excretion of CO_2 that is less than its metabolic production. This net gain in CO_2 causes a rise in the $PaCO_2$. The lungs may be subject to diffuse hypoventilation (global alveolar hypoventilation), or only parts of the lungs may be involved (regional alveolar hypoventilation). As can be seen in the Henderson-Hasselbalch equation, any increase in the $PaCO_2$, if not accompanied by an increase in $[HCO_3^-]$, leads to a measurable drop in the pH.

91. **Describe the treatment of respiratory acidosis.**
Correction of the cause of the hypoventilation. This goal may involve the treatment of airway obstruction or, in respiratory failure, even mechanical ventilation.

92. **What causes respiratory alkalosis?**
Alveolar hyperventilation that leads to a rise in pH. Alveolar hyperventilation, in turn, leads to an increase in the excretion of CO_2 and a drop in the $PaCO_2$. The causes of respiratory alkalosis include:
- CNS stimulation of ventilation: physiologic (voluntary, anxiety, fear, fever, and pregnancy) or pathologic (intracranial hemorrhage, stroke, tumors, brainstem lesions, and salicylates)
- Peripheral stimulation of ventilation: reflex hyperventilation due to abnormal lung or chest wall mechanics (pulmonary emboli, myopathies, and interstitial lung diseases), arterial hypoxemia, high altitudes, pain, congestive heart failure, shock of any etiology, and hypothermia
- Hyperventilation with mechanical ventilation
- Others: severe liver disease and uremia

93. **Are the plasma electrolytes alone (Na^+, K^+, Cl^-, and HCO_3^-) sufficient to determine a patient's acid-base status?**
No. Remember that the regulatory systems of the body work to maintain the pH (or $[H^+]$), and that pH is a function of the ratio of $PaCO_2$ to $[HCO_3^-]$. The pH is not determined by the absolute value of $PaCO_2$ or $[HCO_3^-]$ alone. Thus, a set of plasma electrolytes demonstrating a normal $[HCO_3^-]$ does not necessarily indicate a normal acid-base status.

94. **Give two interpretations of a low $[HCO_3^-]$ and high $[Cl^-]$.**
Either a metabolic acidosis (probably a non–anion-gap [AG] acidosis) or a chronic respiratory alkalosis with an appropriate metabolic response (renal lowering of $[HCO_3^-]$ as a response to the chronically low $PaCO_2$). This is an attempt to maintain a more normal pH.

95. **Give two interpretations of a high [HCO$_3^-$] and low [Cl$^-$].**

A metabolic alkalosis or a chronic respiratory acidosis with an appropriate metabolic response (renal increase in [HCO$_3^-$] in response to chronically high PaCO$_2$) in an attempt to maintain a more normal pH. Note that without an accompanying pH and PaCO$_2$, one cannot tell whether an abnormal [HCO$_3^-$] is due to a metabolic cause (a metabolic acidosis or alkalosis) or to a metabolic response to a primary respiratory disorder. This illustrates the importance of obtaining ABGs (with a pH and PaCO$_2$) in addition to a [HCO$_3^-$] to properly assess a patient's acid-base status.

96. **What is meant by the anion gap (AG)?**

The difference between the routinely measured cations and anions in the plasma. It is usually calculated as follows:

$$AG = [Na^+] - [Cl^- + HCO_3^-]$$

97. **Is the AG really a "gap"?**

No. Because electroneutrality is always maintained in solution, there is no actual anion "gap." The calculated gap is composed predominantly of negatively charged proteins in plasma and averages 12 ± 3 mEq/L. An increase is most commonly caused by addition of an acid salt (H$^+$A$^-$), which reduces plasma HCO$_3^-$ concentration by titration. Electroneutrality is maintained in the face of the reduced plasma HCO$_3^-$ concentration by the accompanying anion. Because the anion is not measured routinely in the electrolyte profile, the routine measurement would reveal only decreased HCO$_3^-$ concentration. With plasma Na$^+$ and Cl$^-$ remaining unchanged, this reduced HCO$_3^-$ concentration leads to an increased AG. Note that the AG would not change if the added acid were HCl. Other circumstances that can increase the AG include increased protein concentration and alkalemia, which increase the net negative charge on plasma proteins. The presence of a large quantity of cationic (positively charged) proteins, as with multiple myeloma, can reduce the AG.

98. **What is the conceptual difference between an AG and a non-AG metabolic acidosis?**

An AG acidosis is caused by the addition of a nonvolatile acid to the ECF. Examples include diabetic ketoacidosis, lactic acidosis, and uremic acidosis. A non-AG acidosis commonly (but not exclusively) represents a loss of HCO$_3^-$. Examples include lower GI losses from diarrhea and urinary losses due to renal tubular acidosis (RTA). Therefore, when approaching a patient with an AG acidosis, one should look for the source and identity of the acid gained. By contrast, when evaluating a patient with a non-AG acidosis, one should begin by looking for the source of the HCO$_3^-$ loss.

99. **What are the causes of AG metabolic acidosis?**

The mnemonic KUSMAL can be used to remember the differential diagnosis of AG metabolic acidosis.

K = **K**etones (diabetic, alcohol, starvation)
U = **U**remia
S = **S**alicylates
M = **M**ethyl alcohol
A = **A**cid poisoning (ethylene glycol, paraldehyde)
L = **L**actate (circulatory/respiratory failure, sepsis, liver disease, tumors, toxins)

Morganroth ML: An analytical approach in the diagnosis of acid-base disorders, *J Crit Illness* 5:138–150, 1990.

100. **What is the significance of plasma osmolal gap? How does it help in the evaluation of a patient with metabolic acidosis?**
The difference between the measured and the calculated plasma osmolality. Plasma osmolal gap of 0.25 mOsm/kg suggests, in a patient with AG metabolic acidosis, the possibility of ingestion of methanol or ethylene glycol. Isopropyl alcohol and ethanol increase the osmolal gap but not the AG, because acetone is not an anion.

101. **What are the common causes of a non-AG metabolic acidosis?**

ASSOCIATED WITH K^+ LOSS	DRUGS
Diarrhea	Acetazolamide
RTA (proximal or distal)	Amphotericin B
Interstitial nephritis	Amiloride
Early renal failure	Spironolactone
Urinary tract obstruction	Toluene ingestion
Posthypocapnia	Urethral diversions
Infusions of HCl (HCl, arginine HCl, lysine HCl)	Ureterosigmoidostomy
	Dual bladder
	Ileal ureter

Toto RD: Metabolic acid-base disorders. In Kokko JP, Tannen RL, editors: *Fluids and Electrolytes*, ed 3, Philadelphia, 1996, WB Saunders.

102. **How does the serum protein level affect the interpretation of AG?**
The AG is significantly influenced by serum albumin level. If the concentration of serum albumin falls to 2 g/dL (which is approximately half the normal), the expected normal AG should be reduced to half. The paraproteins that accumulate in multiple myeloma are usually positively charged because they are rich in lysine and arginine. If there is a significant accumulation of these positively charged particles, the measured cations remain in the normal range. But because these "unmeasured" cations are associated with Cl^- (which is measured), the calculated AG will be reduced proportionately and may even become negative.

103. **Why is ammoniagenesis reduced in renal failure?**
Because in renal failure, the renal mass is reduced and there is a decrease in the ATP stores. Consequently, less ATP can be used to oxidize glutamine to ammonia. Ammonia then combines with H^+ to form ammonium, which is then excreted in the urine. Renal ammoniagenesis is an important mechanism for removal of acid and H^+ from the body.

104. **How is the urine AG useful in the evaluation of metabolic acidosis?**
For the evaluation of some cases of hyperchloremic metabolic acidosis.

Urine anion gap = Unmeasured cations − unmeasured anions = $(Na^+ + K^+) − Cl^-$

In normal subjects excreting 20–40 mEq of NH_4^+/L, the urine AG is positive or near zero. Conversely, in metabolic acidosis, the NH_4^+ excretion increases if the renal acidification mechanisms are intact. Consequently, urinary Cl^- excretion also increases to maintain electroneutrality. Urinary Cl^- therefore exceeds cation ($K^+ + Na^+$) excretion, and the urine AG is negative (often −20 to greater than −50 mEq/L). Conversely, in acidosis in which the renal acidification mechanisms are impaired (as in renal failure and RTA), the urine AG remains positive, as in normal subjects.

Battle DC, Hizon M, Cohen E, et al: The use of the urine anion gap in the diagnosis of hyperchloremic metabolic acidosis, *N Engl J Med* 318:594–599, 1988.

105. **Why is K^+ factored in the calculation of urine AG and not in plasma AG?**
Potassium is predominantly an intracellular cation with the plasma K^+ level being ~ 4 mEq/L under normal conditions. The cations in plasma, therefore, are almost entirely represented by Na^+, because Ca and Mg are also present in very small amounts. Conversely, the urine K^+ is usually much greater because most of the dietary K^+ is excreted daily in the urine with some being excreted in fecal route. Thus, K^+ is a major cation in the urine and used in the calculation of urine AG.

106. **In which two clinical situations should the urine AG not be used?**
   - In **ketoacidosis,** the excretion of ketoacids neutralize the increased excretion of NH_4^+ cations, decreasing the negativity of the AG.
   - In **hypovolemia,** the avid proximal Na^+ reabsorption causes decreased distal Na^+ delivery resulting in a defect in acidification. The Cl^- reabsorption that accompanies Na^+ prevents NH_4Cl excretion, and the urine AG remains positive.

107. **What causes a decreased AG?**
An increase in **unmeasured cations** such as K^+, Ca^{2+}, or Mg^{2+}, the addition of **abnormal** cations (lithium), or an increase in **cationic immunoglobulins** (plasma cell dyscrasias). AG also can be decreased by loss of unmeasured anions such as albumin (serum hypoalbuminemia) or if the effective negative charge on albumin is decreased by acidosis.

108. **What is RTA?**
A disorder of tubular function in which the kidney has a compromised ability to excrete acid and/or recover filtered HCO_3^- in the setting of higher than normal $[H^+]$ in the ECF. The laboratory presentation is that of a non-AG metabolic acidosis. There are four types of RTA.

109. **Describe type I RTA.**
Type I RTA (distal or classic RTA) is characterized by reduced net proton secretion by the distal nephron in the setting of systemic acidemia. Because the distal nephron is largely responsible for net acid excretion, patients with this disorder have continuous net acid retention (less net acid excretion than net acid production) and are, therefore, not in net acid balance. The diagnosis is made by demonstrating an inappropriately alkaline urine (pH > 5.5) in the setting of an acidemic serum (pH < 7.36) and by excluding the presence of drugs that alkalinize the urine (acetazolamide) or urea-splitting bacteria in the urine that can increase the urinary pH.

110. **Describe type II RTA.**
Type II RTA (proximal RTA) is characterized by a reduced capacity for HCO_3^- recovery by the proximal tubule but intact distal nephron function. These patients waste HCO_3^- in the urine until the ECF concentration of HCO_3^- is reduced to a level such that the reduced filtered load of HCO_3^- (GFR $\times$ plasma HCO_3^-) can now be more completely resorbed and the urine becomes nearly bicarbonate-free. The reduction in plasma HCO_3^- concentration results in an increase in $[H^+]$. However, in the steady-state condition of low plasma HCO_3^-, these patients can excrete an appropriately acid urine (pH < 5.5) because distal nephron function is intact, and they are thus in acid balance (amount of acid excreted equals amount of acid produced), unlike the situation described for type I.

111. **What is type III RTA?**
Type III RTA represents a variant of type I, and the term is rarely used.

112. **Describe type IV RTA.**

Type IV RTA is characterized by reduced aldosterone effect on the renal tubules, which may result in insufficient secretion of acid necessary to maintain normal acid-base status. These patients nevertheless can excrete an appropriately acidic urine in the face of acidemic stress. Unlike the other types of RTA, type IV RTA is commonly associated with hyperkalemia due to a coexisting reduction in K^+ secretion. This disorder is commonly seen in patients with hyporenin-hypoaldosteronism but also is seen in isolated aldosterone deficiency and resistance.

KEY POINTS: RENAL TUBULAR ACIDOSIS ✔

1. Type IV is the most common type of RTA in clinical practice.

2. Type IV RTA is often secondary to diabetic or nondiabetic renal disease (e.g., obstructive uropathy, aldosterone deficiency).

3. Drugs (e.g., triamterene and trimethoprim) are another common cause of RTA.

RTA = renal tubular acidosis.

113. **How is type I (distal) RTA managed?**

Alkali is given in amounts necessary (usually 1–2 mEq/kg/day) to correct the acidosis and to buffer the acid being retained. K^+ supplements are commonly required at the initiation of treatment but usually not in the steady-state treatment once the acidosis has been corrected.

114. **How is type II (proximal) RTA managed?**

Alkali is not usually required in adults because they do not have net acid retention and have only mild acidemia. But because the chronic acidemia inhibits bone growth in children, they must be treated with large amounts of alkali (10–20 mEq/kg/day) as well as large K^+ supplements (the increased urinary HCO_3^- losses are accompanied by accelerated urinary K^+ losses).

115. **How is type IV RTA managed?**

The clinically mild degrees of acidemia rarely require alkali treatment. Hyperkalemia is more commonly a clinical concern and dictates whether mineralocorticoid replacements with synthetic steroids are required.

116. **What is lactic acidosis?**

The accumulation of lactic acid, the end product of glycolysis. This accumulation leads to a depletion of the body's buffers and a drop in pH. Lactate, being an unmeasured anion, is one of the causes of an increased anion-gap acidosis.

117. **List the causes of lactic acidosis.**

- Cellular hypoxia
- Decreased hepatic utilization of lactic acid (seen in advanced hepatocellular insufficiency of any cause)
- Cyanide poisoning
- Alcohol consumption
- Neoplasms with a large tumor burden
- Diabetic ketoacidosis (even in the absence of shock or other etiologies)
- Lactic acidosis X (severe lactic acidosis without obvious cause)
- Factitious lactic acidosis

118. **How does cellular hypoxia cause lactic acidosis?**
Oxygen is required for the oxidative phosphorylation of the lactic acid produced by glycolysis. Anything interfering with the available cellular supply of O_2 or its utilization will lead to the accumulation of lactic acid. This category includes respiratory failure, circulatory failure, and CO poisoning. This also can be seen in thiamine deficiency and has been reported in patients on long-term total parenteral nutrition without supplementation with thiamine.

KEY POINTS: LACTIC ACIDOSIS ✔

1. In patients with lactic acidosis, bicarbonate administration is useful only when the pH < 7.15.

2. Alkali may cause paradoxical increase in lactate production in patients with milder acidosis.

3. The most common causes of lactic acidosis are cellular hypoxia, decreased hepatic utilization of lactic acid, alcohol consumption, neoplasms with a large tumor burden, and diabetic ketoacidosis.

4. "Lactic acidosis X" refers to severe lactic acidosis without obvious cause.

119. **How does cyanide poisoning cause lactic acidosis?**
By blocking oxidative phosphorylation, leading to increased glycolysis, decreased utilization of lactic acid, and therefore lactic acid accumulation.

120. **Explain how alcohol consumption may lead to lactic acidosis.**
Alcohol causes a modest increase in lactic acid production. In association with caloric depletion, the lactic acidosis can be severe.

121. **How does large tumor burden lead to lactic acidosis?**
By the increased rates of glycolysis in tumor cells compared to normal cells. This occurs even with sufficient O_2.

122. **What causes factitious lactic acidosis?**
Storage of blood for prolonged periods of time. The red and white cells generate lactic acid in the tube as it is stored and is most commonly seen in patients with high white blood cell counts.

123. **What is D-lactic acidosis and how is it treated?**
An uncommon condition seen in patients with short bowel syndrome, as in patients with a history of small bowel resection, jejunoileal bypass, and other conditions. In these patients, glucose is rapidly transported into the large bowel and is metabolized by lactobacilli into D-lactate. The D-lactate is then rapidly absorbed into plasma and cannot be metabolized, because humans lack the D-lactate dehydrogenase (the enzyme in human body is L-lactate specific). This results in the accumulation of D-lactate and leads to D-lactic acidosis. Clinically, patients present with ataxia, confusion, neurologic deficits, and speech and memory defects, typically after a large meal containing carbohydrates. The condition is diagnosed by measuring lactate using D-lactate dehydrogenase. The treatment usually consists of oral antibiotics to kill lactate-producing bacilli, low-carbohydrate diets using starch polymers rather than glucose, and of course, bicarbonate therapy.

124. **What causes metabolic alkalosis?**
The addition of excess HCO_3^- or alkali or loss of acid. Note that a low Cl^- and a high HCO_3^- concentration can result from both metabolic alkalosis as well as from a metabolic response to a respiratory acidosis. However, the pH and $PaCO_2$ help to differentiate these two disorders.

125. **What are the two categories of metabolic alkalosis?**
Chloride-responsive (urine Cl^- < 10 mEq/L) and **chloride-resistant** (urine Cl^- > 20 mEq/L). Forms of alkalosis responsive to chloride salt administration are generally associated with ECF volume depletion and low urinary Cl^- concentration in spot urine tests, whereas the Cl^--unresponsive alkaloses are associated with ECF volume expansion and urine Cl^- > 20 mEq/L.

126. **What conditions are associated with chloride-responsive metabolic alkalosis?**
   - Gastric fluid loss
   - Postdiuretic therapy
   - Posthypercapnia
   - Congenital chloride diarrhea

127. **List the conditions associated with chloride-resistant metabolic alkalosis.**
   - Primary aldosteronism
   - Primary reninism
   - Hyperglucocorticoidism
   - Hypercalcemia
   - Potassium depletion
   - Liddle's syndrome (an autosomal dominant disorder with increased Na^+ reabsorption in the collecting tubules and, usually, K^+ secretion)
   - Bartter's syndrome (an autosomal recessive disorder with impaired Na^+ in the loop of Henle)
   - Chloruretic diuretics

128. **Which is the most common acid-base disturbance seen in cirrhosis?**
Primary respiratory alkalosis due to centrally mediated hyperventilation, especially with superimposed encephalopathy. The exact etiology is unclear but may be related to the hormonal imbalance associated with liver failure. Estrogens and progesterone have been implicated, a situation somewhat similar to that seen in pregnancy.

129. **How do you treat a patient with metabolic alkalosis and edema?**
Frequently with NaCl with or without potassium. But in patients with edematous conditions presenting with metabolic alkalosis, using saline may be risky. In such patients, using acetazolamide (a carbonic hydrase inhibitor and a diuretic) may be useful. It increases renal $Na-HCO_3^-$ excretion and ameliorates edema and alkalosis. In patients resistant to acetazolamide, isotonic HCl may be given cautiously in a period of 8–24 hours (the amount needed is TBW $\times$ 0.5 $\times$ ΔHCO_3^-). If all measures fail, dialysis can be performed to ameliorate alkalosis.

130. **How do you diagnose a mixed acid-base disorder?**
   1. Define the primary disturbance and the compensatory process involved. The primary disturbance is identified by the direction of the changes in pH, HCO_3^-, and $PaCO_2$ levels.
   2. Determine whether the pulmonary or renal compensation is appropriate (see Table 9–2). Two facts must be kept in mind while making these interpretations. First, adequate compensation takes 12–24 hours to occur, and second, "overcompensation" never occurs in primary acid-base disturbances.
   3. Consider the patient's history and clinical presentation to formulate a differential diagnosis. In general, the underlying clinical condition gives clues to the possible mixed acid-base disturbance, which is then defined using the nomograms of expected compensation.

Narins R, Emmett M: Simple and mixed acid-base disorders: A practical approach, *Medicine* 59:161–187, 1980.

131. **What findings suggest a combined metabolic and respiratory acidosis?**
A distinctly lower pH, even though the HCO_3^- and $PaCO_2$ may not be changed.

132. **What findings suggest combined metabolic acidosis and metabolic alkalosis?**
In combined metabolic acidosis and metabolic alkalosis, the pH and HCO_3^- can be lower, normal, or higher, but an elevated AG with a high or normal HCO_3^- suggests the diagnosis.

133. **What findings suggest combined metabolic alkalosis and respiratory acidosis?**
Combined metabolic alkalosis and respiratory acidosis (which can be seen in patients with adult respiratory distress syndrome [ARDS] or COPD who are vomiting) causes HCO_3^- levels of higher-than-predicted compensation for a given high $PaCO_2$.

134. **A 34-year-old woman is admitted to the hospital because of nausea and vomiting for the last 2 days. She admits to having taken several aspirin pills to alleviate her joint pains before she noticed epigastric pain and vomiting. Her arterial blood gas analysis reveals the following: pH 7.64, $PaCO_2$ 32, and plasma bicarbonate 33 mEq/L. What kind of acid-base disorder is present in this patient?**
The patient has an alkalotic state because the pH is higher than the normal range. Because the patient presented with significant emesis, it is logical to think that the primary disturbance is metabolic alkalosis, which is supported by the fact that plasma bicarbonate is significantly elevated. The expected respiratory compensatory response is to increase $PaCO_2$ by 6–7 mmHg for every 10 mEq/L increase in plasma bicarbonate. However, in this patient, the $PaCO_2$ is actually lower than normal, indicating a primary respiratory alkalosis. Thus, this patient has a mixed acid-base disorder. The combined metabolic and respiratory alkalosis explains why the pH is so disproportionately high.

135. **In what situations are potentially fatal mixed acid-base disorders encountered?**
In general, combined respiratory and metabolic acidosis or metabolic and respiratory alkalosis can result in pH changes that are fatal. Common examples include:
- An alcoholic with ketoacidosis (metabolic acidosis) may have superimposed vomiting from gastritis (metabolic alkalosis) and hyperventilation associated with withdrawal (respiratory alkalosis).
- A combination of metabolic acidosis and respiratory alkalosis is seen typically in patients with sepsis, salicylate intoxication, and severe liver disease.
- Metabolic acidosis can coexist with metabolic alkalosis in patients with renal failure or with alcoholic or diabetic ketoacidosis (acidosis) who are vomiting or having gastric suction (alkalosis).
- Vomiting in a pregnant woman or a patient with liver failure causes a mixture of respiratory and metabolic alkalosis.

CALCIUM, PHOSPHATE, AND MAGNESIUM METABOLISM

136. **How is calcium distributed in the body and in the serum?**
A 70-kg man has approximately 1000 g of calcium in his body. Of this amount, bone contains 99%, whereas the ECF and ICF contain only 1%. Furthermore, only about 1% of skeletal calcium is freely exchangeable with ECF calcium. The routine measurement for serum calcium (normal = 9–10 mg/mL = 4.5–5.0 mEq/L = 2.25–2.5 mM/L) measures total calcium. Approximately 40% is protein-bound, 5–10% is complexed to other substances (e.g., phosphate, sulfate), and 50% is ionized.

137. **Explain the significance of the ionized fraction of calcium.**
The ionized fraction determines the activity of calcium in cellular and membrane function. The concentration of total calcium can vary without changing the ionized fraction by changing the protein concentration. It is also possible to vary the ionized fraction without changing the total calcium by changing serum pH. Increasing serum pH decreases the ionized fraction of calcium and vice versa.

138. **What are the major sites of calcium reabsorption in the nephron?**
About 50% of the filtered calcium is reabsorbed in the proximal tubule, and most of the remainder ($\sim$40% of the total) is reabsorbed in the loop of Henle, primarily the ascending limb of the loop of Henle. A small amount of calcium is reabsorbed in the distal convoluted tubule and an even smaller amount in the collecting tubule.

139. **What are the major hormones involved in calcium metabolism?**
Parathyroid hormone (PTH), vitamin D, and calcitonin.

KEY POINTS: ELECTROLYTE DISTURBANCES ✓

1. Magnesium deficiency must be excluded in patients with resistant hypokalemia.

2. Hyperglycemia is the most common cause of nonhypotonic hyponatremia.

3. Although hypoalbuminemia results in reduction of total serum calcium, ionized calcium remains unchanged (physiologically more important fraction).

140. **Summarize the roles of these hormones in calcium metabolism.**
PTH is secreted in response to a decrease in serum calcium and promotes calcium resorption from bone because it enhances renal resorption of calcium and excretion of phosphate. Low serum calcium concentration stimulates 1-hydroxylation of 25-hydroxyvitamin D by the kidney to form 1,25-dihydroxyvitamin D (the active form of **vitamin D**). This hormone promotes calcium resorption from the gut and mineralization of bone. Increases in serum calcium lead to increased secretion of **calcitonin**. This hormone inhibits bone reabsorption and 1-hydroxylation of 25-hydroxyvitamin D and thereby ameliorates hypercalcemia.

141. **What factors affect renal calcium excretion?**
With some exceptions, renal calcium handling varies directly with renal Na^+ handling. Therefore, renal calcium excretion is increased by saline diuresis, loop diuretics, and volume expansion. In contrast, renal calcium excretion is decreased in volume depletion and other states associated with renal salt retention. One notable exception to this general rule is that the natriuresis associated with thiazide diuretics is accompanied by decreased, rather than increased, urinary calcium excretion.

142. **Define "pseudohypocalcemia" and "pseudohypercalcemia."**
These terms refer to an alteration of the total calcium concentration in the setting of a normal ionized fraction. Because the ionized fraction is normal, such patients are asymptomatic. Abnormalities in the concentration of serum proteins are a common cause of these disorders. Hypoalbuminemia causes a decrease in the total serum calcium level without a change in the level of ionized calcium. For each decrease of 1.0 g/dL in serum albumin, one should expect a drop in the total serum calcium of approximately 0.8 mg/dL.

143. **List the common causes of true hypocalcemia.**
    - Hypoparathyroidism (usually following thyroid or parathyroid surgery)
    - Vitamin D deficiency
    - Magnesium depletion (usually at levels < 0.8 mEq/L)
    - Liver disease (decreased synthesis of 25-hydroxyvitamin D)
    - CKD (hyperphosphatemia and decreased synthesis of 1,25-dihydroxyvitamin D)
    - Acute pancreatitis
    - Tumor lysis syndrome
    - Rhabdomyolysis

144. **What are the signs and symptoms of hypocalcemia?**
    The symptoms depend on the magnitude of the decrease in serum calcium, the rate of the drop, and its duration. The symptoms of hypocalcemia are due to the resultant decrease in the excitation threshold of neural tissue, which causes an increase in excitability, repetitive responses to a single stimulus, reduced accommodation, or even continuous activity of neural tissue. Specific signs and symptoms include:
    - Tetany and paresthesia
    - Altered mental status (lethargy to coma)
    - Seizures
    - QT interval prolongation on the ECG
    - Increased intracranial pressure
    - Lenticular cataracts

145. **What are Trousseau's and Chvostek's signs?**
    Both are indications of the latent tetany caused by hypocalcemia. Of the two signs, Trousseau's is more specific and reliable.
    - **Trousseau's sign:** A sphygmomanometer is placed on the arm and inflated to greater than systolic blood pressure and left in place for at least 2 minutes. A positive response is carpal spasm of the ipsilateral arm. Relaxation takes 5–10 seconds after the pressure is released.
    - **Chvostek's sign:** Tapping the facial nerve between the corner of the mouth and the zygomatic arch produces twitching of the ipsilateral facial muscle, especially the angle of the mouth. This sign may be seen in 10–25% of normal adult patients.

146. **What causes hypercalcemia?**
    Primary hyperparathyroidism (~50% of cases), malignancy, use of thiazide diuretics, vitamin D excess, hyper- and hypothyroidism, granulomatous disorders, immobilization, and milk-alkali syndrome.

147. **What are the signs and symptoms of hypercalcemia?**
    Weakness, constipation, nausea, anorexia, polyuria, polydipsia, and pruritus. Severe hypercalcemia may present with progressive CNS symptoms of lethargy, depression, obtundation, coma, and seizures. Rapid onset is more likely to be symptomatic than a slowly progressive level, regardless of the ultimate level at presentation.

148. **Describe the appropriate treatment for hypercalcemia.**
    Treatment depends on the calcium level and symptoms of the patient. Acute, symptomatic hypercalcemia should be treated aggressively, first with saline infusion to expedite calcium excretion. Most patients with hypercalcemia are significantly volume-depleted as a result of the osmotic diuresis related to the hypercalciuria.

149. **How is normal saline infused for aggressive treatment of hypercalcemia?**
    At a rapid rate, ≥300 mL/hr, with KCl and possibly magnesium added to the solution depending on measured blood values. After the patient is volume-repleted, furosemide may

be given to promote calciuresis. Care must be taken to keep input equal to or greater than output to avoid making the patient hypovolemic again.

150. **How is calcitonin used in the treatment of hypercalcemia?**
Calcitonin is useful for decreasing serum calcium and has the added advantage of rapid onset of action. It may be given in the presence of renal insufficiency or thrombocytopenia or when mithramycin is contraindicated. Its disadvantage is that rapid resistance often develops, probably related to the development of antibodies. This resistance can sometimes be delayed by concomitant administration of prednisone.

151. **Describe the role of bisphosphonates in the treatment of hypercalcemia.**
Bisphosphonates inhibit osteoclast activity and are effective with those cancers in which this mechanism is present. They are given via IV infusion over 5 days or as oral tablets.

152. **What other agents are useful for treatment of less significant levels of hypercalcemia?**
Glucocorticoids (prednisone, 20–40 mg/day), phosphates (1–6 g/day), prostaglandin inhibitors (aspirin and NSAIDs), or oral bisphosphonates. All of these agents are less effective but may suffice for chronic maintenance.

Bilizekian JP: Management of acute hypercalcemia, *N Engl J Med* 326:1196–1203, 1992.

153. **What factors regulate phosphate metabolism in the body?**
Serum phosphate is lowered by insulin, glucose (by stimulating insulin secretion), and alkalosis, which cause transcellular translocation of phosphate from plasma. Phosphate is resorbed predominantly in the proximal tubule, with small amounts being absorbed in the distal tubule. Renal phosphate excretion is increased by PTH, alkalosis, saline diuresis, ketoacidosis, and increased dietary phosphate intake.

154. **In which clinical situations can hypophosphatemia develop?**
- Decreased intake of phosphorus
- Shifts of phosphorus from serum into cells
- Increased excretion of phosphorus into urine
- Spurious hypophosphatemia (mannitol infusion)

155. **What factors may lead to decreased intake of phosphorus?**
- Decreased dietary intake
- Alcoholism
- Decreased intestinal absorption due to vitamin D deficiency, malabsorption, steatorrhea, secretory diarrhea, vomiting, or phosphate binders

156. **What factors may cause shifts of phosphorus from serum into cells?**
- Respiratory alkalosis (e.g., sepsis, heat stroke, hepatic coma, salicylate poisoning, gout)
- Recovery from hypothermia
- Hormonal effects (e.g., insulin, glucagon, androgens)
- Recovery from diabetic ketoacidosis
- Carbohydrate administration (hyperalimentation, fructose or glucose infusions)

157. **List the factors that may lead to increased excretion of phosphorus in urine.**
- Hyperparathyroidism
- Renal tubule defects (as in aldosteronism, SIADH, mineralocorticoid administration, diuretics, corticosteroids)
- Hypomagnesemia

158. **What electrolyte disturbances are commonly seen in progressive renal disease?**
Patients with progressive renal disease develop hyperphosphatemia, hypocalcemia, and secondary hyperparathyroidism. They are also at risk of developing at least two kinds of bone disease.

159. **What are the main disturbances thought to be responsible for the abnormalities of calcium and phosphate metabolism in progressive renal disease?**
- A rise in inorganic phosphate concentration in the serum due to poor renal excretion. This rise leads to a decrease in serum calcium concentration and stimulation of PTH secretion. The increased PTH secretion leads to increased bone resorption and osteitis fibrosa cystica.
- Resistance to the action of vitamin D. One function of this hormone is to promote calcium resorption from the gut. Decreased gut resorption of calcium exacerbates the hypocalcemia and reduces available calcium for bone mineralization.
- Defective synthesis of 1,25-dihydroxyvitamin D (the active form of this hormone). Reduced levels of 1,25-dihydroxyvitamin D result in defective bone mineralization (osteomalacia in adults, rickets in children).

160. **How does magnesium depletion affect calcium and phosphate metabolism?**
Magnesium depletion results in decreased secretion and end-organ responsiveness of PTH. This leads to functional hypoparathyroidism and the resultant effects on the serum level and urinary excretion of calcium and phosphate. This disorder can be corrected with magnesium repletion.

161. **What are some common causes of magnesium deficiency?**
Dietary insufficiency (decreased intake, protein-calorie malnutrition, prolonged IV feeding), intestinal malabsorption, chronic loss of GI fluids, loop diuretics (Mg^{2+} is reabsorbed predominantly in the thick ascending limb of the loop of Henle), other drugs (gentamicin, cisplatin, pentamidine, cyclosporine), alcoholism, hyperparathyroidism, and lactation.

162. **What is the milk-alkali syndrome?**
The presence of hypercalcemia, increased BUN and creatinine, increased serum phosphate, and metabolic alkalosis in a patient ingesting large quantities of milk and calcium carbonate-containing antacids. The patient usually presents with nausea, vomiting, anorexia, weakness, polydipsia, and polyuria. If it continues, metastatic calcification can occur, leading to mental status changes, nephrocalcinosis, band keratopathy, pruritus, and myalgias. The treatment is withdrawal of the milk and antacid.

163. **What electrolyte abnormalities are seen in human immunodeficiency virus (HIV) infection?**
In addition to the main proteinuric syndrome caused by focal sclerosis (so-called HIV nephropathy), a variety of electrolyte disorders are commonly seen in patients with HIV. Asymptomatic **hyperkalemia** is a common manifestation. The hyperkalemia may be due to many possible causes, including hyporenin-hypoaldosteronism, adrenal insufficiency, drugs such as pentamidine and trimethoprim-sulfamethoxazole, and even isolated hypoaldosteronism. **Hyponatremia** is frequently caused by hypovolemia, adrenal insufficiency, and SIADH due to associated pulmonary or cerebral diseases. Other electrolyte abnormalities include hypocalcemia, hypomagnesemia, and hypouricemia. Hypercalcemia is seen in association with lymphomas and cytomegalovirus infection.

Klotman ME, Klotman PE: AIDS and the kidney, *Semin Nephrol* 18:371–372, 1998.

164. **List the electrolyte disturbances associated with alcoholism.**
    - Hypokalemia
    - Hypophosphatemia
    - Hypomagnesemia
    - Hyponatremia

165. **How common is hypokalemia in alcoholics? Explain.**
    Hypokalemia is seen in one half of hospitalized, withdrawing alcoholics. This does not necessarily mean a total body K^+ deficit. Respiratory alkalosis, inadequate dietary intake, and GI losses (vomiting, diarrhea) are the common etiologic factors for hypokalemia. Withdrawal as well as severe liver failure causes respiratory alkalosis.

166. **How common is hypophosphatemia in alcoholics? Explain.**
    Hypophosphatemia (<2.5 mg/dL) is a common finding in hospitalized severe alcoholics, noted in more than half (50%) of patients in some series. The common predisposing factors are respiratory alkalosis, decreased dietary intake, transcellular shifts due to glucose administration, and rarely, associated proximal tubular injury leading to phosphate wasting.

167. **Explain the relationship between chronic alcoholism and hypomagnesemia.**
    Chronic alcoholism is the most common cause of hypomagnesemia in the United States. It is seen in alcoholics who are withdrawing and more commonly in those who had withdrawal seizures. GI losses, cellular uptake, dietary deficiencies, and possibly lipolysis leading to fatty acid-magnesium precipitation are the possible causes.

168. **How may beer contribute to hyponatremia?**
    Beer is virtually solute-free, so when large quantities are ingested, this free-water volume exceeds the excretory capacity of the kidney, and hyponatremia results.

BIBLIOGRAPHY

1. Brenner RM, editor: *Brenner & Rector's The Kidney*, ed 8, Philadelphia, 2008, WB Saunders.
2. Goldman L, Ausiello D, editors. *Cecil Textbook of Medicine*, ed 23, Philadelphia, 2007, WB Saunders.
3. Rose BD, Post T, editors. *Clinical Physiology of Acid-Base and Electrolyte Disorders*, ed 5, New York, 2001, McGraw-Hill.
4. Schrier RW, editor: *Renal and Electrolyte Disorders*, ed 6, Philadelphia, 2003, Lippincott Williams & Wilkins.

CHAPTER 10

RHEUMATOLOGY

Roger Kornu, M.D., Kathryn H. Dao, M.D., F.A.C.P., F.A.C.R., Catalina Orozco, M.D., and Rahul K. Patel, M.D.

The wolf, I'm afraid, is inside tearing up the place.

Flannery O'Connor (1925–1964)
Novelist afflicted with systemic lupus erythematosus (letter)

1. **Give an operational definition of rheumatic diseases.**
   Syndromes of pain or inflammation or both in articular or periarticular tissues.

2. **How common are the rheumatic diseases?**
   Fairly common. Forty-six million (22%) adults have self-reported doctor-diagnosed arthritis according to data from the National Health Interview Survey (2003–2005). By the year 2030, 67 million (25%) adults will have doctor-diagnosed arthritis. Overall, 2% of the general population has an inflammatory arthritis, and half of those have rheumatoid arthritis (RA).

   Centers for Disease Control and Prevention: *Arthritis*. Available at: http://www.cdc.gov/arthritis.

SIGNS AND SYMPTOMS

3. **What are key points in assessing a rheumatic history?**
   - Pain location
   - Symmetry of symptoms
   - Presence of morning stiffness
   - Effect of exercise
   - Additional constitutional symptoms (fatigue, low-grade fever, and weight loss)
   - Daily function
   - Family history (such as positive human leukocyte antigen [HLA]-B27 in ankylosing spondylitis)

4. **What is the "squeeze test"?**
   A physical examination maneuver that assesses the possible presence of inflammatory arthritis. The metacarpophalangeal (MCP) squeeze test is performed by squeezing all four MCPs together to elicit tenderness. The metatarsophalangeal (MTP) squeeze test elicits tenderness across the four MTP joints.

5. **What is Finkelstein's test?**
   A maneuver to demonstrate de Quervain's tenosynovitis in which a fist is made around the thumb and the wrist is moved toward the ulnar side. In a positive test, a sharp pain is felt at the base of the thumb.

6. **Define "Tinel's sign."**
   The sensation of focal pain and electrical sensations occurring when a nerve is tapped at the site of entrapment.

7. **How do you elicit Phalen's sign?**
   Ask the patient to:
   - Raise both arms to shoulder level.
   - Press the back (dorsum) of the hands together.
   - Slightly drop the elbows, causing maximal flexion of the wrist, and maintain for 30–60 seconds.
     If the patient has carpal tunnel syndrome (CTS), the discomfort will be reproduced.

8. **What does the Schober test detect?**
   Limited forward flexion of the lumbar spine. Schober's test is useful in the diagnosis of the spondyloarthropathies. Two points on the patient's lumbar spine (usually the lumbar sacral junction and a point 10 cm above) are marked while the patient is standing. The distance is remeasured after the patient bends to touch the toes (maximal forward flexion). An elongation < 5 cm suggests spine stiffness.

9. **Straight leg raising (SLR) is a useful diagnostic maneuver in what common condition?**
   Back pain. If the pain is due to nerve root compression, the symptoms are reproduced with SLR. To perform the maneuver, lift the lower leg by the calcaneus with the knee remaining straight. The cross-table SLR test additionally brings the heel across the other leg and may increase the sensitivity of this maneuver.

10. **What distinguishes Bouchard's nodes and Heberden's nodes?**
    The location of the bony enlargement. Bouchard's nodes involve the proximal interphalangeal (PIP) joints; Heberden's nodes, the distal interphalangeal (DIP) joints. Both are associated with osteoarthritis (OA) and women are affected more frequently than men in a 10:1 ratio. Heredity plays a particularly strong role in mothers, daughters, and sisters.

11. **What is Jaccoud's deformity?**
    Deformities of the hands secondary to chronic inflammation of the joint capsule, ligaments, and tendons. The changes may mimic those of RA such as ulnar deviation of the fingers and MCP joint subluxation. Erosions are not present on x-ray, although after several recurrences, notches may be seen radiographically on the ulnar side of the metacarpal heads. Although originally described in rheumatic fever, this disorder has been extended to include the arthropathy of other conditions, most commonly systemic lupus erythematosus (SLE).

12. **Name dermatologic findings associated with some rheumatic diseases.**
    See Table 10-1.

13. **Which rheumatic syndromes have been associated with uveitis?**

Ankylosing spondylitis	Psoriasis	Kawasaki disease (KD)
Juvenile idiopathic	Sarcoidosis	Relapsing
arthritis	Inflammatory bowel	polychondritis
Reactive arthritis	disease	
Sjögren's syndrome	Behçet's disease (BD)	

TABLE 10-1. DERMATOLOGIC FINDINGS IN RHEUMATIC DISEASES

Dermatologic Finding	Description	Disease
Malar rash	Butterfly appearance on face which spares the nasolabial folds	Systemic lupus erythematosus
Palpable purpura	Slightly elevated purpuric rash over one or more areas of the skin	Vasculitis
Erythema nodosum	Reddish/violet subcutaneous nodules that tends to develop in a pretibial location	Sarcoidosis, inflammatory bowel disease, tuberculosis, streptococcal infection
Keratoderma blennorrhagicum	Hyperkeratotic skin lesions on soles and palms	Reactive arthritis
Heliotrope rash	Violaceous eruption on the upper eyelids	Dermatomyositis
Gottron's papules	Erythematous rash extensor on the regions of MCP and IP joints	Dermatomyositis
Erythema chronicum migrans	Reddish, central clearing known as a "target lesion"	Lyme disease
Morphea	Small area(s) of skin fibrosis	Systemic sclerosis
Linear scleroderma	Band-like lesion which may expand across dermatomes	Systemic sclerosis
"En coup de sabre"	Specific curvilinear band that resembles a dueling scar that occurs across the face	Systemic sclerosis

IP = interphalangeal; MCP = metacarpophalangeal.

14. **Describe Raynaud's phenomenon.**
The presence of color changes (usually white, blue, then red) in the hands (or any distal part of the body) incited by exposure to cold or intense emotion. Raynaud's phenomenon may present without the classic triphasic color response. When one inquires about Raynaud's, it is sometimes difficult not to suggest a positive answer. Preferably, one should ask, "While grocery shopping, do you notice any problems in the frozen food section?" or "If you look at your hands when you get cold, do they look any different to you?"

15. **Distinguish between primary and secondary Raynaud's phenomenon.**
Primary Raynaud's phenomenon or *Raynaud's disease* occurs without association with another condition. Raynaud's occurring in association with another condition is usually termed *Raynaud's syndrome* or *secondary Raynaud's phenomenon*. The primary/secondary designation seems much easier to remember.

16. **Which rheumatic conditions are typically associated with Raynaud's phenomenon?**

    Systemic lupus erythematosus (SLE)

    Antiphospholipid antibody (APA) syndrome

    CREST (calcinosis cutis, Raynaud's phenomenon, esophageal dysfunction, sclerodactyly, and telangiectasia) syndrome

    Drug-induced lupus

    Reflex sympathetic dystrophy

    Systemic sclerosis

    Idiopathic Raynaud's phenomenon

    Carcinoid syndrome

    Connective tissue disease

    Polymyositis

    Sjögren's syndrome

    Cold agglutinin disease

    Cryoglobulinemia

    Systemic vasculopathies

    Cholesterol emboli

    Drug-induced (especially beta blockers)

17. **What factors predict the development of a systemic autoimmune disease in a patient presenting with Raynaud's phenomenon?**

    Positive antinuclear antibodies (ANAs) (positive predictive value 30%), abnormal nail bed capillaries (positive predictive value 47%), or abnormal pulmonary function studies. One study showed that 12.6% of patients presenting with Raynaud's phenomenon went on to develop a rheumatic disease.

    Spencer-Green G: Outcomes in primary Raynaud's phenomenon: With meta-analysis of frequency rates and predictions of transformation to secondary diseases, *Arch Intern Med* 158:595–600, 1998.

18. **What is erythromelalgia?**

    Intense burning pain, pronounced erythema, and increased skin temperature often in response to mild thermal stimuli or exercise. Erythromelalgia is often thought of as the opposite to Raynaud's phenomenon. The condition is believed to arise from vasomotor abnormalities resulting in abnormal blood flow to the extremities.

LABORATORY AND RADIOGRAPHIC EVALUATION

19. **When is an arthrocentesis (joint aspiration) indicated?**

    When joint infection is suspected. Synovial fluid analysis on patients with a mono- or polyarticular arthropathy of unclear etiology may be helpful in determining the etiology.

20. **Which studies should generally be performed on synovial fluid after arthrocentesis?**

    - Gram stain and bacterial culture
    - Total leukocyte count and differential
    - Crystal evaluation by polarized light microscopy
    - Culture for mycobacteria or fungi, if suspected

21. **What are rice bodies?**

    Aggregates of fibrin frequently found in the synovial fluid of patients with RA.

22. **What is the erythrocyte sedimentation rate (ESR)?**

    A measurement of the distance in millimeters that red blood cells travel in a Westergen or Wintrobe tube over 1 hour that is an indirect measurement of acute-phase reactants in systemic inflammation.

23. **Describe the clinical utility of C-reactive protein (CRP).**
    To monitor disease progression and therapy response in inflammatory conditions.
    CRP is an acute-phase reactant protein that is synthesized in response to tissue injury.
    CRP rises within 4–6 hours with a peak in 24–72 hours and normalization within
    1 week.

24. **What are rheumatoid factors (RFs)?**
    Antibodies directed at the Fc portion of the immunoglobulin G (IgG) molecule. Although IgM
    RFs are the most common, all immunoglobulin isotypes have been reported. IgG RFs are
    associated with a greater likelihood of vasculitis.

25. **Which conditions are associated with circulating RFs?**
    - Hepatitis C, occurring in 70% of patients with active disease. Because chronic hepatitis
      can also produce achiness and occasionally a mild synovitis, hepatitis C should be
      excluded before establishing a diagnosis of RA, even if serum transaminase levels are
      normal.
    - Bacterial endocarditis
    - Viral infections (parvovirus B19)
    - Sarcoidosis
    - Primary biliary cirrhosis
    - SLE

26. **Do all patients with RA have circulating RF?**
    No. RF may be detectable in 50% of RA patients in the first 6 months of diagnosis and
    85% in the first 2 years; however, up to 25% of patients with clinical RA have no circulating
    RF. The titer has little prognostic value in an individual patient, and remeasurements provide
    little added information.

KEY POINTS: SIGNIFICANCE OF LABORATORY VALUES ✔ IN RHEUMATIC DISEASE

1. ANA titers are not associated with intensity of disease.

2. Mixed connective tissue disease is a specific diagnosis which may have associated
   features of SLE, scleroderma, Sjögren's and/or polymyositis in association with anti-RNP
   antibodies.

3. Joint fluid analysis includes cell count, gram stain, culture, and crystals.

4. A patient with low positive RF and arthralgia should be checked for hepatitis C, which can
   produce synovitis and cryoglobulins (which can produce a false-positive RF).

ANA = antinuclear antibody; RF = rheumatoid factor; SLE = systemic lupus erythematosus.

27. **What are anti-CCP antibodies?**
    Anti-cyclic citrullinated peptide (anti-CCPs) antibodies, which are directed against the
    citrullinated residue of certain molecules (such as filaggrin and fibrin). These antibodies
    are found in the sera of patients with RA.

28. **What is the sensitivity and specificity of RF and anti-CCP antibodies?**
    - **RF:** 66% sensitivity, 70% specificity
    - **Anti-CCP antibodies:** 82% sensitivity, 95% specificity
    Measurement of anti-CCP antibodies is superior in specificity compared with RF alone, but the diagnostic yields of both tests are very good in patients suspected with RA. High titers of either RF or anti-CCP antibodies correlate with more severe disease including erosive disease and extra-articular manifestations.

29. **What is the ANA?**
    Antinuclear antibody (ANA) refers to any autoantibody that reacts to certain nuclear antigens (e.g., histones, ribonucleoproteins, DNA, or centromere). With the development of immunofluorescence microscopy techniques, different staining patterns were discovered, and it became clear that many different nuclear antigens can elicit an antibody response. Thus, many antibodies can be classified as ANA (Table 10-2). Detecting the specific antibody reaction requires more refined techniques.

TABLE 10-2. ANTIGENS AND ANTINUCLEAR ANTIBODIES	
Antigen	Antibody
Deoxyribose phosphate backbone of DNA	Anti-DNA (double-stranded or native)
Purine and pyrimidine bases	Anti–single-stranded DNA
H1, H2A, H2B, H3, H2A/H2B complex, H3/H4 complex	Antihistones
DNA topoisomerase I	Anti–SCL-70
Histidyl tRNA transferase	Anti–Jo-1
Kinetochore	Anticentromere
RNA polymerase I	Antinucleolar
Y1–Y5 RNA and protein	Anti-Ro
U1–6 RNA and protein	Anti-RNP (includes anti-Sm)

Adapted from von Mühlen CA, Tan EM: Autoantibodies in the diagnosis of systemic rheumatic diseases. Semin Arthritis Rheum 24:323–358, 1995.

30. **What is the significance of a positive ANA in a patient who is otherwise healthy?**
    Uncertain. ANA positivity is common and may not carry any significance. In 1997, the ANA Subcommittee of the International Union of Immunological Societies (IUIS) Standardization Committee completed a multicenter study with the objective of identifying the range of ANA titers in normal individuals and in patients with certain rheumatic diseases. The study found that a positive ANA can be found in 31.7% of healthy individuals at 1:40 serum dilution, 13.3% at 1:80, 5.0% at 1:160, and 3.3% at 1:320. Despite these frequencies, the ANA titer may be useful in determining the presence of disease. Setting a low cutoff of 1:40 (high sensitivity, low specificity) could aid in diagnosis because it would classify most patients who have SLE, systemic sclerosis (SSc), or Sjögren's syndrome. Conversely, setting a high cutoff at 1:160 serum dilution (high specificity, low sensitivity) could be useful to confirm the presence of disease and would likely exclude 95% of normal individuals

    Tan EM, Feltkamp TE, Smolen JS, et al: Range of antinuclear antibodies in "healthy" individuals, *Arthritis Rheum* 40:1601–1611, 1997.

31. **Do ANA staining patterns detect specific ANAs? What is their clinical relevance?**

    No. The fluorescence test for ANA is performed by incubating the patient's serum with a fixed monolayer of human larynx epithelioma cancer (HEp-2) cell lines. If ANAs are present in the serum, they bind to the nuclear component of the substrate. Next, fluorescent anti-Ig is added, which binds to antibodies (if present) in the test serum. With the fluorescent tag, the ANA can be directly visualized under fluorescent light. Different patterns of staining occur, and although they may provide some information, they do not identify the specific antibody present, nor are they specific for a disease entity or clinically relevant. For example, the rim or peripheral pattern (usually associated with antibodies directed against nuclear membrane proteins) may be obscured if another autoantibody (staining a homogeneous pattern) is present.

KEY POINTS: DIAGNOSING RHEUMATIC DISEASES ✓

1. Inflammatory arthritis tends to involve small joints, has a morning stiffness component, and improves with activity.

2. Joint arthrocentesis is most useful in evaluating for joint infection.

3. Rheumatoid factor and anti-CCP antibodies help improve sensitivity and specificity in diagnosing rheumatoid arthritis.

4. Although ANA positivity may occur in normal patients, its titer and its presence with other autoantibodies are useful in diagnosing connective tissue diseases.

5. The HLA B27 association with arthritis is highest in ankylosing spondylitis and reactive arthritis but lower with the spondylitis associated with psoriasis and inflammatory bowel disease.

ANA = antinuclear antibody; HLA = human leukocyte antigen.

32. **Why is it helpful to know which specific ANA is present in a given patient?**

    To increase the diagnostic likelihood of a specific rheumatic diagnosis and provide prognosis.

33. **What rheumatic diseases are associated with specific ANAs?**

    See Table 10-3.

TABLE 10-3.	SPECIFIC ANTINUCLEAR ANTIBODIES AND DISEASE ASSOCIATION
Antibody	**Associated Diseases**
Ro/SSA	SLE, neonatal lupus syndrome, subacute lupus, Sjögren's syndrome, RA
dsDNA	SLE (with nephritis)
Sm	SLE
Jo-1	Polymyositis (pulmonary involvement)
Centromere	CREST syndrome (limited scleroderma)
SCL-70	Systemic sclerosis
Histone	SLE, drug-induced lupus

(continued)

TABLE 10-3. SPECIFIC ANTINUCLEAR ANTIBODIES AND DISEASE ASSOCIATION—*(continued)*	
Antibody	Associated Diseases
RNP	SLE, MCTD
Ribosomal P	SLE (with psychosis)
Cardiolipin	SLE (with thromboembolic events), antiphospholipid syndrome

CREST = calcinosis cutis, Raynaud's phenomenon, esophageal dysfunction, sclerodactyly, and telangiectasia; MCTD = mixed connective tissue disease; RA = rheumatoid arthritis; SLE = systemic lupus erythematosus.

34. **What are antineutrophil cytoplasmic antibodies (ANCAs)?**
Antibodies directed against enzymes (proteinase-3 [PR-3] and myeloperoxidase) found in primary granules of neutrophils and lysosomes of monocytes. Immunofluorescence detects two principal staining patterns: (1) a fine granular cytoplasmic staining (c-ANCA) and (2) a perinuclear collection of antibody (p-ANCA).

35. **Which diseases are associated with soft tissue calcification on plain x-rays?**

Calcific tendinitis	Ehlers-Danlos	Parathyroid disease
Chondrocalcinosis	syndrome	Renal osteodystrophy
Dermatomyositis	Neoplasia	Sarcoidosis
Diabetes	Neuropathic	Scleroderma
	arthropathy	Trauma

36. **Describe typical radiographic features of inflammatory arthritis in early and progressive disease.**
Soft tissue swelling and juxta-articular osteoporosis in early disease and more diffuse osteoporosis with uniform loss of cartilage in chronic disease. Further inflammation will lead to synovial hypertrophy and erosions with marginal areas of the synovium.

37. **List five classic radiographic findings of OA.**
- Subchondral cyst formation
- New bone formation (osteophytes)
- Bone sclerosis
- Joint space narrowing
- Lack of osteoporosis

38. **Describe the role of magnetic resonance imaging (MRI) and peripheral ultrasound (US) in inflammatory arthritis.**
To detect subtle bony abnormalities that may not be seen on plain radiographs. MRI is able to detect early bony erosions. Peripheral US is also a sensitive test for detecting erosions. US is less expensive than MRI but accurate results are dependent upon the operator's skill.

RHEUMATOID ARTHRITIS

39. **What is the basis for the revised RA classification criteria established in 2010 by the ACR and European League Against Rheumatism (EULAR)?**
Definite RA is based on:
- Presence of synovitis in at least 1 joint

- Absence of an alternative diagnosis to explain the synovitis
- Achievement of a total score ≥ 6 from individual scores from 4 domains:
  - ○ Number and site of involved joints (score range 0-5)
  - ○ Serologic abnormalities (score range 0-5)
  - ○ Elevated acute-phase response (score range 0-1)
  - ○ Symptom duration (2 levels; range 0-1)

Aletaha D, Neogi T, Silman AF, et al: 2010 Rheumatoid arthritis classification criteria: An American College of Rheumatology/European League Against Rheumatism Collaborative Initiative. *Arthritis Rheum* 62(9):2569–2581, 2010.

40. **What is the advantage of these new criteria?**
To identify patients with new symptoms of inflammatory synovitis who are likely to develop persistent or erosive joint disease as seen in RA.

41. **What is the differential diagnosis of RA?**
- Connective tissue disease (SLE, SSc, Sjögren's disease)
- Psoriatic arthritis
- IBD
- Polyarticular gout
- Lyme-related arthropathy
- Viral-induced arthropathies (parvovirus B19, hepatitis C)

42. **Describe the epidemiology of RA.**
RA occurs in up to 1% of the general population worldwide with lower prevalence in parts of Africa (0.1%) and China (0.3%) and higher prevalence in Pima and Chippawa Indians (5%). Peak incidence is in the fourth and fifth decades of life, but almost any age can be affected.

43. **What are the genetic associations in RA?**
First-degree relatives of patients with RA have a 1.5-fold increased risk of developing RA compared with the general population. Monozygotic twin studies found a concordance rate for RA of 12–15%. An increased prevalence of RA is present in a subset of populations with the presence of HLA-DR4 (Western European descent) and HLA-DR1 or HLA-DR10 (Spanish, Basque, and Israeli descent). RA susceptibility is associated with the third hypervariable region of DR1β-chains from amino acids 70–74 referred to as the "shared epitope" (QKRAA, QRRAA or RRRAA) and is associated with both susceptibility and severity of RA.

Nepom GT, Byers P, Seyfried C, et al: HLA gene association with RA: Identification of susceptibility alleles using specific oligopeptide probes, *Arthritis Rheum* 32:15, 1989.

44. **Explain the influence of gender in RA.**
Females have a two to three times increased likelihood of developing RA compared with males. Estrogen has been shown to inhibit T suppressor cell function and enhance T helper function, leading to stimulatory effects on the immune system. In addition, null parity increases RA risk. The last trimester of pregnancy is associated with decreased RA disease activity. Men with RA tend to have lower testosterone levels than other men and later disease onset than women.

45. **What are nongenetic risk factors for RA?**
Smoking and infections (bacterial and viral). A 25 pack-year or more history of tobacco use is associated with more severe disease with greater seropositivity, nodules, and radiographic changes. Bacterial infections have been implicated in initiation of RA through activation of Toll-like receptors on mast cells and stimulation of innate immunity. Viruses have also been considered in etiology of RA. Epstein-Barr virus (EBV), parovirus B19, and retroviruses have similar amino acid sequences to the shared epitope and may trigger an autoimmune response leading to inflammation.

46. **What is the synovium?**

    A 1- to 2-cell-thick lining of the joint made up of two types of synoviocytes: type A (macrophage-like cells probably derived from bone marrow) and type B (fibroblast-like cells that are probably of mesenchymal origin). The subsynovium constitutes the second layer of normal synovium.

47. **How does RA affect the synovium?**

    By inducing intimal lining hyperplasia and subsynovial infiltration with mononuclear cells (especially CD4-negative T cells, macrophages, and B cells). Increased numbers of type A and type B synoviocytes are added to the synovial lining. The lining is the main source of the inflammatory cytokines and proteases thought to lead to the joint destruction in RA. Activated chondrocytes and osteoclasts may also be involved. In addition, other cell types including plasma cells, T and B lymphocytes, and dendritic cells may also accumulate in RA synovium. Synovial fluid has elevated polymorphonuclear leukocytes (PMNs) with lesser cell types including lymphocytes, macrophages, natural killer cells, and fibroblasts present.

48. **What is pannus?**

    A term to describe the area of proliferating synovium that can erode the adjacent cartilage and bone. (*Pannus* means cloth in Latin.) Angiogenesis allows the synovium to hypertrophy leading to enlargement of pannus and an influx of inflammatory cells.

49. **How does pannus contribute to joint destruction in RA?**

    Pannus tissue adheres to articular cartilage, and the cells within the pannus produce proteinases that can destroy cartilage. The marginal erosions on radiographs are likely due to bone invasion by pannus. Synovial tissue analysis also reveals inflammatory mediators including cytokines, enzymes, adhesion molecules, and transcription factors. Notable examples include interleukin-1 (IL-1), tumor necrosis factor-alpha (TNA-alpha), IL-6, IL-8, IL-17, matrix metalloproteinases, cathepsins, and other proteases. Receptor activator for nuclear factor kappa-B ligand (RANK-L) production leads to osteoclast activation, which may be involved in the bone loss in RA.

50. **Which joints are most commonly involved in RA?**

    Multiple diarthrodial joints (with free motion) in a symmetrical distribution. In early disease, the MCP, PIP, wrist, and MTP joints are involved. Larger joints of the upper and lower extremities, such as the elbows, shoulders, ankles, and knees, are also commonly affected, although symptoms may appear later. Less common are cervical spine, temporomandibular, and sternoclavicular joint involvement. Joints that are very uncommon in RA include the distal interphalangeal (DIP) joints and thoracic and lumbar spine.

51. **Describe the typical late joint deformities in RA.**

    - Swan neck deformity typically results from inflammation and flexor contraction of the MCP joints, which causes flexion at the MCP and DIP joints with hyperextension of the PIP joints.
    - Boutonnière deformity is due to flexion contracture at the PIP joint with extension of the DIP joint due to injury or weakening of the extrinsic extensor tendon.
    - Ulnar deviation is due to MCP joint subluxation.
    - The "piano key sign" is characterized by softening of the ulnar styloid due to destruction of the ulnar collateral ligamaent.
    - In the feet, late deformities include claw toe or hammer toe, which is due to subluxation of the metatarsal heads.

52. **Describe cervical spine involvement in RA.**

    Initial symptoms include pain with motion in the neck and occipital headache. Risk factors for cervical spine disease include high RF seropositivity, later onset, active synovitis, and rapid progression of erosive disease. Significant laxity at the atlantoaxial joint with subluxation makes patients prone to slowly progressive, spastic quadriparesis. If this laxity is present, the hyperextension of the neck that occurs during intubation for general anesthesia can produce quadriplegia. Therefore, patients with neck pain or longstanding disease should undergo cervical spine evaluation before any surgical procedure.

53. What are rheumatoid nodules?

Firm, usually movable nodules ranging in size from a few millimeters to 2 cm found over pressure areas. The classic rheumatoid nodule has a central area of necrosis surrounded by a rim of palisading fibroblasts surrounded by a collagenous capsule with perivascular collections of chronic inflammatory cells. Rheumatoid nodules occur in 20–35% of patients with RA and can be found at the elbow, knuckles, wrist, soles, Achilles tendon, head, bridge of the nose (if pressure area from glasses), and sacrum. RF is usually positive, as are anti-CCP antibodies. Accelerated nodule formation has been described in patients receiving methotrexate treatment for RA, even when methotrexate shows efficacy at calming the arthritis and the patient has had no previous nodule formation. Nodulosis goes away when methotrexate is discontinued.

54. What factors suggest an aggressive disease course in RA?

- Acute onset of disease with involvement of multiple joints
- High titers of RF
- Positive ANA
- Presence of nodules
- Lower socioeconomic status
- Fewer years of formal education.

55. List some extra-articular manifestations of RA.

See Table 10-4.

TABLE 10-4. EXTRA-ARTICULAR MANIFESTATIONS OF RHEUMATOID ARTHRITIS

Organ System	Extra-Articular Manifestation
Constitutional	Fever, fatigue, weight loss
Skin	Rheumatoid nodules
Pulmonary	Pulmonary nodules, pleural thickening, pleural effusions, diffuse interstitial lung disease, BOOP
Ophthalmologic	Keratoconjunctivitis sicca, episcleritis, scleritis
Vascular	Small vessel vasculitis
Neurologic	Cervical spine subluxation causing cervical myelopathy, nerve entrapments
Cardiac	Pericarditis, coronary atherosclerosis
Muscular	Muscle atrophy
Hematologic	Anemia of chronic disease, thrombocytosis, lymphoma

BOOP = bronchiolitis obliterans with organizing pneumonia.

56. **What is Felty's syndrome?**

    The triad of RA, splenomegaly, and leukopenia. Felty's occurs in 1% of RA patients with severe disease who typically have RF positivity, rheumatoid nodules, and other extra-articular manifestations. Leukopenia predominantly affects neutrophils with white blood cell (WBC) count $< 2000/mm^3$. Patients are more susceptible to bacterial infections and have a higher risk of development of non-Hodgkin's lymphoma. Patients with Felty's also are susceptible to large granular lymphocyte (LGL) syndrome with CD2, 3, 8, 16, and 57 markers and susceptibility to infections.

57. **What is Caplan's syndrome?**

    The development of lung inflammation and scarring in patients with RA and pneumoconiosis from mining dust exposure. Multiple perihilar lung nodules with pathology similar to rheumatoid nodules are also found. These patients can develop massive fibrosis and are at increased risk of tuberculosis.

58. **Why is functional capacity so important in patients with RA?**

    Because functional status may be one of the best predictors of premature mortality.

59. **Why is early treatment of RA so important?**

    Because the joints can be significantly structurally damaged early in the disease if not treated. The structural damage produces mechanical derangements in the joint leading to deformity and profoundly impaired joint function.

60. **How does pregnancy affect RA?**

    Usually with improvement. Signs and symptoms of RA subside in approximately 70% of women during pregnancy. No data suggest that RA has a detrimental effect on the fetus; however, arthritis should be assessed before pregnancy, if possible, because anesthesia and intubation (if needed) can be problematic and even dangerous when cervical spine disease is present. Delivery also can be difficult if arthritis limits hip motion. Postpartum flares of disease occur in approximately 90% of women who experience improvement during pregnancy.

    Griffin J: Rheumatoid arthritis: Biological effects and management. In Scott JS, Bird HA, editors: *Pregnancy, Autoimmunity and Connective Tissue Disorders*, Oxford, 1990, Oxford University Press, pp 140–162.

61. **Describe the basic mechanism of action of nonsteroidal anti-inflammatory drugs (NSAIDs).**

    Inhibition of production of prostaglandins (and other inflammatory cytokines) through competition with arachidonic acid for cyclooxygenase (COX) binding. There are two main subtypes of COX. COX-1 is often described as a "housekeeping" enzyme and has been associated with regulating normal cellular processes such as gastric cellular protection, platelet aggregation, and kidney function. COX-2 is expressed in the brain, kidney, bone, and possibly, the cardiovascular system. COX-2 seems to be involved more specifically in the synthesis of inflammatory mediators than COX-1. Without COX, there are fewer circulating prostaglandins and, therefore, less inflammation and pain.

62. **What is the advantage of selective COX-2 inhibition over nonselective COX inhibition?**

    Decreased risk of gastrointestinal (GI) injury. COX-1 is known to be involved in gastric cellular protection, so selective inhibition of COX-2 would theoretically lead to less gastric and duodenal injury. Clinical studies do show this, but toxicity still may occur with COX-2 inhibition. Although improved GI tolerance has been shown, there has been no significant improvement in efficacy with selective COX-2 inhibition. Patients at risk of peptic ulcer disease (PUD) who use NSAIDs chronically should be evaluated for proton pump inhibitor (PPI) prophylaxis. (See Chapter 2, General Medicine and Ambulatory Care.)

63. **What side effects are found in both NSAIDs and COX-2 inhibitors?**
    - **Renal:** hypertension, acute renal failure, and papillary necrosis
    - **Hepatic:** elevated transaminases and rarely acute hepatic injury
    - **Nervous system:** dizziness, headache, and cognitive dysfunction
    Also see Chapter 2, General Medicine and Ambulatory Care.

64. **How do the effects of aspirin on platelets differ from those of other NSAIDs?**
    Acetylated salicylates (such as aspirin) **irreversibly** destroy the COX enzyme that leads to decreased platelet aggregation. Other NSAIDs (including nonacetylated salicylates) allow the return of normal enzyme function once the drug level has decreased. Because COX-2 does not regulate platelet aggregation, newer COX-2 NSAIDs have little effect on platelet function.

65. **What is the role of glucocorticoids (GCs) in the management of RA?**
    Mainly for managing disease flares and bridging therapies. GCs reduce synthesis of enzymes involved in the production of prostaglandins and proinflammatory cytokins such as IL-1, IL-6, TNA-alpha. Because of more specific, safer agents, GCs are currently used less often in the long-term management of RA. The relatively quick onset of action (hours to days) make GCs a good agent for disease flare-ups. Low-dose GCs are also used as bridging therapy concurrently with disease-modifying antirheumatic drug (DMARD) therapy.

66. **What are common adverse side effects from long-term use of GCs?**
    - Osteoporosis (secondary)
    - Hyperglycemia
    - Increased incidence of cardiovascular disease
    - Cushing's syndrome
    - Increased risk of cataracts
    - Increased risk of infection

67. **What are DMARDs and how are they used in the treatment of RA?**
    Disease-modifying antirheumatic drugs are thought to alter the natural history of RA, lessening the likelihood of joint destruction and deformity. Nonbiologic DMARDs are typically oral and have been used clinically for many years. Biologic DMARDs are structurally engineered versions of already natural molecules such as monoclonal antibodies and have more specific targets in the inflammatory cascade of disease.

KEY POINTS: TREATMENT OF RHEUMATIC DISEASE ✔

1. COX-2 selective inhibition is safer from GI toxicities than from traditional NSAIDs, but are no more efficacious and may have a higher cardiovascular risk.

2. Patients taking chronic NSAIDs who are at risk of PUD may benefit from prophylactic treatment with PPIs to prevent PUD.

3. Disease-modifying medications including the biologic agents have improved clinical outcomes in rheumatoid arthritis.

4. Although glucocorticoid treatments are common in managing several rheumatic diseases, there are many untoward side effects including osteoporosis, increased cardiovascular disease, elevated glucose, and increased risk of infection.

COX-2 = cyclooxygenase-2; GI = gastrointestinal; NSAIDs = nonsteroidal anti-inflammatory drugs; PPIs = proton pump inhibitors; PUD = peptic ulcer disease.

68. **Name the most commonly used nonbiologic DMARDs, list mechanism of action, and name common side effects.**
    See Table 10-5.

TABLE 10-5. MECHANISM OF ACTION AND SIDE EFFECTS OF NONBIOLOGIC DISEASE MODIFYING ANTIRHEUMATIC DRUGS

Nonbiologic DMARDs	Mechanism of Action	Common Side Effects
Methotrexate	Inhibits dihydrofolate reductase, which leads to anti-inflammatory effects and down-regulation of cytokines, although the exact mechanism is still unclear	Nausea, stomatitis, alopecia, fatigue, elevated liver transaminases, bone marrow suppression, pneumonitis
Sulfasalazine	Suppresses lymphocyte and leukocyte functions	Nausea, rash, leukopenia
Hydroxychloroquine	Accumulation in lysosomes raises the intravesical pH and interferes with antigenic peptides	Nausea, rash, hyperpigmentation, retinopathy
Leflunomide	Inhibits pyrimidine synthesis which inhibits T-cell function	Nausea, stomatitis, alopecia, fatigue, elevated liver transaminases, bone marrow suppression

DMARDs = disease-modifying antirheumatic drugs.

69. **Name other less common nonbiologic DMARDs.**
    Minocycline has shown efficacy in small clinical trials. Gold compounds were used more frequently in the past, but much less frequently now because of high levels of toxicity. Cyclosporine, tacrolimus, and azathioprine have been shown to have efficacy as well.

70. **Name current biologic DMARD therapies, list mechanism of action, and name common side effects.**
    See Table 10-6.

SYSTEMIC LUPUS ERYTHEMATOSUS

71. **What is SLE?**
    An autoimmune inflammatory disease that can affect many organ systems with protean manifestations. The pathogenesis of lupus is largely unknown, but immunologic abnormalities can give rise to excessive autoantibody production that can cause tissue damage.

TABLE 10-6. MECHANISM OF ACTION AND SIDE EFFECTS OF BIOLOGIC DISEASE MODIFYING ANTIRHEUMATIC DRUGS

Biologic DMARDs	Class	Mechanism of Action and Route of Administration	Common Side Effects
Infliximab	TNF-α inhibitor	Chimeric monoclonal antibody that binds to both soluble and membrane bound TNF-α; intravenous administration	Infection (including reactivation of TB and fungal infection), infusion reaction, lymphoma, demyelinating disorder, drug-induced lupus
Entanercept	TNF-α inhibitor	Soluble receptor fusion protein that binds to soluble TNF-α; subcutaneous administration	Infection (including reactivation of latent TB and fungal infection), injection site reaction, lymphoma, demyelinating disorder, drug-induced lupus
Adalimumab	TNF-α inhibitor	Fully humanized monoclonal antibody that binds to both soluble and membrane bound TNF-α; subcutaneous administration	Infection (including reactivation of latent TB and fungal infection), injection site reaction, lymphoma, demyelinating disorder, drug-induced lupus
Golimumab	TNF-α inhibitor	Fully humanized monoclonal antibody that binds to both soluble and membrane bound TNF-α; subcutaneous administration	Infection (including reactivation of latent TB and fungal infection), injection site reaction, lymphoma, demyelinating disorder, drug-induced lupus
Certolizamab pegol	TNF-α inhibitor	Pegulated humanized antibody Fab fragment chemically linked to polyethylene glycol and binds to soluble and membrane bound TNA-α and does not contain an Fc portion unlike the other monoclonal antibodies to TNF-α; subcutanous administration	Infection (including reactivation of latent TB and fungal infection), injection site reaction, lymphoma, demyelinating disorder, drug-induced lupus, pancytopenia

(continued)

TABLE 10-6. MECHANISM OF ACTION AND SIDE EFFECTS OF BIOLOGIC DISEASE MODIFYING ANTIRHEUMATIC DRUGS—*(continued)*

Biologic DMARDs	Class	Mechanism of Action and Route of Administration	Common Side Effects
Abatacept (CTLA-4Ig)	T-cell inhibitor	Recombinant fusion protein that binds to CD80/CD86 on the surface of APC and prevents binding onto CD28 on T cells (blocks T-cell second signals); intravenous administration	Infection, infusion reaction, malignancy, COPD exacerbations
Rituximab	B-cell inhibitor	Chimeric anti-CD20 monoclonal antibody that involves inhibition of T cell activation through reduction of antigen presentation by B cells; intravenous administration	Infection, infusion reactions, headache, fever
Tocilizumab	IL-6 inhibitor	Humanized IL-6 receptor antibody. IL-6 has proinflammatory effects and activates T cells, B cells, and macrophages	Infection, infusion reaction, elevated hepatic function tests, elevated total cholesterol, neutropenia

APC = antigen presenting cell; COPD = chronic obstructive pulmonary disease; DMARDs = disease-modifying antirheumatic drugs; IL = interleukin; TB = tuberculosis; TNF = tumor necrosis factor.

72. **What are the ACR classification criteria for SLE?**
See Table 10-7.

TABLE 10-7. AMERICAN COLLEGE OF RHEUMATOLOGY CRITERIA FOR CLASSIFICATION OF SYSTEMIC LUPUS ERYTHEMATOSUS*

Malar rash	Fixed erythema, flat or raised, over the malar eminences, sparing the nasolabial folds
Discoid rash	Erythematous raised patches with adherent keratotic scaling and follicular plugging: atrophic scarring may occur in older lesions
Photosensitivity	Skin rash as a result of unusual reaction to sunlight, by patient history or physician observation
Oral ulcers	Oral or nasopharyngeal ulceration usually painless, observed by physician

(continued)

TABLE 10-7. AMERICAN COLLEGE OF RHEUMATOLOGY CRITERIA FOR CLASSIFICATION OF SYSTEMIC LUPUS ERYTHEMATOSUS*— *(continued)*

Nonerosive arthritis	Involving two or more peripheral joints, characterized by tenderness, swelling, or effusion
Pleuritis or pericarditis	a. Pleuritis: convincing history of pleuritic pain or rub heard by physician or evidence of pleural effusion *or* b. Pericarditis: documented by electrocardiogram or rub or evidence of pericardial effusion
Renal disorder	a. Persistent proteinuria > 0.5 g/day or > 3+ if quantitative not performed *or* b. Cellular casts: may be red cell, hemoglobin, granular, tubular, or mixed
Seizures or psychosis	a. Seizures: in the absence of offending drugs or known metabolic derangement (e.g., uremia, ketoacidosis, electrolyte imbalance) b. Psychosis: in the absence of offending drugs or known metabolic derangement (e.g., uremia, ketoacidosis, electrolyte imbalance)
Hematologic disorder	a. Hemolytic anemia with reticulocytosis *or* b. Leukopenia: <4000/mm^3 on two occasions *or* c. Lymphopenia: <1500/mm^3 on two occasions *or* d. Thrombocytopenia: <100,000/mm^3 in the absence of offending drugs

Immunologic disorder	a. Anti-DNA: antibody to native DNA in abnormal titer
	or
	b. Anti-Sm: presence of antibody to Sm nuclear antigen
	or
	c. Positive findings of antiphospholipid antibodies based on:
	  1. An abnormal serum concentration of IgG or IgM anticardiolipin antibodies
	  2. A positive test for lupus anticoagulant using standard method
	  or
	  3. A false-positive test for at least 6 mo and confirmed by *Treponema palladium* immobilization fluorescent treponemal antibody absorption test

Positive ANA	An abnormal titer of ANA by immunofluorescence or an equivalent assay at any point in time in the absence of drug

ANA = antinuclear antibody; Ig = immunoglobulin; SLE = systemic lupus erythematosus.
*Four of these criteria must be present in order for the patient to enroll in a SLE research study.
Adapted from Hochberg MC: Updating the American College of Rheumatology revised criteria for the classification of systemic lupus erythematosus [letter]. Arthritis Rheum 40:1725, 1997.

73. **How are these criteria used for the diagnosis of SLE in an individual patient?**
    The ACR classification criteria were proposed to identify SLE patients for enrollment
    into clinical trial, providing a uniform base for which studies can be conducted in lupus
    patients. The ACR criteria are intended to reflect the major clinical features of the disease
    (e.g., dermatologic, renal, neurologic, articular, hematologic, and immunologic findings).
    Although these criteria may be helpful in aiding the diagnosis of lupus, patients who do
    not fulfill the classification criteria may still have the disease. The diagnosis of SLE in
    clinical practice is based upon autoantibody analysis, symptoms, laboratory tests of
    involved organ systems, and physical examination findings.

74. **What are common laboratory and clinical findings in SLE?**
    See Table 10-8.

TABLE 10-8. FREQUENCIES OF VARIOUS MANIFESTATIONS OF SYSTEMIC LUPUS ERYTHEMATOSUS BY DISEASE STAGE

Manifestation	Early Disease (%)	Late Disease (%)
Arthritis	46–53	83–95
Rash	9–11	81–88
Fever	3–5	77
Mucosal ulcers	—	7–23
Alopecia	—	37–45
Serositis	5	63
Pulmonary inflammation	—	9
Liver function test abnormalities	1	—
Vasculitis	—	21–27
Myositis	—	5
Osteoporosis	—	High
Osteonecrosis	—	7–24
Leukopenia	41–66	41–66
Thrombocytopenia	2	19–45
Anemia	2	57–73
CNS abnormalities	3	55–59
Nephritis	6	31–53
Renal failure	<1	20

CNS = central nervous system.
From Lahita RG: The clinical presentation of systemic lupus erythematosus in adults. In Lahita RG (ed): Systemic Lupus Erythematosus, 4th ed. San Diego, CA, Academic Press, 2004, p 435.

75. **When is the peak incidence of SLE?**
    15–44 years of age, which is believed to be related to the hormonal changes that occur
    during puberty and the childbearing years. The incidence of SLE in prepubertal females is
    similar to that of postmenopausal females.

    Masi AT, Kaslow RA: Sex effects in systemic lupus erythematosus: A clue to pathogenesis, *Arthritis Rheum* 21:480–484, 1978.

76. **How can cutaneous lupus be categorized?**
    - Acute cutaneous lupus erythematosus (ACLE)
    - Subacute cutaneous lupus erythematosus (SCLE)
    - Chronic cutaneous lupus erythematosus (CCLE)

77. **Compare and contrast the typical rashes of ACLE with SCLE.**
    The prototypical lesion of ACLE is the malar or butterfly rash, which is an erythematous rash that can be flat or raised. The rash spans the bridge of the nose and extends over the malar eminences. Ultraviolet (UV) light may exacerbate the lesion; hence, the nasolabial folds are often spared because these regions receive less UV rays. The rash of SCLE is also photosensitive and is often located in the upper chest, shoulders, and neck. SCLE may start as erythematous, scaly papules or plaques, often progressing into larger papulosquamous or annular polycyclic lesions that can then coalesce to produce large confluent areas with central hypopigmentation. Neither ACLE nor SCLE results in dermal scarring.

78. **What are some examples of CCLE?**
    - Lupus tumidus
    - Lupus profundus
    - Chilblain lupus
    - Discoid lupus erythematosus (DLE).

79. **Describe DLE and explain the relationship between SLE and DLE.**
    Discrete erythematous plaques covered by scales that extend into hair follicles, causing follicular plugging. The plaques can occur over the face, scalp, pinnae and conchae bowl of the ear, neck, and in areas that may not be exposed to the UV rays. DLE can exist in patients with SLE or in isolation. About 10% of patients with discoid lesions will have SLE.

    Walling HW, Sontheimer RD: Cutaneous lupus erythematosus: Issues in diagnosis and treatment, *Am J Clin Dermatol* 10:365–381, 2009.

80. **What are other cutaneous manifestations of lupus?**

Raynaud's phenomenon	Bullae	Livedo reticularis
Periungual telangiectasia	Livedo reticularis	Alopecia
	Petechiae	
	Vasculitis	

81. **List the differential diagnoses of a lupus patient who presents with musculoskeletal complaints.**

Synovitis	Myopathy	Septic arthritis
Fibromyalgia	Osteonecrosis	Adrenal insufficiency
Myositis	Fractures	

    Some of these disorders are related to the disease itself, whereas others may be related to medication side effects or existing comorbid conditions.

82. **What is the prevalence of lupus nephritis and how is nephritis categorized?**
    About 50%. The Society of Pathology/Renal Pathology Society (ISN/RPS) in 2003 revised the World Health Organization (WHO) classification of lupus nephritis by adding chronicity and activity scores. Classification is based on biopsy:
    - **Class I:** minimal mesangial lupus nephritis
    - **Class II:** mesangial proliferative lupus nephritis
    - **Class III:** focal lupus nephritis, subcategorized as proliferative with activity (class III-A), proliferative and sclerosis with activity and chronicity (class III-A/C), or sclerosing with chronicity (class III-C)

- **Class IV:** diffuse lupus nephritis, subcategorized as segmental and active [class IV-S(A)], global proliferative and active [class IV-G(A)], segmental with activity and chronicity [class IV-S(A/C)], global proliferative with activity and chronicity [class IV–G(A/C)], segmental with chronicity [class IV–S(C)], or global proliferative with chronicity [class IV–G(C)]
- **Class V:** membranous lupus nephritis
- **Class VI:** advanced sclerosis lupus nephritis

Weening JJ, D'Agati VD, Schwartz MM, et al: The classification of glomerulonephritis in systemic lupus erythematosus revisited, *J Am Soc Nephrol* 15:241–250, 2004.

83. **What happens to lupus activity in patients with renal failure?**
Oftentimes, lupus becomes quiescent with the onset of uremia and dialysis. Several studies note the ability to discontinue GCs without a return of extrarenal manifestations once dialysis has been initiated. Although there are reports of subsequent disease exacerbations, disease activity usually does not recur in transplanted kidneys.

84. **How commonly does SLE affect the GI tract?**
Frequently. GI manifestations may be present in up to 50% of patients with SLE. Anorexia, nausea, and vomiting are among the most common symptoms. Oral ulcerations (most commonly painless buccal erosions) were identified in 40% of one group of patients. Esophageal involvement such as esophagitis, esophageal ulceration, or esophageal dysmotility seems to correlate with the presence of Raynaud's phenomenon. Intestinal involvement results in abdominal pain, diarrhea, and occasionally, hemorrhage. Intestinal ischemia may be present and may progress to infarction and perforation. Pneumatosis intestinalis in SLE is usually benign and transient but may represent an irreversible necrotizing enterocolitis. In addition, pancreatitis and abdominal serositis are well-recognized. Abnormal liver functions also occur. A vasculitic process has been implicated in the pathogenesis of GI manifestations.

85. **What is the most common pathologic abnormality in patients with lupus central nervous system (CNS) disease?**
Small infarcts and hemorrhages. Vasculitis is suggested by such commonly used designations as "lupus cerebritis" and occurs in < 15% of patients.

Johnson RT, Richardson EP: The neurological manifestations of systemic lupus erythematosus, *Medicine* 47:337–369, 1968.

86. **What are the neuropsychiatric manifestations of SLE?**
- Psychosis
- Cranial, autonomic, and peripheral neuropathies
- Migraine headaches
- Seizure
- Aseptic meningitis
- Pseudotumor cerebri
- Chorea
- Cerebral infarction
- Transverse myelitis (rare)
- Posterior reversible encephalopathy syndrome (PRES)
- Organic brain syndrome (delirium, mild memory loss, and impaired concentration)
  Because of the difficulty in establishing an unequivocal diagnosis, rates of CNS features in SLE cross a broad range. Neuropsychiatric manifestations of lupus may occur in approximately 70% of patients. The more subtle features of cognitive dysfunction may be the most common CNS finding. Abnormal single-photon emission computed tomography (SPECT) or positron-emission tomography (PET) scanning and decreasing intellectual

function, as measured by a standard battery of neurocognitive function tests, are present. The cause for this problem is not known, but cytokines are believed to play an important role.

87. **What is PRES?**
Posterior reversible encephalopathy syndrome, which is a rare neurologic manifestation that has recently been described in patients with SLE. PRES is often associated with acute hypertension and renal failure. Diagnosis is based on presenting symptoms of headaches, seizures, altered mental status, cortical blindness, focal neurologic deficits, and typical MRI findings of posterior cerebral edema.

Leroux G, Sellam J, Costedoat-Chalumeau N, et al: Posterior reversible encephalopathy syndrome during systemic lupus erythematosus: Four new cases and review of the literature, *Lupus* 17:139–147, 2008.

88. **Describe the pulmonary manifestations of lupus.**
Pleurisy or pleural effusion is most common. Up to 60% of patients may have pleuritic pain over the course of their illness. Effusions can be either transudative or exudative and, in rare cases, are the presenting feature. The so-called shrinking lung syndrome describes dyspnea associated with diaphragmatic dysfunction, probably secondary to chronic pleural scarring. Pulmonary parenchymal involvement or lupus pneumonitis has been described, as have pulmonary hemorrhage, pulmonary emboli, and pulmonary hypertension. Emboli and hypertension are more common when APAs are also present.

89. **Which drugs are commonly associated with the development of a clinical syndrome of lupus and a positive ANA?**

Hydralazine	Methyldopa	D-penicillamine
Procainamide	Minocycline	Chlorpromazine
Quinidine	Isoniazid	TNF inhibitors
Diphenylhydantoin	Sulfasalazine	Diltiazem

So-called slow acetylators more commonly develop clinical symptoms, which typically include fever, rash, and arthritis. The clinical features usually regress fairly promptly, although the laboratory abnormality may persist (sometimes indefinitely) when the drug is discontinued. The clinical features commonly present in drug-induced lupus rarely, if ever, include CNS disease or nephritis. There are numerous published reports of many other drugs inducing lupus symptoms on a small number of patients.

90. **What antibody is often touted to be diagnostic for drug-induced lupus?**
Antihistone. Although antihistone antibody is present in as many as 90% of the cases of drug-induced lupus, the antibody is also present in nearly 75% of patients with SLE, and its presence is not diagnostic for drug-induced lupus.

91. **Summarize the mortality rate associated with SLE.**
Death rates from SLE have declined significantly over the last half of the 20th century. The 5-year survival rate in the 1950s was only 50%, whereas it is now > 90%. Survival in those with late-onset disease seems to be reduced compared with survival among those patients afflicted at an earlier age.

92. **List some factors that may contribute to the morbidity or mortality of patients with SLE.**
- Nonadherence to medical advice and treatment
- Presence of active disease
- Medication toxicity
- Infection
- Cardiovascular events

Death early in the course of disease is usually related to the disease itself. Nephritis and CNS disease are the most ominous prognostic factors. Of the causes of death not directly related to active disease, infection is most common, followed by myocardial infarction, stroke, and other atherosclerotic complications. Two recent studies have shown the presence of accelerated atherosclerosis in SLE.

Asanuma Y, Oeser A, Shintani AK, et al: Premature coronary-artery atherosclerosis in systemic lupus erythematosus, *N Engl J Med* 349:2407–2415, 2003.

Roman MJ, Shanker BA, Davis A, et al: Prevalence and correlates of accelerated atherosclerosis in systemic lupus erythematosus, *N Engl J Med* 349:2399–2340, 2003.

93. **Discuss the interaction of pregnancy and SLE.**
Fertility is unaffected by the disease (i.e., patients become pregnant just as readily as women without lupus), and disease exacerbations can occur during pregnancy. Recent data suggest, though, that pregnant patients with lupus do not have disease flares more frequently than nonpregnant patients. Because such flares can be severe, pregnant patients with SLE should be considered at high risk for complications. Preeclampsia, premature births, spontaneous abortions, intrauterine growth delay, and intrauterine fetal deaths are higher in lupus patients. Active disease during the antecedent 3–6 months may increase the risk of flare during the pregnancy. Pregnancy outcome is optimal if the disease has been under control for at least 6–12 months.

Lockshin MD: Pregnancy does not cause systemic lupus erythematosus to worsen, *Arthritis Rheum* 32:665–670, 1989.

94. **How does neonatal lupus occur?**
Through transplacental passage of maternal Anti-SSA/Ro antibodies to the fetus. These antibodies have been linked to direct tissue injury. Babies born with neonatal lupus can exhibit cutaneous lesions as SCLE, hematologic aberrations, hepatic abnormalities, or congenital heart block (CHB), which potentially can be fatal.

95. **What is the incidence of CHB in neonatal lupus?**
1–2%; it is typically identified between 16 and 24 weeks of gestation. The risk for recurrence is 10 times higher in subsequent pregnancies.

Buyon JP, Hiebert R, Copel J, et al: Autoimmune-associated congenital heart block: Demographics, mortality, morbidity and recurrence rates obtained from a national neonatal lupus registry, *J Am Coll Cardiol* 31:1658–1666, 1998.

96. **What drugs are approved by the FDA for the treatment of SLE?**
   - Low-dose aspirin
   - GCs
   - Hydroxychloroquine

97. **Describe the APA syndrome?**
A symptom complex that occurs in approximately 40% of SLE patients and includes one or more of the following: multiple miscarriages, arterial or venous thrombosis, and thrombocytopenia in association with a laboratory finding of APAs. These antibodies can be specific (such as anticardiolipin antibodies), or they may be identified by their effect on the clotting cascade (lupus anticoagulant). Common laboratory tests indicating the presence of antibodies to various phospholipids include prolonged partial thromboplastin time, false-positive Venereal Disease Research Laboratory (VDRL) test for syphilis, or positive anticardiolipin antibodies. A less common example is the dilute Russell viper venom clotting time. APA syndrome may occur by itself (primary APA syndrome) or in association with an underlying connective tissue syndrome, primarily lupus (secondary APA syndrome).

98. **What is Hughes syndrome?**

Antiphospholipid syndrome. Graham R. V. Hughes, a rheumatologist, originally described antiphospholipid syndrome in 1983.

99. **Describe catastrophic APA syndrome.**

Sudden overwhelming vascular occlusion mediated by APAs. Clinical features result from widespread thrombosis of small vessels and the systemic inflammatory response which may include ischemic bowel, pulmonary emboli, acute respiratory distress syndrome (ARDS), infarctive skin lesions, encephalopathy with altered consciousness, seizure, myocardial infarction, and cardiac valvular lesions. Renal involvement is present in the majority of cases.

100. **What factors increases the risk of catastrophic APA syndrome?**

- Presence of other diseases, such as SLE or BD, even if treated
- Infections
- Vaccination
- Flare of underlying disease
- Withdrawal of anticoagulation

Mortality > 50% even with prompt intervention.

101. **How is catastrophic APA syndrome treated?**

- Anticoagulation
- GCs
- Treatment of underlying conditions such as infection
- IV immunoglobulin
- Plasma exchange
- Cytotoxic agents

Petri M: Management of thrombosis in antiphospholipid antibody syndrome, *Rheum Dis Clin North Am* 27:633–641, 2001.

SYSTEMIC SCLEROSIS

102. **What is scleroderma?**

A connective tissue disease is characterized by abnormal collagen deposition into the skin and other organs. The term "scleroderma" is derived from two Greek words: ***skleros***, meaning hard, and ***derma***, meaning skin. Disease pathogenesis is believed to occur as a consequence of aberrant immune activation causing endothelial damage, followed by fibroblast activation that results in obliterative vasculopathy and fibrosis. Of note, the disease is heralded by a vasculopathy, **not** vasculitis. The term "scleroderma" is being phased out and replaced by the term "systemic sclerosis (SSc)" with subcategories of localized sclerosis (morphea, linear scleroderma) or systemic sclerosis (diffuse SSc or limited SSc).

103. **Describe CREST syndrome.**

Calcinosis, **R**aynaud's, **e**sophageal dysmotility, **s**clerodactyly, and **t**elangiectasias. CREST is often found in patients with limited SSc but can be present in diffuse SSc.

104. **Compare and contrast diffuse SSc and limited SSc.**

Patients with diffuse SSc have truncal skin involvement, higher mortality rates, and greater risks of developing pulmonary fibrosis, tendon friction rubs, and scleroderma renal crisis than those with limited SSc. Anti-Scl 70 antibodies are more often found in diffuse SSc. Patients with limited SSc have a higher incidence of pulmonary hypertension and anticentromere antibodies.

105. **Summarize the genetic component of SSc.**
Family members of SSc patients have a significantly greater risk of developing scleroderma than someone with no family history. One likely culprit is an abnormality in the fibrillin gene. This has been elegantly shown in a population study of Choctaw Indians, in whom a genetic defect has been traced to a single common ancestor.

Tan FK, Arnett FC: Genetic factors in the etiology of systemic sclerosis and Raynaud's phenomenon, *Curr Opin Rheumatol* 12:511–519, 2000.

106. **List the noncutaneous features of SSc.**
- Arthralgia
- Inflammatory muscle disease
- GI dysmotility with malabsorption
- Pulmonary interstitial fibrosis with or without pulmonary hypertension
- Scleroderma renal crisis

107. **Do specific autoantibodies help predict the form of SSc a patient may develop?**
Yes. Although > 80% of patients with scleroderma have a positive ANA, this test adds little specificity. Antitopoisomerase 1 (anti–Scl-70) has a positive predictive value of 70% for developing scleroderma. Centromere antibodies have a positive predictive value of 88% for the development of CREST.

Spencer-Green G: Tests preformed in systemic sclerosis: Anticentromere antibody and anti Scl-70 antibody, *Am J Med* 103:242–248, 1997.

108. **What is scleroderma renal crisis?**
A life-threatening aspect of diffuse SSc manifested by sudden onset of malignant hypertension, hemolytic anemia, hyperreninemia, and renal failure. Angiotensin-converting enzyme inhibition therapy has been shown to improve clinical outcomes.

109. **What are the risk factors for scleroderma renal crisis?**
- Diffuse skin involvement
- Rapid progression of skin thickening
- Disease duration < 4 years
- Anti-RNA-polymerase III antibodies
- New-onset anemia
- New-onset cardiac involvement
- High-dose corticosteroid therapy
- Pregnancy

Steen VD, Medsger TA Jr, Osial TA Jr, et al: Factors predicting development of renal involvement in progressive systemic sclerosis, *Am J Med* 1976:779–786, 1984.

110. **What part of the GI tract can SSc affect?**
Anywhere from mouth to anus. Patients may have small oral aperture, dry mucosal membranes with periodontal disease, esophageal dysmotility, reflux, esophagitis, stricture, dysphagia, delayed stomach emptying, pseudo-obstruction of the small intestines, bacterial overgrowth, malabsorption, wide mouth diverticuli, and fecal incontinence due to rectal sphincter fibrosis.

111. **What abnormalities on pulmonary function testing can be seen with SSc?**
- Decreased diffusing capacity for carbon monoxide (DLCO) (earliest marker of pulmonary hypertension)
- Increased A-a gradient with exercise activity
- Decreased vital capacity and increased forced expiratory volume in 1 second–to–forced vital capacity (FEV_1/FVC) ratio (restrictive pattern)

112. **How does SSc affect the heart?**
   - Myocardial fibrosis
   - Dilated cardiomyopathy
   - Cor pulmonale
   - Arrhythmias
   - Pericarditis
   - Myocarditis
   - Heart failure with preserved ejection fraction (diastolic heart failure)
   - Myocardial infarction

113. **Are scleredema and scleromyxedema related to SSc?**
   No. Scleredema is a dermatosis of unknown etiology characterized by symmetrical truncal skin induration and thickening, sometimes with erythema. A high proportion of cases are associated with diabetes, malignancies, and infections. Skin biopsy of a patient with scleredema may reveal thickened dermal collagen with a mild infiltration of mucin in the deeper regions of the dermis. Scleromyxedema (also called "papular mucinosis") is characterized by raised pale, waxy papules that result from excessive mucin deposition distributed over the face, fingers, arms, and legs. This condition is associated with paraproteins, particularly IgG lambda. Cases of scleromyxedema have been described in patients with multiple myeloma, amyloidosis, and human immunodeficiency virus (HIV) infection. Patients with scleredema and scleromyxedema do not typically exhibit Raynaud's phenomenon and positive autoantibodies as would be found in SSc.

IDIOPATHIC INFLAMMATORY MYOPATHIES

114. **What are the idiopathic inflammatory myopathies (IIMs)?**
   Polymyositis, dermatomyositis, and inclusion body myositis (IBM).

115. **What are the diagnostic criteria for polymyositis and dermatomyositis?**
   - Symmetrical proximal weakness
   - Elevated muscle enzymes (creatine phosphokinase [CPK], aldolase, aspartate aminotransferase [AST], alanine aminotransferase [ALT], lactate dehydrogenase [LDH])
   - Myopathic electromyography (EMG) abnormalities
   - Typical changes on muscle biopsy
   - Typical dermatologic features (Gottron's sign, heliotropic rash)
   To make a definite diagnosis of dermatomyositis, three of four criteria plus the rash must be present. For a definite diagnosis of polymyositis, four criteria must be present without the rash. Note that the criteria do not distinguish polymyositis from inclusion body myositis (IBM).

   Bohan A, Peter JB: Polymyositis and dermatomyositis, *N Engl J Med* 292:344–347, 1975.

116. **Compare and contrast polymyositis with dermatomyositis.**
   Both polymyositis and dermatomyositis are characterized by muscle weakness and abnormal muscle findings, but the disorders differ significantly. In dermatomyositis, the inflammation is perivascular (e.g., surrounding the fascicles) with a predominance of CD4+ cells; whereas in polymyositis, CD8+ lymphocytes invade the muscle fiber (e.g., endomysial infiltration). Dermatomyositis can be associated with cancer and may overlap with SSc or mixed connective tissue disease (MCTD). Sclerotic thickening of the dermis, contractures, esophageal hypomotility, microangiopathy, and calcium deposits may be present in dermatomyositis but typically are not seen with polymyositis.

   Dalakas MC, Hohlfeld R: Polymyositis and dermatomyositis, *Lancet* 362:971–982, 2003.

117. **List some of the characteristic features of IBM.**
- Usually occurs in older people.
- Insidious onset.
- Incidence greater in men than women.
- Muscle involvement may be focal or diffuse with asymmetry.
- Can involve both proximal and distal muscles.
- CPK normal (25%) or only slightly elevated.
- Light microscopy shows ragged red fibers, atrophic fibers, and intracellular lined vacuoles.
- Electron microscopy shows intracytoplasmic, intranuclear tubular or filamentous inclusions.

118. **What is Gottron's sign?**
An erythematous rash that is frequently scaly and occurs over the MCP and IP joints in a symmetrical pattern.

119. **Where does the term "heliotropic" rash come from?**
A South American plant with clusters of rich purple flowers, whose scent is similar to cherry pie, named "heliotrope." The heliotropic rash refers to the violaceous coloration similar to that of the plant seen along the eyelids of a patient with dermatomyositis.

120. **What percentage of patients who have an IIM have normal muscle enzymes?**
$\leq$33%.

121. **Give examples of myositis-associated/-specific antibodies.**
Patients with IIM and anti-Jo-1 can present with arthritis, interstitial lung disease, and Raynaud's phenomenon. Anti-SRP is typically found in patients with polymyositis, and its presence portends a poor prognosis. IIM patients with anti-U1RNP may have myositis overlap with MCTD. Anti-Mi-2 is found in patients with classic dermatomyositis; these patients have good prognoses and will respond well to treatment.

122. **What is the antisynthetase syndrome?**
A subcategory of the IIM defined by the presence of autoantibodies to aminoacyl-tRNA synthetases. Specific clinical manifestations include myositis, interstitial lung disease, arthritis, Raynaud's phenomenon, fever, and mechanics hands. Antibodies to Jo-1, PL-12, OJ, EJ, PL-7, KS, and Zo have been reported.

123. **What further evaluation for an occult malignancy should be undertaken in an adult diagnosed with dermatomyositis?**
Because of the increased risk of malignancy in patients with myositis, particularly dermatomyositis, age-appropriate cancer screening should be pursued. (See Chapter 2, General Medicine and Ambulatory Care.)

SPONDYLOARTHROPATHIES

124. **What is a spondyloarthropathy?**
A group of inflammatory diseases of uncertain etiology that affect the spine and sacroiliac joints characterized by the absence of RF autoantibodies and a high association with class 1 major histocompatability antigen, HLA-B27. Other unifying features include peripheral oligoarthropathy, enthesopathy, and extra-articular foci of inflammation such as uveitis. Diseases classified as spondyloarthropathies include:

Ankylosing
  spondylitis
Reactive
  arthritis
Juvenile
  spondyloarthritis

SAPPHO (synovitis,
  severe acne,
  palmoplantar
  pustulosis,
  hyperostosis, and
  osteitis)

Psoriatic arthritis
Enteropathic arthritis
Arthritis associated with
  Whipple's disease

Arnett FC: Seronegative spondyloarthritis. In Nabel EG, editor: *ACP Medicine*, New York, 2010, BC Decker, www.acpmedicine.com.

125. **What mechanisms may explain the association of HLA-B27 with arthropathy?**
Although the exact mechanism is unknown, one hypothesis suggests that B27 presents an arthritogenic peptide or alters immune repertoire through its antigen presentation role. Another possibility is that the B27 peptide itself may be prone to misfolding, forming homodimers that subsequently trigger an inflammatory response. Lastly, B27 may serve as a surface ligand for other immunomodulatory receptor families, such as KIRs (killer cell immunoglobulin receptors). In addition, we know that individuals who are homozygous for B27 are three times more likely to develop ankylosing spondylitis than heterozygotes, suggesting a gene dosage effect.

Melis L, Elewaut D: Progress in spondylarthritis. Immunopathogenesis of spondyloarthritis: which cells drive disease? *Arthritis Res Ther* 11:233–238, 2009.

126. **Describe the principal clinical features of ankylosing spondylitis.**
- Occurs more often in men than in women in a 3:1 ratio.
- Begins in later adolescence.
- Presents with inflammatory low back pain and stiffness.
- Has inflammatory pain pattern that improves with activity and worsens with rest.
- Has predominantly lower limb peripheral joint involvement.

127. **Name the extra-articular features of ankylosing spondylitis.**
- Anterior uveitis (occurring in ~25%)
- Aortitis (often progressing to aortic valve insufficiency)
- Cardiac conduction defects
- Pulmonary fibrosis (<1%)

128. **What is the difference between a syndesmophyte and an osteophyte?**
Syndesmophytes represent ossification of the outer layers of the annulus fibrosus (Sharpey's fibers), creating an osseous bridge across vertebra at the discovertebral junction. The syndesmophyte is a characteristic radiographic finding in ankylosing spondylitis, though it may be seen in any of the spondyloarthropathies. Spinal **osteophytes** are triangular ossifications, continuous with the vertebral bodies, forming at either the margins of a vertebral body or a few millimeters from the margin of the discovertebral junction. Osteophytes are often associated with degenerative disc disease.

Brower AC: The "phytes" of the spine. In Brower AC, Flemming DJ, editors: *Arthritis in Black and White*, ed 2, Philadelphia, 1997, WB Saunders, pp 175–191.

129. **Describe the mucocutaneous manifestations of reactive arthritis.**
- Small painless areas of **desquamation on the tongue** that may be unnoticed by the patient
- **Circinate balanitis** usually affecting the glans penis that can range from small erythematous macules to large areas of dry, flaking skin
- **Keratoderma blennorrhagica,** a thickening and keratinization of the skin that generally involves the feet, hands, and nails that resemble psoriasis clinically and on histopathology

130. **List the five patterns of joint involvement found in psoriatic arthritis and their relative frequencies.**
    - **DIP joints of hands and/or feet:** 8%
    - **Peripheral asymmetrical oligoarthropathy:** 8%
    - **Symmetrical polyarthritis resembling RA:** 18%
    - **Arthritis mutilans** ("opera glass hands"): 2%
    - **Sacroiliitis with or without higher levels of spinal involvement:** 24%

    Arnett FC: Seronegative spondyloarthropathies, *Bull Rheum Dis* 37:1–12, 1987.

131. **What are the treatment options for ankylosing spondylitis?**
    NSAIDs, either nonselective or selective COX-2 inhibitors. Anti-TNF treatment such as etanercept, infliximab, adalimumab, or golimumab may be considered for those with persistent disease activity. Unlike RA, conventional DMARDs such as methotrexate and sulfasalazine do not have any demonstrable effect on axial disease, though they may have some benefit for peripheral arthritis. Nonpharmacologic treatment, including patient education and exercise programs, should also be part of the treatment approach.

    Zochling J, van der Heijde D, Burgos-Vargas R, et al: ASAS/EULAR recommendations for the management of ankylosing spondylitis, *Ann Rheum Dis* 65:442–452, 2006.

VASCULITIS

132. **What is vasculitis?**
    A varied group of disorders that share a common underlying pathology of inflammation of a single blood vessel or blood vessels. Vasculitis occurs as a primary disorder or secondary to a variety of diseases or drugs.

133. **How are vasculitides classified?**
    By the predominant sizes of the involved blood vessels (large, medium, and small). The presence or absence of ANCA is a more recent addition to proposed classification criteria; however, there is substantial overlap among different vasculitides.

134. **What are the possible immune-pathogenic mechanisms of vasculitis?**
    - Deposition of circulating antigen-antibody complexes or in situ formation of immune complexes within the vessel wall
    - Cell-mediated hypersensitivity
    - Granulomatous tissue reaction

135. **What is polymyalgia rheumatica (PMR)?**
    An inflammatory condition that causes pain or stiffness, usually in the neck, shoulder girdle, and hip girdle with sudden onset and occurrence in patients older than 50 years. Patients typically have elevated ESR or CRP or both, which suggests a systemic inflammatory process.

136. **What are the types of large vessel vasculitis?**
    Giant cell arteritis (GCA) and Takayasu's disease (TD).

137. **What is the association between PMR and GCA?**
    Approximately 15% of patients with PMR develop GCA, and approximately 50% of patients with GCA have associated PMR.

138. **How does the distribution of blood vessels involved in GCA affect the symptoms?**
    If the *extracranial* branches of the aorta (with sparing of the intracranial vessels) are involved, the classic manifestations of blindness, headache, scalp tenderness, and jaw claudication are seen. Vasculitis of the vertebral arteries can impair the posterior cerebral circulation and

cause stroke, transient ischemic attacks, vertigo, and dizziness. Involvement of the subclavian, axillary, and proximal brachial arteries leads to the aortic arch syndrome of claudication of the arms and absent or asymmetric pulses.

139. **What is TD?**
A large vessel vasculitis affecting blood vessels with elastic lamina. The populations at highest risk include women who are adolescent or in the second and third decades of life. The syndrome is most commonly seen in Japan, Southeast Asia, India, and Mexico. Clinical manifestations range from asymptomatic disease with nonpalpable pulses to catastrophic neurologic impairment (stroke, postural dizziness, seizures, and amaurosis).

140. **What are the medium vessel vasculitides?**
   - Polyarteritis nodosa (PAN)
   - KD
   - Primary CNS vacuities

141. **What is PAN?**
A vasculitis characterized by necrotizing inflammation of medium-sized or small arteries. Patients typically present with systemic symptoms involving the kidneys, skin, joints, muscles, nerves, and GI tract.

142. **Which are the characteristics of KD?**
Fever, bilateral nonexudative conjunctivitis, erythema of the lips and oral mucosa, rash, extremity changes, and lymphadenopathy. The most serious complication is severe coronary aneurysmal dilations. KD is one of the most common vasculitides of childhood and usually occurs in children < 5 years old.

143. **Compare the common clinical presentations and laboratory findings of GCA, TD, KD, and PAN.**
See Table 10-9.

144. **With which diseases are ANCAs associated?**
   - Wegener's granulomatosis (WG)
   - Microscopic polyarteritis (MPA)
   - A pauci-immune (meaning lack of immune complex deposition or complement consumption) crescentic glomerulonephritis, limited to the kidneys

TABLE 10-9. CHARACTERISTICS OF GIANT CELL ARTERITIS, TAKAYASU'S DISEASE, KAWASAKI'S DISEASE, AND POLYARTERITIS NODOSA		
	Vessels Affected	**Clinical Manifestations**	**Laboratory Data**
GCA	Large extracranial vessels	Visual changes, headache, scalp tenderness and jaw claudication	Elevated ESR and CRP
TD	Large blood vessels with elastic lamina	From asymptomatic to severe neurological impairment	Elevated ESR
KD	Medium vessel vasculitis	Fever, rash, conjunctivitis, erythema (lips/mucosa), LAD	Elevated ESR

(continued)

TABLE 10-9. CHARACTERISTICS OF GIANT CELL ARTERITIS, TAKAYASU'S DISEASE, KAWASAKI'S DISEASE, AND POLYARTERITIS NODOSA— *(continued)*

	Vessels Affected	Clinical Manifestations	Laboratory Data
PAN	Predominantly medium-sized venules	Systemic symptoms, HTN, renal insufficiency, abdominal pain, neurologic dysfunction	Possible hepatitis B Aneurysms on angiography

CRP = C-reactive protein; ESR = erythrocyte sedimentation rate; GCA = giant cell arteritis; HTN = hypertension; KD = Kawasaki disease; LAD = lymphadenopathy; PAN = polyarteritis nodosa; TD = Takayasu's disease.

- Churg-Strauss syndrome (CSS)
- Drug-induced vasculitis: propylthiouracil, hydralazine, minocycline, and others
- Inflammatory rheumatic disease: RA, SLE, Sjögren's syndrome, SSc, inflammatory myopathies, and APA syndrome
- Autoimmune gastrointestinal disorders: ulcerative colitis and primary sclerosing cholangitis

145. **What is WG?**
One of the systemic necrotizing vasculitis characterized by granulomatous inflammation of the small vessels of the upper respiratory tract, lungs, and kidneys commonly associated with c-ANCA. Over 80–90% of WG patients have PR3-ANCA.

146. **Which organs are primarily affected in WG?**
Respiratory tract (upper and/or lower) and kidneys. Respiratory tract involvement can manifest as recurrent sinusitis, otitis media, tracheobronchial inflammation and erosions, lung nodules, or pneumonitis with cavitation. Renal involvement occurs in the form of a pauci-immune glomerulonephritis.

147. **What are other symptoms in WG?**
- Arthritis
- Neurologic symptoms including polyneuritis, meningitis and mononeuritis multiplex
- Skin ulcerations in the distal portions of arms or legs
- Eye inflammation due to contiguous granulomatous sinus disease (nasolacrimal duct obstruction, proptosis, and ocular muscle or optic nerve involvement) or due to focal vasculitis (conjunctivitis, episcleritis, scleritis, corneoscleral ulceration, uveitis, and granulomatous vasculitis of the retina and optic nerve).

148. **What is CSS?**
A granulomatous small vessel vasculitis that involves mainly the blood vessels of the lungs, GI system, and peripheral nerves and is associated with p-ANCA (myeloperoxidase) antibodies. The heart, skin, and kidneys may also be affected, and eosinophilia and severe asthma are very characteristic.

149. **How is MPA characterized?**
By pauci-immune necrotizing small vessel vasculitis of the lungs and kidneys without clinical or pathologic evidence of necrotizing granulomatous inflammation. MPA is the most common pulmonary-renal syndrome. Other organs involved include the skin, musculoskeletal system, and GI tract. Over 80% of patients with MPA are ANCA-positive, most often p-ANCA (MPO-ANCA).

150. **What is cryoglobulinemic vasculitis (CV)?**
Small vessel vasculitis caused by the localization of mixed cryoglobulins in vessel walls, which incites acute inflammation. The most frequent manifestations are purpura, arthralgias, and nephritis. Mixed cryoglobulins and RF are often positive. Most patients have an associated infection with hepatitis C virus.

151. **Define "Henoch-Schönlein purpura (HSP)"?**
As a small vessel vasculitis characterized by vascular deposition of IgA-dominant immune complexes. Purpura, arthralgias, and colicky abdominal pain are the most frequent manifestations. Approximately half the patients have hematuria and proteinuria, but only 10–20% have renal insufficiency. HSP is the most common vasculitis in childhood and has an excellent prognosis.

152. **Compare the common clinical presentations and laboratory findings of MPA, WG, CSS, CV, and HSP.**
See Table 10-10.

TABLE 10-10. CHARACTERISTICS OF MICROSCOPIC POLYANGIITIS, WEGENER GRANULOMATOSIS, CHURG-STRAUSS SYNDROME, CRYOGLOBULINEMIC VASCULITIS, AND HENOCH–SCHÖNLEIN PURPURA

Disease	Vessel Size Affected	Clinical Feature	Frequency (%)	Laboratory
MPA	Small to medium-sized vessels	Glomerulonephritis	>90	Usually p-ANCA (anti-MPO)
		Pulmonary and skin	50	
		Neurologic, GI	Less common	
WG	Small to medium-sized vessels	Pulmonary, ENT	90	Usually c-ANCA (anti-PR3)
		Glomerulonephritis	80	
		Neurologic, GI and skin	50	
CSS	Small to medium-sized vessels	Pulmonary and peripheral nerve.	70–80	Eosinophilia
		Skin, ENT, GI, renal and musculoskeletal	50	Usually p-ANCA (anti-MPO)
CV	Small vessels	Skin	90	Cryoglobulins, RF
		Musculoskeletal	70	
		Renal	55	
		Neurologic, GI	30–40	
HSP	Small vessels	Skin	90	IgA deposition
		Musculoskeletal	75	
		GI	60	

c-ANCA = cytoplasmic antineutrophil cytoplasmic antibody; CSS = Churg-Strauss syndrome; CV = cryoglobulinemic vasculitis; ENT = ear, nose, and throat; GI = gastrointestinal; HSP = Henoch-Schönlein purpura; MPA = microscopic polyangiitis; MPO = myeloperoxidase; p-ANCA = perinuclear antineutrophil cytoplasmic antibody; RF = rheumatoid factor; WG = Wegener's granulomatosis.

153. **What is BD?**
A systemic vasculitic disorder of unknown etiology, characterized by relapsing episodes of oral aphthous ulcers, genital ulcers, skin lesions, and ocular lesions (retinal vasculitis, anterior and posterior uveitis). Other symptoms include arthralgia/arthritis, CNS vasculitis, meningitis, thrombosis, and GI ulcerations. BD affects blood vessels of all sizes and is most common along the "Old Silk Route," which spans the region from Japan and China in the Far East to the Mediterranean Sea, including countries such as Turkey and Iran.

154. **What are the skin lesions of BD?**
- Folliculitis
- Acneiform lesions
- Erythema nodosum lesions that may ulcerate
- Pathergy (pustular reaction to skin injury)
- Palpable purpura
- Pyoderma gangrenosum type lesions

155. **What are the ocular findings associated with BD?**
- Retinal vasculitis
- Anterior and posterior uveitis
- Hypopyon (severe anterior uveitis with purulent material in the anterior chamber)
- Cataracts
- Glaucoma
- Neovascularization
- Conjunctival ulceration

156. **What treatments are available for the management of vasculitis?**
Corticosteroids and immunosuppressive medications. The treatment choices for vasculitis will be determined by the type and severity of the manifestations of the disease. Some commonly used immunosuppressants include cyclophosphamide, azathioprine, and methotrexate.

OSTEOARTHRITIS

157. **Is OA a genetic disease?**
Yes, in that there is a hereditary component. Perhaps the most recognized inherited feature is the presence of Heberden's nodes in mothers and sisters of affected patients. Studies have uncovered a mutation in a type II collagen gene (Arg519 to Cys) that predisposes to early OA.

> Pun YL, Moskowitz RW, Lie S, et al: Clinical correlations of osteoarthritis associated with a single-base mutation (arginine 519 to cysteine) in type II procollagen gene: A newly defined pathogenesis, *Arthritis Rheum* 37:264–269, 1994.

158. **Compare the biochemical changes of the aged joint with the osteoarthritic joint.**
See Table 10-11.

159. **What is spinal stenosis syndrome?**
The progressive narrowing of the spinal canal, most commonly from OA of the lumbar or cervical spine. With cervical disease, patients typically present with pain and limitation of motion. Hyperreflexia is common. Other signs may include muscle weakness, spastic gait, and Babinski's sign. In the lumbar region, the clinical manifestations are mostly those of neurogenic claudication and compression of the cauda equina when severe.

TABLE 10-11. BIOCHEMICAL DIFFERENCES BETWEEN THE AGING JOINT AND OSTEOARTHRITIS

	Aging Joint	Osteoarthritis
Bone	Osteoporosis	Thickened cortices, osteophytes, subchondral cysts, remodeling
Chondrocyte activity	Normal	Increased
Collagen	Increased cross-linking of fibrils	Irregular weave Smaller fibrils
Water	Slight decrease	Significant increase
Proteoglycan	Normal total content Decreased chondroitins Increased keratin Normal aggregation	Decreased total proteoglycan component Increased chondroitins Decreased keratin Decreased aggregation

From Brandt KD, Fife RS: Aging in relation to the pathogenesis of osteoarthritis. Clin Rheum Dis 12:117–130, 1986.

160. **What is DISH?**
Diffuse idiopathic skeletal hyperostosis characterized by extensive ossification of tendinous and ligamentous attachments to the bone. Spine involvement with flowing calcification over the anterior longitudinal ligament is among the most common findings. Extraspinal manifestations also are reported. DISH has been associated with obesity, increased waist circumference, hypertension, dyslipidemia, diabetes mellitus, hyperuricemia, metabolic syndrome, and an increased risk for cardiovascular diseases.

161. **What radiographic features help to distinguish DISH from ankylosing spondylitis, degenerative spine disease, and spondylosis deformans?**
   - Flowing calcification along the anterolateral aspect of at least four contiguous vertebral bodies
   - Relative preservation of intervertebral disc height in the involved vertebral segment and absence of extensive radiographic changes of "degenerative" disc disease (disc space narrowing with vacuum phenomena, vertebral body marginal sclerosis)
   - Absence of apophyseal joint ankylosis and sacroiliac joint erosion, sclerosis, and intra-articular osseous fusion

162. **What is the vacuum phenomenon?**
A radiographic finding seen in degeneration of the intervertebral disc that has the appearance of a radiolucent stripe in an intervertebral disc. Radiolucencies represent gas or nitrogen that appears at the site of negative pressure produced by abnormal spaces of clefts.

INFECTIOUS ARTHRITIS

163. **What is the mechanism for acute rheumatic fever?**
Antibody formation to group A streptococcus that occurs after pharyngeal infection, which may be asymptomatic. The antibodies cross-react with human antigens, leading to a

persistent autoimmune reaction with tissue destruction (molecular mimicry) and development of immune complexes. Arthritis is one of the earliest manifestations of rheumatic fever and has a migratory pattern.

164. **What is St. Vitus' dance?**
A neurologic disorder consisting of abrupt, purposeless involuntary movements that disappear during sleep. The disorder is found in patients with rheumatic fever and is also called "Syndenham's chorea" or "chorea minor."

165. **What viral illnesses may be associated with arthropathy?**
- Hepatitis B and C
- Parvovirus B19
- EBV
- Cytomegalovirus (CMV)
- Enteroviruses (ECHO [enteropathic cytopathogenic human orphan], coxsackievirus)
- HIV
- Mumps
- Rubella
- Smallpox (vaccinia)
- Group A arboviruses (Ross River virus, chikungunya, o'ynong-nyong, sindbis, Mayaro)

   Naides SJ: Viral arthritis including HIV, *Curr Opin Rheumatol* 7:337–342, 1995.

166. **What arthropathy is associated with chronic hepatitis B infection?**
Polyarteritis nodosa, likely associated with persistent circulating hepatitis B antigen.

167. **What are the articular manifestations of hepatitis C infection?**
- Arthropathy
- Nondestructive RA-like arthritis
- Monoarthritis
- Oligoarthritis
Hepatitis C can also be part of the mixed cryoglobulinemia syndrome.

168. **What arthropathy is associated with active parvovirus infection?**
Nondestructive RA-like picture with positive RF. The arthropathy clears with no chronic or destructive sequelae.

169. **Summarize the association of rubella infection with arthropathy.**
Joint symptoms usually begin within 1 week of the onset of the rash of rubella and include arthralgia and arthritis, especially in adult women. In the past, arthritis and arthralgias often were seen after rubella vaccination, but they are less common because a less arthrogenic strain of virus is used for the vaccine.

170. **What are the common articular problems experienced by patients infected with HIV?**
- Arthralgia
- Reactive arthritis associated with HLA-B27 (but axial disease and sacroiliitis are unusual)
- Psoriatic arthritis with asymmetrical polyarticular inflammatory arthritis that may be more severe than in non-HIV patients
- "Painful articular syndrome" describing an exquisitely painful, asymmetrical, minimally inflammatory arthritis involving the large joints of the lower extremities
- Septic arthritis, typically *Staphylococcus aureus* but also with *Streptococcus, Salmonella,* atypical *Mycobacteria,* and other opportunistic infections

   Solomon G, Brancato L, Winchester R: An approach to the human immunodeficiency virus–positive patient with a spondyloarthropathic disease, *Rheum Dis Clin North Am* 17:43–58, 1991.

171. **What are the specific muscle problems encountered by patients infected with HIV?**
- IIM (polymyositis and dermatomyositis)
- Nemaline rod myopathy with findings of nemaline rods without inflammation on muscle biopsy
- Noninflammatory myopathy associated with severe wasting
- Pyomyositis or direct muscle infection with small muscle abscesses frequently caused by *S. aureus*, *Mycobacterium avium*, cryptococci, *Microsporidia*, and other organisms
- Medication-associated myopathy seen with zidovudine (AZT) and other nucleoside and nucleotide reverse transcriptase inhibitors (NRTIs)

172. **What is DILS?**
Diffuse infiltrative lymphocytosis syndrome, a condition occurring in 3–8% of HIV-infected patients, producing prominent salivary gland involvement and sicca symptoms due to CD8 infiltration. In addition to salivary glands, other organs may be involved in DILS resulting in neuropathy, interstitial pneumonitis, interstitial nephritis, and hepatitis.

173. **Is DILS the same as Sjögren's syndrome?**
No. DILS is a distinct entity with different immunogenetics and pathophysiology from Sjögren's syndrome. DILS is a predominantly CD8 disease whereas Sjögren's syndrome is a CD4 disease. In addition, African American DILS sufferers show a high incidence of HLA-DR8, whereas DR6 and DR7 are more prevalent in Caucasians. By contrast, in patients with Sjögren's syndrome, HLA-DR2 and DR3 predominate.

174. **Which bacterial pathogens are most commonly responsible for septic arthritis?**
- *Neisseria gonorrhoeae*
- *Staphylococcus* spp.
- *Streptococcus* spp.
- Gram-negative bacilli

175. **What are the common clinical manifestations of gonococcal arthritis?**
Migratory tenosynovitis and macular or papular rash on a distal extremity. Gonococcal arthritis occurs in approximately 0.1–0.5% of patients with gonorrhea, but synovial fluid cultures are positive in < 50% of cases.

176. **What are the clinical manifestations of Lyme disease and the time of their occurrence in the untreated disease course?**
Early localized:
- Erythema chronicum migrans (ECM)
- Flulike illness
Early disseminated:
- Neurologic findings (meningitis, cranial neuropathies such as Bell's palsy, peripheral neuropathy)
- Cardiac findings (arteriovenous block, myopericarditis)
Late:
- Inflammatory arthritis with chronic inflammatory synovitis

177. **What is the classic skin manifestation of Lyme disease?**
ECM, an expanding erythematous ring (often asymptomatic) with central clearing beginning at the sight of the tick bite. The *Borrelia* organism can be cultured from the margin of the lesion. In endemic regions, ECM is the most common presenting feature of early Lyme disease. Other skin manifestations include benign lymphocytoma and acrodermatitis chronica atrophicans.

178. **Is chronic arthritis of Lyme disease produced by active joint infection?**
Likely not. Live spirochetes have rarely been documented. In addition, spirochetal DNA has not been reliably discovered after amplification with polymerase chain reaction (PCR) technology.

CRYSTAL ARTHROPATHY

179. **What three principal crystals are associated with joint inflammation?**
■ Urate (gout)
■ Calcium pyrophosphate (CPP; "pseudogout")
■ Hydroxyapatite

   Dieppe P, Calvert P: *Crystals and Joint Disease*, London, 1983, Chapman & Hall.

180. **What conditions have been associated with calcium pyrophosphate dihydrate (CPPD) disease?**

Hemochromatosis	Hypophosphatasia	Hypomagnesemia
Hypothyroidism	Amyloidosis (likely)	Gout
Aging	Trauma, including	
Hyperparathyroidism	surgery	
Gene mutations (ANKH)	OA (likely)	

181. **Why is the polarizing microscope important in the diagnosis of rheumatic diseases?**
To analyze synovial fluid and identify the specific etiologies of inflammatory arthritis, in particular crystal-induced arthritis. The microscopy operates on the relatively simple observation that some crystals refract light into fast and slow rays (i.e., they are birefringent). Polarized light passing through a crystal is no longer parallel to light not passing through the crystal. If a second polarizer is added so that its axis is rotated 90° (extinction) to the light as it emerges from the first polarizer but after some light is bent (rotated) by the crystal in between the polarizers, the only light reaching the observer's eye is the light that the crystal has rotated. Monosodium urate crystals have a strongly negative birefringent appearance on polarized light microscopy and appear yellow when oriented parallel to the axis of the compensator. Calcium pyrophosphate crystals are weakly positively birefringent and appear blue when oriented parallel to the axis of the compensator. Polarized microscopy requires operator expertise for accuracy.

   Rosenthal AK, Mandel N: Identification of crystals in synovial fluids and joint tissues, *Curr Rheumatol Rep* 3:11–16, 2001.

182. **Where is chondrocalcinosis commonly demonstrated roentgenographically?**
In the joint cartilages. The cartilages appear punctate or stippled with linear densities within the articular hyaline or fibrocartilage in knee menisci, radiocarpal joints, annulus fibrosus of intervertebral discs, and symphysis pubis. When present in peripheral joints, the findings are usually bilateral. The prevalence in the general population (as assessed by multiple radiologic studies) is 10–15% in people aged 65–75 years but rises above 40% in people older than 80 years.

183. **What are the four stages of gout?**
■ **Stage 1:** asymptomatic hyperuricemia
■ **Stage 2:** acute gouty arthritis
■ **Stage 3:** intercritical gout or the period between attacks
■ **Stage 4:** chronic tophaceous gout

184. **Describe stage 1 gout.**
Elevated serum urate levels in the absence of symptomatic articular disease or nephrolithiasis. Not all patients with asymptomatic hyperuricemia progress to gout, but the higher the serum level, the greater the likelihood of developing articular disease. With serum urate > 9 mg/dL, the annual incidence of gout is 4.9%, with 5-year incidence of 22%. In most cases, 20–30 years of sustained hyperuricemia pass before an attack of nephrolithiasis or arthropathy.

Campion EW, Glynn RJ, DeLabry LO: Asymptomatic hyperuricemia. Risks and consequences in the Normative Aging Study, *Am J Med* 82:421–426, 1987.

185. **Describe the characteristics of the first attack of acute gouty arthritis (stage 2).**
Exquisite pain usually occurring in a single joint (monoarticular). Fever, swelling, erythema, and skin sloughing may be associated findings, suggesting cellulitis. Fifty percent of initial attacks occur as podagra (involving the great toe or MTP joint), and 90% of patients with gout have podagra at some stage of disease without treatment. Typical sites of acute gout attacks include feet, ankles, knees, and less commonly, upper extremity joints such as elbows, wrists, and fingers.

186. **What are the symptoms of stage 3 gout?**
None. Stage 3 gout refers to the asymptomatic period between attacks. However, 62% of patients have a second attack of articular disease within 1 year of the first attack, 16% within 1–2 years, 11% within 2–5 years, 4% after 5–10 years, and 7% after > 10 years.

187. **What is chronic tophaceous gout (stage 4)?**
Chronic arthritis with extra-articular tissue deposition of urate. Gout flares in this stage are often polyarticular, with longer duration and severity. In some cases, chronic tophaceous gout may have an appearance mimicking RA (pseudorheumatoid pattern), with chronic, nearly symmetrical arthritis with nodules (tophi in gout). The principal determinant of the rate of urate deposition is the serum urate concentration. Tophi are often observed on finger pads, olecranon bursae, pinnae of the ear, and pressure points.

Teng GG, Nair R, Saag KG: Pathophysiology, clinical presentation and treatment of gout, *Drugs* 66:1547–1563, 2006.

188. **What are the treatment options for acute gout flares?**
NSAIDs, colchicine, and corticosteroids, either oral or intra-articular. Ideally, acute gout flares are treated within 12 hours of symptom onset to reduce the severity. Oral NSAIDs can be given at high dose for 2–3 days, then tapered off within 5–7 days. NSAIDs have potential GI and renal toxicities, especially in elderly patients and those with comorbidities such as congestive heart failure or anticoagulation use. Oral colchicine at lower doses (1.2 mg initially, followed by 0.6 mg 1 hr later) was shown in a recent randomized study to have equal efficacy but better tolerability than traditional higher dose colchicines (1.2 mg initially, then 0.6 mg every hour for 6 hr) for acute gout flares. Severe diarrhea, nausea, and vomiting are among the common side effects of colchicine, especially with a higher dose regimen.

Terkeltaub R: Update on gout: New therapeutic strategies and options, *Nat Rev Rheumatol* 6:30–38, 2010.

189. **What are the treatment options for chronic gout?**
Allopurinol, probenecid, and febuxostat. New evidence-based guidelines focus on treating chronic gout to a target uric acid level < 6 mg/dL. Allopurinol is commonly used in uric acid overproducers and undersecreters. Uricosuric agents similar to probenecid are

limited to undersecreters with normal renal function. Allopurinol can be initiated at a dose of 100 mg daily, titrating higher to a maximum approved dose of 800 mg/day. Allopurinol dosing should be more cautious in patients with renal insufficiency (CrCl < 50 mL/min) or elderly patients. Febuxostat, a nonpurine inhibitor of xanthine oxidase, could be used for treatment in those patients with allopurinol hypersensitivity, intolerance, or treatment failure. Febuxostat is dosed at 40 mg daily, or 80 mg daily for those who do not attain adequate uric acid suppression at the lower dose. Chronic urate-lowering therapy should not be started during acute gout flares, but can be continued through acute flares in those already taking urate-lowering treatment. Also, it is not uncommon for patients starting chronic urate-lowering therapy to have more frequent acute gout flares due to mobilization and destabilization of urate deposits in tissues and joints. These patients should receive acute gout prophylaxis with low-dose daily colchicine (0.6 mg daily or twice daily) or NSAIDs for the first 6 months of therapy.

Teng GG, Nair R, Saag KG: Pathophysiology, clinical presentation and treatment of gout, *Drugs* 66:1547–1563, 2006.

Terkeltaub R: Update on gout: New therapeutic strategies and options, *Nat Rev Rheumatol* 6:30–38, 2010.

SOFT TISSUE RHEUMATISM

190. **What is fibromyalgia (FM)?**
A chronic nondestructive illness characterized by fatigue, generalized pain, sleep disturbance (sometimes termed "nonrestorative" sleep), and tender points in a characteristic distribution (see Fig. 10-1). Eighteen reproducible tender points have been established, and diagnosis of FM requires the presence of at least 11. Patients may have FM alone or in association with other diseases such as RA, OA, Lyme disease, and sleep apnea. The disease is often mimicked by hypothyroidism.

Wolfe F, Smythe HA, Yunus MB, et al: The American College of Rheumatology 1990 criteria for the classification of fibromyalgia: Report of the Multicenter Criteria Committee, *Arthritis Rheum* 33:160–172, 1990.

191. **What other symptoms and syndromes may be associated with FM?**
- IBS
- Tension headaches
- Irritable bladder (daytime urinary frequency, nocturia, dysuria, urgency, urge incontinence)
- Chronic cough

192. **How is FM treated?**
With muscle reconditioning (slow but consistent physical training), restoration of more normal sleep patterns, and pain control. Low-dose tricyclic antidepressants may help with sleep and non-narcotic medications such as NSAIDs or acetaminophen may be used for pain control. Biofeedback may also be of use. More recent U.S. Food and Drug Administration (FDA)–approved medications include duloxetin, pregabalin, and milnacipran.

193. **Define the following disorders named after occupations.**
- **Housemaid's knee:** prepatellar bursitis
- **Tailor's seat** (also called "weaver's bottom"): inflammation of the ischial bursa (the bursa that separates the gluteus maximus from the ischial tuberosity)

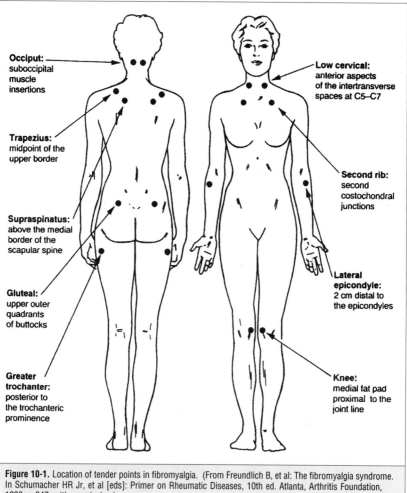

Occiput: suboccipital muscle insertions

Trapezius: midpoint of the upper border

Supraspinatus: above the medial border of the scapular spine

Gluteal: upper outer quadrants of buttocks

Greater trochanter: posterior to the trochanteric prominence

Low cervical: anterior aspects of the intertransverse spaces at C5–C7

Second rib: second costochondral junctions

Lateral epicondyle: 2 cm distal to the epicondyles

Knee: medial fat pad proximal to the joint line

Figure 10-1. Location of tender points in fibromyalgia. (From Freundlich B, et al: The fibromyalgia syndrome. In Schumacher HR Jr, et al [eds]: Primer on Rheumatic Diseases, 10th ed. Atlanta, Arthritis Foundation, 1993, p 247, with permission.)

194. **Define the following disorders named after specific sports and activities.**
   - **Little Leaguer's shoulder:** separation of the proximal humeral epiphysis, probably secondary to the repetitive motion associated with pitching
   - **Tennis elbow:** lateral epicondylitis
   - **Golfer's elbow:** medial epicondylitis
   - **Jumper's knee:** Sinding-Larsen-Johannson (SLJ) syndrome or patellar tendinopathy usually seen in basketball and volleyball athletes but also in ballet dancers

195. **What is deQuervain's tenosynovitis?**
   Inflammation of the synovial lining and subsequent narrowing of the membrane (stenosing tenosynovitis) of the abductor pollicis longus and extensor pollicis brevis tendons at the radial styloid.

196. **What is patellofemoral syndrome (PFS)?**
Knee pain that worsens with activity, while descending stairs and after long periods of inactivity. PFS occurs when the patella does not move or "track" in a correct fashion when the knee is being bent and straightened. This movement can lead to damage of the surrounding tissues, such as the cartilage on the underside of the patella itself, which can lead to pain in the region. This injury is quite common in people who play sports, in particular adolescent girls.

OTHER RHEUMATIC CONDITIONS

197. **What is pyoderma gangrenosum?**
Skin lesions that begin as pustules or erythematous nodules and break down to form spreading ulcers with necrotic, undermined edges. Pyoderma gangrenosum is frequently associated with inflammatory bowel disease (IBD) but also occurs in chronic active hepatitis, seropositive RA (without evidence of vasculopathy), leukemia, and polycythemia vera. Differential diagnosis of the lesions includes necrotizing vasculitis, bacterial infection, and spider bites.

198. **What is Sjögren's syndrome?**
An exocrinopathy manifested by sicca (dryness) symptoms. The lacrimal and salivary glands are primarily affected, but the urogenital and GI systems may be involved as well.

199. **What are the revised ACR criteria for Sjögren's syndrome?**
I. Presence of ocular symptoms (dry eyes, recurrent feeling of sand or gravel in the eyes, or use of tear substitutes more than three times a day)
II. Presence of oral symptoms (feeling of dry mouth daily, recurrent or persistent swollen salivary glands, frequent use of liquids to help swallow dry food)
III. Objective evidence of ocular dryness (e.g., the Schirmer's test or rose Bengal score)
IV. Objective evidence of salivary gland involvement (e.g., sialogram, salivary scintigraphy or salivary flow test)
V. Positive histopathology on salivary gland biopsy
VI. Presence of Sjögren's specific autoantibodies, SSA/Ro or SSB/La.

Patients are considered to have Sjögren's if:

1. Four out of six criteria are present and either V or VI is present or
2. Three out of four objective criteria are present (III, IV, V, and VI).

Vitali C, Bombardieri S, Jonsson R, et al: Classification criteria for Sjögren's syndrome: A revised version of the European criteria proposed by the American-European Consensus Group, *Ann Rheum Dis* 61:554–558, 2002.

200. **How do you treat Sjögren's syndrome?**
Primarily with symptom relief using ductal plugs, preservative-free artificial tears, and cholinergic agonists or other secretagogues There is limited evidence to support the use of immunomodulatory agents in treating primary Sjögren's syndrome, but anecdotal published reports have reported that hydroxychloroquine may help with the arthralgias and dermatologic conditions. Patients benefit from regular dental and ophthalmologic evaluation.

201. **What is undifferentiated connective tissue disease (UCTD)?**
A syndrome with clinical and laboratory features that are suggestive of an autoimmune etiology but the diagnosis is unable to be confirmed. An exact diagnosis of a rheumatic disease is not always possible at initial presentation. The clinical manifestations of a given rheumatic disease may not develop at once but may unfold over time, and many features are shared among different rheumatic diseases. Myositis, for example, can be found as a primary condition (polymyositis) or as part of other systemic diseases (e.g., dermatomyositis, SSc, and SLE). In addition to shared clinical features, rheumatic diseases may have shared serologic features.

The most obvious example is ANA, which may be found in various diseases, including SLE, SSc, Sjögren's syndrome, inflammatory myopathies, Hashimoto's thyroiditis, and IBD. When clinical and laboratory features suggest an autoimmune etiology but clinical and serologic heterogeneity make the diagnosis uncertain, the designation UCTD may be used.

KEY POINTS: SPECIFIC RHEUMATIC DISEASES ✓

1. Rheumatoid arthritis is a chronic, symmetrical inflammatory disease that will lead to joint damage and destruction. Early diagnosis and early initiation of disease-modifying treatment lead to better outcomes.

2. SLE is a heterogeneous, autoimmune disease more common in premenopausal females and is associated with ANA autoantibodies.

3. Undifferentiated connective tissue disease is a description commonly applied to a patient with signs and symptoms definitive enough to be clearly autoimmune and inflammatory in nature, but not sufficient to render a more exact diagnosis.

4. Spondyloarthropathies are characterized by inflammatory symptoms of the axial skeleton and have associated symptoms of enthesopathy and uveitis.

ANA = antinuclear antibody; SLE = systemic lupus erythematosus.

202. **How is UCTD different from MCTD?**
MCTD is defined by specific characteristics and was first described as a separate entity in 1972. MCTD is used specifically when features of SLE and SSc are present with high titers of antibody to U_1RNP.

203. **What diseases are associated with complement deficiencies?**
See Table 10-12.

TABLE 10-12. CLINICAL MANIFESTATIONS OF COMPLEMENT COMPONENT DEFICIENCY	
Deficient Component	Clinical Syndrome*
Classic Pathway	
C1q	SLE, infections
C1r/C1s	SLE, infections
C4	SLE, infections
C2	SLE, infections
Lectin Pathway	
MBL	Infections
Central component	
C3	Severe infections, GN, SLE
Membrane attack component	
C5, C6, C7, C8 or C9	*Neisseria* infections

(continued)

> **TABLE 10-12.** CLINICAL MANIFESTATIONS OF COMPLEMENT COMPONENT DEFICIENCY—*(continued)*
>
> | Deficient Component | Clinical Syndrome* |
> |---|---|
> | **Alternative Pathway** | |
> | Properdin, factor D | *Neisseria* infections |
>
> GN = glomerulonephritis; MBL = mannan-binding lectin; SLE = systemic lupus erythematosus.
> *With early component deficiencies of the classic pathway (C1, C4, or C2), infections are caused by the commonly encountered pyogenic organisms. With a late component (C5–9) or an alternative pathway component deficiency, *Neisseria* infections predominate, especially meningococcal infections.
> From Atkinson JD: Complement system. In Firestein GS, Budd RS, Harris ED, et al (eds): Kelley's Textbook of Rheumatology, 8th ed. Philadelphia, WB Saunders, 2008.

204. **Describe Still's disease.**
A syndrome characterized by high spiking fevers ($\leq$104°F), polyarthritis, evanescent rash typically on the trunk, leukocytosis, and elevated inflammatory markers and ferritin that occurs in children and adults. Fevers may occur only once or twice a day and patients typically have a negative RF and ANA.

205. **What is sarcoidosis?**
A systemic inflammatory disease characterized by a noncaseating granulomatous reaction in affected organs. The lungs are most commonly affected, but the skin (typically as erythema nodosum), eyes (potentially all compartments), joints (arthralgias or synovitis), upper respiratory tract (nasal congestion), and lymph nodes (enlargement) are also affected. Asymptomatic sarcoid granulomas have been found in muscle biopsy and may occur in bones, appearing radiographically as cysts. Osteolysis also has been described.

206. **What is Löfgren's syndrome?**
An acute presentation of sarcoidosis that consists of fever, bilateral hilar adenopathy, erythema nodosum, symmetrical polyarthritis, and uveitis. This syndrome is more common in Scandinavians.

207. **What is Ehlers-Danlos syndrome?**
A group of disorders characterized by hyperextensibility of skin and hypermobility of joints, predisposing to early development of osteoarthritis.

208. **Distinguish between Legg-Calvé-Perthes disease and Osgood-Schlatter disease.**
   - **Legg-Calvé-Perthes disease:** idiopathic osteonecrosis of the femoral capital epiphysis usually in boys ages 3–8 that may result in a large flat femoral head
   - **Osgood-Schlatter disease** (also called "tibial tubercle apophysitis"): inflammation at the site where the patellar tendon inserts onto the tibial tubercle that is probably due to a repetitive motion injury, usually occurring in adolescents

209. **Describe RS3PE syndrome.**
Remitting **s**eronegative **s**ymmetrical **s**ynovitis with **p**itting **e**dema (RS3PE). Mostly affecting men older than 70 years, the syndrome is characterized by an acute onset of severe synovitis of the small joints with pitting edema of the dorsal aspect of the hand. Symptoms respond to low-dose prednisone and the syndrome can mimic conditions like RA and PMR.

210. **Define "Cogan's syndrome."**
An unusual vasculopathy associated with interstitial keratitis, sensorineural hearing loss, tinnitus, and vertigo. Systemic features such as fever, weight loss, and fatigue are present in about one half of patients.

211. **What is pigment villonodular synovitis (PVNS)?**
A proliferative disorder of unknown etiology characterized by inflammation and hemosiderin of the synovium. The knee is most commonly affected, and clinically, the patient presents with monoarticular joint swelling. MRI is the diagnostic modality of choice because it may detect the hemosiderin that will show nodular foci.

212. **Describe Paget's disease of bone.**
A chronic disorder of bone remodeling in which there is increased osteoclast-mediated bone resorption leading to increased bone formation; however, this reorganization leads to a disorganized bone matrix and mechanical weakness of the bone. Patients are older than 40 years with a 2:1 incidence in men compared with women. Most patients are asymptomatic, but bone pain and joint pain at night tends to occur. Paget's disease is typically found through serendipitous testing such as an elevated alkaline phosphatase or noted on x-rays ordered for other reasons. Radionuclide bone scan can show the extent of disease. Treatments include analgesics, bisphosphonates, and calcitonin.

213. **What conditions are associated with avascular necrosis of bone?**
   - Trauma (femoral head fracture)
   - Gaucher's disease
   - Hemoglobinopathies
   - Pregnancy
   - Exogenous or endogenous overproduction of glucocorticoids
   - SLE
   - Alcoholism
   - Lymphoproliferative diseases
   - HIV
   - Anticardiolipin antibody
   - Kidney transplantation

214. **What mechanisms contribute to bone loss with the use of GCs?**
Inhibition of osteoblast proliferation and stimulation of osteoblast and osteocyte apoptosis (physiologic cell death). Increased bone resorption also occurs by increasing osteoclast proliferation via stimulating production of receptor activator of nuclear factor kappa-B (RANK) leading to osteoclastogenesis. Corticosteroids have also been shown to decrease intestinal absorption of calcium and increase urinary calcium excretion. The calcium loss stimulates parathyroid hormone (PTH) production and PTH levels are often elevated. The severity of bone loss parallels the dose and duration of treatment. Patients at doses of > 7.5 mg/day will generally have some bone loss, usually in trabecular bone.

   Sambrook PN, Jones G: Corticosteroid osteoporosis, *Br J Rheum* 34:8–12, 1995.

   Khosla S: Minireview: The OPG/RANKL/RANK system, *Endocrinology* 2:5050–5055, 2001.

215. **Describe nephrogenic systemic fibrosis (NSF).**
Large areas of hardened skin in patients with chronic kidney disease that is likely associated with gadolinium-based MRI contrast agents. Histopathology reveals disruption of normal collagen bundles with increased dermal mucin deposition.

ACKNOWLEDGMENT

The editor gratefully acknowledges contributions by Dr. Richard A. Rubin that were retained from the previous edition of *Medical Secrets*.

WEBSITES

1. www.rheumatology.org
2. www.niams.nih.gov

BIBLIOGRAPHY

1. Ball GV, Gay RM: Vasculitis. In *Arthritis and Allied Conditions*, ed 14, Baltimore, 2001, Williams & Wilkins.

2. Firestein GS, Budd RC, Harris ED, et al, editors: *Kelley's Textbook of Rheumatology*, ed 8, Philadelphia, 2008, WB Saunders.

3. Hochberg MC, editor: *Rheumatology*, ed 3, St. Louis, 2003, Mosby.

4. Klippel JH, editor: *Primer on the Rheumatic Diseases*, ed 13, Atlanta, 2008, Arthritis Foundation.

5. Koopman WJ, editor: *Arthritis and Allied Conditions: A Textbook of Rheumatology*, ed 15, Philadelphia, 2005, Lippincott Williams & Wilkins.

6. Resnick D, editor: *Diagnosis of Bone and Joint Disorders*, ed 4, Philadelphia, 2002, WB Saunders.

7. Sheon RP, et al, editors: *Soft Tissue Rheumatic Pain: Recognition, Management and Prevention*, ed 3, Philadelphia, 1996, Lippincott Williams & Wilkins.

8. Wallace DJ, et al, editors: *Dubois' Lupus Erythematosus*, ed 7, Philadelphia, 2007, Lea & Febiger.

CHAPTER 11

ALLERGY AND IMMUNOLOGY

Roger D. Rossen, M.D., and Holly H. Birdsall, M.D., Ph.D.

> *Some men also have strange antipathies in their natures against that sort of food which others love and live upon. I have read of one that could not endure to eat either bread or flesh; of another that fell in a swooning fit at the smell of a rose .... [T]here are some who, if a cat accidentally come into the room, though they neither see it, nor are told it, will presently be in a sweat, and ready to die away.*
>
> Increase Mather (1639–1723), *Remarkable Providence*

THE IMMUNE SYSTEM AND ANTIBODIES

1. **Name the two major divisions of the immune system. Which is older?**

   The **innate immune system** and the **adaptive** or **cognitive immune system**. The innate immune system is phylogenetically older.

2. **Which is the first line of defense against infection?**

   Innate immunity is the first line of defense against infection because its elements are already present in the circulation and can respond immediately to microbial invasion. However, the innate system has no memory; on subsequent exposure to the same antigen, the response is no greater, no faster, and no more effective than it was on first exposure to antigen.

3. **What are the major components of the innate immune system?**

   Neutrophils, monocytes, macrophages, eosinophils, basophils, mast cells, natural killer (NK) cells, complement proteins, and acute-phase reactants. All of these elements have germline-encoded receptors that recognize motifs commonly present on microbes.

4. **What are the types of mast cells in humans?**

   Humans also appear to have two major mast cell populations that are identified by differences in neutral protease content of their cytoplasmic granules. Both populations contain tryptase, but only one contains both tryptase and chymase. The tryptase-only mast cells (MC^T) are located primarily at mucosal surfaces, whereas the tryptase- and chymase-positive mast cells (MC^{TC}) are located primarily in connective tissue, around blood vessels, and at serosal surfaces. The factors responsible for human mast cell growth remain to be clearly defined. Although human interleukin-3 (IL-3) appears to have some mast cell growth-promoting activity, its effects are less well defined. Of interest is that MC^Ts, but not MC^{TC}s, appear to be T lymphocyte–dependent. This is suggested by a marked decrease in MC^Ts, but not MC^{TC}s, mast cell numbers in the tissues of patients with severe T-cell immunodeficiency disorders.

5. **Are all mast cells alike?**

   No. Mast cell heterogeneity exists in both animals and humans. Differences have been most extensively studied in mice, which appear to have two major mast cell populations, labeled "mucosal mast cells (MMCs)" and "connective tissue mast cells (CTMCs)." MMCs are found principally at mucosal surfaces, whereas CTMCs are found within connective tissue, lining blood vessels, and at serosal surfaces. They differ with respect to histamine content, the extent to which they degranulate following non–immunoglobulin E (IgE) stimuli, arachidonic acid metabolite production, and histochemical-staining characteristics. MMCs respond to stimulation by the T-cell cytokine IL-3. In contrast, expression of the CTMC phenotype depends on stimulation by fibroblasts.

6. **What are the major differences between mast cells and basophils?**
See Table 11-1.

TABLE 11-1. COMPARISON OF MAST CELLS AND BASOPHILS

Parameter	Mast Cells	Basophils
Life span	Weeks to years	Days
Origin	Probably bone marrow	Bone marrow
Location	Tissues, noncirculating	Normally circulating
Size	8–20 mm	5–7 mm
Nucleus	Round to oval, may be indented	Multilobulated
Cytoplasmic granules	Smaller, more numerous	Larger, fewer granules
High-affinity IgE receptor	Present	Present
Histamine release	Yes	Yes
Major arachidonic acid metabolites	PGD_2, LTC_4, $-D_4$, $-E_4$	LTC_4
Staining characteristics		
Toluidine blue	Yes	Yes
Tryptase	Yes	No
Chloroacetate esterase	Yes	No

IgE = immunoglobulin E; LT = leukotriene; PG = prostaglandin.

7. **What are the major components of the adaptive immune system? How do they work?**
B lymphocytes that make antibodies and T lymphocytes that provide the effector elements of antigen-specific cell-mediated immune responses. Elements of the adaptive immune system display a large repertoire (e.g., tens of millions) of specific antigen receptors that are generated by DNA rearrangements. Each lymphocyte and its clonal descendants express one of the millions of possible antigen receptors. because numerically there are very few cells at any one time that can recognize newly introduced antigens, B cells and T cells must be appropriately stimulated and induced to divide and produce multiple copies of themselves.

8. **What is the major advantage of the adaptive immune system?**
The ability to select B cells and T cells that have high-affinity receptors for new antigens and to stimulate them to replicate and provide a specific, fine-tuned response to foreign invaders.

9. **What is the major disadvantage of the adaptive immune system?**
The required expansion process takes time after the first encounter with antigen, in some cases more than 2 weeks. Many infectious agents can cause death or severe disability in less time than it takes the adaptive immune system to mobilize a specific response. This disadvantage leaves a gap in the host defense system.

10. **Explain the role of vaccines in the adaptive immune system.**
To stimulate specific immune responses in advance of an encounter with a pathogenic microorganism so that an appropriate immune recognition system is in place before any real-life encounters take place.

11. **Explain immunologic memory.**
Although circulating antibodies and T cells produced during the initial response to a foreign substance may be lost with time, a second encounter with the same antigen typically induces a much more vigorous response that comes into play often within only a day or two after the second encounter. The innate and adaptive immune systems work together. For instance, T cells activate macrophages, allowing them to more effectively kill the organisms they ingest. Phagocytic cells ingest microbes coated by antibodies from the adaptive immune system. In order to mount an immune response, naive lymphocytes require costimulatory signals that are typically provided either by microbes or by cells of the innate system after encounter with microbial products.

12. **What are the major divisions of the adaptive immune system?**
Humoral immunity and **cell-mediated immunity.** The effector functions that they mediate often involve cells of the innate immune system.

13. **How does humoral immunity work?**
Through antibodies, produced by B cells. Terminally differentiated B cells, called "plasma cells," produce most of the antibodies. Humoral immune responses defend the host against extracellular bacteria and toxins. Blocking antibodies can prevent the adherence of bacteria, viruses, or toxins to host cells. Antibodies can activate complement through the classical pathway and lyse cells. Complement activation also generates chemotactic fragments that activate mast cells and phagocytes and chemotactically attract phagocytic cells into sites of inflammation. NK cells can bind to antibody-coated targets and lyse them in antibody-mediated cytotoxicity. Antibodies can also opsonize; in other words, their binding facilitates uptake of the antigen by phagocytic cells.

14. **How does cell-mediated immunity work?**
Through the action of T cells. CD8+ cytolytic T cells can kill target cells directly. CD4+ helper cells can activate macrophages to become more effective at killing the organisms they ingest. This process is also considered to be cell-mediated immunity, although, again, a cell of the innate system carries out the ultimate effector function. Cells of the innate system are also needed to initiate humoral and cell-mediated responses. Dendritic cells and macrophages ingest organisms, digest them into peptides, and present them to T cells and B cells in a way that causes antigen-specific lymphocytes to proliferate and differentiate into effector cells.

15. **What is the major histocompatibility complex (MHC)?**
A cluster of genes (located on chromosome 6 in humans) that play a critical role in directing the activities of T cells.

16. **Name the two major classes of MHC molecules and their subtypes.**
MHC class I molecules, which are found on all somatic cells, and MHC class II molecules, which are found on a group of cells called "antigen-presenting cells (APCs)" (e.g., dendritic

cells, monocytes, macrophages, B cells). Humans have three major types of class I MHC molecules: human leukocyte antigen (HLA)–A, HLA-B, and HLA-C. The class II MHC molecules include HLA-DR, HLA-DQ, and HLA-DP.

17. **How do MHC molecules function in the immune system?**
The antigen receptor of T cells can recognize only peptides displayed in MHC molecules. CD8+ T cells (cytolytic T cells) bind only to antigenic peptides displayed within the antigen-presenting cleft of MHC class I molecules. CD4+ T cells bind only to antigenic peptides displayed in MHC class II molecules.

18. **Describe the process by which antigens are displayed in MHC class I molecules.**
Under normal conditions, host proteins in the cytoplasm are broken down in an intracellular recycling process. Peptide fragments, generated by enzymes in an intracellular structure called a "proteasome," are loaded into MHC class I molecules and displayed on the cell membrane. If an infecting virus has usurped the host synthetic machinery, some of the proteins displayed in MHC class I as a result of this process will be of viral origin. These proteins can be recognized by specific CD8 cells, which then lyse the infected host cell.

19. **Describe the process by which antigens are displayed in the MHC class II molecules.**
Extracellular antigens ingested by phagocytic cells and B cells are digested within endosomal vesicles by proteolytic enzymes; peptides generated here are loaded into MHC class II molecules. CD4 T cells recognize peptides displayed in MHC class II molecules on APCs. If the CD4 cells simultaneously receive additional signals from costimulatory molecules that are also displayed by these APCs, they become activated. Activated helper T (Th) cells produce messenger molecules called "cytokines" that further activate B cells to produce antibodies, CD8 T cells to become killer cells, and macrophages to produce molecules that can kill ingested microorganisms.

20. **What two signals are required to activate naive T cells?**
Initially, antigenic peptides displayed in MHC molecules. The second signal is provided by one or more costimulatory molecule produced by the APC, in response to molecules displayed by pathogens. If these costimulatory signaling molecules are not present, the T cell–MHC interaction may alternatively cause the T cell to undergo programmed cell death, a process known as "apoptosis."

21. **What are MHC class III genes?**
Included within the stretch of chromosome 6 that contains the genes for MHC class I and class II molecules are genes for complement components C2, C4, and factor B as well as other molecules with immunoregulatory properties, including the genes for tumor necrosis factor (TNF)–α and TNF-β, also known as "lymphotoxin." These additional genes within the MHC region of chromosome 6 are also known, in aggregate, as "MHC class III genes."

22. **What are B lymphocytes (B cells)?**
Cells derived from hematopoietic stem cells that are the precursors of plasma cells, the antibody- or Ig-producing cells in the body. They differentiate from stem cells in the bone marrow, migrate through the blood, and eventually come to reside in the B-cell areas of the spleen, lymph nodes, and submucosal tissues of the respiratory tree and the gut. The B designation comes from the discovery that antibody-producing cells develop in the bursa of Fabricius, an anatomic structure located in the cloaca of birds.

23. **Define and explain the basic structure of an antibody.**
A protein (or IgG molecule) produced by B cells that binds to antigen. Ig molecules are composed of two identical heavy chains and two identical light chains. Each light and heavy chain combine to form an antigen-binding cleft at their amino terminus, and the two heavy chains associate with each other at their carboxy end. Overall, the structure resembles a lobster with the claws representing the two antigen-binding sites. The tail of the lobster is composed only of heavy chains and is called the "Fc piece." This end can bind to Fc receptors, structures that are largely found on phagocytes, and certain other effector cells of the immune system such as mast cells and eosinophils.

24. **Summarize the classes of the heavy chains and light chains of Ig.**
There are five classes of heavy chains (mu, gamma, alpha, epsilon, and delta) that form the five isotypes or Ig classes: IgM, IgG, IgA, IgE, and IgD, respectively. There are two types of light chains, kappa and lambda, that are used by all Ig classes. IgA can polymerize into dimers and higher multimers. Secreted IgM is a pentamer of five basic subunits joined by a protein called "J," the joining piece.

25. **What are the seven domains of the heavy-chain constant region?**
Three domains in IgG, IgD, and IgA and four domains in IgE and IgM. These constant regions are responsible for the functional aspects of the Ig molecules (i.e., complement binding to the CH2 region, half-life in the circulation, ability to be transported across the placenta [IgG] or across mucous membranes [IgA]).

26. **Explain the heavy-chain variable region.**
The amino terminal half is the variable region: V_L and V_H have three regions where the amino acid sequences are highly variable. The variation in sequence within these regions determines the ability of antibodies to bind to one but not another antigen. That is, the variable regions confer specificity. A given B cell produces antibodies of a single specificity. However, during isotype switching, progeny of a given B cell may stop making IgM and begin producing IgG, IgA, or IgE. In that case, the gene sequence encoding the V_H domain is transferred to genes encoding the C_H domains of the new Ig class (Fig. 11-1).

27. **What are the features of primary and secondary antibody responses?**
A primary antibody response occurs after the first exposure to an antigen, whereas a secondary antibody response occurs with the second and subsequent exposures. A secondary response is faster and bigger and contains antibodies that bind with higher affinity to antigen and a greater diversity of T cells that react with the target antigens. In a secondary response, the antibody levels increase and new effector T cells enter the circulation within 1–2 days. In contrast, during a primary response, the emergence of these elements of an adaptive response can take a week or more. During a secondary response, the quantity of antibodies and the number of effector T cells is increased 10-fold or higher. The average affinity of the antigen-binding sites is also higher in a secondary response. Finally, during a secondary response, more of the antibodies belong to the IgG class, whereas in a primary response most of the antibodies are IgM. Major features of these two responses are illustrated in Figures 11-2 and 11-3.

28. **Why are IgG antibodies "better" than IgM antibodies?**
Because IgG antibodies enable neutrophils and monocyte/macrophages to phagocytose antibody-coated particles. This process is called "opsonization." They can also direct the killing of infected cells, tumors, and parasites in a process called "antibody-dependent

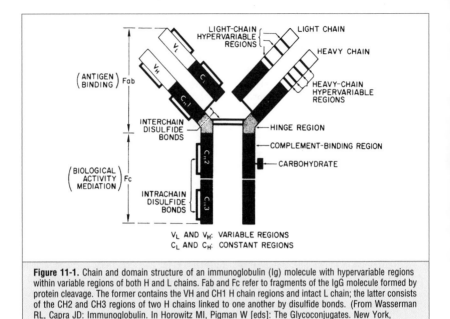

Figure 11-1. Chain and domain structure of an immunoglobulin (Ig) molecule with hypervariable regions within variable regions of both H and L chains. Fab and Fc refer to fragments of the IgG molecule formed by protein cleavage. The former contains the VH and CH1 H chain regions and intact L chain; the latter consists of the CH2 and CH3 regions of two H chains linked to one another by disulfide bonds. (From Wasserman RL, Capra JD: Immunoglobulin. In Horowitz MI, Pigman W [eds]: The Glycoconjugates. New York, Academic Press, 1977, pp 323–348, with permission.)

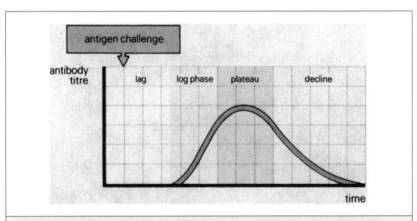

Figure 11-2. After antigen challenge, the primary antibody response proceeds in four phases: (1) a lag phase when no antibody is detected; (2) a log phase in which the antibody titer rises logarithmically; (3) a plateau phase during which the antibody titer stabilizes; and (4) a decline phase during which the antibody is cleared or catabolized. (From Roitt IM, Brostoff J, Male DK: Immunology. New York, Gower Medical, 1989, p 8.1, with permission.)

cellular cytotoxicity." IgG molecules, because of their smaller size, can more readily enter interstitial fluids, and in contrast to IgM molecules, they can be transported across the placenta.

29. **What are the physical and biologic properties of the different classes of Ig?**
See Table 11-2.

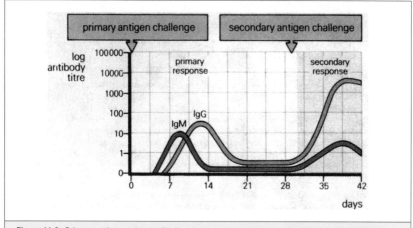

Figure 11-3. Primary and secondary antibody responses. In comparison with the antibody response to primary antigenic challenge, the antibody level after secondary antigenic challenge in a typical immune response (1) appears more quickly and persists for longer, (2) attains a high titer, and (3) consists predominantly of IgG. In the primary response the appearance of IgG is preceded by IgM. (From Roitt IM, Brostoff J, Male DK: Immunology. New York, Gower Medical, 1989, p 8.1, with permission.)

TABLE 11-2. PHYSICAL AND BIOLOGIC PROPERTIES OF HUMAN IMMUNOGLOBULINS*

Property	IgG	IgA	IgM	IgD	IgE
Molecular form	Monomer	Monomer, polymer	Pentamer	Monomer	Monomer
Subclasses	IgG 1,2,3,4	IgA 1,2	None	None	None
Molecular weight	150,000 for IgG 1,2,4 180,000 for IgG3	160,000 + polymers	950,000	175,000	190,000
Serum level (mg/mL)	9,3,1,0.5	2.1	1.5	4	0.03
Serum half-life (days)	23D for IgG 1,2,4 7D for IgG3	6	5	3	3
Complement fixation	IgG 1,2,3 +	(−)	+	(−)	(−)
Alternative pathway activation	IgG4	+	(−)	+	?
Placental transfer	+	(−)	(−)	(−)	(−)

(continued)

**TABLE 11-2.   PHYSICAL AND BIOLOGIC PROPERTIES OF HUMAN IMMUNOGLOBULINS*—*(continued)*

Property	IgG	IgA	IgM	IgD	IgE
Other properties	Secondary response	Abundant in mucous secretions	Primary response, rheumatoid factor	–	Binds to mast cells

Ig = immunoglobulin.
*The plus and minus signs indicate whether the molecules have or do not have the indicated property.
Modified from Paul WE: Fundamental Immunology, 2nd ed. New York, Raven Press, 1989; and Samter M, Talmage MM, Frank DF, et al (eds): Immunological Diseases, 4th ed. Boston, Little, Brown, 1988, p 44.

COMPLEMENT SYSTEM

30. **Summarize the functions of the complement system.**
The complement system functions as the innate part of humoral immunity by promoting inflammatory reactions, and it facilitates the effector functions of antibodies, especially IgM and IgG antibodies. C3b, generated by the cleavage of C3, binds to the surface of antigens, including microbes, and facilitates their uptake by neutrophils and monocytes that express a C3b receptor. C5a and, to some extent, C3a are chemotactic for neutrophils and monocytes and serve to recruit leukocytes into sites of inflammation. C3a and C5a are also known as "anaphylatoxins" because of their ability to induce mast cell degranulation. The terminal complement components, C6, C7, C8, and C9, form the membrane attack complex, a tubular structure that inserts through the plasma membrane of cells and microbes and kills them. Figure 11-4 summarizes specific functions of the complement system.

31. **Summarize the activation sequences of the classical complement pathways.**
Initiation of classical complement pathway activation starts with binding of the C1 complex and proceeds through the activation cascade shown in Figure 11-5. C1 is composed of C1q, C1r, and C1s. To be activated, two of the five arms of C1q must interact with binding sites located near the hinge region of IgG and IgM molecules. Therefore, C1q activation requires two adjacent IgG molecules or a single IgM molecule.

32. **Summarize the activation sequences of the alternative complement pathways.**
Activation of the alternative pathway is initiated by binding of C3b to the surface of antigens, particularly microbial membranes. The alternative pathway bypasses C1, C2, and C4. Therefore, measurement of C3 and C4 can give some indication as to whether the activation has been via the classical (immune complex) or the alternative (pathogen) pathway. The activation of C3 and the downstream participation of C5, C6, C7, C8, and C9 is the same for both pathways, and the biologic activities of opsonization, recruitment of inflammatory cells, mast cell degranulation, and cell lysis are identical for both pathways. The alternative pathways are also diagrammed in Figure 11-5.

33. **What is mannose-binding protein?**
A protein utilized in a third mechanism for activation of the complement cascade that is structurally similar to C1q of the classical pathway. This protein, called the "mannose-binding lectin," reacts with repeating carbohydrate residues on bacterial surfaces that are commonly

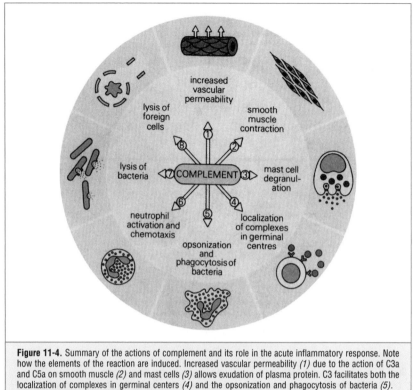

Figure 11-4. Summary of the actions of complement and its role in the acute inflammatory response. Note how the elements of the reaction are induced. Increased vascular permeability *(1)* due to the action of C3a and C5a on smooth muscle *(2)* and mast cells *(3)* allows exudation of plasma protein. C3 facilitates both the localization of complexes in germinal centers *(4)* and the opsonization and phagocytosis of bacteria *(5)*. Neutrophils, which are attracted to the area of inflammation by chemotaxis *(6)*, phagocytose the opsonized microorganisms. The membrane attack complex, C5–9, is responsible for lysis of bacteria *(7)* and other cells recognized as foreign *(8)*. (From Roitt IM, Brostoff J, Male DK: Immunology. New York, Gower Medical, 1989, p 13.11, with permission.)

displayed by a wide array of microbes. Mannose-binding lectin employs C4 and C2 in an activation pathway that is closely homologous to that utilized by the classical complement activation pathway.

34. **What is the common purpose of all of these activation cascades?**
To assemble an enzyme that cleaves and activates C3 so that C3 can bind covalently to a microbial surface and provide a template for the assembly of an enzyme that cleaves and activates C5 and the remaining elements of complement (C6–9).

35. **What factors cause activation of the classical complement pathway?**
Antibody-antigen (immune) complexes. When bound to antigens, a single IgM or two IgG molecules (IgG doublet) of the IgG subclasses 1, 2, and 3, but not 4, can bind C1 and initiate complement activation. The binding site for C1q in the Ig molecule is not exposed until the antibody binds antigen. Therefore, soluble antibodies in the circulation do not activate complement. Certain viruses, urate crystals, DNA, and mitochondria that are released by damaged cells also activate the classical pathway by binding C1q, the ligand protein of the C1 complex. Progression of the cascade through C3, 5, 6, 7, 8, and 9 requires assembly of these components on planar surfaces, as are provided by target cell membranes.

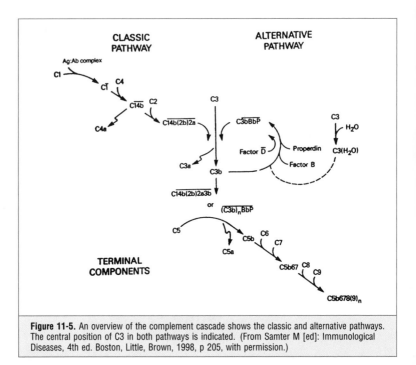

Figure 11-5. An overview of the complement cascade shows the classic and alternative pathways. The central position of C3 in both pathways is indicated. (From Samter M [ed]: Immunological Diseases, 4th ed. Boston, Little, Brown, 1998, p 205, with permission.)

36. **What factors protect the body cells against the complement cascade?**
Enzymes in the blood promptly degrade activated C3 that is not covalently attached to a membrane structure or an antigen-antibody complex. Activation of the complement cascade does not proceed in fluids such as blood plasma beyond C3 because of these enzymes. In addition, mammalian somatic cells, but not red blood cells (RBCs), are protected against injury by activated complement by three proteins: decay-accelerating factor; membrane cofactor protein; and CD59, also called "protectin." These proteins interfere with the assembly of the enzymes that could otherwise complete the complement cascade and lyse the cell.

37. **What factors cause activation of the alternative complement pathway?**
Substances found on bacterial and yeast cell walls. Aggregates of Ig and cells whose surfaces are poor in sialic acid residues can also activate the alternative pathway. C3 has a highly reactive thioester bond that allows activated C3 to bind covalently to a wide variety of substrates. Most bacteria, some parasites, and virtually all plant cells display these residues.

38. **When evaluating patients, does it help to measure serum complement levels?**
Sometimes. Hospital clinical laboratories can usually measure serum C3 and C4. When the differential diagnosis includes sepsis, an active collagen vascular disease, or an allergic reaction, measurements of C3 and C4 are sometimes helpful. If the disease process is more than 24 hours old, one must realize that the complement proteins are among the acute-phase reactants and complement biosynthesis is stimulated by acute inflammation. Although complement may have been consumed in the first hours of the disease, new protein synthesis will cause a prompt rebound in plasma levels to normal or even supernormal levels. When interpreting serum complement levels (C3 and C4), one must realize that a normal level does not rule out either complement activation or complement-mediated tissue damage.

39. **How does liver disease affect complement levels?**
Severe liver disease leads to persistently low complement protein levels. Complement proteins are made in the liver.

40. **What patterns of serum C3 and C4 levels are seen with activation of the classical and alternative complement pathways? Name at least one disease associated with each pattern.**
See Table 11-3.

TABLE 11-3. SERUM COMPLEMENT LEVELS IN DISEASE			
Pathway	C4	C3	Disease
Classical	↓	↓	Systemic lupus erythematosus, serum sickness
Classical (fluid phase)	↓	N	Hereditary angioedema
Alternative	N	↓	Endotoxemia (gram-negative sepsis)
Alternative (fluid phase)	N	↓	Type II membranoproliferative glomerulonephritis (C3 nephritic factor)
↓ = Decreased; N = normal.			

INTERFERONS

41. **What are α, β, and γ interferons (IFNs)?**
Interferons have been divided into three classes: IFN-α, IFN-β, and IFN-γ. IFN-α and IFN-β were previously classified as type I and IFN-γ as type II. IFN-β is divided into two major subtypes: IFN-β_1 and IFN-β_2.

42. **How are IFN-α, IFN-β_1, and IFN-β_2 produced?**
   - **IFN-α** is produced by leukocytes, fibroblasts (to a lesser degree) and other cells and is composed of 20 or more subtypes.
   - **IFN-β_1** is produced by fibroblasts, leukocytes (to a lesser degree), and many other cells.
   - **IFN-β_2 (IL-6)** is produced by fibroblasts, T cells, monocytes, and endothelial cells.

43. **Summarize the major functions of IFN-α, IFN-β_1, and IFN-β_2.**
Both IFN-α and IFN-β_1 modulate antibody production, graft rejection, and delayed-type hypersensitivity (DTH) reactions. They can induce autoimmune and inflammatory reactions, and they have important antiviral, antibacterial, antifungal, and antitumor activities. IFN-β_2 has important immunomodulatory activity and poor antiviral activity. It has also been called "B-cell differentiation factor" because it stimulates mature B to differentiate into Ig-secreting plasma cells. It also plays a role in early hematopoiesis and may be an important autocrine growth factor for B cell malignancies.

44. **What produces IFN-γ? Summarize its functions.**
Activated T lymphocytes, NK cells, and lymphokine-activated killer (LAK) cells. IFN-γ is unrelated to the other IFNs in either structure or function. Its biologic effects include enhancing cytotoxic T-cell and NK-cell activity, induction of class II antigen expression on B cells and other APCs, and induction of IL-2 receptor expression on T cells. It down-regulates collagen synthesis and inhibits IL-4–induced IgE synthesis.

B CELLS AND T CELLS

45. **Outline B cell ontogeny from stem cell to plasma cell.**
    Stem cell → pre-B → immature B → mature B → activated B → secretory B → plasma cell.
    Immature B cells can be identified by the expression of IgM on their surface. Encounters with
    cognate antigen at this stage can lead to clonal deletion or anergy. Mature B cells have both
    IgM and IgD on their surface, and interaction with cognate antigen stimulates cell
    differentiation and survival.

46. **What is the role of surface Ig on B cells?**
    To provide antigen-binding sites on the B cell membrane. Before active secretion of Ig begins,
    B cells produce Ig with an added polypeptide tail at the carboxy terminus that anchors Ig
    in the B cell membrane. Binding of antigen to these cell surface Ig molecules activates the
    B cells. If the B cell receives additional costimulatory signals via specific cell surface
    molecules on T cells (e.g., from molecules called "CD40 ligand" or "CD154"), the B cell
    differentiates into an antibody-producing cell. In the absence of costimulatory signals, it does
    not differentiate further nor does it produce antibody.

47. **Summarize the role of T cells. Where do they mature?**
    T cells function as both effectors and regulators of the immune response. Like B cells, they
    are derived from embryonic hematopoietic stem cells in the bone marrow. Unlike B cells,
    T cells mature in the thymus, hence their name. In the thymus, T cells are selected for their
    ability to interact weakly with either MHC class I or class II molecules (positive selection).
    However, cells that react strongly with these molecules are deleted (negative selection).
    Because antigenic peptides expressed in the thymus are from self-proteins, negative selection
    removes potential autoreactive cells. Thymic epithelial cells have the ability to express
    many self-proteins normally produced only in specialized tissues (such as insulin), allowing
    the thymus to screen for T cells that might react with a wide diversity of host antigens.

48. **What are the major subtypes of T cells?**
    CD4 T cells and CD8 T cells.

49. **Describe the principal function of CD4 T cells.**
    CD4 cells function primarily as helper/inducer T cells that provide soluble and cognate signals
    to (1) B cells to stimulate antibody production, (2) CD8 cytolytic T cells, and (3) monocytes
    and macrophages to facilitate their ability to carry out cell-mediated immune responses.
    Recently, it has been recognized that CD4 T cells can also act as killer cells or even as
    suppressor cells—that is, cells that can suppress cell-mediated responses carried out by
    other T cells. These immunomodulatory CD4 cells express high levels of the IL-2 receptor
    protein called "CD25Y."
    The incontrovertible fact about CD4 T cells is that they are stimulated to recognize and
    react against antigen presented by MHC class II molecules displayed on APCs.

50. **Describe the principal function of CD8 T cells.**
    CD8 T cells classically are considered to carry out killer functions; for example, they kill
    virus-infected cells. As was noted with the CD4 T cell, many functional restrictions no longer
    apply because numerous exceptions have been noted. What is important is that they
    recognize antigen only when presented by MHC class I molecules.

51. **What is the CD nomenclature for phenotyping cells?**
    The CD (cluster designation) nomenclature is a system for the identification of cell
    surface antigens that have been defined by monoclonal antibodies. Development of a
    monoclonal antibody to a cell surface protein is one important step in its characterization.

These antibodies allow identification of target proteins on cell surfaces. They can be used to help purify the proteins and illuminate their function. Over 200 CD antigens have been recognized thus far by international committees that assign these numbers. CD markers identify targets that can be used to remove whole classes of cells from the circulation by means of cytolytic monoclonal antibodies or by machines, called "cell sorters," that recognize and segregate cells expressing specific molecules identified by monoclonal antibodies.

52. **How is the CD nomenclature used in clinical medicine?**
    Antibodies to CD3 and CD4 have been used to help control transplant rejection reactions by removing and inactivating the effector T cells. A few important CD markers are listed in Table 11-4.

TABLE 11-4. CD MARKERS, ISOFORMS, SITES OF EXPRESSION, AND FUNCTION

Surface Marker	Isoforms	Sites of Expression	Comments
CD2	50-kD protein	Thymocytes, T cells, NK cells (large granular lymphocytes)	Adhesion molecule that binds to LFA-3, a ligand on APC. Ligation with LFA-3 activates T cells.
CD3	γ: 25-kD glycoprotein δ: 20-kD glycoprotein ε: 20-kD protein	Thymocytes, T cells	Associated with TCR. Required for cell surface expression of TCR.
CD4	57-kD glycoprotein	Thymocytes, TH1 and Th2 T cells, monocytes, and some macrophages	Coreceptor for MHC class II, and for HIV-1 + HIV-2 gp120.
CD8	α: 32-kD glycoprotein β: 32–34 kD	Thymocytes, CD8 T cells	Coreceptor for MHC class I; anti-CD8 blocks cytotoxic T-cell responses.
CD16	50–80 kD	NK cells, granulocytes, macrophages	Low-affinity Fcγ receptor that plays a role in antibody-dependent cell mediated cytotoxicity and activation of NK cells.
CD19	95 kD	B cells	Coreceptor for B cells involved in B-cell activation.
CD28	44-kD homodimer	T-cell subsets Activated B cells	Binding to CD80 (on B cells) or CD86 (on macrophages or dendritic cells) sends costimulatory, differentiation-inducing signal.

(continued)

TABLE 11-4. CD MARKERS, ISOFORMS, SITES OF EXPRESSION, AND FUNCTION—*(continued)*

Surface Marker	Isoforms	Sites of Expression	Comments
CD45RO	180-kD glycoprotein	Memory T cells, B-cell subsets, monocytes	See CD45RA.
CD45RA	205–220-kD glycoprotein	Naive T cells, B cells, monocytes	Role in signal transduction, tyrosine phosphatase.
CD56	135–220-kD heterodimer	NK cells	Promotes adhesion of NK cells.
CD80	60-kD protein	B-cell subset Ligand for CD28 on T cells	Costimulator involved in antigen presentation.
CD86	80-kD protein	Activated B cells Monocytes, dendritic cells	Costimulatory ligand for CD28 on T cells, during antigen presentation.

APC = antigen-presenting cell; HIV = human immunodeficiency virus; LFA = leukocyte function-associated antigen; MHC = major histocompatibility complex; NK = natural killer; TCR = T-cell receptor; Th2 = T helper 2 cell.
From David J: Immunology. In Dale DC, Federman DD (eds): Scientific American Medicine. New York, Scientific American, 1996, p 6; and Janeway CA, Travers P, Walport M, Capra JD (eds): Immunobiology, 4th ed. London, Current Biology Publications, and New York, Garland Publishing, 1999.

53. **What are cytokines, where are they made, and what do they do?**
Proteins produced by many cells, not necessarily only cells of the immune system, that function as intracellular signaling molecules, usually within the radius of a few cell diameters. There are at present more than 38 cytokines (Table 11-5).

TABLE 11-5. ACTIONS OF CYTOKINES RELEVANT TO ALLERGIC AND IMMUNE RESPONSES

Cytokine	Effects
GM-CSF	Secreted by activated macrophages, T cells, mast cells, eosinophils, and other cells. Promotes differentiation of neutrophils and macrophages. Activates mature eosinophils. Prolongs eosinophil survival.

(continued)

TABLE 11-5. ACTIONS OF CYTOKINES RELEVANT TO ALLERGIC AND IMMUNE RESPONSES—*(continued)*

Cytokine	Effects
IFN-γ	Derived mainly from Th1 lymphocytes, cytotoxic T cells, NK cells, but also macrophages.
	Represents the most important cytokine activator of macrophages.
	Increases expression of class I and II MHC antigens.
	Stimulates B-cell proliferation and differentiation.
	Inhibits IL-4–induced IgE synthesis.
	Inhibits Th2 lymphocytes.
	Induces ICAM-1 expression.
IL-1	IL-1 family contains IL-1α, IL-1β, the IL-1 receptor antagonist (IL-1ra), and IL-18.
	Produced mainly by monocytes and macrophages, but also by lymphocytes and other cells.
	Induced by endotoxin, microorganisms, antigens, and cytokines.
	Increases proliferation of B cells and antibody synthesis.
	Promotes growth of Th cells in response to APCs.
	Stimulates production of T-cell cytokines and IL-2 receptors.
	Without IL-1, tolerance develops or immune response is impaired.
	Promotes formation of arachidonic acid metabolites, including PGE$_2$ and LTB$_4$.
	Induces proliferation of fibroblasts and synthesis of fibronectin and collagen.
	Increases ICAM-1, VCAM-1, E-selectin, and P-selectin expression.
	IL-1ra antagonizes proinflammatory effects of IL-1.
IL-2	Induces clonal T cell proliferation.
	Enhances proliferation of cytotoxic T cells, B cells, NK cells, macrophages.
IL-3	Derived primarily from Th cells, but also from mast cells and eosinophils.
	Stimulates development of mast cells, lymphocytes, macrophages.
	Activates eosinophils.
	Prolongs eosinophil survival.
IL-4	Preformed peptide in mast cells and eosinophils.
	Also secreted by Th2 cells, cytotoxic T cells, and basophils.
	Promotes growth of Th2 cells, cytotoxic T cells, mast cells, eosinophils, basophils.
IL-4	Initiates IgE isotype switching.
	Up-regulates expression of high- and low-affinity IgE receptors.
	Increases expression of class I and II MHC antigens on macrophages.
	Stimulates VCAM-1 expression.
IL-5	Produced by Th2 cells and mast cells.
	Attracts eosinophils.

(continued)

TABLE 11-5.	ACTIONS OF CYTOKINES RELEVANT TO ALLERGIC AND IMMUNE RESPONSES—*(continued)*
Cytokine	**Effects**
	Activates eosinophils.
	Prolongs eosinophil survival.
IL-6	Synthesized primarily by monocytes and macrophages, but also by T, B, and other cells.
	Mediates T-cell activation, growth, differentiation.
	Induces B-cell differentiation into plasma cells.
	Inhibits TNF and IL-1 synthesis and stimulates IL-1ra synthesis.
IL-7	Necessary for development of B and T cells.
	Enhances growth of cytotoxic T and NK cells.
	Increases tumor killing by monocytes and macrophages.
IL-8	Produced mainly by monocytes, phagocytes, and endothelial cells.
	Exerts potent chemoattraction for neutrophils.
	Attracts activated eosinophils.
	Induces neutrophil degranulation and activation.
	Inhibits IL-4–mediated IgE synthesis.
IL-9	Produced by Th2 cells.
	Promotes mast cell and T-cell proliferation.
	Stimulates IgE synthesis.
	Produces eosinophilia.
	Induces bronchial hyperreactivity.
IL-10	Secreted primarily by monocytes and B cells.
	Inhibits monocyte/macrophage function.
	Stimulates growth of mast cells, B cells, and cytotoxic T cells.
	Induces permanent tolerance in Th lymphocytes.
	Decreases synthesis of IFN-γ and IL-2 by Th1 cells.
	Inhibits IL-4–induced IgE synthesis and promotes IgG4 production.
	Decreases eosinophil survival.
IL-11	Produced in response to respiratory viral infections.
	Promotes generation of mast cells and B cells.
	Induces bronchial hyperreactivity.
IL-12	Synthesized by monocytes/macrophages, dendritic cells, B cells, neutrophils, mast cells.
	Induced by IFN-γ and microorganisms.
IL-12	Promotes Th1 and inhibits Th2 cell development.
	Inhibits IL-4–induced IgE synthesis.
	Enhances activity of cytotoxic T cells and NK cells.
IL-13	Produced by Th1 and Th2 cells, mast cells, and dendritic cells.
	Exerts effects similar to IL-4 on B cells and macrophages but does not affect T cells.

(continued)

TABLE 11-5. ACTIONS OF CYTOKINES RELEVANT TO ALLERGIC AND IMMUNE RESPONSES—(continued)

Cytokine	Effects
	Induces IgE isotype switching.
	Increases VCAM-1 expression.
	Promotes airway hyperreactivity and mucus hypersecretion.
	Suppresses production of proinflammatory cytokines and chemokines.
	Decreases synthesis of nitric oxide.
IL-16	Secreted by CD8+ T cells, eosinophils, mast cells, and epithelial cells.
	Promotes growth of CD4+ T cells.
	Provides major source of CD4+ T-cell chemotactic activity after antigen challenge.
	Induces IL-2 receptors and class II MHC expression on CD4+ T cells.
IL-18	Produced by lung, liver, and other tissues, but not by lymphocytes.
	Stimulates secretion of IFN-γ and GM-CSF.
	Enhances IgE synthesis.
	Promotes Th1 responses and activates NK cells (similar to IL-12).
	Induces synthesis of TNF, IL-1, Fas ligand.
	Decreases IL-10 synthesis.
IL-23	Induces secretion of IFN-γ.
TGF-α	Synthesized by macrophages and keratinocytes.
	Stimulates proliferation of fibroblasts.
	Promotes angiogenesis.
TGF-β	Secreted by platelets, monocytes, some T cells (Th3), and fibroblasts.
	Stimulates monocytes and fibroblasts, inducing fibrosis and extracellular matrix formation.
	Attracts mast cells, macrophages, fibroblasts.
	Inhibits B cells, Th cells, cytotoxic T cells, NK cells, mast cells.
	Induces IgA isotype switching and secretory IgA synthesis in gut lymphoid tissue.
	Inhibits airway smooth muscle cell proliferation.
TNF-α	Produced primarily by mononuclear phagocytes; stored preformed in mast cells.
	Induced by endotoxin, GM-CSF, IFN-γ, IL-1, and IL-3.
	Binds to cell surface receptors TNFR I and TNFR II.
	Enhances class I and II MHC expression.
	Activates neutrophils, modulating adherence, chemotaxis, degranulation, respiratory burst.
	Increases cytokine production by monocytes and airway epithelial cells.
TNF-α	Promotes ICAM-1, VCAM-1, and E-selectin expression.
	Stimulates COX-2 expression in airway smooth muscle.
	Induces bronchial hyperreactivity.

(continued)

TABLE 11-5.	ACTIONS OF CYTOKINES RELEVANT TO ALLERGIC AND IMMUNE RESPONSES—*(continued)*
Cytokine	Effects
TNF-β	Mediates toxic shock and sepsis. Produces cachexia associated with chronic infection and cancer. Synthesized primarily by lymphocytes. Binds to cell surface receptors TNFR I and TNFR II. Mediates functions similar to TNF-α.

APC = antigen-presenting cell; COX-2 = cyclooxygenase-2; GM-CSF = granulocyte macrophage–stimulating factor; ICAM-1 = intercellular adhesion molecule-1; IFN = interferon; Ig = immunoglobulin; IL = interleukin; IL-1ra = interleukin-1 receptor antagonist; LT = leukotriene; MHC = major histocompatibility complex; NK = natural killer; PG = prostaglandin; TGF = tumor growth factor; Th = T helper cell; TNF = tumor necrosis factor; VCAM = vascular cell adhesion protein.
From Hamilton ME: Immunology and pathophysiology of allergic disease. In Naguwa SM, Gershwin ME (eds): Allergy and Immunology Secrets. Philadelphia, Hanley & Belfus, 2001.

TESTS OF IMMUNOLOGIC FUNCTION AND ALLERGY DIAGNOSIS

54. Name common diseases associated with elevation of the total serum IgE level.
   - **Atopic (allergic) diseases:** allergic rhinitis, allergic asthma, allergic bronchopulmonary aspergillosis
   - **Primary immunodeficiency disorders:** Wiskott-Aldrich syndrome, Nezelhof's syndrome (cellular immunodeficiency with IgE), selective IgA deficiency with concomitant atopic disease, Job's syndrome
   - **Infections:** parasitic; viral, including infectious mononucleosis; and fungal, including candidiasis
   - **Malignancies:** Hodgkin's disease, bronchial carcinoma, IgE myeloma
   - **Dermatologic disorders:** atopic dermatitis and bullous pemphigoid, eczema
   - **Acute graft-versus-host disease (GVHD)**

55. How useful is measurement of total serum IgE in such diseases?
   Limited. In many of these diseases, IgE levels may be normal, mildly elevated, or markedly elevated. The clinical usefulness of measurement of total serum IgE is usually limited to diagnosis and monitoring of exacerbations, remissions, and/or treatment of allergic bronchopulmonary aspergillosis, parasitic infections, and immunodeficiency disorders.

56. How can antibody measurements be used to indicate an active infection?
   IgG antibodies can persist for years after an infection has resolved and cannot be used to prove active infection. However, IgM antibodies are produced as new B cells are stimulated by the infection; their development indicates an active ongoing infection. The presence of a rising titer of antibodies also indicates an active response, regardless of antibody class. The first serum sample, typically called the "acute sample," and a second sample, drawn 1 or more weeks later, typically called the "convalescent sample," should be sent to the laboratory together for simultaneous testing. Many titrations, that is, antibody measurements, are done using serial twofold dilutions of serum. Results are not considered significant until there is a fourfold or greater rise in titer.

57. **How would 2 weeks of treatment with H_1 or H_2 antihistamines be expected to affect the results of allergy and DTH skin testing?**

Marked inhibition of positive skin test reactivity. The wheal-and-flare reaction of a positive skin test is primarily due to histamine stimulation of H_1 receptors in small blood vessels. H_2 antihistamines may occasionally depress skin test reactivity as well and should also be avoided before skin testing. To guard against the chance that the patient has forgotten to stop these drugs, a histamine standard should be used as a positive control in performing allergy skin testing. Antihistamines must be discontinued, usually 2 days before skin testing.

58. **How would 2 weeks of treatment with corticosteroids affect the results of allergy and DTH skin testing?**

Corticosteroids do not affect mast cell degranulation, nor do they affect the biologic effects of histamine. Thus, corticosteroids do not alter allergy skin test results. In contrast, DTH skin testing is a type IV reaction and is a sensitive measurement of T-cell function. Histamine does not play a significant role in DTH, and antihistamines (both H_1 and H_2) do not affect DTH skin testing. However, corticosteroids may substantially depress cell-mediated responses, including the mobilization of T cells to specific antigen depots. Thus, DTH reactions (e.g., purified protein derivative [PPD] skin tests) may be profoundly depressed by treatment with corticosteroids.

59. **When is the radioallergosorbent test (RAST) useful?**

For measurement of antigen-specific IgE antibody in serum, but the test is only semiquantitative.

60. **How is the RAST performed?**

Initially, by coupling purified allergen to a carrier (particles, paper discs, or plastic wells), then incubating the allergen/carrier with the patient's serum. After washing, ^{125}I-labeled anti-IgE is added and radioactivity present on the immunoabsorbent material (carrier) is measured. The RAST is used less often and replaced with an enzyme-linked immunosorbent assay (ELISA) system that uses enzymatic color change rather than radioactivity.

61. **How does the RAST compare with skin testing in the diagnosis of allergy?**

The RAST is less sensitive, and its correlation with the clinical history of allergy to specific agents is less clear-cut than with skin testing. Furthermore, validity of the RAST is highly dependent on proper controls and interpretation of the results by the reporting laboratory. However, the RAST may be useful in patients in whom skin testing cannot be done for one reason or another, such as patients with extensive skin diseases or dermatographism, urticaria pigmentosa, or cutaneous mastocytosis. It may also be useful in patients receiving H_1 antihistamines and patients in whom skin testing is considered to carry a high risk of severe anaphylaxis.

62. **Is a positive RAST result diagnostic of allergy?**

No. No test of immediate hypersensitivity, whether skin testing or the RAST, is by itself diagnostic and cannot be taken as evidence of allergy to a specific agent unless the clinical history also suggests that the patient is highly reactive to the same substance. In practice, although the specificity of the RAST (and skin testing, for that matter) is low, the sensitivity is relatively high and a negative RAST (or, for that matter, negative intradermal testing) is good evidence that the patient is not sensitive to a specific allergen.

63. **Describe the advantages of ELISA.**

The ELISA has, to a great extent, replaced the radioimmunoassay (RIA) in diagnostic testing. The ELISA eliminates the radioactive hazards of RIA and has a sensitivity that is comparable or better (sensitivity of ≤ 1 ng, depending on test substance and components used in the assay).

64. **How is the ELISA performed?**
The ELISA is typically performed in plastic, flat-bottomed, 96-well, microtiter plates. The concentration of the substance to be measured is determined by comparing the optical density of the test samples against negative controls and a standard curve. The basic ELISA procedure used to test for antibody against specific antigen is:
1. Coat wells with antigen (by incubating appropriate concentration of antigen in the wells) and then wash.
2. Add test sample and incubate.
3. Wash.
4. Add enzyme-linked antispecies Ig and incubate.
5. Wash.
6. Add developing substrate and measure optical density.

65. **How is anergy established?**
With DTH skin testing, Typically, one employs four or five recall antigens to ensure a > 90% chance of using at least one antigen against which normal age-matched individuals would mount a DTH response. Recall antigens are antigens that a person has already encountered before; thus, during the test, the immune responses are asked to mount a secondary response.

66. **Which antigens are available for anergy testing?**
- Trichophyton (1:30 dilution)
- Tetanus toxoid (10 Lf/mL)
- Mumps antigen (40 cfu/mL)
- *Candida* extract (500 PNU/mL)
- PPD (50 TU/mL)

67. **How is the test performed?**
0.1 mL of each antigen is injected intradermally at widely spaced sites, usually on the volar surface of the forearms. Mean diameter of induration is read at 48 hours. There is disagreement as to whether a 5- or 10-mm-diameter indurated lesion represents a positive result. To assess nonspecific reactions, one can use 0.1 mL of saline as a negative control, but most forego this procedure because there is nothing to show at 48 hours unless the tester inadvertently triggers a capillary bleed at the site of the injection.

IMMUNOGLOBULIN AND OTHER IMMUNE–RELATED DEFICIENCY DISORDERS

68. **Name some of the characteristics of antibody-deficiency disorders.**
See Table 11-6.

TABLE 11-6. CHARACTERISTICS OF ANTIBODY DEFICIENCY DISORDERS

1. Recurrent infections with extracellular encapsulated pathogens.
2. Relatively few problems with fungal or viral (except enteroviral) infections.
3. Chronic sinusitis and pulmonary disease; some patients may develop bronchiectasis.
4. Growth retardation is not a striking feature.
5. Low antibody levels measured in serum and secretions. Low Ig levels by themselves are not sufficient evidence of an antibody deficiency syndrome, and titers of specific antibodies should be measured.

(continued)

> **TABLE 11-6. CHARACTERISTICS OF ANTIBODY DEFICIENCY DISORDERS—** *(continued)*
>
> 6. The hallmark of these deficiency syndromes is the inability to make antibodies to new antigens when challenged with vaccines or following infection with one or another microbe.
> 7. Patients may or may not lack B lymphocytes. If they have B lymphocytes, these may lack surface Igs or complement receptors, indicating that they are arrested relatively early in ontogeny.
> 8. Absence of cortical follicles in lymph nodes and spleen are seen in X-linked agammaglobulinemia.
> 9. Scanty cervical lymph nodes and small or absent tonsils and adenoids are characteristic of X-linked agammaglobulinemia.
> 10. Replacement therapy with IV Ig has greatly increased lifespan and reduced morbidity.
>
> Ig = immunoglobulin; IV = intravenous.
> From Wyngaarden JB, Smith LH (eds): Cecil Textbook of Medicine, 18th ed. Philadelphia, WB Saunders, 1988, p 1943.

69. **What is the most common Ig deficiency disorder?**
Selective IgA deficiency, which has a frequency of approximately 1 in 500–700 persons.

70. **Describe the clinical significance of selective IgA deficiency.**
Many patients are asymptomatic, but some have recurrent infections, particularly of the respiratory tract. IgG_2 deficiency sometimes accompanies IgA deficiency, and these patients are particularly prone to infectious complications with encapsulated bacteria (such as *Streptococcus pneumoniae*, or *Haemophilus influenzae*) because the principal IgG antibody response against bacterial polysaccharide is usually IgG_2. In selective IgA deficiency, the serum IgA level is less than 5 mg/dL (0.05 mg/mL). IgA in secretions is almost always depressed as well. IgG and IgM levels are normal. A few patients have autoimmune disorders (including systemic lupus erythematosus [SLE] and rheumatoid arthritis [RA]).

71. **How is selective IgA deficiency treated?**
With supportive treatment. Even if patients have an increased incidence of infections, intravenous immunoglobulin (IVIG) therapy is unlikely to be effective because infused IgG will not be transported into secretions. Ig infusions also pose a risk because 50% of these patients may have the ability to develop antibodies to the small quantities of IgA present in most IVIG preparations. Life-threatening anaphylaxis can occur with the second and subsequent infusion of IVIG. A similar risk is associated with blood transfusions. IgA-deficient patients can develop antibodies to IgA in the plasma that accompanies packed RBCs. Subsequent transfusions, if needed, should be performed with well-washed RBCs to remove all traces of IgA.

72. **What is common variable immunodeficiency disease (CVID)?**
A heterogeneous group of disorders characterized by hypogammaglobulinemia (total IgG < 250 mg/dL and total Ig usually < 350 mg/dL), decreased ability to produce antibody after antigenic challenge, and recurrent infections. A significant fraction of patients whose serum IgG level is depressed, but still greater than 250 mg/dL, may have a similar clinical presentation. The most common serum Ig pattern, however, is panhypogammaglobulinemia—a deficiency of IgG, IgM, and IgA.

73. **How does CVID present?**
In late childhood or early adulthood but may present at any age. Recurrent bacterial infections of the upper and lower respiratory tract with encapsulated bacteria (e.g., *S. pneumoniae*, *H. influenzae*) are common pathogens, and bronchiectasis may develop. Patients may also have defective cell-mediated immunity and may have mycobacterial, fungal, and protozoal (i.e., *Giardia lamblia*) infections. Patients with CVID have an increased frequency of autoimmune disorders, including pernicious anemia, Coombs-positive hemolytic anemia, autoimmune thrombocytopenia, and thyroiditis. Gastrointestinal (GI) disorders are common, including diarrhea, malabsorption, and nodular lymphoid hyperplasia of the small intestine. Finally, there is an increased incidence of malignancy, particularly of the lymphoreticular system and the GI tract.

74. **Identify the principal immunologic defects in CVID.**
A defect in B-cell maturation. The B cells cannot terminally differentiate into antibody-producing plasma cells. This subset of patients generally has normal numbers of circulating, surface Ig-positive B cells. Up to 20% of patients may have increased suppressor cell activity, causing decreased antibody production. But a host of other immunologic defects are seen in some patients, including T-cell immunoregulatory defects. Depressed cell-mediated immunity, as demonstrated by cutaneous anergy, may be present in up to 30% of patients.

75. **Discuss treatment for CVID.**
The principal therapy for CVID is IVIG replacement and aggressive management of infections with appropriate antibiotics. IVIG is given every 3–4 weeks. The usual dose is 200 mg/kg, and the infusion is given slowly over several hours. Adverse reactions consisting of pruritus, headache, and nausea usually resolve with slowing or stopping of the infusion. IVIG often dramatically decreases the frequency and severity of infections and may also alleviate some of the symptoms, such as arthralgias, that sometimes accompany CVID.

76. **List the common secondary causes of hypogammaglobulinemia and the mechanism by which they cause disease.**
See Table 11-7.

TABLE 11-7. SECONDARY CAUSES OF HYPOGAMMAGLOBULINEMIA

Cause	Mechanism
Drugs	Drugs
a. Anticonvulsants (especially with phenytoin)	a. Decreased B and T cells responses, often hypogammaglobulinemia
b. Cytotoxic agents as used in cancer chemotherapy	b. Decreased Ig production and T-cell activity
Multiple myeloma	Decreased Ig production
Chronic lymphocytic leukemia	Decreased Ig production and T-cell activity
Myotonic dystrophy	Selective hypercatabolism of IgG
Nephrotic syndrome	Ig loss in urine (particularly IgG)
Intestinal lymphangiectasia	Ig loss through GI tract, increased Ig catabolism
Radiation therapy	Decreased Ig production

GI = gastrointestinal; Ig = immunoglobulin.

77. **What immunologic defects are heralded by recurrent bacterial infections?**
    Before the emergence of human immunodeficiency virus-1 (HIV-1), development of serial severe bacterial infections, defined as three or more episodes of bacterial sinusitis, pneumonia, or sepsis within the span of 1 year, was an indication to evaluate patients for a congenital or acquired antibody-deficiency syndrome. Less commonly, recurrent bacterial infections may suggest complement deficiency or defective neutrophil function. Patients with antibody-deficiency syndromes commonly experience repeated infections with encapsulated organisms (e.g., *H. influenzae, S. pneumoniae*) that are common upper respiratory tract commensals.

78. **How are patients screened for antibody deficiencies?**
    With the measurement of serum Ig levels (IgG, IgM, and IgA) and IgG subclasses. Further evaluation may include measuring serum isohemagglutinin titers (IgM antibodies) and serum IgG antibody levels after immunization with protein (tetanus toxoid) and carbohydrate antigen-containing vaccines. Ideally, antibody levels found in preimmunization and 3-week postimmunization sera are compared to accurately measure the antibody response to a specific antigen challenge.

79. **What are the clinical characteristics of disorders of cell-mediated immunity?**
    - Recurrent infections with low-grade or opportunistic infectious agents, such as fungi, viruses, or protozoa (e.g., *Pneumocystis carinii*)
    - T-cell anergy, defined as a general lack of T-cell–mediated immune responses
    - Growth retardation, a dramatically shortened life span, wasting, and diarrhea in children
    - GVHD if patients are given fresh blood or unmatched allogeneic bone marrow
    - Fatal infections after live virus vaccines and after vaccination with other attenuated microorganisms including bacille Calmette-Guérin (BCG)
    - High incidence of malignancy

80. **How do complement deficiencies present?**
    Isolated C3 deficiency typically presents at a very early age, most often shortly after birth. Because C3 deficiency has such a profound negative effect on leukocyte phagocytic function, patients experience recurrent life-threatening pyogenic infections. Deficiencies of the terminal complement components, with the possible exception of C9 deficiency, increase susceptibility to bacteremia with neisserial species, typically *Neiserria gonorrhoeae*. Deficiency of properdin, an alternative complement pathway component, may also be accompanied by recurrent pyogenic and neisserial infections. Complement deficiency can be evaluated by obtaining a CH50 (or CH100) and by measuring levels of specific complement components thereafter as indicated.

81. **Chronic or recurrent meningococcemia or gonococcemia are commonly associated with which host immune defects?**
    Deficiencies of the late components of complement (C6, C7, and C8) are the predominant defects associated with these disorders. Low C3, absent C5, or properdin deficiency has also been associated with such infections.

82. **What complication of gonococcal infection is of special concern in sexually active adults?**
    Acute monoarticular arthritis may be a consequence of bacteremia with *N. gonorrhoeae*. Such patients must be evaluated for complement deficiency after treatment of the septic joint. The intense neutrophilic infiltrate triggered by these infections is considered an orthopedic emergency requiring immediate drainage of the pus and irrigation of the joint to reduce the residence time of the inflammatory leukocytes in the joint space. The aim of this emergency

treatment is to reduce the damage to the articular cartilage caused by leukocyte proteases and reactive oxygen products.

Ross S, Densen P: Complement deficiency and infection: Epidemiology, pathogenesis and consequences of neisserial and other infections in an immune deficiency, *Medicine* 63:243–273, 1984.

83. **What clinical conditions are associated with deficiencies of the various components of the complement system?**
See Table 11-8.

TABLE 11-8. DISEASES ASSOCIATED WITH INHERITED COMPLEMENT DEFICIENCIES

Deficient Component	Reported Cases	Associated Diseases
C1	31	Autoimmune diseases, SLE-like syndromes
C4	20	Autoimmune diseases, SLE-like syndromes
C2	109	Autoimmune diseases, SLE-like syndromes
C3	20	Bacterial infections, mild glomerulonephritis
C5	28	Gram-negative coccal infections
C6	76	Gram-negative coccal infections
C7	67	Gram-negative coccal infections
C8	68	Gram-negative coccal infections
C9	18	Gram-negative coccal infections
Properdin	70	Gram-negative coccal infections
Factor I	17	Bacterial infections
Factor H	13	Bacterial infections
Factor D	3	Bacterial infections
C4-binding protein	3	—
C1 Inhibitor	100	Hereditary angioedema

SLE = systemic lupus erythematosus.
From David J: Immunology. In Dale DC, Federman DD (eds): Scientific American Medicine. New York, Scientific American, 1996. Section 6, Subsection VII, Table 6-9, p 26.

84. **How do defects of neutrophil function present?**
With recurrent infections occurring in the pediatric age group. However, some adults may have a variant of chronic granulomatous disease of childhood (CGD) in which the defect in respiratory burst is qualitatively less than in typical CGD.

85. **How is neutrophil function evaluated?**
Specialty reference laboratories can provide diverse functional tests that identify defects in the ability of leukocytes to traverse endothelial barriers, phagocytose bacteria, and generate antimicrobial substances intracellularly. This testing can be usually arranged by community hospital laboratories by sending appropriately collected blood samples to experienced laboratories. For example, a nitroblue tetrazolium test can be performed to assess neutrophil

respiratory burst in patients with a clinical history suggestive of CGD. Leukocyte adhesion deficiency syndrome can be assessed functionally and by flow cytometric analysis for defects in cell surface expression of CD18-dependent beta integrins. Patients with neutrophil functional defects are particularly susceptible to catalase-positive organisms.

ALLERGIC RESPONSES

86. **What is anergy?**
The lack of an immunologic response to an antigen under circumstances in which one would normally expect to see one. T-cell anergy, for example, is demonstrated by the lack of reaction to common DTH recall antigens. Clinically, this is seen frequently in patients with miliary tuberculosis, Hodgkin's disease, or HIV infection. B-cell anergy is failure to develop a specific antibody response in a person who has been immunized with antigens that are known to routinely stimulate antibody responses in other individuals of the same species. Anergy may be temporary, as occurs during measles infection, or of indeterminate duration, as in sarcoidosis, acquired immunodeficiency syndrome (AIDS), and certain disseminated malignancies and overwhelming infectious diseases, including lepromatous leprosy.

87. **Summarize the clinical significance of anergy.**
Anergic individuals have increased susceptibility to infections that require cell-mediated immune responses for adequate host defense.

88. **What are APCs? What is their role in the immune response?**
Cells that present antigen principally to T lymphocytes, as a result of which the T cells are activated and stimulated to perform one of their many functions. Classic APCs are dendritic cells, B cells, and monocyte/macrophages (including those specialized forms found in specific tissues such as microglial cells and Kupffer cells). All three of these express MHC class II molecules so that they can display antigens to CD4 T cells. Like all somatic cells, they also express MHC class I molecules and can display antigen peptides to CD8 T cells.

89. **How do APCs activate naive T cells?**
By presenting costimulatory signals to the T cell along with antigen. These costimulatory molecules include CD80 and CD86 (also known as "B7.1" and "B7.2"), which interact with CD28 on T cells. Dendritic cells are often considered to be the most effective APC because of their constitutive expression of costimulatory molecules. The other APCs tend to up-regulate their expression of costimulatory molecules after encounter with microbes or microbially induced molecules. Stimuli with cytokines such as IFN-δ can up-regulate MHC molecules on these cells.

90. **What is major basic protein (MBP)?**
The principal bioactive protein in the cytoplasmic granules of eosinophils. MBP is the only one localized to the crystalline core and is also present in much smaller amounts in basophils. The "MBP" abbreviation should not be confused with myelin basic protein from Schwann cells, which is also abbreviated "MBP."

91. **List the biologic effects of MBP.**
- Is highly toxic to many parasites (including *Schistosoma mansoni*, *Trichinella spiralis*, and *Trypanosoma cruzi*).
- Is toxic to a wide variety of mammalian cells (including human cells).
- Stimulates histamine release from basophils and mast cells.
- Neutralizes heparin.
- Causes bronchospasm.

92. **Describe the mechanism of immediate hypersensitivity reactions and give some clinical examples.**
Type I, or immediate hypersensitivity, reactions are classic allergic reactions initiated by degranulation and activation of mast cells. There are several mechanisms by which mast cells can be induced to degranulate. One is by cross-linking of several IgE molecules bound in Fc receptors on the mast cell membrane. Cross-linking can also be achieved by autoantibodies that react with either IgE or the mast cell receptor for the Fc of IgE. Autoantibodies specific for these antigens have recently been recognized as the agents responsible for 20% or more of cases with chronic idiopathic urticaria/angioedema. Mast cells can also be degranulated by the anaphylatoxins C3a and C5a. Both are products of complement activation. Finally, mast cells can be degranulated by direct chemical and physical stimuli, such as those provided by iodinated radiocontrast dyes and opioids.

93. **Distinguish between an anaphylactic reaction and an anaphylactoid reaction.**
Degranulation resulting from cross-linking of cell-bound IgE is called an **anaphylactic reaction**. Degranulation caused by activation of antigen-nonspecific receptors like those for C3a or C5a, which does not involve the IgE receptors, is called an **anaphylactoid reaction**.

94. **Explain the clinical significance of immediate hypersensitivity reactions.**
Mast cells release granules containing preformed mediators, including histamine, heparin, and tryptase. They also mobilize arachidonic acid to generate prostaglandins (PGs) and leukotrienes (LTs). Several hours later, the mast cell begins to release cytokines such as TNF-α. Immediate reactions resulting in release of preformed mediators like histamine become clinically evident within seconds to minutes. Clinical examples include anaphylaxis, allergic rhinitis (hay fever), food allergy, extrinsic (allergic) asthma, immediate drug allergy (such as to penicillin), and acute urticaria (hives).

95. **What are the four types of hypersensitivity reactions?**
See Table 11-9.

Type	Mechanism	Timing to Onset	Clinical Example
I	Mast cells and basophils, often involving IgE.	1–15 min	Atopy, hay fever, urticaria
II	Antibody reacts with host cells leading to phagocytosis or lysis. Stimulatory or blocking antibodies may also cause disease.	Hours	Autoimmune hemolytic anemia (lysis), diabetes (blocking antibodies), Graves' disease (stimulatory antibodies)
III	Immune complexes of any specificity deposit in tissues (typically the walls of small vessels, and the kidney) leading to frustrated phagocytosis and complement activation.	Hours	Arthus reaction, polyarteritis nodosa, serum sickness, small vessel vasculitis

TABLE 11-9. FOUR TYPES OF HYPERSENSITIVITY REACTIONS

(continued)

TABLE 11-9. FOUR TYPES OF HYPERSENSITIVITY REACTIONS—*(continued)*

Type	Mechanism	Timing to Onset	Clinical Example
IV	T-cell–mediated either by CD4 cells activating macrophages or by cytolytic CD8 cells.	36–48 hr	Granulomatous reactions in tuberculosis and sarcoidosis; PPD reaction

PPD = purified protein derivative.

96. How do type IV, or DTH, reactions differ from types I–III?

Type IV reactions are a reflection of cell-mediated immunity and initiated by T cells. Unlike reaction types I–III, DTH can be transferred by T cells, but not by serum.

97. Describe the mechanism of type IV reactions.

When antigen-sensitized T cells are re-exposed to the same antigen by APCs, T-cell activation occurs. Activated T cells secrete IFN-γ, IL-2, and other cytokines, causing monocytes to accumulate at the site of the reaction and differentiate into macrophages. Over 90% of the T cells that accumulate at the site of a DTH reaction are not antigen-specific; rather, they have been called to that site by the activity of the chemokines and cytokines produced by the infiltrating monocytes and few antigen-specific T cells that have localized in the vicinity of the APCs.

98. Summarize the clinical effects of type IV reactions.

Additional inflammatory mediators and cytokines are released that cause edema and sometimes necrosis of bystander cells. If the antigen persists or can be degraded only with difficulty, as is the case with the antigenic lipids of *Mycobacterium tuberculosis*, lymphocyte and macrophage activation continues and may result in granuloma formation. DTH reactions differ in tempo, depending on the cells involved (Table 11-10).

TABLE 11-10. EXAMPLES OF DELAYED HYPERSENSITIVITY REACTIONS

Time to Type	Inducing Antigen	Peak	External Signs	Histologic Appearance
Tuberculin	Tuberculin	48 hr	Indurated, painful skin swelling	Intradermal lymphocyte and monocyte infiltration
Jones-Mote	Foreign proteins such as ovalbumin	24 hr	Slight skin thickening	Intradermal, lymphocyte and basophil infiltration
Contact	Urushiol, the antigen of poison ivy	48 hr	Eczema	Same as tuberculin

(continued)

TABLE 11-10.   EXAMPLES OF DELAYED HYPERSENSITIVITY REACTIONS— *(continued)*

Time to Type	Inducing Antigen	Peak	External Signs	Histologic Appearance
Granulomatous	Talcum powder silica, and other substances that stimulate phagocytosis but cannot be metabolized	4 wk	Skin induration	Epithelioid cell granuloma formation, giant cells, macrophages, fibrosis, necrosis

Modified from Klein J: Immunology. Oxford, Blackwell Scientific Publications, 1990.

99.   **Describe the mechanism of type II or cytotoxic reactions.**
Type II reactions occur when antibody binds to specific antigens on circulating cells or antigens fixed in tissues. Antibody binding activates complement. If the target site lacks decay-accelerating factor or other complement regulatory proteins, as is the case with RBCs, the complement cascade can go to completion, causing lysis of the target cell. Target cells coated with both antibody and bound complement fragments can be opsonized for phagocytosis by macrophages that reside within the reticuloendothelial system and by circulating phagocytes.

100.   **Give a clinical example of a type II reaction.**
Goodpasture's syndrome. Rarely, antigens localized in basement membranes can become a target of autoantibodies. In Goodpasture's syndrome, the antigen is localized in the basement membranes of the renal glomeruli and the lung. Deposition of antibody binds and activates complement and induces leukocytes to localize at the sites of antigen-antibody and complement deposition with the result that the leukocyte proteases break down the basement membranes.

101.   **Describe the mechanism of type III, or immune complex reactions.**
Type III reactions are caused by the formation of soluble or not-so-soluble antigen and antibody complexes in the circulation. These deposit preferentially in (1) fenestrated endothelia, as are found in the choroid plexus and in the renal glomeruli and (2) bifurcations of postcapillary venules where eddy currents slow the flow of blood. Immune complexes usually activate complement in situ. This activation causes neutrophils to accumulate and these cause tissue damage.

102.   **Give clinical examples of type III reactions.**
Arthus reaction, such as happens in hyperimmunized people who receive a tetanus toxoid booster, and generalized serum sickness that occurs after the injection of foreign proteins into the circulation in people who have preformed antibodies to that protein.

103.   **What is an Arthus reaction?**
An acute inflammatory response at the site of deposition of antigen in tissue. Arthus reactions are caused by antigen-antibody complexes (immune complexes) and were first described by Nicolas-Maurice Arthus, a French physiologist, in 1903. The common site of the reaction is skin near a site of subcutaneous injection of an antigen.

104. **When does an Arthus reaction occur in the clinical setting?**
When there are high serum levels of complement-fixing antibodies. Immune complexes form in the blood vessel walls of the dermis and subcutaneous tissues causing a localized vasculitis. Arthus reactions depend on both neutrophil and complement function. In humans, localized Arthus reactions have been reported at the sites of injection of second and subsequent tetanus and diphtheria immunizations and, rarely, at the site of injection of insulin in diabetics.

105. **What is an allergen?**
A special type of antigen that commonly induces synthesis of IgE antibodies that sensitize mast cells and basophils. Whether the host makes IgE depends on multiple factors, but most particularly, it depends on the type of cytokines that the Th cells make after the injection of the antigen.

COMMON ALLERGIC DISORDERS AND THEIR TREATMENT

106. **Which principal components of house dust have been implicated in causing allergic disease?**
Antigens from dust mites, cockroaches, cats, dogs, pollens, molds, and other environmental substances. Dust mites and cockroach-related antigens are often the most important sources of offending allergens in the home and are particularly prevalent in clothing, carpets, and mattresses. Both species of dust mite (*Dermatophagoides pteronyssinus* and *Dermatophagoides farinae*) can be found in bedding, upholstered furniture, and carpets in offices and homes in the United States. The allergens are released into the excretions of the mites. Dust mites thrive optimally at 25°C and 80% relative humidity. Human epidermal scales are a major substrate for dust mite growth.

107. **Describe the approach to treatment of house dust allergy.**
Efforts to minimize exposure to dust and to decrease favorable environments available for dust mite growth may be highly beneficial for allergic patients. Antiallergic medications and, when necessary, immunotherapy (allergy shots) are effective forms of therapy. In practice, symptoms of allergic rhinitis can be controlled in 90% of patients if the patients use prescribed medications regularly for prophylaxis as well as treatment and if proper attention is given to eliminating sources of dust mite and other allergens from the home.

108. **Which biologic functions are mediated via H_1, H_2, or a combination of H_1 and H_2 histamine receptors?**
See Table 11-11.

109. **List the modes of therapy for allergic rhinitis.**
- Avoidance of the offending allergens
- Medical therapy
- Allergen-specific immunotherapy

110. **List the options for medical therapy.**
- **H_1 antihistamines.**
- **Topical corticosteroid nasal sprays:** Highly effective but must often be used for 1–2 weeks before there is evidence of efficacy, and they must be used continuously through the

TABLE 11-11.   BIOLOGIC FUNCTIONS MEDIATED BY H1, H2, OR A COMBINATION
                OF H1 AND H2 RECEPTORS

H1 Receptors	H2 Receptors	H1 and H2 Receptors
Smooth muscle contraction	Gastric acid secretion	Hypotension
↑ Vascular permeability	↑ Cyclic AMP	Tachycardia
Pruritus	Mucous secretion	Flushing
Stimulation of prostaglandin synthesis	Inhibits basophil, but not mast cell histamine release	Headache
Tachycardia	Stimulates IL-5 production by Th2 cells	
↑ Cyclic GMP production		

↑ = increased; AMP = adenosine monophosphate; GMP = guanosine monophosphate; IL = interleukin; TH = T helper cells.
Note that although the majority of histamine receptors in the skin are H1, some H2 receptors and recalcitrant cases of urticaria may require treatment with both H1- and H2-specific antihistamines.

patient's allergy season. They are very safe even with continuous year-round use and can be used even during an upper respiratory infection.

- **Cromolyn sodium:** In patients who have ocular pruritus as part of their symptom complex, cromolyn sodium eyedrops or some other mast cell stabilizer are necessary to control the problem fully. Nasal sodium cromolyn is a useful adjunct to control nasal symptoms of allergic rhinitis.
- **Parasympathetic blockers (ipratropium bromide) nasal spray:** Can be used to control troublesome rhinorrhea.
- **Sympathomimetics:** Among the most effective is nasal inhalation of topical oxymetazoline, but it must be used only intermittently to avoid rhinitis medicamentosa.
- **Omalizumab.**

111. **Does systemic corticosteroid therapy have a role in the treatment of allergic rhinitis?**
Rarely. Systemic therapy with corticosteroids is indicated only for severe acute exacerbations and for control of nasal polyps.

112. **How does allergy immunotherapy work?**
The mechanisms are not definitively known. Allergen-specific immunotherapy involves the subcutaneous injection of extracts of the specific allergens responsible for a patient's symptoms. Patients do produce more IgG specific for the allergen, which may have a blocking function. There is a decrease in IgE antibodies specific for the allergen, and there may be some induction of T-cell anergy. Recruitment of effector cells is reduced. There is also a shift of T-cell cytokine production from those produced by Th2 cells (i.e., IL-4, IL-5, and IL-13) to those produced by Th1 cells (IL-2 and IFN-δ). Immunotherapy with bacterial vaccines has no proven efficacy.

113. **What immunologic changes occur in patients who undergo allergen-specific immunotherapy?**
- Diminished seasonal increases of allergen-specific IgE
- Increased allergen-specific IgG

- Decreased basophil histamine release
- Development of allergen-specific suppressor T cells

114. **What causes rhinitis medicamentosa?**
Long-term use of inhaled topical vasoconstrictors to treat symptoms of allergic rhinitis that may have been complicated by recurrent episodes. Rhinitis medicamentosa results in intense nasal congestion, often with complete obstruction of the nasal airway due to rebound vasodilatation. The causative agents are typically over-the-counter medications such as oxymetazoline nasal spray that patients have used to excess before seeking professional help.

115. **How is rhinitis medicamentosa treated?**
With discontinuation of the offending drug and a short course of oral corticosteroids for severe cases.

116. **Should alpha adrenergic topical vascoconstrictors be avoided in the treatment of allergic rhinitis?**
No. The risk of rhinitis medicamentosa should not preclude the use of alpha adrenergic topical vasoconstrictors such as oxymetazoline in treatment of allergic rhinitis. When used correctly, these agents help to open up the nasal passages and increase nasal airflow for 8–12 hours to ensure that inhaled topical corticosteroids can be effectively delivered throughout the nasal passages and as far as the posterior nasopharynx.

117. **How can the risk of rhinitis medicamentosa be minimized with use of these agents?**
To be certain that there are no complications from the use of these potent vasoconstrictors, treatment must be interrupted from time to time. This can be achieved by taking a drug holiday every 3 or 4 days. Some patients may be able to use these drugs daily if treatment is limited to once per day, preferably in the evening or at bedtime.

ASTHMA

See also Chapter 6, Pulmonary Medicine.

118. **Which types of infections play a role in the exacerbation of asthma?**
Upper respiratory infections caused by viruses and *Mycoplasma pneumonia*. Respiratory syncytial virus parainfluenza, influenza A, rhinovirus, and adenovirus have also been implicated.

119. **What factors determine the severity of the exacerbation?**
Multiple factors, including age, severity of the underlying asthma, concurrent medical problems, site and severity of the infection, and specific infectious agent.

120. **Do bacterial infections play a role in the exacerbation of asthma?**
Not usually. Bacterial infections of the respiratory tract, except as causative agents for chronic sinusitis, have not been commonly associated with exacerbations of asthma, but they may be a significant cause of exacerbation in patients with chronic obstructive pulmonary disease (COPD), in whom bronchospasm is triggered by allergenic stimuli. Considering these relationships, empirical antibiotic therapy, although often used during exacerbations of asthma in children and adults, frequently does not result in a remission of symptoms. More important in such cases is increased use of inhaled corticosteroids.

121. **Discuss the role of circadian rhythms in a patient who complains of nocturnal worsening of asthma.**

Considerable attention has been directed toward the role of circadian rhythms in nocturnal exacerbations of asthma (usually between 3 AM and 7 AM). Cortisol levels decrease, plasma histamine levels increase, and epinephrine levels decrease during the night. The decrease in plasma cortisol is not thought to be a major factor because administration of corticosteroids in the evening is ineffective in preventing nocturnal exacerbations. Plasma histamine levels do not correlate with changes in pulmonary function tests (PFTs). However, epinephrine levels do correlate, suggesting a possible important physiologic role. Circadian changes in the airways themselves are also important. Both airway caliber and reactivity change at night, with an overall 5–10% decrease in flow rates in normal individuals, but up to a 50% decrease in asthmatics. Increased vagal tone, impaired mucociliary clearance, and airway cooling and drying have also been reported as contributing factors in nocturnal asthma.

122. **How does gastroesophageal reflux disease (GERD) affect nocturnal exacerbations of asthma?**

GERD may also exacerbate asthma at night by microaspiration or reflex bronchoconstriction caused by stimulation of nerve endings by acid in the lower esophagus. GERD may be exacerbated by theophylline, which decreases lower esophageal sphincter tone. (See also Chapter 7, Gastroenterology.)

123. **How can adjustment in beta agonist therapy improve nocturnal worsening of asthma?**

The patient's pharmacologic regimen should be carefully reviewed and compliance assured. Use of longer-acting, inhaled beta agonists should be encouraged. The introduction of the long-acting form of albuterol, salmeterol, has a beneficial effect on nocturnal asthma in some patients. A recent randomized trial suggests that simultaneous administration of salmeterol and fluticasone by means of a Diskus inhaler significantly reduced nocturnal symptoms in patients with moderate-to-severe asthma. The comparison group received conventional therapy with corticosteroids and the long-acting beta agonist delivered by separate inhalers. Some patients also benefit from the use of LT receptor antagonists.

Ringdal N, Chuchalin A, Chovan L, et al: for the PJ EDICT Investigators: Evaluation of Different Inhaled Combination Therapies (EDICT): A randomized, double-blind comparison of seretide (50/250 microg bd) diskus versus formoterol (12 microg bd) and budesonide (800 microg bd) given concurrently (both via Turbuhaler) in patients with moderate-to-severe asthma, *Respir Med* 96:851–861, 2002.

124. **How can adjustment of theophylline therapy improve nocturnal asthma?**

Theophylline absorption may be decreased at night, leading to lower serum levels. If necessary, the evening dose should be adjusted so that peak levels occur approximately 6 hours later.

125. **Do corticosteroids help in the treatment of nocturnal asthma?**

Oral corticosteroids should not be given in the evening because the hypothalamic-pituitary-adrenal axis is more readily suppressed at that time of day by exogenous corticosteroids. There is also no evidence that differences in the time of administration either improve or reduce the benefits associated with the use of these drugs.

126. **What other measures may improve the symptoms of nocturnal asthma?**

Patients who have an allergic component to their asthma and who are on maximal pharmacologic therapy should be considered for immunotherapy. Potential environmental and dietary agents should be considered as exacerbating factors. For example, dust mites may cause immediate hypersensitivity reactions during the night. Allergen or irritant exposure several hours before going to sleep can also be important. The late-phase response that may occur after such exposure typically peaks 6–12 hours later and may cause severe, prolonged bronchospasm.

127. **Which nonasthmatic factors may lead to nocturnal worsening of symptoms?**
Cardiac diseases and sleep apnea. Older patients who by other criteria are at risk for atherosclerotic cardiovascular disease should be systematically evaluated to be certain that the nocturnal asthma is not an early or subtle manifestation of paroxysmal nocturnal dyspnea. One also should consider that what the patient perceives to be nocturnal asthma may actually be sleep apnea. Nocturnal asthma is not related to any particular stage of sleep. The patient's sleep partner should be interviewed to describe what type of sleep problems the patient is having and, if indicated, a formal sleep study should be performed.

128. **Why is it critical that nocturnal asthma be treated aggressively?**
Because the majority of fatalities due to asthma occur during the early morning hours.

129. **A 22-year-old patient complains of symptoms of asthma after playing basketball. What is a likely explanation?**
The patient probably has exercise-induced asthma (EIA). Bronchoconstriction typically begins after cessation of exercise and is usually maximal 3–12 minutes later. The severity varies, but it is almost always short-lived.

130. **What causes EIA?**
The cause of EIA is believed to be water loss from the bronchial mucosa, resulting in hyperosmolarity in the bronchial tissue. This mechanism has been demonstrated by prevention of EIA during exercise by means of air that is fully saturated with water vapor at body temperature. Water content of the inspired air is probably the single most important factor affecting bronchospasm, but the level of ventilation achieved, the temperature of the inspired air, and the interval since the previous episode of EIA are also contributing factors. The severity of EIA cannot be predicted by baseline PFTs.

131. **Why is the interval since the previous episode of EIA an important factor?**
Because a refractory period usually occurs for as long as 2 hours after the previous episode. During this period, a second challenge invokes less than half of the initial airway response.

132. **What exercise should be recommended for asthmatics?**
Swimming, whenever possible.

133. **What is aspirin-exacerbated respiratory disease?**
This condition is most dramatically evident in patients who in adult life have developed three manifestations of atopic disease sometimes known as Samter's triad: (1) rhinosinusitis, (2) nasal polyposis, and (3) asthma that is typically severe and exacerbated by aspirin and other nonsteroidal cyclooxygenase-1 (COX-1) inhibitors. In such people, COX-1 inhibitor therapy is sometimes also associated with hives, flushing, and abdominal pain. Because selective inhibition of COX-2 does not provoke these responses, patients can be treated with COX-2 inhibitors with impunity.

134. **What causes aspirin-exacerbated respiratory disease?**
The underlying mechanism remains unknown, but there are several distinctive features of arachidonic acid metabolism in people who are aspirin sensitive. Their mast cells and eosinophils produce cysteinyl LTs at a very high rate. PGE_2, a product of the COX pathway, inhibits 5-lipoxygenase, the enzyme that is responsible for the production of LTs from arachidonic acid. One explanation is that aspirin-induced reduction in synthesis of PGE_2 disinhibits synthesis of downstream bronchospastic metabolites in the 5-lipoxygenase pathway (Fig. 11-6). Indeed, during aspirin-induced asthma, one can measure increased quantities of LTE_4 in the urine and LTC_4 in nasal and bronchial secretions. Recent studies indicate that patients also have increased numbers of receptors for cysteinyl LTs in the nasal mucosa.

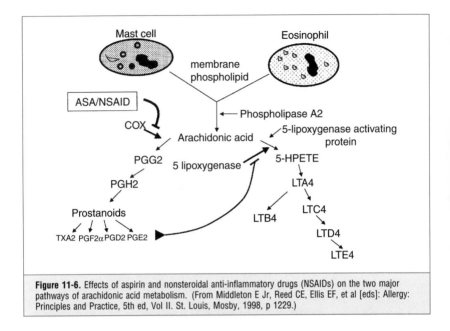

Figure 11-6. Effects of aspirin and nonsteroidal anti-inflammatory drugs (NSAIDs) on the two major pathways of arachidonic acid metabolism. (From Middleton E Jr, Reed CE, Ellis EF, et al [eds]: Allergy: Principles and Practice, 5th ed, Vol II. St. Louis, Mosby, 1998, p 1229.)

Sousa AR, Parikh A, Scadding G, et al: Leukotriene-receptor expression on nasal mucosal inflammatory cells in aspirin-sensitive rhinosinusitis, *N Engl J Med* 347:1493–1499, 2002.

135. **What are the two major pathways of arachidonic acid metabolism?**
PGD_2 and thromboxanes A_2 and B_2 are the major products of the **COX pathway** of arachidonic acid metabolism. LTs, especially LTC_4, LTD_4, and LTE_4, are major products of the **lipoxygenase pathway.** These eicosanoids exhibit an array of potent inflammatory and immunoregulatory properties.

136. **What effects do aspirin, nonsteroidal anti-inflammatory drugs (NSAIDs), eicosapentaenoic acid (fish oil), and corticosteroids have on mediator production by these pathways?**
Aspirin and NSAIDs inhibit COX; that is, they inhibit PG and thromboxane but not LT production. Eicosapentaenoic acid (fish oil) inhibits both PG/thromboxane and LT formation by preferential fatty acid substitution for arachidonic acid in the cell membranes of eicosanoid-producing cells. Corticosteroids also inhibit both PG/thromboxane and LT generation by stimulating production of the intracellular protein, lipocortin, which inhibits the activity of phospholipase A.

137. **How is aspirin-exacerbated respiratory disease treated?**
Treatment options include strict avoidance of aspirin and other NSAIDs and desensitization therapy, which is typically attempted by treating patients with as much as 650 mg of aspirin twice daily on a continuous basis. Whereas long-term desensitization therapy has been reported to reduce disease activity in many aspirin-sensitive patients, as shown by a reduced need for surgery for nasal polyps and reduced requirements for corticosteroids, in others, the gastric irritation caused by aspirin has prevented them from continuing with the therapy.

138. **What are Charcot-Leyden crystals, Creola bodies, and Curschmann's spirals?**
   - **Charcot-Leyden crystals:** Composed of lysophospholipase, and their presence in tissue or secretions has been considered as specific for eosinophil activity; however, lysophospholipase is also found in basophils.
   - **Creola bodies:** Clumps of epithelial cells that suggest a desquamating disease process.
   - **Curschmann's spirals:** Mucus plugs composed of mucus, proteinaceous material, and inflammatory cells in a swirling, spiraling pattern. They usually conform to the configuration of the involved airways.

   These three entities may be found alone or together as part of the clinical presentation of asthma. They are characteristically seen in patients who have died from status asthmaticus.

FOOD ALLERGY

139. **When does a food allergy occur?**
   When ingested food antigens bind to IgE on the surface of intestinal mast cells, causing an immediate hypersensitivity reaction. Basophils may also participate if food antigens appear in the circulation. Foods that commonly cause true food allergies include peanuts, true nuts, shellfish, eggs, milk proteins, and wheat. Cooking may destroy allergenic substances in some foods.

140. **Summarize the symptoms of food allergy.**
   - **GI tract:** nausea, vomiting, diarrhea, bloating, and pain
   - **Symptoms:** urticaria, angioedema, headache, wheezing, hypotension, and other manifestations of anaphylaxis

141. **What can mimic a food allergy?**
   Examples include allergic as well as pharmacologic reactions to food additives, preservatives, dyes, and toxins. GI disorders such as eosinophilic gastroenteritis, malabsorption syndromes, enzyme deficiencies, gluten-sensitive enteropathy, gallbladder disease, peptic ulcer disease, and scrombroid poisoning are among a long list of important, nonimmunologic causes of adverse food reactions. Finally, the psychological aspect of food intolerance may be important, particularly in patients who are convinced that allergy is the cause of their GI symptoms.

142. **How is a food allergy generally diagnosed?**
   By a careful history and physical examination to rule out other potential causes of adverse reactions to food. In an allergic reaction, symptoms should occur after each ingestion of the specific food. This and the resolution of symptoms with elimination of the food from the diet support a diagnosis of food allergy. The onset of symptoms may be delayed for up to 2 hours. The longer time until onset of symptoms with some GI reactions compared with the typical 15–20 minutes for most immediate hypersensitivity reactions may be due to the need to transport the antigen into the GI tract or other processes related to digestion and absorption. In practice, the patient's own experience is frequently the best guide. If the symptoms have been truly dramatic, the patient will tell you straight out, "Doctor, I think I'm allergic to peanuts." If the history is that of an acute GI or systemic allergic response, further tests for all practical purposes are not necessary.

143. **Which test is the gold standard for diagnosis of food allergy?**
   A double-blind, placebo-controlled ingestion of the suspected food. To disguise the food's appearance, it is often desirable to put the food in gelatin capsules.

Bock SA: Double-blind, placebo-controlled food challenge (DBPCFC) as an office procedure: A manual, *J Allergy Clin Immunol* 82:986, 1988.

144. **Discuss the role of skin testing for food allergy.**
Skin testing by means of a prick/puncture test with extracts of the suspected foods is also useful but mainly when the result is negative. Like skin testing for inhaled allergens, skin testing for food has a high sensitivity. If the result is negative, it is unlikely that a particular food, at least in the form that was used for testing, is the offending agent. By itself, a positive skin test is not diagnostic of food allergy unless the history independently suggests that this particular food has caused allergic symptoms. Skin testing can be used to narrow the choices of foods to be used for a double-blind, placebo-controlled trial of ingestion.

145. **Discuss the role of RAST in the diagnosis of food allergy.**
The RAST and other more quantitative in vitro tests may also be used, but they should be reserved for patients in whom skin testing cannot be properly performed and interpreted and patients thought to be at particular risk of a severe anaphylactic reaction to skin testing.

146. **Is a direct food challenge safe?**
Food challenge should be performed only in an appropriate medical setting, because life-threatening anaphylaxis may occur. In some patients, such as those with a low probability of a positive reaction, an open challenge may be useful. If positive, then a double-blinded, placebo-controlled challenge can be used to confirm the diagnosis.

147. **Define "Chinese restaurant syndrome."**
A reaction to glutamate ingested as MSG (monosodium glutamate), a flavoring agent commonly used in Chinese cooking. It occurs within 15–30 minutes of ingestion and consists of a sensation of warmth and tightness on the face and anterior chest. It is occasionally confused with angina pectoris but is benign and requires no therapy except avoidance of foods cooked with MSG.

Kwok RHN: Chinese restaurant syndrome, *N Engl J Med* 278:1122, 1968.

148. **What is the treatment for food allergy?**
Avoidance. Treatment with antiallergic medications, such as antihistamines or oral cromolyn, cannot be expected to decrease the risk of life-threatening reactions. Anaphylaxis caused by food ingestion should be treated like any other anaphylactic reaction, except that nasogastric (NG) tube placement and lavage may be useful to remove residual food antigen. Immunotherapy has no place in the treatment of food allergy.

DRUG ALLERGIES

149. **Compare drug allergy, drug intolerance, and idiosyncratic drug reaction.**
All three are types of adverse drug reactions. A true **drug allergy** is an immunologically mediated adverse reaction to a drug. It can occur with very small doses of the offending agent and accounts for only 54% of all adverse drug reactions. **Drug intolerance,** which also can occur with very small doses, is the result of an undesirable pharmacologic effect of the drug. An **idiosyncratic drug reaction** is based on the individual patient's biochemical alterations of a drug's metabolism.

150. **What confounding factors may complicate the diagnosis of adverse drug reactions?**
Be aware that the listed drug is only one of many ingredients in a pill or capsule. Patients may develop allergic reactions to the dyes used as colorants, excipients, and other agents that either stabilize the medication, slow its absorption, or make it resistant to stomach acids. The tip-off to this type of problem is the patient who confidently states that he or she is allergic to a long list of pharmacologically unrelated oral medications. Further investigation reveals that what they all have in common is the same colorant. One can test this hypothesis by giving the patient the intravenous (IV) form of the offending drug by mouth in a gelatin capsule. If the reaction is to the additives, there will be no reaction to the pure drug.

151. **What are the indications for skin testing for penicillin allergy?**
- Possible or definite past history consistent with immediate hypersensitivity to penicillin, and
- Need for penicillin therapy, and
- Lack of effective alternative antibiotic therapy.

152. **How does penicillin hypersensitivity develop?**
By haptenation of host serum proteins or cell proteins. It may involve a number of structural components (or "determinants") of the penicillin molecule. The penicilloyl determinant is referred to as the "major determinant," and other degradation products of penicillin G, including penicilloate, are referred to as "minor determinants." This "major" and "minor" nomenclature refers only to the abundance of the breakdown product and does not necessarily indicate relative clinical importance. Indeed, some reports suggest that the minor determinants may be responsible for the majority of life-threatening anaphylactic reactions.

153. **How do you test for penicillin hypersensitivity?**
One can purchase the major determinant antigens for immediate hypersensitivity skin testing purposes as penicilloyl-polylysine. The minor determinants are not available except in a research setting. The next best option is to prepare dilutions of the particular formulation of penicillin that you need to use to treat the patient and proceed to use serial dilutions for skin testing, if the test with penicilloyl-polylysine is negative.

154. **A patient has a history of hypotension after an intravenous pyelogram (IVP). What is the likely explanation?**
Systemic reactions to the older hyperosmolar radiocontrast media occur in 1% of patients with a fatality rate of about 0.0009%. The reaction may begin just after the onset of the infusion or up to 30 minutes after its completion. Cardiovascular collapse can result in death. The cause is unknown. It does not appear to be a true IgE-mediated immediate hypersensitivity reaction. It has been suggested that these anaphylactoid reactions result from the ability of the dyes to initiate acute degranulation of mast cells and basophils by activating the alternative complement pathway. A method for detecting patients at risk is not available. Specifically, skin testing with IV contrast material or iodine is of no value.

155. **The same patient now requires a radiocontrast study. What procedure should be followed?**
The considerable risk of a repeat reaction on re-exposure can be minimized by use of the newer lower osmolar radiocontrast agents and by appropriate prophylaxis. Management of patients who require the radiocontrast procedure includes careful evaluation and documentation of the essential nature of the procedure. Informed consent should be obtained from the patient and the family (especially with regard to the small but definite risk of a fatal outcome). Necessary personnel and supplies for emergency treatment, adequate patient hydration, and preprocedure medical prophylaxis are also necessary.

156. **Summarize the usual prophylactic regimen.**
    - Steroids (usually methylprednisolone, 32 mg orally at 13, 7, and 1 hr before the procedure).
    - H$_1$ antihistamines (diphenhydramine, 50 mg parenterally or orally 1 hr before radiocontrast media administration).
    - Ephedrine, 25 mg orally, may, if not contraindicated, offer additional benefit.

    Reactions after prophylactic therapy are usually mild. However, it is important that the procedure be started at the scheduled time or the efficacy of the prophylaxis may be decreased. It has been suggested that in patients with a history of radiocontrast media reactions, nonionic radiocontrast media do not seem to offer a significant protective advantage over medical prophylaxis, but because the consequences of an adverse reaction are life-threatening, it is wise to err on the side of caution and use both prophylaxis and the newer low-osmolar reagents.

    Patterson R, DeSwarte RD, Greenberger PA, et al: Drug allergy and protocols for the management of drug allergies, *N Engl Reg Allergy Proc* 7:325–342, 1986.

ANGIOEDEMA AND CHRONIC URTICARIA

157. **What clinical and laboratory findings are most important in illuminating the cause of angioedema?**
    The majority of angioedema cases are idiopathic, and an extensive evaluation fails to reveal a specific cause or associated underlying disease. However, a careful history is of the utmost importance. For example, allergic angioedema may be suggested by a temporal relationship to exposure to specific allergens (such as food). Cold urticaria/angioedema is indicated by onset after exposure to cold temperatures. A number of findings may indicate hereditary angioedema (HAE), including a positive family history, low C4 during and between attacks, and low antigenic or functional activity of C1 esterase inhibitor (C1INH). Because patients may have one gene producing functional C1INH and one gene producing a nonfunctional C1INH, it may be necessary to measure the quantity of functional or biologically active inhibitor as opposed to just the total quantity of C1INH protein.

158. **What other diseases may be associated with angioedema?**
    Connective tissue diseases, malignancies, thyroid disease, and liver disease (such as hepatitis B). Not infrequently, angiotensin-converting enzyme (ACE) inhibitors may increase the risk of angioedema. Patients who have an episode of angioneurotic edema after use of one ACE inhibitor should not be treated with another ACE inhibitor nor should they be treated with angiotensin receptor blockers (ARBs).

159. **What is the cause of angioedema in the HAE?**
    Deficiency of C1INH (C1-inhibitor). Eighty-five percent of HAE patients have depressed serum levels of C1INH (by antigenic assay), whereas the remaining 15% have normal enzyme levels but lack functional activity. The clinical presentation and inheritance patterns are similar for both groups. Decreased C1INH leads to unchecked activation of the classical complement pathway and decreased inhibition of Hageman factor–dependent activation of the kinin and plasmin pathways. This results in increased generation of C2 kinin, bradykinin, and other molecules that can increase vascular permeability. C1INH is an inhibitor of multiple enzymes, including many in the clotting cascade. Tissue injury can lead to angioedema because consumption of C1INH during clotting leaves the conversion of bradykinin to kinin unchecked.

160. **What are some of the most important clinical characteristics of HAE?**
- Variable age of onset
- Involvement of nonlaryngeal sites, such as the abdominal viscera that can cause abdominal pain
- Inability to clearly identify inciting cause
- Presence of propensity of life-threatening laryngeal edema that is due to other causes

161. **How is HAE distinguished from urticaria?**
Urticaria, although commonly seen in association with other causes of angioedema, is not part of the HAE syndrome. Pain, not pruritus, is typical of HAE lesions. If pruritus is intense, it is likely that one is dealing with urticarial angioedema. Patients typically have depressed serum C4 levels even when they are asymptomatic between attacks.

162. **Summarize the treatment of HAE.**
Attenuated androgen (i.e., stanazolol) therapy dramatically decreases the severity and frequency of attacks. Androgens should be tapered to the lowest dose that adequately controls disease activity in order to minimize potential adverse effects such as virilization and hepatic toxicity.

163. **What elements in the history are important in the evaluation of a previously healthy 26-year-old patient who presents with an 8-week history of daily urticaria?**
A careful history should be obtained to determine whether the urticaria is related to the ingestion of a specific food or liquid, environmental exposure, animal exposure, physical condition (e.g., heat, cold, water, sunlight, pressure, exercise), or stress. The history should also seek to rule out symptoms suggestive of an underlying systemic disease. A careful medication history should also be obtained for the ingestion of both prescription and over-the-counter medications (particularly aspirin and aspirin-containing compounds). Urticaria persisting for longer than 6 weeks is deemed chronic.

164. **What elements of the physical examination are important in evaluating chronic urticaria?**
A thorough physical examination should be performed to identify potential underlying illnesses, such as thyroid disease, malignancy, infection, and rheumatic diseases.

165. **Summarize the role of imaging modalities in the evaluation of chronic urticaria.**
A chest x-ray usually should be obtained, particularly if the patient has not had one within the past 6 months. Computed tomography (CT) scanning may help to detect more difficult to diagnose and treat malignancies such as pancreatic cancer. If the patient has poor dental health or findings suggestive of a dental abscess, dental x-rays may reveal the source of an occult infection.

166. **What laboratory tests may be useful in patients with chronic urticaria?**
Complete blood count (CBC) with differential, urinalysis, erythrocyte sedimentation rate (ESR), and liver function tests. In patients older than 40 years, a serum protein electrophoresis should be obtained to rule out paraproteinemia.

167. **Which other tests may be helpful in specific cases?**
Cryoglobulins, screening for antinuclear antibodies (ANAs), thyroid function studies, complement C3 and C4, and rheumatoid factor (RF). In patients who have traveled abroad recently to Third World countries, testing stool for ova and parasites may be helpful. Hepatitis B and C testing may be indicated. In patients from South or Central America, American trypanosomiasis (Chagas' disease) should also be considered. Whether these and other tests

for the evaluation for systemic diseases are obtained depends on the degree of clinical suspicion based on the history, physical examination, and initial laboratory results. Tests for specific types of the physical urticarias can be performed as indicated. Some investigations attribute a significant fraction of chronic urticaria cases to the development of autoantibodies either to the mast cell receptor for IgE or to IgE itself.

168. **Describe the first-line treatment for chronic urticaria.**
A combination of nonsedating H_1 antagonists and H_2 antagonists (e.g., 60 mg fexofenadine and 150 mg ranitidine q12h). In the great majority of cases, this treatment is sufficient to reduce the frequency and duration of the urticarial episodes to a tolerable level. Despite extensive evaluation, more than 90% of the cases of chronic urticaria are ultimately classified as idiopathic. Appropriate therapy can be provided if an underlying treatable cause of the urticaria is identified.

169. **What other alternatives are available for treatment of chronic urticaria?**
Systemic corticosteroids at the lowest dose needed to control symptoms. Typical urticarial lesions do not usually require biopsy. However, in particularly severe, persistent cases, and especially when urticarial lesions are very painful (as opposed to pruritic), very erythematous, or persist longer than 24 hours, a skin biopsy may reveal urticarial vasculitis. Some of these cases are accompanied by hypocomplementemia and may require more aggressive medical therapy.

ANAPHYLAXIS

170. **List the clinical manifestations of anaphylaxis.**
   - **General:** flushing and sense of foreboding
   - **Skin:** urticaria/angioedema, flushing, and pruritus
   - **Eyes:** lacrimation and pruritus
   - **Upper respiratory tract:** sneezing, nasal pruritus, discharge and congestion, hoarseness, laryngeal edema, and stridor
   - **Lower respiratory tract:** bronchospasm, tachypnea, intercostal retractions, and use of accessory muscles of respiration
   - **Cardiovascular:** hypotension, tachycardia, and arrhythmia
   - **GI:** nausea, vomiting, abdominal pain, and diarrhea
   - **Neurologic:** headache, syncope, and seizure

171. **A 20-year-old man presents with hypotension, wheezing, and urticaria 30 minutes after a bee sting. What is the likely diagnosis?**
Systemic anaphylaxis, an immediate hypersensitivity reaction, triggered by bee venom, that results in mast cell/basophil release of mediators like histamine, PGs, and LTs, into tissues and the circulation.

172. **What is the first priority of treatment?**
Maintenance of cardiovascular and pulmonary function and immediate treatment with epinephrine by either subcutaneous or intramuscular routes (0.3–0.5 mL of a 1:1000 dilution). With cardiovascular collapse, IV epinephrine may be indicated.

173. **What other immediate steps should be taken?**
   - Application of a tourniquet proximal to the site of allergen inoculation (e.g., a bee sting or allergen injection in the forearm).
   - If the anaphylaxis is due to oral intake of an allergen, an NG tube may be inserted and residual gastric contents removed to prevent further antigen absorption.

- Leg elevation.
- Oxygen, airway support, and IV fluids for blood pressure.

174. **Summarize the pharmacologic treatment of systemic anaphylaxis.**
   - Parenteral H_1 and H_2 antihistamines.
   - Inhaled beta$_i$ agonists, especially when bronchospasm occurs.
   - Vasopressor agents when indicated.
   - Steroids to attenuate a subsequent late-phase response.
     The aggressiveness of therapy depends on the severity of the anaphylaxis and the response to treatment.

175. **Which class of medications should be used with particular caution in patients prone to develop anaphylaxis?**
   Beta blockers, which should be avoided whenever possible, because they may accentuate the severity of anaphylaxis, prolong its cardiovascular and pulmonary manifestations, and greatly decrease the effectiveness of epinephrine in reversing the life-threatening manifestations of anaphylaxis. For similar reasons, this class of drugs should be avoided in patients with asthma who require treatment with selective beta agonists.

176. **When should a patient be desensitized to a needed drug (e.g., penicillin)?**
   Only in patients with life-threatening conditions for which the drug is so necessary for a favorable therapeutic result that this potential benefit outweighs the risks associated with desensitization therapy. The patient should be skin tested to verify the presence of an IgE-mediated hypersensitivity to the drug. Desensitization should be done in a highly monitored situation, typically an intensive care unit, where cardiopulmonary resuscitation can be carried out under optimal conditions, if necessary.

177. **How is desensitization performed?**
   Initially by starting treatment with a minute quantity of a drug that, if given in the full therapeutic dose, all at once, would cause anaphylaxis. After the initial test dose, serial, closely spaced injections of systematically increasing quantities of the drug are given at approximately 20-minute intervals. The aim of this treatment is to slowly discharge the anaphylactogenic mediators of mast cells that display surface IgE antibodies to the drug. Essentially, the treatment is designed to cause a controlled anaphylaxis. Patients should not be premedicated with antihistamines or glucocorticoids that mask the allergic reaction because it is necessary to titrate the rate of desensitization based on the patient's response. Once a patient has been desensitized, it is critical that there be no lapse in therapy because any significant interruption could allow the patient's mast cells to regenerate mast cell mediators such as histamine that upon resumption of therapy would be discharged and induce anaphylaxis.

VASCULITIS AND OTHER IMMUNE-MEDIATED DISORDERS
See also Chapter 10, Rheumatology.

178. **What are the major distinguishing factors between Churg-Strauss syndrome (allergic angiitis and granulomatosis) and classic polyarteritis nodosa (PAN)?**
   See Table 11-12. Both are systemic necrotizing vasculitides. Patients who have characteristics of both Churg-Strauss and PAN are classified as having polyangiitis overlap syndrome. Patients who fail corticosteroid therapy or who have fulminant disease should receive cytotoxic drug therapy.

TABLE 11-12. COMPARISON OF CHURG-STRAUSS SYNDROME AND PAN

	Churg-Strauss	PAN
Pulmonary involvement	Yes	No
Histology	Necrotizing vasculitis with granulomas	Necrotizing vasculitis
Vessel involvement	Small-to-medium arteries	Medium muscular arteries; veins, venules with aneurysmal dilatation
Asthma/atopic disease	Yes*	No
Eosinophilia (blood and/or tissue)	Yes	No
Association with HBsAg	No	Yes

HBsAg = serum hepatitis B surface antigen; PAN = polyarteritis nodosa.
*Often present for years before onset of vasculitis.

179. **What does palpable purpura indicate?**
Palpable purpura indicates cutaneous vasculitis.

180. **What is the classic triad of Wegener's granulomatosis (WG)? Describe the clinical presentation and laboratory findings.**
WG is a systemic necrotizing vasculopathy of unknown etiology. The classic triad includes necrotizing granulomatous vasculitis of (1) the upper respiratory tract and (2) the lungs as well as (3) glomerulonephritis. Vasculitis of many other organs, including the skin, ears, eyes, joints, and central nervous system (CNS), may also be present. Vasculitis typically involves both small arteries and veins. The glomerulonephritis is usually focal or crescentic without vasculitis or granulomas. Since the original description by Wegener in Germany in 1939, many more limited forms of the disease have been recognized.

181. **Which laboratory tests help in the diagnosis of WG?**
Laboratory data are generally nonspecific, although recently an antibody to cytoplasmic components of the polymorphonuclear leukocyte (antineutrophil cytoplasmic antibody [ANCA], also known as "antibody to proteinase-3") has been associated with active disease. The ESR is markedly elevated (often > 100 mm/hr) and is a sensitive indicator of disease activity. Mild anemia, leukocytosis, and an increase in serum IgG and IgA levels are commonly seen. Chest x-ray patterns include multiple nodules (which frequently cavitate), infiltrates, and solitary nodules. The mean age of onset is 40 years with a male predominance.

182. **Describe the general approach to treatment for WG.**
Before the use of cytotoxic drugs, specifically cyclophosphamide, WG was an almost uniformly fatal disease, with a mean survival of 5 months. Corticosteroid therapy did not significantly alter the disease's outcome. However, treatment with cyclophosphamide results in complete remission in over 90% of patients. Combination treatment with corticosteroids

and cyclophosphamide should be given initially to gain benefits from the rapid anti-inflammatory effects of the steroid while the cytotoxic actions of the cyclophosphamide are taking effect.

183. **How should cyclophosphamide and corticosteroid therapy be administered?**
Prednisone may be started at 1 mg/kg daily, maintained for 1 month, tapered to alternate-day therapy, and then gradually discontinued, depending on the patient's response. Cyclophosphamide should be started at 2 mg/kg orally and continued for at least a year. If, at the end of the year, clinical remission has been obtained, the cyclophosphamide may be tapered and discontinued. The patient's hematologic parameters should be closely monitored for cyclophosphamide toxicity. The patient's WBC count should be maintained $> 3000/mm^3$ with a neutrophil count $> 1000/mm^3$ to lessen the risk of infectious complications.

184. **Are any other drugs helpful in the treatment of WG?**
Other cytotoxic drugs, such as azathioprine, are less effective than cyclophosphamide in the treatment of WG. In a recent study of patients who had a partial or complete remission after cyclophosphamide/prednisolone induction therapy, leflunomide together with low-dose prednisone was used for maintenance therapy.

185. **What are the major differences between WG and Goodpasture's syndrome?**
See Table 11-13.

TABLE 11-13. WEGENER'S GRANULOMATOSIS VERSUS GOODPASTURE'S SYNDROME		
	Wegener's	**Goodpasture's**
Etiology	Unknown.	Unknown, but hydrocarbon exposure increases risk.
Patients	Male > female. Fifth decade.	Male >> female. Young adults.
Histopathology	Necrotizing granulomatous vasculitis of upper/lower respiratory tract.	Linear deposition of IgG along basement membrane of lung and kidney demonstrated by immunofluorescence, vasculitis absent.
Target organs	Lung > kidney; may also affect: CNS, eyes, ears, joints, skin, heart, others.	Kidney > lung.
Primary symptoms	Chronic sinusitis/rhinitis, fever, weight loss, cough, chest pain, hemoptysis may occur.	Hemoptysis, dyspnea, easy fatigability.
Typical chest x-ray findings	Pulmonary nodule(s) with or without cavitation.	Diffuse bilateral infiltrates.

(continued)

TABLE 11-13. WEGENER'S GRANULOMATOSIS VERSUS GOODPASTURE'S SYNDROME—(continued)

	Wegener's	Goodpasture's
Diagnosis	Clinical picture with biopsy showing necrotizing vasculitis with granulomas of small arteries and veins.	Demonstration of circulating or tissue-bound anti–basement membrane antibodies, pulmonary hemorrhage, glomerulonephritis.
Treatment	Cyclophosphamide, corticosteroids.	Vigorous plasmapheresis, corticosteroids, cyclophosphamide.

CNS = central nervous system; Ig = immunoglobulin.

186. **Hepatitis B surface antigenemia is associated with which of the vasculitides?**
PAN, which is seen in 40% of hepatitis B surface antigen (HBsAg)–positive patients. The severity of the vasculitis and hepatitis is not correlated.

187. **An 18-year-old male presents with abdominal pain, bloody diarrhea, peripheral neuropathy, and demonstration of IgA deposits on biopsy of the GI tract. What is the most likely diagnosis?**
Henoch-Schönlein purpura, although the age of onset is typically younger. The disease is almost always limited to males. This type of hypersensitivity vasculitis principally involves the skin, joints, intestine, and kidney. The disease is usually self-limited, although chronic renal failure may rarely occur. A history of recent infection, usually of the upper respiratory tract, is often reported. Circulating IgA immune complexes are common. Serum IgA levels may be elevated and IgA deposition can be demonstrated in the affected tissues.

188. **Which other laboratory and clinical findings distinguish the CREST (calcinosis cutis, Raynaud's phenomenon, esophageal dysfunction, sclerodactyly, and telangiectasia) syndrome from diffuse scleroderma?**
In CREST syndrome, skin involvement is principally limited to the extremities, and internal organ involvement generally develops more slowly and is less severe than in diffuse scleroderma. Particularly noteworthy of the CREST syndrome (but very rarely seen in diffuse scleroderma) is the development of pulmonary arterial hypertension in the absence of pulmonary fibrosis. This occurs in somewhat less than 10% of patients with limited systemic sclerosis or CREST. Intimal proliferation of the small and medium-sized pulmonary arteries is prominent. Pulmonary hypertension may be progressive and is almost uniformly fatal. Biliary cirrhosis also may occur in the CREST syndrome but is uncommon in systemic sclerosis.

189. **In a patient who complains of fatigue with hair-combing and stair-climbing, what are the most likely diagnoses?**
Diseases characterized by proximal muscle weakness, such as myasthenia gravis, Eaton-Lambert syndrome (myasthenic syndrome), polymyositis, dermatomyositis, and polymyalgia rheumatica.

190. **What is the usefulness of RFs in the diagnosis of RA?**
RFs are autoantibodies (most commonly IgM) that react with the Fc portion of IgG. The presence of RF is not diagnostic of RA and may not be detected in approximately 20% of patients with this disease. When present, RF may be detected in blood, synovial fluid, and pleural fluid. Neither on the basis of specificity nor on the basis of sensitivity is RF warranted as a screening test for collagen vascular disease. In cases of RA documented by clinical criteria, it may be useful to follow RF titers because high titers of RF are found mainly in patients who have more aggressive joint and extra-articular manifestations of disease.

KEY POINTS: ALLERGY AND IMMUNOLOGY ✔

1. The biologic effects of glucocorticoids are not synchronized with blood levels of the drug; effects do not start until a minimum of 4–6 hr after administration.

2. The presence of specific IgM antibodies is indicative of an active infection.

3. The kinetics of a hypersensitivity response is an important diagnostic clue to the underlying mechanism.

4. Corticosteroids are anti-inflammatory, not immunosuppressive.

5. Chronic sinusitis may in fact represent allergic rhinitis.

6. Smoking cessation is critical for successful management of asthma, COPD, and allergic rhinitis.

7. Classification of collagen vascular diseases is based on clinical criteria, with laboratory testing playing a useful but subsidiary role.

COPD = chronic obstructive pulmonary disease; Ig = immunoglobulin.

191. **What is the single best diagnostic test for Sjögren's syndrome?**
Biopsy of the labial minor salivary glands is the most specific diagnostic procedure available.

192. **How can eye involvement in Sjögren's disease be confirmed?**
Eye involvement may be confirmed by the Schirmer test. This test measures tear production very simply. If the patient's tears wet only 10 mm of the filter paper in 5 minutes, tear production is poor and the test is considered positive. Other ophthalmologic tests include rose Bengal staining of the conjunctivae and/or the finding of keratitis on slit lamp examination.

193. **What other tests are useful in Sjögren's disease?**
Parotid salivary flow rates and salivary radionuclide scanning may be used to assess salivary gland function. Autoantibodies in sera may include Ro (SS-A), La (SS-B), RF, and Epstein-Barr–related nuclear antigen.

194. **Describe the presentation of drug-induced lupus.**
With many of the same symptoms as idiopathic SLE, although they are generally milder. However, lupus nephritis and cerebritis rarely, if ever, complicate the syndrome. Drug-induced lupus is more frequent in women than men and in people with HLA-DR4 phenotype. Symptoms resolve shortly after discontinuation of the drug, although laboratory abnormalities may persist for months or years. The ANA pattern in drug-induced lupus is

usually homogeneous or speckled and is caused by antihistone antibodies. Antibodies to double-stranded DNA, as seen in SLE, are not found in drug-induced lupus.

195. **A patient with SLE asks whether she should be vaccinated against measles. What is your recommendation?**
Live, attenuated vaccines currently available are measles, mumps, rubella, oral influenza, oral typhoid, varicella, shingles, BCG, and yellow fever. Vaccinia (smallpox) is no longer given, and oral live polio vaccine is only used in special circumstances. Live vaccines should not be administered to immunologically compromised patients, particularly those with depressed cell-mediated immunity, including SLE. Conditions in which live vaccination of patients should be avoided are listed in Table 11-14. In addition, household contacts of immunocompromised patients should not receive oral live polio vaccine because the live, attenuated strain may revert to the wild type in the GI tract and spread by the fecal-oral route.

TABLE 11-14. PATIENTS IN WHOM USE OF LIVE VACCINES SHOULD BE AVOIDED

- Patients with primary immunodeficiency disorders (especially those with defective cell-mediated immunity such as SCID)
- Patients given immunosuppressive therapy (e.g., corticosteroids, cytotoxic drugs, radiation therapy)
- Patients with malignancies that cause immunosuppression (e.g., leukemia, lymphoma, Hodgkin's disease)
- Patients with systemic immunoregulatory, inflammatory, or infectious diseases associated with defective cell-mediated immunity (e.g., SLE, diabetes mellitus, sarcoidosis, HIV-1 infections, atopic dermatitis)
- Children < 1 year of age
- Patients with severe malnutrition or burns
- Pregnant women (because of potential harm to fetus)*

HIV = human immunodeficiency virus; SCID = severe combined immunodeficiency disease; SLE = systemic lupus erythematosus.
*The exception is yellow fever vaccine when the mother must travel to an endemic area. The risks of infection and detrimental effects without the vaccine are greater than the risks of receiving immunization.

---

196. **What is erythema multiforme (EM)?**
An immunologic reaction of the skin and mucous membranes to a variety of antigenic stimuli. The specific antigen cannot be identified in up to 50% of cases. The lesions may be localized or widespread and consist of bullae, erythematous plaques, and epidermal cell necrosis. The lesions are usually bilaterally and symmetrically distributed on the extensor surfaces of the limbs, on the dorsal and volar aspects of the hands and feet, and on the trunk. The lesions, which resemble "targets" or "bull's eyes," are diagnostic. They appear as a central vesicle or dark purple papule, surrounded by a round, pale zone that is in turn surrounded by a round area of erythema.

197. **List the precipitating factors in EM.**
- **Viral diseases:** herpes simplex, hepatitis, influenza A, vaccinia, mumps
- **Fungal diseases:** dermatophytoses, histoplasmosis, coccidioidomycosis

- **Bacterial diseases:** hemolytic streptococcal infections, tuberculosis, leprosy, typhoid
- **Collagen vascular diseases:** RA, SLE, dermatomyositis, allergic vasculitis, PAN
- **Malignant tumors:** carcinoma, lymphoma after radiation therapy
- **Hormonal changes:** pregnancy, menstruation
- **Drugs:** penicillins, sulfonamides, barbiturates, salicylates, halogens, phenolphthalein
- **Miscellaneous:** rhus dermatitis, dental extractions, *M. pneumoniae* infection

198. **What is the Stevens-Johnson syndrome?**
A severe form of EM with fulminant, disseminated, multisystem involvement. Patients appear toxic, with fever, chills, malaise, tachycardia, tachypnea, and prostration. Diffuse vesicular, bullous, and ulcerative lesions of the skin and mucous membranes develop and desquamate, leading to secondary infections, which in turn may lead to sepsis and even death. It is associated with all causes of EM.

199. **What is Guillain-Barré syndrome (GBS)?**
The acute form of the acquired demyelinating neuropathies. In patients who do not spontaneously remit within 4–6 weeks and develop chronic weakness, the condition is called "chronic inflammatory demyelinating polyradiculopathy." The causes of these conditions remain obscure and the principal therapy is supportive, particularly with regard to decreased respiratory function. But there is a growing consensus that these conditions are immunologically mediated.

200. **Summarize the recommended treatment for GBS.**
Management involves a carefully orchestrated mix of anti-inflammatory and immunomodulatory therapy. Agents that have been used include azathioprine, cyclosporine, and cyclophosphamide as well as plasmapheresis or high-dose IVIG. Dramatic but often unsustained remissions have been observed with these treatments, particularly if instituted within 7 days of the onset of symptoms, when the disease process is still classified as acute GBS.

201. **How is plasmapheresis used for treatment of GBS?**
Because plasmapheresis is an inefficient procedure for reducing circulating Ig levels, typically 6–10 plasmapheresis procedures or more are performed at the rate of 2 or 3/wk. Each procedure consists of the exchange of total plasma volume (usually 2–3 L in an adult) with an albumin/saline/electrolyte solution. The frequency of procedures varies with the overall medical condition of the patient and the availability of venous access.

202. **Explain the role of IVIG in the treatment of GBS.**
Plasmapheresis can theoretically be followed by IV infusions of Ig to prevent rebound synthesis of autoantibodies, but this strategy would add significantly to the expense. At present, it is not clear that the added cost would be worth it. However, a recent report suggests that IVIG treatment may be superior for the subset of patients who have IgG autoantibodies to GM1 gangliosides.

Kuwabara S, Mori M, Ogawara K, et al: Intravenous immunoglobulin therapy for Guillain-Barré syndrome with IgG anti-GM1 antibody, *Muscle Nerve* 24:54–58, 2001.

203. **What are the target organs of the common autoantibodies that characterize organ-specific autoimmune diseases?**
- **Myasthenia gravis:** acetylcholine receptors
- **Graves' disease:** thyroid-stimulating hormone receptor
- **Thyroiditis:** thyroid (often involves T cells as well)
- **Insulin-resistant diabetes with acanthosis nigricans:** insulin receptor
- **Insulin-resistant diabetes with ataxia telangiectasia:** insulin receptor
- **Allergic rhinitis, asthma, and autoimmune abnormalities:** beta$_2$ adrenergic receptors

- **Juvenile insulin-dependent diabetes:** pancreative islet cells, insulin
- **Pernicious anemia:** gastric parietal cells, vitamin B_{12}–binding site of intrinsic factor
- **Addison's disease:** adrenal cells
- **Idiopathic hypoparathyroidism:** parathyroid cells
- **Spontaneous infertility:** sperm
- **Premature ovarian failure:** interstitial cells, corpus luteum cells
- **Pemphigus:** intercellular substance of skin and mucosa
- **Bullous pemphigoid:** basement membrane zone of skin and mucosa
- **Primary biliary cirrhosis:** mitochondria
- **Autoimmune hemolytic anemia:** erythrocytes
- **Idiopathic thrombocytopenic purpura:** platelets
- **Idiopathic neutropenia:** neutrophils
- **Vitiligo:** melanocytes
- **Chronic active hepatitis:** nuclei of hepatocytes

204. **What is the cold agglutinin syndrome? How is it diagnosed?**
The cold agglutinin syndrome is characterized by hemolytic anemia secondary usually to IgM antibodies, although low-affinity IgG antibodies have also been implicated. The IgM antibodies can cause RBC lysis with decreasing temperature. IgG antibodies can, in addition, facilitate uptake of the antibody-coated RBC by phagocytes. Agglutination of normal RBCs at 20°C occurs with serum from virtually all patients with the cold agglutinin syndrome. (See also Chapter 14, Hematology.)

205. **How is the cold agglutinin syndrome diagnosed?**
The direct Coombs' test is typically positive for complement and negative for Ig. This finding reflects the fact that the antibody involved has a high affinity for RBC only in the cold. Warming the antibody causes it to dissociate. Hence, only RBCs in cold extremities (e.g., fingers, toes, tip of the nose) are likely to show a positive direct Coombs' test.

206. **What causes cold agglutinin syndrome?**
The cold agglutinin syndrome is typically idiopathic, with the presentation of hemolytic anemia in the sixth or seventh decade of life. Despite the monoclonal nature of the antibody response, patients typically do not develop multiple myeloma or Waldenstrom's macroglobulinemia. Cold agglutinin syndrome may also occur in association with the lymphoproliferative disorders (i.e., non-Hodgkin's lymphoma), infections (*M. pneumoniae*, infectious mononucleosis), and rarely in connective tissue disorders such as SLE. The cold agglutinins in these disorders may be anti-I, or directed at other RBC antigens. Determination of antibody specificity is not necessary for either diagnosis or blood transfusion.

207. **What is the "innocent bystander" mechanism of drug-induced hemolysis?**
Some drugs can cause an immune hemolytic anemia even though they do not bind to RBCs. These drugs, bound to plasma proteins, stimulate the formation of complement-fixing antibodies that activate the classical complement pathway. The C3b generated by these reactions in the plasma binds covalently to nearby RBCs. Occasionally, this process leads to full assembly of the terminal components of the complement cascade, causing intravascular hemolysis of these "innocent bystanders."

THERAPIES FOR IMMUNOLOGIC AND ALLERGIC DISORDERS

208. **When is cromolyn sodium particularly useful?**
As a prophylactic agent in patients with sufficiently frequent symptoms to justify continuous therapy because it is most effective when administered before exposure

to an allergen (i.e., before mast cell degranulation). Cromolyn inhibits both immediate hypersensitivity and late-phase reactions. It requires a run-in period of 3 weeks to reach maximum effectiveness.

209. **Describe the mechanism of action of cromolyn sodium.**
Inhibition of the degranulation of mucosal mast cells, thereby preventing the release of the mediators of immediate hypersensitivity. The mechanism by which this occurs is unknown, although inhibition of calcium influx is one of several proposed explanations. This drug has no intrinsic antihistamine, bronchodilator, or anti-inflammatory activity and is available for use via inhalational, intranasal, and topical ophthalmic routes.

210. **What are the limitations of using monoclonal antibodies as therapeutic agents?**
Monoclonal antibodies are almost always made in mice, and the mouse Ig is sufficiently different from human immunoglobulin that it triggers production of human antibodies in recipients. Although serum sickness is a possibility, as was seen after infusion of horse antitoxins in the past, this problem is vanishingly rare. The main limitation is the shortened half-life of the mouse monoclonal after it complexes with human antimouse antibodies in the recipient.

211. **How can monoclonal antibodies be "humanized"?**
By using genetic engineering techniques so that almost all of the molecule, with the exception of the antigen-binding site, becomes a human IgG. Whereas unmodified murine monoclonal antibodies may have a half-life of less than 2 days, humanized antibodies can circulate with a half-life of 20 days, which is close to that of human IgG. Monoclonal antibodies are now used to help control allergic reactions, transplant rejection, and autoimmune responses and as an adjunct to cancer chemotherapy.

212. **What is omalizumab?**
An anti-IgE monoclonal antibody containing a mouse antibody against human IgE that has been "humanized."

213. **How is omalizumab used in treatment of allergies?**
Biweekly or monthly subcutaneous injections of omalizumab have been shown to reduce symptoms of allergic rhinitis and improve airway function in patient with moderate-to-severe asthma. Currently, the therapy is administered for 12 weeks, but its high cost may make its use prohibitive for most patients.

Casale TB, Condemi J, LaForce C, et al: Effect of omalizumab on symptoms of seasonal allergic rhinitis: A randomized controlled trial, *JAMA* 286:2956–2967, 2001.

214. **Give the serum half-lives and relative potencies of the common glucocorticoids.**
See Table 11-15.

215. **What are the effects of corticosteroids on circulating leukocytes?**
The short answer is that neutrophil numbers increase, partly owing to accelerated release from the bone marrow and partly owing to the decreased ability of neutrophils to migrate out of the circulation during corticosteroid treatment. The numbers of circulating lymphocytes, monocytes, and particularly eosinophils decreases. Overall, the total white count is increased. Table 11-16 offers a more detailed answer.

TABLE 11–15. RELATIVE POTENCIES AND EFFECTS OF COMMON GLUCOCORTICOIDS

Preparation	Potency Relative to Hydrocortisone	Relative Sodium-Retaining Potency	Approximately Equivalent Dose of Action (mg)	Duration of Action
Hydrocortisone	1	1	20	Short
Cortisone	0.8	0.8	25	Short
Prednisolone	4	0.8	5	Intermediate
Prednisone	4	0.8	5	Intermediate
6α-Methylprednisolone	5	0.5	4	Intermediate
Triamcinolone	5	0	4	Intermediate
Dexamethasone	25	0	0.75	Long
Betamethasone	25	0	0.75	Long

From Schleimer RP: Glucocorticosteroids. In Middleton E, et al (eds): Allergy: Principles and Practice, 3rd ed. St. Louis, Mosby, 1988, p 742.

TABLE 11–16. EFFECTS OF CORTICOSTEROIDS ON THE NUMBERS OF LEUKOCYTES IN THE BLOOD

Cell Type	Effect on Numbers	Effect on Function	Comment
Neutrophil	Increase	Minimal effect on chemotaxis, phagocytosis, bactericidal activity; transendothelial migration in response to chemotactic stimuli is almost abolished.	Decrease in numbers sequestered in marginating pools, increased production and release from bone marrow, increased half-life in circulation.
Lymphocytes	Decrease	Decreased proliferative response, inhibition of mediator production and release, altered helper and suppressor function.	Greater effect on T cells than on B cells; priming for antibody formation to new antigens is unaffected.

(continued)

TABLE 11–16. EFFECTS OF CORTICOSTEROIDS ON THE NUMBERS OF LEUKOCYTES IN THE BLOOD—*(continued)*

Cell Type	Effect on Numbers	Effect on Function	Comment
Lymphocytes			
T cells	Decrease a. Helper/ inducer (CD4)— decrease b. Cytotoxic/ suppressor (CD8)—no change		
B cells	Minimal decrease or no change		
Monocytes	Decrease	Depressed chemotaxis, suppression of cytotoxic activity, decreased transendothelial migration.	Possible sequestration.
Eosinophils	Decrease	Inhibition of mediator production and release.	Possible sequestration.
Basophils	Decrease	Inhibition of degranulation.	Possible sequestration.
NK cells	No effect	No effect.	
Null cells	No effect	Unknown.	

NK = natural killer.

TRANSPLANTATION IMMUNOLOGY

216. **Explain the importance of HLA typing in solid organ and bone marrow transplantation (BMT).**
HLA compatibility of donor and recipient affects graft outcome in both solid organ transplantation (such as kidney, heart, lung, and liver) and BMT. For solid organs, matching for the HLA-D or MHC type II antigens is more important than matching at HLA-A or HLA-B, the MHC type I antigens, because MHC class II molecules are involved in activating CD4 Th cells that are needed for both humoral and cell-mediated effector functions that attack the graft. HLA incompatibility may lead to graft rejection of solid organ transplantation and to GVHD in BMT.

217. **Is HLA compatibility a major graft survival factor in corneal transplants?**
HLA compatibility is not a major graft survival factor for first-time, nonvascularized corneal transplants.

218. **Explain how the mechanism of graft rejection differs from the mechanism of GVHD in BMT.**
In graft rejection, the graft is attacked by the recipient's immune system. In contrast, in BMT with GVHD, the immunocompetent cells from the donor attack the recipient, whose own immune system has been ablated prior to the transplant.

219. **Explain the importance of ABO typing in solid organ transplantation and BMT.**
ABO blood typing is critical in solid organ transplants because ABO antigens are expressed on all tissue cells of the transplanted organ, and because type O, type A, or type B recipients almost always have preformed antibodies to these blood group antigens. Thus, transplantation of solid organ grafts at a minimum requires compatibility at ABO. However, ABO compatibility, oddly enough, is not a requirement for bone marrow grafting because the donor graft will thereafter supply all blood cells.

220. **List the four types of graft rejection and their immunologic mechanisms.**
See Table 11-17.

TABLE 11-17. TYPES OF SOLID ORGAN GRAFT REJECTION		
Type	Onset	Major Effector Mechanisms
Hyperacute	Minutes to hours	Humoral: preformed cytotoxic antibody in the recipient against donor graft antigen(s) a. ABO system b. Anti-HLA class I
Accelerated	2–5 days	Cell-mediated: due to prior T-cell sensitization against donor antigen(s)
Acute	7–28 days	Principally cell-mediated immunity: allogeneic reactivity by recipient T cells against donor antigen(s) Humoral immunity to HLA antigens
Chronic	>3 mo	Principally cell-mediated immunity allogeneic reactivity by recipient T cells against donor antigen(s) Humoral immunity to HLA antigens

HLA = human leukocyte antigen

221. **What is the mechanism of action of cyclosporine? What are its principal adverse effects?**
Cyclosporine inhibits calcineurin-dependent signal transduction and binds to cytoplasmic immunophilins. This interaction inhibits the phosphatase activity of calcineurin, resulting in a reduction of IL-2 production and T-cell activation.

222. **List the principal side effects of cyclosporine.**
- Nephrotoxicity (25–75% of patients)
- Hypertension
- Hirsutism
- Hepatotoxicity
- Gingival hyperplasia
- Seizures (5% of patients)
- Tremor (>50% of patients)

BIBLIOGRAPHY

1. Abbas AK, Lichtman AH, Pillai S: *Cellular and Molecular Immunology*, ed 6, Philadelphia, 2009, WB Saunders.
2. Adkinson NF, Middleton E, Busse W, et al, editors: *Middleton's Allergy: Principles and Practice*, ed 7, St. Louis, 2008, Mosby.
3. Murphy KP, Murphy KM, Travers P, et al, editors: *Janeway's Immunobiology*, ed 7, New York, 2008, Garland.
4. Klein J: *Immunology*, ed 2, Oxford, 1997, Blackwell Scientific Publications.
5. Paul WE, editor: *Fundamental Immunology*, ed 6, Philadelphia, 2008, Lippincott Williams & Wilkins.
6. Rich RR, Fleisher TA, Shearer WT, et al, editors: *Clinical Immunology, Principles and Practice*, ed 3, St. Louis, 2008, Mosby.

CHAPTER 12

INFECTIOUS DISEASES

Harrinarine Madhosingh, M.D., and Frederick S. Southwick, M.D.

> . . . for various reasons, it [syphilis] remained a horror, aside from the fact that no one wants to be
> infected by millions of Treponema pallidum, *the causative microbe, whose wriggling corkscrew can
> reach the bone marrow and spleen within forty-eight hours of infection, and produce a persistent
> malaise, rashes, ulcerous skin lesions, and other debilitating symptoms.*
> William Styron (1925–2006)
> "The Case of the Great Pox" from
> *Havanas in Camelot*, 2006

FEVER

1. **What is the definition of fever of unknown origin (FUO)?**
   - Fever of $\geq$ 38.3°C on several occasions
   - Illness lasting at least 3 weeks
   - No diagnosis after inpatient work-up for 3 days or after two or more outpatient visits

   Petersdorf RG, Beeson PB: Fever of unexplained origin: Report on 100 cases, *Medicine (Baltimore)*
   40:1–30, 1961.

2. **What are the three major causes of FUO?**
   Infection, malignancy, and autoimmune disease.

3. **What are some of the infectious etiologies of FUO?**
   - Cholangitis
   - Intra-abdominal or pelvic abscess
   - Acalculous cholecystitis
   - Tuberculosis
   - Typhoid fever
   - Epstein-Barr virus (EBV)
   - Cytomegalovirus (CMV)
   - Cat-scratch disease (due to *Bartonella henselae*)
   - Visceral leishmaniasis
   - Endocarditis (especially subacute bacterial endocarditis)
   - Toxoplasmosis
   - Q-fever (*Coxiella burnetii*)
   - Brucellosis
   - Trichinosis
   - Histoplasmosis
   - Lymphogranuloma venereum (LGV)
   - Whipple's disease

4. **List the noninfectious causes of FUO.**
   See Table 12-1.

TABLE 12-1. NONINFECTIOUS CAUSES OF FEVER OF UNKNOWN ORIGIN

Autoimmune	Malignancies	Miscellaneous
Temporal arteritis (giant cell arteritis)	Leukemia	Medications (drug fever)
	Lymphoma (especially Hodgkin's)	Venous thromboembolism and pulmonary embolism
Systemic lupus erythematosus	Myeloid metaplasis	Sarcoidosis
	Renal cell carcinoma	Crohn's disease
Adult Still's disease	Hepatoma	Granulomatous disease
Polymyalgia rheumatica		Familial Mediterranean fever (FMF)
		Adrenal insufficiency
Polyarteritis nodosa		Thyrotoxicosis
Mixed connective tissue disease		Factious sources
Wegener's granulomatosis		
Relapsing polychondritis		
Subacute thyroiditis		

5. **Is the etiology of FUO always found?**
No. Up to 10–30% of these patients do not have an identified etiology, but the fever usually resolves with full recovery. Reevaluation of these patients will sometimes reveal an etiology after an initial negative work-up.

KEY POINTS: MOST COMMON ETIOLOGIES OF FEVER OF UNKNOWN ORIGIN ✔

1. Infectious: tuberculosis and abscesses

2. Autoimmune: Still's disease and temporal arteritis

3. Malignancies: lymphomas, leukemia, renal cell carcinoma, and hepatocellular carcinomas

6. **What is the difference between sepsis and systemic inflammatory response syndrome (SIRS)?**
SIRS is defined by the presence of two or more of the following criteria:
- Temperature > 38.5 or $< 35°C$
- Heart rate > 90 beats/min (bpm)
- Respiratory rate > 20 or arterial carbon dioxide pressure ($PaCO_2$) < 32 mmHg
- White blood count $> 12,000$ or < 4000 or $> 10\%$ bands
In **sepsis,** the clinical signs of SIRS are present but there is evidence of infection (either by cultures or on examination).

SELECTED GRAM-POSITIVE BACTERIA

7. **What is PVL?**
   Panton-Valentine leukocidin, a toxin produced by methicillin-resistant *Staphylococcus aureus*
   (MRSA) that has been proposed as a major determinant of disease. This toxin, although
   epidemiologically linked to community-associated methicillin-resistant *Staphylococcus
   aureus* (CA-MRSA) infections, has not been definitively proven to be a major virulence
   determinant for this organism.

   Voyich JM, Otto M, Mathema B, et al: Is Panton-Valentine leukocidin the major virulence determinant
   in community-associated methicillin-resistant *Staphylococcus aureus disease? J Infect Dis*
   194:1761–1770, 2006.

8. **What are the mechanisms of resistance to antibiotics with *S. aureus*?**
   - Enzyme production (β-lactamases) that leads to resistance to β-lactam antibiotics
   - Chromosomally mediated production of altered penicillin-binding proteins (PBPs), which
     have lower affinity to binding of β-lactam antibiotics
   - Altered cell wall thickness
   - Acquisition of VanA gene from enterococci

   Hiramatsu K, Okuma K, Ma XX, et al: New trends in *Staphylococcus aureus* infections: Glycopeptide
   resistance in hospital and methicillin resistance in the community, *Curr Opin Infect Dis* 15:407–413, 2002.

   Sieradzki K, Tomasz A: Alterations of cell wall structure and metabolism accompany reduced
   susceptibility to vancomycin in an isogenic series of clinical isolates of *Staphylococcus aureus, J Bacteriol*
   185:7103–7110, 2003.

9. **How does CA-MRSA differ from hospital-acquired MRSA?**
   The mecA gene of CA-MRSA is packaged in a type IV staphylococcal cassette cartridge
   (SCCmec) and CA-MRSA is usually sensitive to antibiotics such as quinolones, clindamycin,
   and erythromycin, to which hospital-acquired MRSA is usually resistant.

10. **What types of infections does CA-MRSA cause?**
    - Skin and soft tissue infections (abscess, cellulitis, necrotizing fasciitis)
    - Infective endocarditis
    - Necrotizing pneumonia

    Kowalsk T, Berbari E, Osmon D: Epidemiology, treatment and prevention of community-acquired
    methicillin-resistant *Staphylococcus aureus* infections, *Mayo Clin Proc* 80:1201–1208, 2005.

11. **Which of the coagulase-negative staphylococci has been reported to behave
    as virulently as *S. aureus*?**
    Staphylococcus lugdunensis, which has been reported in cases of native valve endocarditis,
    wound infection and abscess, and infection of intravascular catheters and other medical
    devices. A clue to this species is the antibiotic susceptibility pattern that shows sensitivity to
    beta-lactam antibiotics including oxacillin. Many of the other coagulase-negative
    staphylococci are resistant to beta-lactams.

    Frank KL, Del Pozo JL, Patel R: From clinical microbiology to infection pathogenesis: How daring to be
    different works for *Staphylococcus lugdunensis, Clin Microbiol Rev* 21:111–133, 2008.

12. **Which form of *Staphylococcus* causes urinary tract infections (UTIs) in young
    women?**
    Staphylococcus saprophyticus, a coagulase-negative organism that accounts for up to 15%
    of cases of cystitis in young, sexually active women. Clinical findings are identical to those
    found in UTIs caused by other typical pathogens such as *Escherichia coli, Proteus,* and
    Klebsiella.

13. **Which coagulase-negative *Staphylococcus* may have higher minimal inhibitory concentrations (MICs) to vancomycin and resistance to multiple other antibiotics?**
Staphylococcus haemolyticus, occurring in approximately 10% of clinical coagulase-negative staphylococcus isolates. Studies have shown relative resistance to vancomycin, teicoplanin, and other antibiotics. Newer agents such as linezolid and daptomycin may be useful in treating infections caused by this organism.

> Frogatt JW, Johnston JL, Galetto DW, et al: Antimicrobial resistance in nosocomial isolates of *Staphylococcus haemolyticus, Antimicrob Agents Chemother* 33:460–466, 1989.

14. **What are the toxin-mediated syndromes caused by *S. aureus*?**
 - **Toxic shock syndrome:** a syndrome of fever, rash with desquamation, hypotension and abnormalities in the gastrointestinal, central nervous, musculoskeletal, renal, hepatic, or hematologic systems associated with toxin 1 (TSST-1)
 - **Scalded skin syndrome:** separation of the epidermis from the dermis (which is the basis for the Nikolsky sign), caused by exfoliative toxins (A and B)
 - **Food poisoning:** severe gastroenteritis that is usually self-resolving caused by enterotoxins of *S. aureus*

15. **What other bacteria causes toxic shock syndrome?**
Streptococcus pyogenes.

16. **What is the role of clindamycin in treating toxic shock syndrome?**
To shut down bacterial protein synthesis and, thus, toxin production.

17. **What is necrotizing fasciitis?**
An infection of the deep fascia that rapidly progresses and can lead to necrosis of subcutaneous tissue, typically preceded by trauma. Organisms causing this infection include *S. pyogenes* and *S. aureus*. Other organisms such as *Clostridium* spp. and anaerobes may also be present. Therapy consists of urgent surgical debridement in conjunction with antibiotics.

18. **What are the most common causes of nodular lymphangitis?**
 - *Sporothrix schenckii*
 - *Mycobacterium marinum*
 - *Nocardia brasiliensis*

> Kostman JR, DiNubile MJ: Nodular lymphangitis: A distinctive but often unrecognized syndrome, *Ann Intern Med* 118:883–888, 1993.

19. **List the clinically relevant gram-positive bacilli (rods).**

Clostridium spp.	*Bacillus*	*Erysipelothrix*
Listeria	*Corynebacteria*	*rhusiopathiae*
Actinomyces		*Nocardia*

20. **List the diseases caused by the various *Bartonella* species.**
 - ***Bartonella bacilliformis:*** veruga peruana
 - ***Bartonella quintana:*** Oroya fever (Carrion's disease), trench fever, bacillary angiomatosis/visceral peliosis, fever/bacteremia, endocarditis
 - ***Bartonella henselae:*** lymphadenopathy, fever/bacteremia, bacillary angiomatosis/visceral peliosis, cat-scratch disease, endocarditis
 - ***Bartonella elizabethae:*** endocarditis
 - ***Bartonella clarridgeiae:*** cat-scratch disease
 - ***Bartonella vinsonii* subsp. *berkhoffi:*** endocarditis

- *Bartonella vinsonii* **subsp.** *arupensis:* fever
- *Bartonella grahamii:* neuroretinitis

SELECTED GRAM-NEGATIVE INFECTIONS

21. List the infections classically attributed to *Pseudomonas.*
    - **Malignant (necrotizing) otitis externa:** usually seen in diabetics with symptoms of pain and discharge from the ear
    - **Otitis externa** (swimmer's ear): usually seen in children
    - **Endocarditis:** usually seen in intravenous (IV) drug abusers owing to contamination of drug paraphernalia
    - **Osteomyelitis:** due to puncture wounds of the foot through sneakers, usually seen in young, healthy patients with calcaneal bone osteomyelitis
    - **Cystic fibrosis exacerbations:** due to chronic airway colonization
    - **Nosomocomial:** including ventilator-associated pneumonia
    - **Noma neonaturum:** necrotizing mucosal and perianal infection of newborns
    - **"Green nail syndrome":** paronychia caused by frequent immersion of hands into water

22. What is ecthyma gangrenosum?
    Skin lesions associated with gram-negative bacteremia, most commonly in neutropenic patients. *Pseudomonas aeruginosa* is the most commonly implicated bacteria, but other species have produced this lesion, including *Aeromonas hydrophila* and *E. coli*. The lesions typically begin as painless erythematous macules that rapidly progress to papules and develop central vesicles or bullae. Eventually, they ulcerate to form gangrenous ulcers. The characteristic histologic appearance demonstrates large numbers of bacteria in and around blood vessels, but with an absence of an inflammatory response.

23. List three clinically relevant species of *Burkholderia.*
    - *Burkholderia cepacia:* associated with exacerbation of disease on cystic fibrosis patients
    - *Burkholderia pseudomallei:* the agent of melioidosis, a disease of both humans and animals with a wide variety of clinical symptoms such as skin ulcer, abscess, chronic pneumonia, fulminant septic shock with abscesses in internal organs
    - *Burkholderia mallei:* the cause of glanders, a disease of animals, but a potential zoonosis

VIRUSES

24. What causes hand, foot, mouth disease (HFMD)?
    Usually a virus of the picornavirus family, most often coxsackievirus A16. Outbreaks have occurred with coxsackieviruses A4, A5, A9, A10, B2, and B5 and enterovirus 71.

25. What are the clinical findings of HFMD?
    An ulcerative exanthem, usually occurring on the buccal mucosa, followed by a vesicular exanthem on the hands and feet

26. What animal is the reservoir for the agent causing the hantavirus pulmonary syndrome?
    The deer mouse, *Peromyscus maniculatus,* is the reservoir for the Sin Nombre virus that causes the hantavirus pulmonary syndrome.

    Childs JE, Ksiazek TJ, Spiropoulou CF, et al: Serologic and genetic identification of *Peromyscus maniculatus* as the primary rodent reservoir for a new hantavirus in the southwestern United States, *J Infect Dis* 169:1271–1280, 1994.

27. **With what syndromes are the various herpesviruses associated?**
    - **Herpes simplex virus (HSV):** Mucocutaneous lesions and encephalitis.
    - **Varicella-zoster virus:** Chickenpox and shingles.
    - **CMV:** Mononucleosis syndrome, meningoencephalitis, transverse myelitis, hepatitis, myocarditis, pneumonitis, esophagitis, colitis, and retinitis, usually in immunocompromised patients.
    - **Epstein-Barr virus:** Infectious mononucleosis, Burkitt's lymphoma, nasopharyngeal carcinoma, and Epstein-Barr virus–related lymphoproliferative syndromes.
    - **Human herpesvirus 6 (HHV-6):** Roseola (exanthem subitum) and nonspecific febrile illnesses in young children; mononucleosis-like syndrome in adults; febrile seizures, meningoencephalitis and encephalitis, hepatitis, opportunistic infections (interstitial pneumonitis) in immunocompromised patients. There may be a possible association with chronic fatigue syndrome, lymphoproliferative disorders, and histiocytic necrotizing lymphadenitis (Kikuchi's syndrome).
    - **HHV-7:** Possibly exanthum subitum–like illness, hepatitis, and encephalitis.
    - **HHV-8:** Kaposi's sarcoma, primary effusion (body cavity based), lymphoma, multicentric Castleman's disease. There may be a possible association with primary pulmonary hypertension.
    - **Herpes B virus:** Myelitis and hemorrhagic encephalitis following primate bites and scratches.

28. **List the more common viral hemorrhagic fevers.**

Rift Valley fever	Ebola hemorrhagic	Dengue hemorrhagic
Crimean-Congo	fever	fever
hemorrhagic fever	Marburg hemorrhagic	
Lassa fever	fever	

29. **What is the distribution and clinical presentation of Dengue fever?**
    Tropics and subtropics, including most countries of the South Pacific, Asia, the Caribbean, and Africa. Dengue fever is transmitted by the *Aedes aegypti* mosquito and is also known as "breakbone fever" because of the severe arthralgias.
    Two syndromes are seen:
    1. Dengue fever characterized by fever, headache, rash, myalgia, and arthralgia, which can be severe
    2. Dengue hemorrhagic fever (DHF) associated with thrombocytopenia, neutropenia, elevated liver enzymes, disseminated intravascular coagulation, and hemorrhagic phenomena such as microscopic hematuria.

30. **What is a prion?**
    An infectious misfolded protein.

31. **What are the human prion diseases and their clinical manifestations?**
    See Table 12-2.

32. **How can you differentiate the dementia of Creutzfeld-Jakob disease (CJD) from Alzheimer's disease (AD)?**
    By careful assessment of associated movement disturbances. Ataxia is most often associated with CJD and hypokinesis with AD.

    Edlar J, Mollenhauer B, Heinemann U, et al: Movement disturbance in the differential diagnosis of Creutzfeld-Jakob disease, *Mov Disord* 24:350–356, 2009.

33. **What are the clinical manifestations of infection due to parvovirus B19?**
    - Erythema infectiousum ("fifth disease")
    - Arthropathy (particularly in adults)

TABLE 12-2. CLINICAL MANIFESTATIONS OF HUMAN PRION DISEASE

Disease	Clinical Manifestations
Sporadic Creutzfeldt-Jakob disease	Rapid mental decline toward dementia
	Myoclonus
Variant Creutzfeldt-Jakob	Sensory disturbances (paresthesia)
	Psychiatric symptoms (depression, anxiety, psychosis)
	Neurologic symptoms (ataxia, mental decline)
Gerstmann-Straussler-Scheinker	Cerebellar degeneration (ataxia, lack of coordination)
	Dementia
	Myoclonus
	Dysarthria
	Nystagmus
	Visual disturbances
Fatal familial insomnia	Progressive insomnia
	Disturbances in autonomic nervous system (hyperthermia and tachycardia)
	Endocrine disorders (decreased ACTH secretion and increased cortisol)
Kuru	Tremors
	Ataxia
	Myoclonus
	Choreoatheotosis
	Dementia
	Indifference

ACTH = adrenocorticotropic hormone.

- Transient aplastic crisis (e.g., in patients with sickle cell anemia)
- Pure red cell aplasia (e.g., in patients with acquired immunodeficiency syndrome [AIDS])
- Virus-associated hemophagocytic syndrome
- Hydrops fetalis

34. **What microbial agents are considered potential biologic warfare agents?**
See Table 12-3.

FUNGAL INFECTIONS

35. **Which species of *Candida* are considered resistant to the -azole class of antifungals?**
Candida krusei, which is inherently resistant, and *Candida glabarata,* which demonstrates dose-dependent resistance.

36. **Which species of *Candida* is considered resistant to amphotericin B?**
Candida lusitaniae.

TABLE 12-3. INFECTIOUS AGENTS WITH POTENTIAL USE IN BIOLOGICAL WARFARE AND THEIR SYMPTOMS AND DISEASES

Infectious Agent	Symptoms and Diseases
Bacteria	
Bacillus anthracis	Inhalational and cutaneous anthrax
Brucella spp.	Debilitating flulike illness
Burkholderia mallei	Usually causes glanders in horses but can cause skin and pulmonary infections and sepsis
Coxiella burnetii	Flulike illness, pneumonia, hepatitis
Francisella tularensis	Various forms including pneumonic
Clostridium botulinum	Visual symptoms and muscle weakness leading to respiratory muscle paralysis
C. perfringens	Watery diarrhea, gangrene
Salmonella spp.	Inflammatory diarrhea, typhoid fever
Shigella dysenteriae	Inflammatory diarrhea
Yersinia pestis	Plague (bubonic, pneumonic, septicemic)
Escherichia coli O157:H7	Bloody diarrhea, hemolytic uremic syndrome
Vibrio cholera	Cholera with severe diarrhea and dehydration
Cryptosporidium parvum	Diarrhea, cholecystitis
Multidrug-resistant tuberculosis	Tuberculosis symptoms
Viruses	
Alphaviruses (Venezuelan and eastern and western equine)	Encephalitis
Hantaviruses	Hemorrhagic fever with renal syndrome, Hantavirus cardiopulmonary syndrome
Tick-borne encephalitis	Fever, myalgia, meningitis, encephalitis
Nipah virus	Encephalitis
Arenaviruses (Lassa, Junin)	Lassa fever, hemorrhagic fever
Filoviruses (Ebola and Marburg)	Hemorrhagic fever
Smallpox	Rash, following prodrome of fever and headache/myalgia
Yellow fever	Fever, jaundice, renal failure, and hemorrhage

From Centers for Disease Control and Prevention: Biological and chemical terrorism: Strategic plan for preparedness and response. Recommendations of the CDC Strategic Planning Workgroup. MMWR Morb Mortal Wkly Rep 49(RR-4):1–14, 2000.

37. **What disease should be considered in a diabetic with ketoacidosis and black eschar in the nasal mucosa?**
Rhinocerebral mucormycosis. The zygomycete fungi (*Rhizopus, Mucor, Rhizomucor,* and *Absidia*) can cause this clinical entity that is rapidly progressive with a mortality up to 50%. Therapy includes aggressive surgical debridement and amphotericin B.

38. **List the clinical settings and risk factors associated with *Candida* infections.**
Chronic mucocutaneous infections:
- Defects in T-lymphocyte immunity, either congenital or acquired (e.g., AIDS)

Deeply invasive, disseminated infections:
- Peripheral neutrophil count < 500/mm^3
- Mucosal barrier breakdown (burn, cytotoxic agents, gastrointestinal surgery, or IV catheter sites)
- Broad-spectrum antibiotic use with *Candida* overgrowth
- Indwelling catheter

    Pappas PG, Rex JH, Sobel JD, et al: Guidelines for the treatment of candidiasis, *Clin Infect Dis* 38:161–189, 2004.

39. **What is a dimorphic fungus?**
One that grows both mycelia and yeast forms depending on conditions.

40. **List the clinically important dimorphic fungi and the diseases they cause.**
See Table 12-4.

TABLE 12-4. DISEASES CAUSED BY DIMORPHIC FUNGI	
Fungus	**Disease**
Histoplasma	Pneumonia
	Disseminated disease with bone marrow and adrenal involvement
	Ulcers and polyploidy masses in mouth, esophagus, stomach, small and large intestines, and colon; cutaneous lesions
	Meningitis, encephalitis
Blastomyces	Pneumonia
	Skin lesions (typically a verrucous lesion), osteomyelitis
	Prostatitis
	Disseminated disease
Coccidioides	Valley fever
	Pneumonia (with symptoms similar to community-acquired pneumonia)
	Cutaneous disease
	Meningitis
	Osteomyelitis
	Arthritis
Sporothrix	Cutaneous (lymphocutaneous) disease
	Pneumonia (with symptoms similar to tuberculosis)
	Joint infection
Paracoccidioides	Pneumonia with or without cavitary lesions
	Cutaneous disease (ulcerative lesions that may infiltrate the skin)
	Ulcerative lesions of the mucosa of the mouth, nose, or larynx
Penicillium	Pneumonia
	Cutaneous lesions
	Keratitis, endophthalmitis

KEY POINTS: INFECTIONS CAUSED BY DIMORPHIC FUNGI ✓

1. *Penicillium marneffei* can cause disease in patients with AIDS and other immunosuppressions.

2. Consider histoplasmosis in patients with adrenal insufficiency.

3. Sporotrichosis is also called "alcoholic rose gardener's disease."

AIDS = acquired immunodeficiency virus.

41. **What are the major pulmonary syndromes associated with *Aspergillus* spp.?**
    - **Allergic bronchopulmonary aspergillosis** (ABPA): Occurs in patients with asthma who have eosinophilia, transient pulmonary infiltrates thought to be due to bronchial plugging, and elevated serum IgE and IgG antibody to aspergillus.
    - **Aspergilloma** (fungus ball): Results from colonization and growth of aspergillus, usually within a preexisting pulmonary cavity.
    - **Invasive aspergillosis:** Usually occurs in individuals with profound granulocytopenia and it is being described more frequently in patients with AIDS.
    - **Chronic necrotizing aspergillosis:** Slowly progressive form of invasive aspergillosis that occurs in patients with an underlying lung disease (chronic obstructive pulmonary disease, sarcoid, pneumoconiosis, or inactive tuberculosis) or mild systemic immunocompromising illness (low-dose corticosteroids, diabetes mellitus, alcoholism). These patients usually have a chronic infiltrate that may slowly progress to cavitation of aspergilloma formation.

    Latge JP: Aspergillus fumigatus and aspergillosis, *Clin Microbiol Rev* 12:310–350, 1999.

42. **How are pulmonary syndromes associated with *Aspergillus* spp. treated?**
    - **ABPA:** Corticosteroids have been used traditionally, although anecdotal reports suggest itraconazole may have a role.
    - **Aspergilloma:** No specific treatment is usually given unless significant hemoptysis occurs, in which case surgical excision is performed.
    - **Invasive aspergillosis:** Amphotericin B or one of the newer liposomal preparations, caspofungin or voriconazole, with or without surgical excision, are options for therapy. Many experts recommend the newer -azole, voriconazole, as preferred therapy for *Aspergillus* infections.

PARASITIC INFECTIONS

43. **Which species of *Plasmodium* have a dormant phase in the liver (hypnozoites)?**
    Plasmodium vivax and *Plasmodium ovale*. These species also need to be treated differently to avoid relapse as a result of the hypnozoites.

44. **Why is malaria caused by *Plasmodium falciparum* more severe than other species?**
    Because *Plasmodium falciparum* can infect red blood cells of any age and size, leading to red cell clumping and blockage of small vessel blood flow. The diminished blood flow can lead to severe hypoxic damage, especially in the brain and kidneys.

45. **What is "blackwater fever"?**
Intravascular hemolysis, hemoglobulinuria, and renal failure due to tubular necrosis seen in patients with falciparum malaria exposed to quinine. The urine appears dark owing to hemoglobin deposition.

46. **What chronic infection appears as linear calcifications seen in the wall of the urinary bladder on a roentgenogram?**
Schistosoma haematobium. The eggs are deposited in the submucosa and mucosa of the bladder. The subsequent inflammatory response leads to scarring and calcium deposition.

47. **What is the "hyperinfection" syndrome associated with *Strongyloides stercoralis*?**
The symptoms of abdominal pain, diarrhea, vomiting, shock, fever, cough, and decreased mental status due to dissemination of the filariform larval stage. Hyperinfection syndrome due to *S. stercoralis* is the result of systemic dissemination by the filariform larva in individuals who are immunocompromised, primarily with defects in cell-mediated immunity. Bacteremia occurs frequently, usually with enteric organisms that are thought to accompany the larvae as they migrate through the bowel wall.

48. **What is kala-azar?**
Visceral leishmaniasis, caused by various species of *Leishmania* (*Leishmania donovani, Leishmania infantum,* and *Leishmania chagasi*). The *Leishmania* are transmitted by the bite of a sandfly, which transfers promastigotes of the organism to the host. Clinical findings include fever and splenomegaly with or without hepatomegaly. The diagnosis is made by a splenic or bone marrow aspirate showing amastigotes.

49. **Infection with which species of *Trypanosoma* can lead to dilated cardiomyopathy, conduction abnormalities, and megacolon?**
Trypanosoma cruzi, the causative agent of Chagas' disease, which can lead to the complications described if untreated. In addition, megaesophagus and achalasia have been described. *Trypanosoma brucei* causes African sleeping sickness.

50. **Which nematodes (roundworms) are able to infect the host by penetration of the skin?**
S. stercoralis, Ancylostoma duodenale, and *Necator americanus.*

51. **What is the clinical manifestation of pinworm infection?**
Rectal or perirectal area itching that is worse at night. Infection by *Enterobius vermicularis* is usually acquired by ingestion of eggs. The eggs hatch and mature in the host and the adult female worm migrates to the rectal area to lay eggs.

52. **What is Katayama fever?**
A manifestation of acute schistosomiasis that includes fever, urticarial rash, and hepatosplenomegaly. *Schistosoma japonicum* is most commonly associated with this clinical syndrome.

53. **List the tissue flukes and their typical associations.**
   - ***Fasciolopsis buski:*** The infectious stage (metacercariae) is found in aquatic plants such as water chestnuts, lotus roots, and water bamboo.

- *Fasciola hepatica:* A large liver fluke of sheep that can infect humans through ingestion of a meal that contains infected watercress, chestnuts, or bamboo shoots.
- *Clonorchis sinensis:* A liver fluke that can block bile ducts and lead to jaundice and cholangitis, just as caused by *Fasciola. Clonorchis* is acquired by ingestion of metacercaria in undercooked or raw freshwater fish.
- *Paragonimus westermani:* A lung fluke, acquired by ingestion of the organism in raw or pickled crawfish or freshwater crabs.

54. **What is tungiasis?**
A disease of the skin, caused by infestation by the flea, *Tunga penetrans*. The disease is endemic in areas of Africa and South and Central America. Treatment consists of surgical removal of the flea; antiparasitic medications are not effective.

55. **What is the causative agent of "river blindness"?**
Onchocerca volvulus, which is transmitted by the bite of a black fly that deposits the larvae onto the skin. Onchocerciasis initially presents with an itchy, erythematous rash with formation of fibrous skin nodules later in the disease. Eye lesions also occur that lead to blindness. The incidence of onchocerciasis has been markedly reduced in central African countries through vector control and oral medication use.

56. **Which infectious agents have been reported to be transmitted by blood transfusion?**
See Table 12-5.

TABLE 12-5. INFECTIOUS AGENTS THAT CAN TRANSMIT DISEASE THROUGH BLOOD TRANSFUSION

Viral	Nonviral
Hepatitis (A, B, C and D)	*Treponema pallidum*
Hepatitis G	(syphilis)
HIV-1 and HIV-2	*Babesia microti*
HTLV I and II	*Plasmodium* spp. (malaria)
CMV	*Trypanosoma cruzi* (Chagas' disease)
Human herpes virus 8	*Leishmania* spp.
West Nile virus	*Toxoplasma gondii*
Anelloviridiae (TT virus or	*Yersini enterocolitica*
Thetatorqueirus and its variant,	*Serratia* spp.
SEN virus)	*Pseudomonas* spp.
EBV	*Bacillus cereus*

CMV = cytomegalovirus; EBV = Epstein-Barr virus; HIV = human immunodeficiency virus; HTLV = human T-lymphotrophic virus.
Adapted from Chamberland ME: Emerging infectious agents: Do they pose a risk to the safety of transfused blood and blood products? Clin Infect Dis 34:e797–e805, 2002.

57. **What occupations are associated with an increased risk of** *Chlamydia psittaci* **infection?**
    - Pet shop employees
    - Pigeon fanciers
    - Zoo workers
    - Veterinarians
    - Poultry processors
    These workers usually present with fever, headache, myalgias, and dry cough that can progress to severe disease involving multiple organ systems.

58. **Extrusion of "sulfur granules" from a draining wound is characteristic of which infection?**
    Actinomyces spp. These organisms characteristically form external sinuses, which discharge "sulfur granules" consisting of conglomerate masses of branching filaments cemented together and mineralized by host calcium phosphate stimulated by tissue inflammation. The granules do not contain sulfur.

59. **List the infectious causes of adrenal insufficiency.**
    - *Mycobacterium tuberculosis*
    - Fungi (*Histoplasma capsulatum, Cryptococcus neoformans, Cryptococcus immitis, S. schenckii, Blastomyces dermatitidis, Paracoccidioides brasiliensis*)
    - *Neisseria meningitidis* (in Waterhouse-Friderichsen syndrome) and other organisms causing shock
    - Human immunodeficiency virus (HIV) infection
    - *Mycobacterium avium* complex (MAI)
    - CMV

    Painter BF: Infectious causes of adrenal insufficiency, *Infect Med* 11:515–520, 1994.

60. **Which organisms most commonly cause infectious complications after bites?**
    Human bites:
    - Streptococci (alpha and group A beta-hemolytic)
    - *S. aureus*
    - *Eikenella corrodens*
    - *Peptostreptococcus* spp.
    - *Bacteroides* spp.
    - *Fusobacterium* spp.
    Cat or dog bites:
    - *Pasteurella multocida*
    - *Capnocytophaga canimorsus* (DF-2)
    - Rabies
    Cat bites:
    - Tularemia
    Dog bites:
    - Brucellosis
    - EF-4
    - Blastomycosis

    Goldstein EJC: Bite wounds and infection, *Clin Infect Dis* 14:633–640, 1992.

61. What are the infectious causes of parotitis?

VIRAL

Mumps
Influenza
Parainfluenza types 1 and 3
Coxsackievirus A and B
ECHO (enteropathic cytopathogenic
human orphan virus)
Lymphocytic choriomeningitis
Anaerobic organisms
HIV

BACTERIAL

S. aureus
Streptococcus pneumoniae
Enteric gram-negative bacilli
Haemophilus influenzae
Actinomyces spp.
M. tuberculosis
Salmonella typhi
B. pseudomallei

62. What is the differential diagnosis of exudative pharyngitis?

Streptococci groups A,
C, and G
*Arcanobacterium
hemolyticum*
N. gonorrhoeae

*Corynebacterium
diphtheriae*
Anaerobic bacteria
HIV-1
Yersinia enterocolitica

*Mycoplasma
pneumonia*
Adenovirus
HSV
Epstein-Barr virus

63. What are the most common pathogens seen in months 2–6 after solid organ transplantation?

VIRUSES

CMV
Epstein-Barr virus
Varicella-zoster virus
Papovavirus (BK and JC)
Adenovirus
HSV
Non-A, non-B hepatitis

MISCELLANEOUS

Aspergillus
Nocardia
Toxoplasma
Cryptococcus
Pneumocystis jiroveci
Legionella spp.
Listeria monocytogenes

64. What is the differential diagnosis of monocytosis?

INFECTIOUS

Tuberculosis
Epstein-Barr virus mononucleosis
Rocky Mountain spotted fever (RMSF)
Diphtheria
Subacute bacterial endocarditis
Histoplasmosis
Typhus
Brucellosis
Kala-azar
Malaria
Syphilis
Recovery from neutropenia
Recovery from chronic infection

NONINFECTIOUS

Myeloproliferative disorders
Lymphomas
Solid tumors
Gaucher's disease
Regional enteritis
Ulcerative colitis
Sprue
Rheumatoid arthritis
Systemic lupus erythematosus
Polyarteritis nodosa
Post-splenectomy
Sarcoidosis

65. **What is the differential diagnosis of atypical lymphocytosis in patients with > 20% atypical lymphocytes?**
Mononucleosis caused by Epstein-Barr virus or CMV.

66. **What is the differential diagnosis of atypical lymphocytosis in patients with < 20% atypical lymphocytes?**

INFECTIOUS	NONINFECTIOUS
Rubella	Drug fever
HSV	Dermatitis herpetiformis
Varicella-zoster	Radiation therapy
Tuberculosis	Stress
Brucellosis	Lead intoxication
Smallpox	Drug hypersensitivity reaction
Babesiosis	
Ehrlichiosis	
Rubeola	
Roseola infantum (HHV-6)	
Influenza	
Syphilis	
Toxoplasmosis	
Malaria	
RMSF	

67. **If a patient with no prior history of tetanus vaccination recovers from an episode of tetanus, is she or he at risk for a second episode?**
Yes. The occurrence of tetanus does not prevent second episodes of clinical disease from occurring because the amount of toxin needed to produce the clinical syndrome is so small that it is usually not immunogenic. Persons recovering from tetanus should be vaccinated with tetanus toxoid against future episodes of the disease (see also Chapter 2, General Medicine and Ambulatory Care).

MYCOBACTERIAL INFECTIONS

68. **What is scrofula?**
Cervical lymphadenitis, which is the most common presentation of extrapulmonary tuberculosis. Scrofula refers to painless swelling of the cervical and supraclavicular lymph nodes that is most often caused by *M. tuberculosis* in adults and nontuberculous mycobacteria in children. *Mycobacterium avium-intracellulare* (MAI), *Mycobacterium scrofulaceum,* and *Mycobacterium bovis* have been reported in cases on scrofula.

69. **What is a Ghon complex?**
The lung lesion of primary tuberculosis that consists of the area of initial infection with the bacilli and associated lymphadenopathy. The lesion will decrease in size over time and may become calcified, allowing it to be visible on chest x-ray.

70. **Which mycobacterial species should be considered when a patient who works in an aquarium presents with nodular skin lesions?**
Mycobacteriuim marinum. This organism is found in both salt and fresh water environments and can cause localized granulomas, often associated with lymphangitic spread. Treatment

is usually prolonged (several weeks) and includes surgical débridement when necessary. The organism is notably resistant to isoniazid, which is a mainstay of therapy for other mycobacteria, particularly *M. tuberculosis*.

71. **What is Lady Windermere syndrome?**
A specific pulmonary syndrome caused by MAI. The syndrome is named after the title character of Oscar Wilde's play, "Lady Windermere's Fan," who was extremely genteel and unlikely to cough in public. The syndrome results from cough suppression and is more commonly seen in women. Pulmonary involvement is typically limited to lingula or middle lobe. These patients usually have no underlying lung disease and present with symptoms of bronchitis.

   Tryfon S, Angelis N, Klein L, et al: Lady Windermere syndrome after cardiac surgery procedure: A case of *Mycobacterium avium* complex pneumonia, *Ann Thorac Surg* 89:1296–1299, 2010.

72. **List the mycobacteria that most commonly cause pulmonary disease in patients with HIV.**
   - *M. tuberculosis*
   - MAI
   - *Mycobacteriuim kansasii*

73. **What is Pott's disease?**
An extrapulmonary manifestation of *M. tuberculosis* infection that affects the spine. Complications of this disease include collapse of vertebral bodies (gibbus) as well as chest wall and psoas abscesses.

74. **What is XDR tuberculosis?**
Extensively drug-resistant tuberculosis, which includes resistance to the first-line agents (isoniazid, rifampin, pyrazinamide, and ethambutol) as well as resistance to second-line agents (fluoroquinolones) and at least one of three other agents (amikacin, kanamycin, or capreomycin).

KEY POINTS: TUBERCULOSIS ✓

1. Consider genitourinary tuberculosis in the patient with sterile pyuria.
2. Most tuberculosis cases are due to reactivation of primary infection.
3. John Keats, Frederick Chopin, and Robert Louis Stevenson all had tuberculosis.

75. **What is Hansen's disease?**
Leprosy, caused by *Mycobacterium leprae*, a disease with a variety of clinical manifestations. Patients have visible skin lesions as well as lesions of the peripheral nervous system.

ANTI-INFECTIVE AGENTS

76. **What is the antimicrobial spectrum of penicillins?**
Narrow spectrum for penicillin G including:
   - *S. pyogenes*
   - *S. pneumoniae* (except for those strains with beta-lactam resistance)
   - Oropharyngeal anaerobes
   - *Treponema pallidum*

Broad spectrum for ticarcillin-clavulinate and piperacillin-clavulinate including:
- Gram-positives
- Gram-negatives
- Anaerobes

77. **How do the penicillins work?**
By binding to PBPs and inhibiting cell wall synthesis. Cephalosporins, carbapenems, and monobactams have a similar mechanism of action.

78. **First- and second-generation cephalosporins are more effective than third-generation cephalosporins against which organisms?**
Gram-positives.

79. **List the cephalosporins and the generation to which they belong.**
- **First:** cefazolin, cephalexin, cephradine, cefadroxil
- **Second:** cefoxitin, cefotetan, cefuroxime, cefaclor
- **Third:** ceftriaxone, cefotaxime, ceftizoxime, ceftazidime, cefixime, cefpodoxim
- **Fourth:** cefepime

80. **What is the spectrum of carbapenems?**
Broad-spectrum, including gram-positive, gram-negative, and anaerobic organisms.

81. **Which antibiotics cross-react with penicillins and can lead to allergic reactions in patients with type I immunoglobulin E (IgE)–mediated penicillin allergy?**
Cephalosporins and carbapenems.

82. **What beta-lactam antibiotic could be safely used in patients allergic to penicillins?**
Aztreonam, which covers only aerobic gram-negative organisms.

> Patriarca G, Shiavino D, Altomonto G, et al: Tolerability of aztreonam in patients with IgE-mediated hypersensitivity to beta-lactams, *Int J Immunopathol Pharmacol* 21:357–359, 2008.

> Kishiyama JL, Adelman DC: The cross-reactivity and immunology of beta-lactam antibiotics, *Drug Saf* 10:318–327, 1994.

83. **Which antibiotics inhibit protein synthesis at the *50S* ribosomal subunit?**
- Macrolides and ketolides
- Clindamycin
- Chloramphenicol
- Oxazolidones (linezolid)
- Streptogramins (quinupristin, dalfopristin)

84. **Which antibiotics inhibit protein synthesis by binding to the *30S* ribosomal subunit?**
Tetracyclines and aminoglycosides, through interaction with DNA and other anionic components.

85. **Which antibiotics inhibit DNA gyrase and topoisomerase?**
Fluoroquinolones, which are bactericidal with a relatively broad spectrum but limited anaerobic activity. Gatifloxacin has been removed from the U.S. market owing to problems with blood glucose levels. Ciprofloxacin has little activity against *S. pneumoniae* and is not indicated for treatment of community-acquired pneumonia.

86. **Which antibiotics typically have activity against CA-MRSA?**

Rifampin
Trimethoprim-
   sulfamethoxazole
Clindamycin (but may
   have inducible

clindamycin
   resistance)
Linezolid
Doxycycline
Synercid

Vancomycin
Daptomycin
Tigecycline

87. **What are the major classes of antifungals and their mechanisms of action?**
Azoles, echinocandins, and polyenes. **Azoles** (including fluconazole, itraconazole, and voriconazole) are considered fungistatic agents. These antifungals interact with 14-α-demythlase, which prevents conversion of lanosterol to ergosterol, an integral part of the cell membrane. **Echinocandins** (including caspofungin, anidulafungin, and micafungin) are fungicidal through inhibition of 1-3-β-D-glucan synthase. Although active against many *Candida* species, they have limited activity against *Aspergillus* species. **Polyenes** (including amphotericin B) are fungicidal and bind to ergosterol in the fungal membrane to form channels that allow the efflux (leakage) of intracellular potassium, leading to fungal cell death. These agents are very broad spectrum and cover a variety of fungi.

88. **What is an ESBL?**
Extended-spectrum beta-lactamase. These enzymes can hydrolyze penicillins, broad-spectrum cephalosporins, and monobactams and are typically produced by members of the family *Enterobacteriacae*, which includes *E. coli* and *Klebsiella pneumonia*. Infections caused by organisms producing ESBLs are treated with carbapenems as a general rule.

Shah AA, Hasan F, Ahmed S, et al: Extended-spectrum β-lactamases (ESBLs): Characterization, epidemiology and detection, *Crit Rev Microbiol* 30:25–32, 2004.

89. **What antibiotic causes linear IgA bullous dermatosis?**
Vancomycin. Bullous dermatosis is an autoimmune disease caused by IgA deposition at the basement membrane zone, which eventually leads to loss of adhesion at the dermal-epidermal junction and blister formation. Vancomycin has also been reported to cause "red-man" syndrome (flushing/red rash affecting the face, neck, and torso), neutropenia, thrombocytopenia, nephro- and ototoxicity, toxic epidermal necrolysis, and fever.

Bernstein E, Schuster M: Linear IgA bullous dermatosis associated with vancomycin, *Ann Intern Med* 129:508–509, 1998.

Rocha JL, Kondo W, Baptista MI, et al: Uncommon vancomycin-induced side effects, *Braz J Infect Dis* 6:196–200, 2002.

90. **What electrolytes should be closely monitored with amphotericin B administration?**
Potassium, magnesium, and to a lesser extent, calcium. Amphotericin B is well known to cause both hypokalemia and hypomagnesemia. Other severe reactions that occur during infusion include fever, chills, hypotension, headache, nausea, and tachypnea.

91. **What are the pleuromutilin antibiotics?**
A newer class of antibiotics that bind to the *50S* subunit of bacteria, inhibit peptidyl transferase, and interact with domain V of 23S RNA. Their spectrum includes gram-positive bacteria (including *S. aureus* and *S. pyogenes*) but no activity against *Enterococcus* or gram-negative bacilli. Pleuromutilin antibiotics were developed to provide activity against organisms that are resistant to various antibiotics. Agents in this class include retapamulin, taimulin, and valnemulin.

Yang LP, Keam SJ: Spotlight on retapamulin in impetigo and other uncomplicated superficial skin infections, *Am J Clin Dermatol* 9:411–413, 2008.

HEAD AND NECK INFECTIONS

92. **What is Ludwig's angina?**
Cellulitis involving the sublingual and submaxillary spaces, usually arising from a dental infection. Patients often appear quite ill with swelling below the angle of the jaw. Airway obstruction is frequently a concern due to edema in the sublingual space that forces the tongue into a superior and posterior position. Cervical lymphadenopathy does not usually occur.

93. **What is Vincent's angina?**
A severe form of gingivitis (also called "acute ulcerative gingivitis" or "trench mouth") that leads to ulceration and necrosis of the gingiva with pain and bleeding of the gums. Unlike Ludwig's angina, lymphadenopathy is common. The causative organisms are usually oral anaerobes that are treated with penicillin plus metronidazole.

94. **What is Lemierre's syndrome?**
Jugular vein septic thrombophlebitis. Also called "postanginal sepsis," this syndrome typically starts with tonsillitis or a peritonsillar abscess that affects the deep pharyngeal space and drains into the lateral pharyngeal space. Septic emboli to the lung and other sites may occur. The initial infection is classically associated with *Fusobacterium necrophorum*, although other organisms, including *S. aureus, Bacteroides fragilis, Peptostreptococcus,* and anaerobic streptococci, have been reported.

> Riordan T: Human infection with *Fusobacterium necrophorum* (necrobacillosis), with a focus on Lemierre's syndrome, *Clin Microbiol* 20:622–659, 2007.

> Puymirat E, Biais M, et al: A Lemierre syndrome variant caused by *Staphylococcus aureus, Am J Emerg Med* 26:380, e5–e7, 2008.

95. **What infection, associated with airway compromise, has decreased since the advent of *Haemophilus influenzae* type B (HiB) vaccine?**
Acute epiglottitis, a rapidly progressive cellulitis of the epiglottis classically caused by *H. influenzae.*

96. **What is Pott's puffy tumor?**
Subperiosteal abscess that results from edema of the frontal bone as a complication of frontal sinusitis.

97. **List the complications of frontal, ethmoid, and sphenoid sinusitis.**
See Table 12-6.

TABLE 12-6. COMPLICATIONS OF SINUSITIS	
Sinus Involved	**Complication**
Frontal	Pott's puffy tumor; epidural, subdural or brain abscess
Ethmoid	Periorbital and orbital cellulitis, orbital abscess, cavernous sinus thrombosis, meningitis
Sphenoid	Septic cavernous sinus thrombosis, meningitis

98. **What are the clinical manifestations of sinusitis?**
- Nasal congestion
- Rhinorrhea (which may be purulent)
- Facial pain or pressure
- Maxillary tooth pain

99. **What is the most common cause of acute sinusitis?**
Viruses including adenoviruses, influenza virus, and parainfluenza virus, making antibiotics generally ineffective.

Gwaltney JM Jr: Acute community-acquired sinusitis, *Clin Infect Dis* 23:1209–1223, 1996.

100. **List the frequency of the most common bacterial causes of acute sinusitis in adults.**
See Table 12-7.

TABLE 12-7.   FREQUENCY OF ISOLATION OF BACTERIA IN SINUSITIS

Organism	Frequency (%)
Streptococcus pneumoniae	31–35
Haemophilus influenzae (unencapsulated)	12–40
Moraxella catarrhalis	8–20
Mixed	5
Staphylococcus aureus	4
Anaerobic bacteria (*Bacteroides, Peptococcus, Fusobacterium*)	2–6
Streptococcus pyogenes	2

From Brook I: Acute and chronic bacterial sinusitis. Infect Dis Clin North Am 21:427–428, 2007.

101. **What are causes of eosinophilic meningitis?**
See Table 12-8.

TABLE 12-8.   CAUSES OF EOSINOPHILIC MENINGITIS

Infectious

Bacterial	*Mycobacterium tuberculosis, Rickettsia rickettsii, Treponema pallidum*
Viral	LCM, Coxsackie B4
Fungal	*Coccidioides immitis*
Parasitic	*Angiostrongylus catonensis, Gnathstoma, Baylisascaris, Paragonimus westermanii, Trichinella spiralis, Toxocara canis, Taenia soleum, Fasciola hepatica, Trypanosoma, Toxoplasma gondii, Schistosoma japonicum*

Noninfectious

Drugs	Ciprofloxacin, intraventricular vancomycin, gentamicin, ibuprofen
Malignancy	Non-Hodgkin's lymphoma, Hodgkin's disease, leukemia
Other	Sarcoidosis, ventriculoperitoneal shunts

LCM = lymphocytic choriomeningitis virus.
From Re V, Lo II, Gluckman SJ: Eosinophilic meningitis. Am J Med 144:217–223, 2003.

102. **What drugs cause aseptic meningitis?**
- Antibiotics (trimethoprim-sulfamethoxazole, trimethoprim, sulfamethoxazole, penicillin, cephalosporins, metronidazole)
- Cetuxamib
- Carbamazepine
- Intravenous immunoglobublin (IVIG)
- Nonsteroidal anti-inflammatory drugs (NSAIDs)
- OKT3 antibodies
- Ranitidine
- Rofecoxib

103. **Which bacteria most commonly cause community-acquired meningitis?**

S. pneumonia	Streptococci	S. aureus
N. meningitides	other than	H. influenzae
L. monocytogenes	S. pneumonia	

104. **Who should receive adjunctive steroids when being treated for meningitis?**
Patients with meningitis due to *S. pneumoniae* and admitted with a Glasgow Coma Scale (GCS) of 8–11 (see Chapter 17, Neurology). Note that steroids may be harmful in some subsets of patients and many experts would not use steroids in meningitis caused by other bacteria.

Van De Beek D, de Gans J, Tunkel AR, et al: Community-acquired bacterial meningitis in adults, *N Engl J Med* 354:44–53, 2006.

105. **What antibiotic could be used to treat *Listeria* meningitis in a patient allergic to penicillin?**
Trimethoprim-sulfamethoxazole.

106. **Who should receive postexposure prophylaxis for *Neisseria* meningitis?**
- Health-care workers with close contact to the infected patient or exposure to oral secretions (i.e., intubation)
- Household contacts
- Contacts residing in close quarters such as military barracks, nursery schools, and college dormitories

107. **What are some characteristics of human cestode infections?**
See Table 12-9.

TABLE 12-9. COMMON HUMAN CESTODE INFECTIONS

Species	Stage Found in Humans	Common Name	Pathology	Therapy
Diphyllobothrium latum	Adult	Fish tapeworm	Pernicious anemia	Niclosamide, praziquantel
Hymenolepis nana	Adult	Dwarf tapeworm	Rarely symptomatic	Niclosamide, praziquantel
Taenia saginata	Adult	Beef tapeworm	Rarely symptomatic	Niclosamide, praziquantel

(continued)

TABLE 12-9.   COMMON HUMAN CESTODE INFECTIONS—*(continued)*

Species	Stage Found in Humans	Common Name	Pathology	Therapy
T. solium	Adult	Pork tapeworm	Rarely symptomatic	Niclosamide, praziquantel
	Larva	Cysticercosis	Brain and tissue cysts	Albendazole, praziquantel, surgery
Echinococcus granulosus	Larva	Hydatid cyst disease	Solitary tissue cysts	Surgery, albendazole
E. multilocularis	Larva	Alveolar cyst disease	Multilocular cysts	Surgery, albendazole
Taenia multiceps	Larva	Bladderworm, coenurosis	Brain and eye cysts	Surgery
Spirometra mansonoides	Larva	Sparganosis	Subcutaneous larvae	Surgery

From King CK: Cestode Infections. In Goldman L, Ausiello D (eds): Cecil Textbook of Medicine, 23rd ed. Philadelphia, WB Saunders, 2008.

ENDOCARDITIS

108. **What are the major and minor Duke criteria for diagnosing infective endocarditis?**

Major
- Positive blood cultures with an organism typical for endocarditis (viridans streptococci, *S. aureus*, enterococci, or HACEK [see Question 111]) in at least two separate cultures drawn 12 hours apart
- Evidence of endocardial involvement (positive echocardiogram or new/worsening regurgitant murmur)

Minor
- Predisposition (predisposing heart condition or IV drug abuse)
- Fever
- Vascular phenomena: Janeway lesions, septic pulmonary emboli, major arterial emboli, mycotic aneurysm, conjunctival hemorrhages
- Immunologic phenomena: Osler's nodes, glomerulonephritis, positive rheumatoid factor, Roth spots
- Microbiologic evidence: positive blood culture not meeting major criteria

Endocarditis is **definitely** diagnosed by the presence of:
1. Histologic evidence of endocarditis from abscess or valve vegetations or
2. Gram stain or culture evidence of endocarditis from surgical or autopsy specimen or
3. Presence of two major clinical criteria or
4. Presence of one major and three minor clinical criteria or
5. Five minor criteria

Endocarditis is **possibly** diagnosed by the presence of:
1. One major and one or two minor criteria or
2. Three minor criteria

109. **Endocarditis with which organisms should prompt a work-up for a gastrointestinal malignancy?**
Streptococcus bovis (now called *"Streptococcus gallolyticus"*) and *Clostridium septicum.*

Ridgway EJ, Grech ED: Clostridial endocarditis: report of a case caused by *Clostridium septicum* and review of the literature, *J Infect* 26:309–313, 1993.

110. **What organisms are most commonly associated with prosthetic valve endocarditis?**
Late (>12 mo after surgery)
- *Staphylococcus epidermidis*
- *Streptococci*
- HACEK
Early (<12 mo after surgery)
- *S. aureus*
- Gram-negative bacilli

111. **What are the HACEK organisms?**
- *Haemophilus arphrophilus*
- *Actinobacillus actinomycetemcomitans*
- *Cardiobacterium hominis*
- *Eikenella corrodens*
- *Kingella kingae*

Recently, *A. actinomycetemcomitans* and *H. arphrophilus* have been placed into the new genus *Aggregatibacter*. These organisms can be isolated from blood cultures that are held for at least 5 days.

112. **Which organism is associated with endocarditis in IV drug users?**
P. aeruginosa. The organism is thought to contaminate water used to mix drugs or store drug paraphernalia. Right-sided endocarditis with *S. aureus* is also well described in IV drug abusers.

113. **What organisms have been implicated in culture-negative endocarditis?**

Coxiella burnetti (also the agent of Q fever)	*Granulicatella*	Intracellular organisms (*Rickettsia* and
Tropheryma whippeli	*Mycoplasma hominis* Nutritionally deficient streptococci	*Chlamydia* spp.)
Aiotrophia elegans	*Brucella* spp.	Fungi Anaerobic organisms

Houpikian P, Raoult D: Blood culture-negative endocarditis in a reference center: Etiologic diagnosis of 348 cases, *Medicine (Baltimore)* 84:162–173, 2005.

PULMONARY INFECTIONS

114. **Which organisms cause severe disease in asplenic patients?**
Encapsulated organisms such as *S. pneumoniae, H. influenzae,* and *N. meningitides.*
Asplenic patients have decreased ability to clear opsonized antigens, decreased IgM levels,

and poor antibody production. Gram-negative organisms such as *Klebsiella* and *E. coli,* *Capnocytophaga canimorsus, Babesia microti,* and *Plasmodium falciparum* may all pose a higher risk in this patient population.

Cadili A, de Gara C: Complications of splenectomy, *Am J Med* 121:371–375, 2008.

115. **What organisms most frequently cause community-acquired pneumonia?**

S. pneumoniae	Anaerobic bacteria	Respiratory viruses
M. pneumoniae	*H. influenzae*	*S. aureus*
Chlamydophila	*Legionella pneumophila*	
pneumoniae		

116. **What organisms cause post-influenza bacterial pneumonia?**
    - *S. pneumonia*
    - *S. aureus* (including CA-MRSA)
    - *H. influenzae*

    Rothberg MB, Haessler SD, Brown RB: Complications of viral influenza, *Am J Med* 121:258–264, 2008.

117. **What constitutes an adequate sputum sample in the diagnosis of pneumonia?**
    One with < 10 epithelial cells and > 25 polymorphonuclear leukocytes (PMNs) on Gram stain per low-power field.

118. **What are the clinical findings and treatment of diphtheria?**
    Fever, pharyngitis, and cervical adenopathy associated with adherent pharyngeal membranes. Patients may present with stridor, hoarseness, and paralysis of the palate as well. Cultures on special media (Tindale's media that reveals black colonies with halos) and detection of toxin are used to confirm the diagnosis. Erythromycin and penicillin G are recommended antibiotics.

KEY POINTS: CLNICAL CLUES FOR DIPHTHERIA ✓

1. Mildly painful tonsillitis or pharyngitis associated with gray palatal membrane.

2. Cervical lymphadenopathy and neck swelling.

3. Hoarseness and stridor.

4. Unilateral palatal paralysis.

5. Moderate temperature elevation.

6. Serosanguineous nasal discharge with associated mucosal membrane.

119. **What organisms are responsible for most infections in patients with cystic fibrosis?**
    S. aureus and *P. aeruginosa. B. cepacia* is also commonly seen, particularly in adult patients with cystic fibrosis. Various other bacteria, including non-typeable *H. influenzae*, *S. pneumoniae*, and some of the *Enterobacteriaceae*, are occasionally isolated. The most important fungal pathogen is *Aspergillus fumigatus*, which causes ABPA in this patient population.

    Gilligan PH: Microbiology of airway disease in patients with cystic fibrosis, *Clin Microbiol Rev* 4:35–51, 1991.

GASTROINTESTINAL INFECTIONS

120. **Which organisms most frequently cause traveler's diarrhea?**
See Table 12-10.

TABLE 12-10. FREQUENCY OF ORGANISMS ISOLATED IN CASES OF TRAVELER'S DIARRHEA	
Organism	Frequency Isolated (%)
Bacteria	
Enterotoxigenic *Escherichia coli*	20–50
Enteroinvasive *E. coli*	5–15
Enteroaggregative *E. coli*	5–15
Campylobacter jejuni	5–30
Salmonella spp.	5–25
Shigella spp.	5–15
Aeromonas spp.	0–10
Plesiomonas shigelloides	0–5 (very rare)
Vibrio spp.	≤ 5
Viruses	
Norovirus	0–10
Rotavirus	0–10
Protozoa	
Giardia spp.	0–10
Entamoeba histolytica	0–10
Cryptosporidium parvum	1–5
Cyclospora cayetanensis	0–5
No Pathogen	
	10–50

Adapted from Diemert DJ: Prevention and self-treatment of traveler's diarrhea. Clin Microbiol Rev 19:583–594, 2006.

121. **Which patients should be treated with antibiotics for diarrhea caused by *Salmonella*?**
Those with:
- Severe diarrhea (>10 stools/day)
- Hospitalization
- Immunosuppression due to HIV infection, organ transplantation, chemotherapy, corticosteroids, or other immunosuppressive agents
- Age > 50 years
- Sickle cell disease and other hemoglobinopathies

122. **List the strains of *E. coli* and associated toxins and the diarrheal disease each causes.**
See Table 12-11.

TABLE 12-11. STRAINS OF *ESCHERICHIA COLI* AND THE ASSOCIATED TOXINS AND ILLNESSES

Strain	Toxin	Illness	Other Features
Enterotoxigenic (ETEC)	Cholera-like	Traveler's diarrhea	
Enteroaggregative (EAggEC)	Enterotoxin	Watery diarrhea	Adheres to colonic mucosa
Enteropathogenic (EPEC)	Secretes proteins, not toxins	Diarrhea	Adheres and binds to colonic mucosa
Enterohemorrhagic (EHEC)	Shiga-like cytotoxins and verotoxins	Hemorrhagic colitis; hemolytic uremic syndrome	Most pathogenic strain (OI57:H7)
Enteroinvasive (EIEC)	None	Inflammatory colitis	Requires large inoculum to cause illness

123. **What is the infectious agent causing cholera?**
Vibrio cholerae, a small, curved, gram-negative rod, which produces an enterotoxin. Patients typically develop a profuse watery diarrhea (often described as "rice-water" stool) that can lead to life-threatening dehydration.

124. **What other species of *Vibrio* cause significant disease in humans?**
- ***Vibrio parahaemolyticus:*** Diarrheal illness in the U.S. Gulf Coast, Florida, Japan, Taiwan, and developing when ingested, may lead to severe gastroenteritis that is typically self-resolving.
- ***Vibrio vulnificus:*** Severe cellulitis, necrotizing fasciitis, ulcers, and sepsis, especially in patients with cirrhosis.
- ***Vibrio alginolyticus:*** Cellulitis and acute otitis media or otitis externa.

125. **What are the clinically relevant microsporidia?**
Enterocytozoon bienusi and *Encephalitozoon intestinalis.* Both can cause chronic diarrhea in patients with AIDS.

126. **List the more common parasitic causes of diarrhea.**

Cryptosporidium	*Cyclospora*	*Giardia*
Isospora	*Microsporidium*	*Entamoeba histolytica*

127. **What organism causes diarrhea, mesenteric adenitis, and reactive arthritis and has been the cause of needless appendectomy in the past?**
Y. enterolitica. This organism can cause mesenteric adenitis, which clinically mimics appendicitis—fever, leukocytosis, and right lower quadrant abdominal pain.

128. **What organism causes diarrhea, malabsorption, and endocarditis?**
Tropheryma whippelii, a gram-positive organism that is the causative agent of Whipple's disease. Whipple's disease is a multisystem disorder characterized by migratory polyarthritis,

diarrhea, malabsorption, weight loss, generalized lymphadenopathy, hyperpigmentation, and occasional neurologic abnormalities. Cases of endocarditis alone have been reported.

Dutly F, Altwegg M: Whipple's disease and *Tropheryma whippelii*, *Clin Microbiol Rev* 14:561–583, 2001.

Marin M, Sanchez M, del Rosal M, et al: *Tropheryma whipplei* infective endocarditis as the only manifestation of Whipple's disease, *J Clin Microbiol* 45:2078–2081, 2007.

129. **What pathogens are associated with consumption of contaminated fish and shellfish?**

Hepatitis A virus	*Vibrio*	Norwalk virus
Vibrio cholera O-1 and non O-1	*parahaemolyticus*	*Giardia lamblia*
	Vibrio vulnificus	Diphyllobothriasis
	Clostridium botulinum	Aniskiasis

130. **What toxin-induced syndromes are caused by ingestion of seafood?**
    - Ciguatera poisoning
    - Paralytic shellfish poisoning due to *Gonyaulax* spp. of dinoflagellates
    - Scombroid poisoning
    - Tetrodotoxication due to eating puffer fish (also called "Fugu" or "blowfish")
    - Neurotoxic shellfish poisoning due to the toxic dinoflagellate *Ptychodiscus brevis*
    - Diarrheic shellfish poisoning

    Eastaugh J, Shepherd S: Infectious and toxic syndromes from fish and shellfish consumption: A review, *Arch Intern Med* 149:1735–1740, 1989.

131. **What is possible estuary-associated syndrome (PEAS)?**
    A toxin-mediated illness due to dinoflagellates such as *Pfiesteria* that are found in the estuaries of the Tar-Pamlico and Neuse Rivers in North Carolina and the Maryland Eastern Shore.

    Morris JG Jr: *Pfiesteria*, "the cell from hell," and other toxic algal nightmares, *Clin Infect Dis* 28:1191–1196, 1999.

132. **What laboratory test predicts spontaneous bacterial peritonitis (SBP)?**
    A PMN count of 250 in an ascetic fluid sample has > 90% specificity and sensitivity in diagnosing SBP.

SEXUALLY TRANSMITTED DISEASES

133. **What is the causative agent of condyloma accuminata?**
    Human papillomavirus (HPV), a double-stranded DNA virus with multiple serotypes. Type 6 and 11 are more commonly associated with anogenital warts. Type 16 and 18 are strongly linked to cervical cancer.

134. **What is the causative agent of condyloma lata?**
    Treponema pallidum. Condyloma lata is a manifestation of secondary syphilis in which the generalized maculopapular rash becomes flat and broad with whitish lesions.

135. **What is the difference between nontreponemal and treponemal tests?**
    Nontreponemal tests (reactive plasma reagin [RPR] and Venereal Disease Research Laboratory [VDRL]) are **not specific** for syphilis and can be falsely positive under many conditions. These tests are used to screen for syphilis and to assess therapeutic response because the titers return to normal over time after therapy is initiated. **Treponemal** tests are **specific** for syphilis and include the microhemagglutination assay for *Treponema pallidum*

(MHA-TP) and the fluorescent treponemal antibody absorption test (FTA-Abs). These tests are used to confirm the diagnosis of syphilis and, once positive, will remain positive for life and never return to normal.

136. **What are the causes of false-positive serologic tests for syphilis?**
See Table 12-12.

TABLE 12-12. CAUSES OF FALSE–POSITIVE NONTREPONEMAL AND TREPONEMAL TESTS FOR SYPHILIS	
<6 MO After Exposure	**>6 MO From Exposure**
Nontreponemal Tests (RPR, VDRL)	
Pneumonia (viral, mycoplasma, pneumococcal)	Liver disease
Hepatitis	Malignancy
Tuberculosis	Intravenous drug abuse
Mononucleosis	Aging
Chancroid	Connective tissue disorders
Chickenpox	Multiple blood transfusions
HIV	
Measles	
Malaria	
Immunizations	
Pregnancy	
Laboratory error	
Treponemal tests (FTA, MHA-TP)	
Mononucleosis	SLE
Lyme disease	
Malaria	
Leprosy	

FTA = fluorescent treponemal antibody; HIV = human immunodeficiency virus; MHA-TP = microhemagglutination assay—*Treponema pallidum*; RPR = reactive plasma reagin; SLE = systemic lupus erythematosus; VDRL = Venereal Disease Research Laboratory.

137. **What are the indications for lumbar puncture in a patient with latent syphilis?**
   - Neurologic signs or symptoms
   - Ophthalmic signs or symptoms
   - Tertiary syphilis without neurologic symptoms
   - Treatment failure of secondary syphilis
   - HIV infection and late latent syphilis or syphilis of unknown duration
   - Patient preference (in immunocompetent patients)

138. **What is the earliest manifestation of syphilis?**
Painless ulceration at the site of inoculation (penis, vagina, anus, and throat) often associated with regional lymphadenopathy.

139. **What other sexually transmitted diseases (STDs) present as ulcers with lymphadenopathy?**
    - **Chancroid:** *Haemophilus ducreyi* causes these ulcers and is usually associated with suppurative inguinal lymphadenopathy.
    - **Genital herpes:** HSV type 1 or type 2 causes multiple vesicular or ulcerative painful genital ulcers, often associated with inguinal lymphadenopathy. HSV-2 is classically associated with this presentation, but HSV-1 may be causative in up to 50% of cases.
    - **Granuloma inguinale:** *Klebsiella granulomatis* (formerly *Calymmatobacterium granulomatis*) causes painless, genital ulcerative disease. The lesions are highly vascular, bleed easily on contact, and rarely occur in the United States.
    - **LGV:** *Chlamydia trachomatis* serovars L1, L2, L3 causes tender inguinal or femoral lymphadenopathy that is typically unilateral.

    Division of STD Prevention National Center for HIV/AIDS, Viral Hepatitis, STD, and TB Prevention: Sexually transmitted diseases treatment guidelines, 2010. *MMWR Morb Mortal Weekly Rep* 59:1–110, 2010.

140. **What is a Bartholin's cyst?**
    An obstruction of the Bartholin glands leading to cystic dilatation. Bartholin's glands are located on each side of the vaginal opening. Bartholin's cyst abscess can occur and usually develops rapidly over 2–4 days. Symptoms include acute vulvar pain, dyspareunia, and pain during walking. Local symptoms of acute pain and tenderness are secondary to rapid enlargement, hemorrhage, or secondary infection. The signs are those of a classic abscess: erythema, acute tenderness, edema, and occasionally, cellulitis of the surrounding subcutaneous tissue. Without therapy, most abscesses tend to rupture spontaneously by the third or fourth day.

141. **How is a Bartholin's cyst treated?**
    By observation or antibiotics, depending on the severity of symptoms. Asymptomatic cysts in women older than 40 years do not need treatment. The therapy for acute adenitis without abscess formation is broad-spectrum antibiotics and frequent hot sitz baths. In one series, 80% of cultures from the abscess was sterile; however, organisms such as *C. trachomatis* and *E. coli* have been reported. STDs do not play a major role in causing Bartholin's abscess.

142. **What is the Fitz-Hugh–Curtis syndrome? What organisms cause it?**
    Perihepatitis usually caused by either *N. gonorrhoeae* or *C. trachomatis,* thought to occur by spread of organisms from the fallopian tubes to the surface of the liver. Fitz-Hugh-Curtis syndrome is part of the differential diagnosis of right upper quadrant pain in young, sexually active women, and has been occasionally reported in males, probably as a result of bacteremic spread.

ZOONOSES

143. **What tick-borne diseases are found in the United States?**
    - Lyme disease (*Borrelia burgdorferi*)
    - Q fever (*Coxiella burnetii*)
    - Human ehrlichiosis (*Ehrlichia chaffeensis, Ehrlichia ewingii, Anaplasma phagocytophila*)
    - RMSF (*Rickettsia rickettsii*)
    - Tularemia (*Francisella tularensis*)
    - Babesiosis (*Babesia microti*)
    - Relapsing fever (*Borrelia hermsii*)
    - Tick-borne encephalitis (flavivirus)
    - Colorado tick fever (orbivirus)

144. **What organism shares a common epidemiologic niche and the same tick vector as *B. burgdorferi*?**
B. microti, a protozoan that parasitizes human erythrocytes. *Ixodes scapularis* is the most important tick vector, with *Dermacentor variabilis* being a less frequent vector. Some of this same geographic distribution is also shared by one of the agents causing human granulocyte ehrlichiosis, *A. phagocytophilum,* for which *I. scapularis* (the black-legged tick) is also the vector. Consequently, it is theoretically possible to see simultaneous infection with all three agents.

145. **What organism causes louse-borne relapsing fever?**
Borrelia recurrentis, which is frequently found in areas of overcrowding and poverty. Relapsing fever transmitted by the body louse is not seen in the United States and is more frequent in Africa or South America.

146. **What organism causes tick-borne relapsing fever?**
Borrelia hermsii, found in the United States in Western mountain states typically during late spring and summer. *Borrelia turicatae* has also been reported in the Southwest.

   Davis H, Vincent JM, Lynch J: Tick-borne relapsing fever caused by *Borrelia turicatae, Pediatr Infect Dis J* 21:703–705, 2002.

147. **List the *Rickettsia* species, the diseases they cause, and the common geographic distribution.**
See Table 12-13.

TABLE 12-13. DISEASES CAUSED BY RICKETTSIAL SPECIES AND THEIR GEOGRAPHIC DISTRIBUTION

Disease	Rickettsial Species	Geographic Distribution
African tick-bite fever	*Rickettsia africae*	Sub-Saharan Africa, Caribbean
Boutonneusse fever (Mediterranean spotted fever)	*R. conorii*	Southern Europe, Africa, southern and western Asia
Murine typhus	*R. typhi*	Coastal tropical and subtropical regions
Scrub typhus	*Orientia Tsutsugamushi*	Southern and eastern Asia, western Pacific islands, northern Australia
Louse-borne typhus	*R. prowazekii*	Potentially worldwide
Queensland tick typhus	*R. australis*	Eastern Australia
North Asian tick typhus	*R. sibirica*	North Asia
Rocky Mountain spotted fever	*R. rickettsii*	North, Central, and South America

148. **What questions are helpful in determining the risk of acquiring Lyme disease from a tick bite?**
   - **What is the size of the tick?** Disease is typically spread by the nymph stage of *I. scapularis,* which is quite small.
   - **Was the tick attached and for how long?** Ticks that do not attach to the skin cannot transmit disease; therefore, the risk of transmission is low with ticks that have been attached for < 24 hours.
   - **Was the tick engorged when removed?** Engorgement suggests a prolonged attachment and thus higher risk of transmission.

149. **What organism causes tick paralysis?**
None. Tick paralysis is not caused by an infectious agent but rather by a toxin secreted in tick saliva. Patients present with ascending flaccid paralysis that may be mistaken for other neurologic disorders. Treatment for this condition is quite simple—remove the tick.

   Edlow JA, McGillicuddy DC: Tick paralysis, *Infect Dis Clin North Am* 22:397–413, 2008.

150. **What species of *Ehrlichia* have been associated with human disease?**
   - ***Ehrlichia chaffeensis:*** human monocytic ehrlichiosis (HME)
   - ***Ehrlichia ewingii:*** human granulocytic ehrlichiosis (HGE)
   - ***Anaplasma phagocytophilum:*** human granulocytic anaplasmosis (HGA)
   - ***Ehrlichia sennetsu:*** mononucleosis-like illness in Japan and Malaysia
   - ***Ehrlichia canis:*** one case report in Venezuela

151. **How does human disease due to *Dirofilaria immitis* usually present?**
As a solitary, noncalcified pulmonary nodule. Because humans are an unsuitable host for *D. immitis*, the dog heartworm, larvae that mature in subcutaneous tissues after inoculation by infected mosquitoes enter veins and travel to the heart. From the heart, they embolize to the pulmonary arteries, resulting in infarcts.

   Nicholson CP, Allen MS, Trastek VF, et al: *Dirofilaria immitis:* A rare, increasing cause of pulmonary nodules, *Mayo Clin Proc* 67:646–650, 1992.

152. **Most cases of RMSF occur in what regions of the United States?**
The south Atlantic states (most frequently in North Carolina) and south-central region (Oklahoma, Missouri, and Arkansas). Despite its name, few cases of RMSF occur in the Rocky Mountain states.

153. **What is the Jarisch-Herxheimer reaction?**
A self-limited systemic reaction occurring within 1–2 hours after the initial treatment of syphilis with antimicrobial agents. The reaction occurs most frequently in patients treated for secondary syphilis but can occur during treatment of any syphilitic stage and with other spirochete infections. The reaction consists of the abrupt onset of chills, fever, myalgias, tachycardia, hyperventilation, vasodilatation with associated flushing, and mild hypotension. The symptoms are probably due to the release of pyrogens from the spirochetes and one study found elevated levels of tumor necrosis factor (TNF), interleukin 6 (IL-6), and IL-8.

   Negussie Y, Remick DG, DeForg LE, et al: Detection of plasma tumor necrosis factor, interleukins 6, and 8 during the Jarisch-Herxheimer reaction of relapsing fever, *J Exp Med* 175:1207–1212, 1992.

MISCELLANEOUS INFECTIONS

154. **What infections can occur with medicinal use of leeches?**
Aeromonas hydrophila, which has the same freshwater habitat as the medicinal leech, *Hirudo medicinalis*. Leeches are used in microvascular surgical procedures where because of their anticoagulant properties and *Aeromonas* infections may occur as postoperative infections.

   Abrutyn E: Hospital-associated infection from leeches, *Ann Intern Med* 109:356–358, 1988.

155. **What is typhlitis?**
Necrotizing enterocolitis or neutropenic enterocolitis, a fulminate, necrotizing process that occurs in the gastrointestinal tract of individuals with profound neutropenia. Symptoms of the disease include fever, abdominal pain and distention, rebound tenderness in the right lower quadrant, and diarrhea. The cecum and terminal are characteristically involved.

WEBSITES

1. Centers for Diseases Control: www.cdc.gov
2. Infectious Diseases Society of America: www.idsociety.org
3. National Institute of Allergy and Infectious Diseases: www.niaid.nih.gov

BIBLIOGRAPHY

1. Fauci AS, Braunwald E, Kaspar DL, et al, editors: *Harrison's Principles of Internal Medicine*, ed 17, New York, 2008, McGraw-Hill Medical.
2. Gorbach SL, Bartlett JG, Blacklow NR, editors. *Infectious Diseases*, ed 3, Philadelphia, 2004, Lippincott Williams & Wilkins.
3. Mandell GL, editor: *Mandell, Douglas, and Bennett's Principles and Practice of Infectious Diseases*, ed 7, Philadelphia, 2009, Churchill-Livingstone/Elsevier.
4. Southwick F: *Infectious Diseases: A Clinical Short Course*, New York, 2007, McGraw-Hill Professional.

ACQUIRED IMMUNODEFICIENCY SYNDROME AND HUMAN IMMUNODEFICIENCY VIRUS INFECTION

Joseph Caperna, M.D., Amy M. Sitapati, M.D., and Alfredo Tiu, D.O., F.A.C.P., F.A.S.N.

Drawing largely on the work that Donna Mildvan and Dan Williams started in New York City in early 1981, the Morbidity and Mortality Weekly Report *[May 12, 1982] on "Generalized Lymphadenopathy Among Homosexual Males" was released from Atlanta, the first* MMWR *publication on any aspect of the epidemic in nine months.... Doctors should be alert for the symptoms, the article concluded, most notably fatigue, fever, unexplained weight loss, and, of course, night sweats.*

Randy Shilts
And the Band Played On (1987)

BASIC PRINCIPLES AND EPIDEMIOLOGY

1. **What is human immunodeficiency virus (HIV) and how many virions are typically made per day?**
   HIV is a single-stranded RNA lentivirus that integrates into the host cell DNA. If not treated, approximately 10^{12} virions are produced each day.

2. **Describe the difference between HIV infection and acquired immunodeficiency syndrome (AIDS).**
   HIV infection refers to the detection of HIV antibodies or HIV RNA in a person's serum. In order to make the diagnosis of AIDS in a person with HIV infection, at least 1 of 21 indicator diseases must be diagnosed. **AIDS** is also diagnosed in the presence of HIV infection if the CD4 count < 200 cells/mL or CD4 < 14% even if symptoms of the indicator diseases are absent.

3. **What are the AIDS indicator diseases?**
   See Table 13-1.

4. **What is a T-cell count? What is its use?**
   A laboratory measurement of the CD4+ lymphocyte or the helper-inducer cells in the peripheral blood that is used to assess the degree of immunosuppression. HIV targets these T cells and their progressive death accounts for the immunosuppression of HIV infection. By measuring the T-cell count, a clinician can place a patient along the spectrum of HIV infection. A normal T-cell count (CD4 or CD4+) is 500–1600/mm^3. The World Health Organization (WHO) suggests using a total lymphocyte count of 1200 to approximate a CD4 count of 200. Because various opportunistic infections occur at or below certain CD4 counts, a T-cell count can be used to identify patients at high risk for opportunistic infection who require prophylactic treatment against specific infections. The CD4 count thus has prognostic and therapeutic value.

TABLE 13-1. ACQUIRED IMMUNODEFICIENCY SYNDROME INDICATOR DISEASES

Candidiasis

Cervical cancer (invasive)

Coccidioidomycosis, cryptococcosis, cryptosporidiosis

Cytomegalovirus disease

Encephalopathy (HIV-related)

Herpes simplex (severe infection)

Histoplasmosis

Isosporiasis

Kaposi's sarcoma

Lymphoma (certain types)

Mycobacterium avium complex

Pneumocystis jiroveci pneumonia

Pneumonia (recurrent)

Progressive multifocal leukoencephalopathy

Salmonella septicemia (recurrent)

Toxoplasmosis of the brain

Tuberculosis

Wasting syndrome

HIV = human immunodeficiency virus.
Data from Centers for Diseases Control and Prevention: 1993 Revised classification system for HIV infection and expanded surveillance case definition for AIDS among adolescents and adults. MMWR Morb Mortal Wkly Rep 41(RR-17), 1992. Available at: http://wonder.cdc.gov/wonder/help/AIDS/MMWR-12-18-1992.html

5. **How much time elapses between HIV infection and the diagnosis of AIDS?**
   This period is not easily defined. Studies of large patient cohorts indicate that in the absence of treatment, 50% of HIV-positive patients progress to AIDS in approximately 10 years. The rate of disease progression is not stable over this period because few develop disease early after exposure and proportionally more develop AIDS with each passing year. Several studies indicate that the average loss of CD4+ lymphocytes is 80 cells/yr. Not all persons with HIV infection progress or suffer immune destruction. Rarely, some persons maintain immune function and are called "long-term nonprogressors." It is not certain at this time that 100% of HIV-infected individuals will develop AIDS, even without specific antiretroviral therapy (ART).

   Lifson AR, Rutherford GW, Jaffe HW: The natural history of human immunodeficiency virus infection, *J Infect Dis* 158:1360–1367, 1988.

6. **Have the number of new HIV infections increased in the past few years?**
   Yes. The Centers for Disease Control and Prevention (CDC) estimate for 2006 showed an increase in new HIV infections from 40,000 to 56,300. A disproportionate number of these new HIV cases represent minorities including blacks/African Americans and Hispanics/Latinos.

Centers for Disease Control and Prevention: Cases of HIV infection and AIDS in urban and rural areas of the United States. *HIV/AIDS Surveillance Supplemental Report* 13:1–25, 2008. Available at: www.cdc.gov/hiv/topics/surveillance/resources/reports/#supplemental.

Hall HI, Song R, Rhodes P, et al: Estimation of HIV incidence in the United States, *JAMA* 300:520–529, 2008.

7. **True or false: In 2008, there were more adults who died from HIV globally than live in the United States with HIV infection.**
True. According to the WHO, about 2.3 million new infections occurred worldwide and another 2 million people living with HIV died. The United States shares a fraction of the global burden of disease with an estimated of 1.9 million of the 31.3 million adults living with HIV worldwide.

UNAIDS/WHO Epidemiological Fact Sheets on HIV and AIDS, 2008 Update. Available at: www.who.int/hiv/data/2009_global_summary.gif.

TRANSMISSION, PREVENTION, AND DIAGNOSIS

8. **What is the most common form of HIV transmission?**
Unprotected vaginal or anal sex. In the United States, nearly half (48%) of new infections of HIV are reported in men who have sex with men (MSM). In addition, infection can be spread via sexual intercourse (vaginal, anal, and oral), percutaneous blood exposure (injection use and needlesticks), blood transfusion, perinatal maternal-fetal transmission, and breast feeding.

Centers for Disease Control and Prevention: HIV prevalence estimates—United States, *MMWR Morb Mortal Wkly Rep* 57:1073–1076, 2008.

9. **What increases the risk of HIV transmission between heterosexual partners?**
HIV viral load. Other risk factors found to increase the risk for HIV transmission include exposure volume; presence of other sexually transmitted diseases (STDs) such as syphilis, herpes simplex, gonorrhea, and chlamydia; and lack of circumcision. Although circumcision appears to be protective in heterosexuals in Africa, circumcision has not been found to be protective in MSM.

Quinn TC, Wawer MJ, Sewankambo N, et al: Viral load and heterosexual transmission of human immunodeficiency virus type 1. Rakai Project Study Group, *N Engl J Med* 342:921–929, 2000.

Galvin SR, Cohen MS: The role of sexually transmitted diseases in HIV transmission, *Nat Rev Microbiol* 2:33–42, 2004.

10. **Have studies definitively shown that treatment of other STDs reduces the risk of HIV transmission?**
No. Treatment of STDs has not been found to effectively reduce the risk for HIV transmission, but this may be related to the inclusion in the current studies of controls with asymptomatic syphilis and gonorrhea infections. According to the Study to Understand the Natural History of HIV/AIDS in the Era of Effective Therapy (SUN), a significant percentage of patients with STDs are asymptomatic and have infections that are not urethral but rectal.

Vellozzi C, Brooks JT, Bush TJ, et al: The Study to Understand the Natural History of HIV and AIDS in the Era of Effective Therapy (SUN study), *Am J Epidemiol* 169:642–652, 2009.

Mayer K, Bush T, Conley L, et al: Clinical and behavioral characteristics of HIV-infected American patients in care at increased risk of transmission to others [poster]. Presented at the XVII International AIDS Conference, Mexico City, Mexico, August 3–8, 2008.

11. **Should HIV treatment reduce the risk for HIV transmission?**
Yes. One study used mathematical modeling to predict infections and found that increasing the number of individuals on highly active antiretroviral therapy (HAART) from 50% to 75%,

90%, and 100% would reduce the number of annual new HIV infections by 30%, 50%, and 60%, respectively.

Lima VD, Johnson TK, Hogg RS, et al: Expanded access to highly active antiretroviral therapy: A potentially powerful strategy to curb the growth of the HIV epidemic, *J Infect Dis* 198:56–67, 2008.

12. **Is HIV treatment effective in preventing perinatal HIV transmission from mother to child (vertical transmission)?**
Yes. All pregnant women should be tested for HIV infection so early treatment can be initiated. Without treatment, perinatal transmission rates are 20–33%. With combination therapy treatment of the pregnant mother, transmission rates were lowered to less than 2%. In general, therapy recommendations are the same during pregnancy as in the nonpregnant patient, but efavirenz should be avoided in the first trimester owing to significant teratogenicity manifested as neural tube defects. Zalcitabine and delavirdine are also potential teratogens. The combination of didanosine and stavudine can lead to fatal lactic acidosis and should be avoided in pregnancy unless there are no alternative regimens. When used as part of combination therapy in pregnant women with CD4 counts > 250 cell/mm^3, nevirapine has been associated with fatal hepatotoxicity.

13. **What is the risk of HIV transmission via needlestick?**
$\sim$0.3% among health-care workers. However, each exposure needs to be evaluated individually. There is tremendous variation in the degree of exposure, which affects the likelihood of infection. Exposure to a large volume of infectious material (or material with a high viral load), a deep injury, visible blood on the device causing the injury, prolonged contact with the infectious material, and the portal of entry are important factors. Intramuscular injection, exposures via hollow needles (as opposed to suture needles and pins), and exposure to material from a viremic HIV-infected patient also increase the transmission risk.

Tokars JI, Marcus R, Culver DH, et al: Surveillance of HIV infection and zidovudine use among health-care workers after occupational exposure to HIV-infected blood, *Ann Intern Med* 118:913–919, 1993.

14. **What is PEP, when do you give it, what do you give, and for how long?**
Postexposure prophylaxis. Animal studies have shown optimal benefit when ART is administered within the initial 3 hours, but the benefit of PEP continues for the initial 72 hours after exposure. No randomized, controlled trial has been performed, and most likely, none will be done in the future. However, a retrospective case-control study involving 31 exposed and infected health-care workers and 679 exposed, uninfected workers found that postexposure zidovudine reduced the risk of HIV infection by 79%. Therapy recommendations include combination ART given for 28 days based on the treatment status of the source patient including consideration for possible drug resistance.

Centers for Disease Control and Prevention: Case-control study of HIV seroconversion in health-care workers after percutaneous exposure to HIV-infected blood—France, United Kingdom, and United States, January 1988–August 1994, *MMWR Morb Mortal Wkly Rep* 44:929–933, 1995.

Centers for Disease Control and Prevention: Updated U.S. Public Health Service Guidelines for the management of occupational exposures to HBV, HCV, and HIV and recommendations for postexposure prophylaxis, *MMWR Morb Mortal Wkly Rep* 50:1–67, 2001.

15. **A discordant couple (i.e., one partner is HIV-positive and the other partner is HIV-negative) experiences a condom break during sexual intercourse. What window of time has been shown to be effective for initiating ART and reducing the risk of HIV transmission?**
72 hours. ART given to reduce the risk for sexual transmission of HIV is called "n-PEP" or nonoccupational postexposure prophylaxis, and includes individuals exposed during

intercourse, sexual abuse, and rape and follows a similar guideline as outlined for occupational PEP.

Centers for Disease Control and Prevention: Antiretroviral postexposure prophylaxis after sexual, injection-drug use, or other nonoccupational exposure to HIV in the United States, *MMWR Morb Mortal Wkly Rep* 54:1–20, 2005.

16. **Is there a vaccine available that might reduce the risk for HIV transmission?**
    No. Despite much global research and effort, an effective HIV vaccine has not yet been developed. A placebo-controlled trial involving over 3000 subjects was halted in 2007 because of lack of vaccine efficacy at the interim analysis (the Step Study). Subsequent data analysis suggests that certain populations may actually have an increased risk of HIV acquisition after vaccination. The data from the STEP trial did have a few confounding factors in their analysis. A more recent study shows some possible efficacy of a vaccine and plans for future trials continue.

    Buchbinder SP, Mehrota DV, Duerr A, et al: Efficacy assessment of a cell-mediated immunity HIV-1 vaccine (the Step Study): A double-blind, randomised, placebo-controlled, test-of-concept trial, *Lancet* 372:1881–1893, 2008.

    McElrath MJ, De Rosa SC, Moodie Z, et al: HIV-1 vaccine-induced immunity in the test-of-concept Step Study: A case-cohort analysis, *Lancet* 372:1894–1905, 2008.

    Rerks-Ngarm S, Pitisuttithum P, Nitayaphan S, et al: Vaccination with ALVAC and AIDSVAC to prevent HIV-1 infection in Thailand, *N Engl J Med* 361:2209–2226, 2009.

17. **Who should have HIV testing? How might testing reduce HIV transmission?**
    All persons older than 13 years should be routinely tested for HIV according to the most recent recommendations from the American College of Physicians and the HIV Medicine Association. The CDC recommends screening all patients aged 13–64 years in all health-care settings. Currently, about 25% of patients with HIV are unaware of their status. Once patients are aware of their HIV status, 53% will modify their high-risk behavior. Up to 20,000 HIV infections are transmitted each year from persons who are unaware of their infection. Early identification of HIV infection can lead to early treatment of transmission prevention. At this time, the U.S. Preventive Services Task Force (USPSTF) strongly recommends screening all adolescents and adults who are at high-risk, but does not yet suggest universal screening.

    Chou R, Hoyt L, Huffman HS, et al: U.S. Preventive Services Task Force (USPSTF): Screening for HIV, *Ann Intern Med* 14:55–73, 2005.

    Centers for Disease Control and Prevention: Revised recommendations for HIV testing of adults, adolescents, and pregnant women in health-care settings, *MMWR Morb Mortal Wkly Rep* 55:1–17, 2006.

    Qassem A, Snow V, Shekella P, et al: Screening for HIV in health care settings: A guidance statement from the American College of Physicians and HIV Medicine Association, *Ann Intern Med* 150:125–131, 2009.

18. **What are the problems with rapid tests for HIV?**
    Possible false-positive results. Rapid HIV tests are available using saliva, serum, or whole blood samples, and an increased number of false-positive results have been reported with the oral rapid tests. Any positive rapid test must be confirmed by traditional tests including enzyme immunoassay (EIA) followed by a confirmatory Western blot test.

ACUTE HIV INFECTION

19. **List the symptoms of acute HIV infection along with their frequency.**
    - **Fatigue:** 80%
    - **Lymphadenopathy:** 75%

- **Pharyngitis:** 70%
- **Rash:** 70%
- **Myalgias/arthralgias:** 55%
- **Nausea, vomiting, diarrhea:** 30%
- **Headache:** 30%
- **Weight loss:** 15%
- **Oral candidiasis (thrush):** 15%
- **Central/peripheral neurologic symptoms:** 10%

20. **How soon after acute HIV infection do symptoms develop? How long do the symptoms persist?**
    Symptoms develop 1–8 weeks after the initial infection and are believed to result from specific immune responses to HIV. Patients presenting with these symptoms should have a specific risk history taken for possible recent exposure to HIV. The symptoms that develop are transient and generally are present for 1–3 weeks; however, cases have been reported with symptoms lasting up to 8 weeks.

21. **How can acute primary HIV infection be diagnosed?**
    With nucleic acid–based testing (NAT), which identifies HIV nucleic acid sequences. Early in HIV infection, the host has not yet made antibodies that can be detected reliably in routine antibody-based screening. Traditionally, NAT practice has relied on pooling groups of 8–20 patient-based plasma samples to identify nucleic acid presence for HIV. One could think of this process as grouping samples of HIV antibody–negative specimens and then backtracking to an individual level any batch that is found to have a positive test. Other tests include p24 antigen and HIV RNA viral load levels. False-positive RNA viral load levels have been reported with viral loads up to 1000 copies/mL and are less common at higher RNA levels.

    Fiebig EW, Wright DJ, Rawal BD, et al: Dynamics of HIV viremia and antibody seroconversion in plasma donors: Implication for diagnosis and staging of primary HIV infection, *AIDS* 17:1871–1879, 2003.

VIRAL LOAD AND HIV LIFE CYCLE

22. **What is a "viral load" test? How is it used in patients with HIV?**
    A test that measures the amount of HIV RNA in the plasma and indicates the degree of viral replication. Viral load testing is the single best prognostic indicator in HIV infection, with a higher level of mRNA indicative of a poorer prognosis. The test is routinely performed as part of the initial assessment of newly diagnosed HIV infection. Once therapy has been initiated, the viral load is used to assess the efficacy and durability of ART. There should be at least a 1.0-log decrease in the viral load within 8 weeks of the start of therapy. Within 24 weeks, the viral load should be below detectable limits.

23. **Does "undetectable" viral load mean "cured" or "not infectious"?**
    No. An undetectable viral load means only that the ART has effectively halted viral replication below the threshold that can be detected by the assay being used.

24. **Do patients with undetectable HIV still need to use condoms to prevent HIV transmission during sexual activity?**
    Yes. HIV infection is still present, and HIV infection is, most importantly, still transmissible even though the risk for transmission may be reduced. This appears to be true for sexual, needlestick, and perinatal transmissions.

KEY POINTS: HUMAN IMMUNODEFICIENCY VIRUS INFECTION ✓

1. HIV infection is currently a life-long condition without cure.

2. Persons living with HIV infection are infectious regardless of HIV viral load.

3. Adherence to lifestyle changes (including condom use and clean needles) should be complete and life-long.

4. Many persons living with HIV live long and healthy lives; but delayed diagnosis and poor adherence to therapy can increase the risk for AIDS-related illnesses and mortality.

5. HIV testing can evaluate HIV antibodies yet NAT may detect HIV when antibodies have not yet developed or when immunity is poor.

6. HIV resistance testing should be done early in the disease.

7. Initiation of therapy is individualized but recommended for CD4 < 350.

AIDS = acquired immunodeficiency syndrome; HIV = human immunodeficiency virus; NAT = nucleic acid–based testing.

25. **Describe the HIV life cycle.**
    See Figure 13-1.

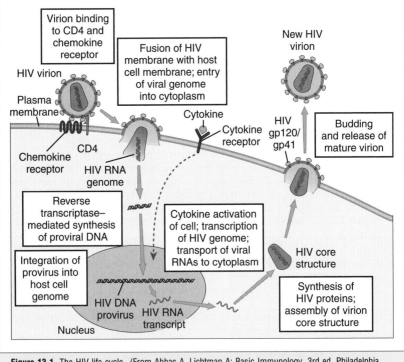

Figure 13-1. The HIV life cycle. (From Abbas A, Lichtman A: Basic Immunology, 3rd ed. Philadelphia, Saunders, 2010.)

26. **What stages of the HIV life cycle are targets of currently available therapy?**
   - Cell entry
   - Reverse transcription
   - Integrase and maturation
   - Protease

   Current therapy can attack these steps in the HIV life cycle. The first point of contact preceding entry of a virion into a new cell is the CD4 receptor and CXCR4 or CCR5 co-receptor. Cell entry can be blocked by an injectable fusion inhibitor, which binds gp41, thereby preventing fusion of viral and cellular membranes or an oral CCR5 receptor antagonist. Reverse transcription enzyme inhibition can be achieved through either nucleoside analogue (NRTI or "nucs") or non-nucleoside analogue reverse transcriptase inhibitors (NNRTI or "non-nucs"). Next, the insertion of HIV proviral DNA into the host can by inhibited by a newer class of therapeutics called "integrase inhibitors." Finally, protease inhibitors (PIs) can interrupt mature cleavage of virions.

HIV TREATMENT AND RESISTANCE TESTING

27. **Describe the mechanism of action of the reverse transcriptase inhibitors (RTIs).**
   The RTIs block the function of viral reverse transcriptase during the transcription of viral RNA to host complementary DNA. There are two kinds of RTIs: NRTIs and NNRTIs. NRTIs mimic nucleoside bases and are incorporated into the DNA chain stopping further chain extension. The NNRTIs bind to the enzyme reverse transcriptase near the active site, sterically obstructing function of the enzyme.

28. **How do PIs work?**
   By preventing the cleavage of HIV polyproteins by HIV-1 protease that is required to make a mature viral core during the final stages of virion synthesis. Virions that subsequently bud from the surface of the cell in the presence of PIs lack a mature developed core. These immature virions are unable to infect new host cells.

29. **What is HAART?**
   Highly active antiretroviral therapy. The term originated from the development of combination of at least three medications that could suppress HIV viral replication below the level of detection by a viral load test. Optimally, targeted ART should include three active drugs from at least two different classes. Traditional HAART has included two NRTIs combined with either an NNRTI or a PI. The Department of Health and Human Services (DHHS) regularly updates a list of recommended guidelines for the prescription of HAART therapy.

   Panel on Antiretroviral Guidelines for Adults and Adolescents: *Guidelines for the use of antiretroviral agents in HIV-1–infected adults and adolescents*, January 10, 2011, Department of Health and Human Services, pp 1–166. Available at: www.aidsinfo.nih.gov/ContentFiles/AdultandAdolescentGL.pdf. Accessed January 26, 2011.

30. **What antiretroviral drugs are currently available?**
   See Table 13-2.

31. **At what threshold of CD4 cell count in an HIV-infected individual should one consider initiating ART?**
   At CD4 cell counts of 350 cells/mm^3. Coexistent chronic hepatitis B virus (HBV), hepatitis C virus (HCV), pregnancy, AIDS-defining illnesses, and HIV-associated nephropathy are also indications to start ART regardless of CD4. With CD4 cell counts between 350 and 500 cells/mm^3, providers should discuss with the patient the benefits and risks of initiating early ART.

TABLE 13-2.	ANTIRETROVIRAL DRUGS FOR TREATMENT OF HUMAN IMMUNODEFICIENCY VIRUS INFECTION
Drug	**Abbreviation**
NRTIs	
Abacavir	ABC
Didanosine	ddI
Emtricitabine	FTC
Lamivudine	3TC
Stavudine	d4T
Tenofovir	TDF
Zalcitabine	ddC
Zidovudine	ZDV, AZT
NNRTIs	
Delavirdine	DLV
Efavirenz	EFV
Nevirapine	NVP
PIs	
Amprenavir	APV
Atazanavir	ATV
Darunavir	DRV
Fosamprenavir	FPV
Indinavir	IDV
Nelfinavir	NFV
Ritonavir	RTV
Saquinavir	SQV
Tipranavir	TPV
Fusion Inhibitor	
Enfuvirtide	T-20
INSTI	
Raltegravir	RAL
CCR5 Antagonist	
Maraviroc	MVC

INSTI = integrase strand transfer inhibitor; NNRTIs = non-nucleoside reverse transcriptase inhibitors; NRTIs = nucleoside reverse transcriptase inhibitors; PIs = protease inhibitors.

32. **Why consider early treatment of HIV infection?**
    To reduce the risk for HIV transmission and theoretically reduce the risk for AIDS-defining illnesses, malignancy, and cardiovascular disease. Newer data suggest that earlier treatment is possibly better before further decline in CD4 cell counts. Earlier suppression of viral replication may also preserve immune function.

33. **What are the preferred initial treatments for HIV infection?**
Individualized selection of two NRTIs with:
- an NNRTI or
- a PI (preferably boosted with ritonavir) or
- an INSTI or
- a CCR5 antagonist

    Panel on Antiretroviral Guidelines for Adults and Adolescents: *Guidelines for the use of antiretroviral agents in HIV-1–infected adults and adolescents*, January 10, 2011, Department of Health and Human Services, pp 1–166. Available at: www.aidsinfo.nih.gov/ContentFiles/AdultandAdolescentGL.pdf. Accessed January 26, 2011.

34. **What are the goals of HIV treatment?**
To reduce HIV RNA to < 50 copies. This level of HIV RNA predicts successful ART. The lower limits of the approved ranges are currently between 40 for an ultrasensitive assay (geared at looking at the lower end of detection for patients on therapy) and 400 for a standard assay (equipped to look at the upper end of detection for patients not on therapy) copies of mRNA/mL. If a specimen has an amount of mRNA below this lower limit, it is said to be "undetectable" or, more accurately, "below the limits of detection." A repeat viral load should be performed within 2–4 weeks, and not more than 8 weeks, of initiation of therapy and should be at least 1.0-log less (down by 90%) than the baseline level. At 48 weeks after beginning treatment, the viral load should be < 50 copies.

35. **List the predictors of long-term virologic success (or reduction of viral load to < 50 copies) in HIV therapy.**
- Low baseline viral load
- High baseline CD4 count
- Rapid reduction of viral load to undetectable levels
- Patient adherence to prescribed therapy

36. **How does patient adherence to prescribed ART affect treatment efficacy?**
See Table 13-3.

TABLE 13-3. LEVEL OF ADHERENCE IN RELATION TO EFFICACY OF THERAPY	
Level of Adherence (%)	Patients with Undetectable Viral Load at 48 wk (%)
95–100	84
90–95	64
80–90	47
70–80	24
<70	12

37. **List the reasons for virologic or treatment failure of ART.**
- Insufficient drug potency
- Poor adherence to ART
- Pharmacokinetics including lack of adequate penetration into compartments such as central nervous system (CNS)
- Decline of immunologic function
- Emergence of resistance to one or more drugs in ART regimen

38. **Is there evidence that interrupted therapy (taking a break from ART) is poor for health?**
Yes. The Strategies for Management of Antiretroviral Therapy (SMART) study clearly showed that the risk of disease progression and death was increased by 2.6 times in the group that interrupted therapy.

   The Strategies for Management of Antiretroviral Therapy (SMART) Study Group: CD4+ count–guided interruption of antiretroviral treatment, *N Engl J Med* 55:2283–2296, 2006.

39. **What is tropism?**
The identification of the specific co-receptor used by the infecting virus in an individual patient and use of that knowledge to select antiviral therapy for that patient. HIV primarily binds to the CD4 receptor on the cell surface, but also requires a chemokine (CCR5 or CXCR4) co-receptor for cell entry that resides beside the CD4 receptor on the cell surface. When HIV envelope glycoprotein gp120 attaches to the CD4 receptor, the virus uses the CCR5 or CXCR4 co-receptors to facilitate cell entry. Some HIV viruses use the CCR5 co-receptor (particularly in early HIV infection), some use the CXCR4 co-receptor, and some use both. Currently, a drug called maraviroc is effective only against HIV viruses which use the CCR5 co-receptor.

KEY POINTS: HUMAN IMMUNODEFICIENCY VIRUS THERAPY ✔

1. HIV therapy is complicated but generally well tolerated despite toxicities.

2. Good adherence ($\geq$95%) is required to secure durable viral control.

3. Suboptimal adherence promotes viral replication and resistance to anti-HIV medications.

4. Optimal time to initiate HIV therapy is clearly before the development of AIDS but often controversial at exactly what level of CD4 count.

AIDS = acquired immunodeficiency syndrome; HIV = human immunodeficiency virus.

40. **How can HIV resistance be measured?**
Through genotypic or phenotypic resistance testing and tropism testing. A genotypic resistance test will report specific sequences of mutations in the form of letters and numbers such as an M184V (lamuvidine resistance) and K103N (efavirenz and nevirapine resistance). A phenotypic resistance test will report a fold-change for a medication to report whether a specific medication may have activity. Phenotypes tend to provide more useful information when complex genetic evolution of the virus has occurred. Tropism assays are similar to resistance tests but look at the co-receptors used by the virus to enter CD4+ cells.

41. **When should an HIV resistance test be ordered?**
At the time of initial HIV diagnosis. ~8–23% of untreated HIV-infected patients already have resistant HIV at the time of diagnosis. The resistance test cannot be accurately done when a viral load is suppressed on therapy to < 500 copies/mL. After treatment begins, failure of a patient to suppress viral load to undetectable by 48 weeks on a new regimen or failure to maintain a viral load < 400 copies/mL on two consecutive tests would also indicate the need for resistance testing.

42. **If the HIV virus develops resistance to one medication, will other medications have increased activity or effectiveness?**
Yes. In the push-and-pull antagonistic development of mutations by the HIV virus, some mutations can increase the effectiveness of specific medications. For example, zidovudine becomes more effective in the presence of lamuvidine resistance with an M184V mutation.

PULMONARY INFECTIONS

43. **What is PCP?**
Pneumocystis jiroveci pneumonia (previously called "*Pneumocystis carinii* pneumonia"). Before routine prophylactic treatments for PCP in HIV infected patients, PCP was the presenting diagnosis in > 60% of patients with AIDS and eventually seen in 80% of patients with AIDS at some time during their illness. Without secondary prophylaxis after initial PCP diagnosis and effective HIV therapy, the recurrence rate of PCP is 40% within 6 months. With more proactive HIV testing before depletion of immune function and the initiation of effective primary PCP prophylaxis, the incidence of PCP should approach zero.

44. **What clinical features in an HIV-infected patient indicate increased risk for PCP?**
   - CD4 count < 200 or < 14% of total lymphocyte count
   - Diagnosis of thrush
   - Concomitant use of immunosuppressive medications for conditions such as organ transplantation

45. **Describe the typical signs and symptoms of PCP.**
   - Nonproductive cough or cough productive of clear sputum
   - Dyspnea on exertion (may have insidious onset)
   - Fever
   - Malaise
   - Sensation of chest tightness or inability to deeply inspire
   - Normal physical examination or signs of tachypnea or dry rales.

   Krajicek BJ, Thomas CF, Limper AH: *Pneumocystis* pneumonia: Current concepts in pathogenesis, diagnosis, and treatment, *Clin Chest Med* 30:265–278, vi, 2009.

46. **What laboratory findings are associated with PCP?**
Hypoxemia with an elevated alveolar-arterial oxygen pressure (PAO_2–PaO_2) gradient and elevated serum lactate dehydrogenase (LDH) levels, although these findings lack sensitivity and specificity. High or rising LDH in PCP suggests increased mortality.

   Zaman MK, White DA: Serum lactate dehydrogenase levels and *Pneumocystis carinii* pneumonia: Diagnostic and prognostic significance, *Am Rev Respir Dis* 137:796–800, 1988.

47. **How is PCP diagnosed?**
By sputum analysis for *P. jiroveci*, with Giemsa stain, cytologic silver stain, or direct fluorescence antibody (DFA). Sputum is sometimes induced, but most centers rely on bronchoscopy with bronchoalveolar lavage (BAL) for diagnosis. Lavage alone has a sensitivity of > 95% and is considered the gold standard. An experienced HIV clinician may make an empirical diagnosis of PCP in HIV-infected patients with appropriate signs and symptoms.

KEY POINTS: *PNEUMOCYSTIS JIROVECI* PNEUMONIA ✓

1. PCP is preventable.

2. Diagnosis of PCP represents a failed opportunity to diagnose HIV infection or use appropriate prophylaxis.

3. Onset of PCP is insidious and progressive.

4. Typical community-acquired "broad-spectrum" antibiotic coverage will not cover PCP.

HIV = human immunodeficiency virus; PCP = *Pneumocystis carinii* (former name of *P. jiroveci*) pneumonia.

48. **Describe the chest x-ray findings in PCP.**
    Diffuse, bilateral, and interstitial infiltrates, often more pronounced in the hilar region (called a "butterfly distribution"). Areas of focal consolidation are less common, as are cystic and cavitary changes. Normal chest x-rays are common, especially in patients presenting early in the illness. Pleural effusion and hilar adenopathy are rare and, if present, should raise the suspicion of another diagnosis.

49. **How is PCP treated?**
    See Table 13-4. For primary treatment, oral trimethoprim-sulfamethoxazole (TMP-SMX) for 21 days is considered the best first-line therapy. In severe infection with hypoxia as determined by a $PaO_2 < 70$ mmHg or an A–a gradient > 35 mmHg, corticosteroids may be needed in addition to antibiotics.

TABLE 13-4. STANDARD AND ALTERNATIVE THERAPIES FOR *PNEUMOCYSTIS JIROVECI* PNEUMONIA		
Drug	**Dosage**	**Additional Information**
Standard Therapy		
TMP-SMX	TMP: 15–20 mg/kg plus SMX: 75–100 mg/kg divided into three or four doses daily IV or orally for 21 days	Preferred treatment. Desensitization available for patients with sulfa allergy. Adjust dose in renal insufficiency.
Alternative Therapies		
Pentamidine	4 mg/kg IV daily for 21 days	Similar efficacy to TMP-SMX but greater toxicity (nephrotoxicity, pancreatitis, glucose dysregulation, cardiac arrhythmias). Reserved for patients with severe disease who require IV therapy.

(continued)

TABLE 13-4. STANDARD AND ALTERNATIVE THERAPIES FOR *PNEUMOCYSTIS JIROVECI* PNEUMONIA—*(continued)*

Drug	Dosage	Additional Information
Dapsone + trimethoprim	Dapsone* 100 mg orally daily plus trimethoprim 15 mg/kg orally daily for 21 days	Appropriate for mild-to-moderate disease. *Confirm G6PD status prior to use when appropriate.
Clindamycin + primaquine	Clindamycin 600–900 mg IV every 6–8 hr (or 300–450 mg orally every 6–8 hr) plus Primaquine* base 15–30 mg orally once daily for 21 days	Appropriate for mild-to-moderate disease.
Atovaquone	750 mg orally twice daily for 21 days	For mild-to-moderate PCP only; not as potent as TMP-SMX.
Trimetrexate (+ leucovorin)	Trimetrexate 45 mg/m^2 (or 1.2 mg/kg) IV daily plus leucovorin 25 mg orally every 6 hr for 21 days	Not as potent as TMP-SMX. Leucovorin must be continued for 3 days beyond completion of trimetrexate.

G6PD = glucose-6-phosphate dehydrogenase; IV = intravenously; PCP = *Pneumocystis carinii* (former name of *P. jiroveci*) pneumonia; TMP-SMX = trimethoprim-sulfamethoxazole.
From Centers for Disease Control and Prevention: Guidelines for prevention and treatment of opportunistic infections in HIV-infected adults and adolescents. Recommended from CDC, the National Institutes of Health, and the HIV Medicine Association of the Infectious Diseases Society of America. MMWR Morb Mortal Wkly Rep 58, 2009. Available at: www.cdc.gov/mmwr/pdf/rr/rr5804.pdf

50. **When is atovaquone used?**
When patients have mild-to-moderate PCP and are allergic or intolerant of TMP-SMX. Compared with TMP-SMX, atovaquone has less bone marrow suppression and rash; however, it is also less effective than TMP-SMX and must be taken with food to ensure absorption. The dosing regimen with the oral suspension is 750 mg twice daily, taken with a fatty meal, for 21 days.

51. **What are the side effects of medications used to treat moderate to severe PCP?**
TMP-SMX:
- Rash
- Stevens-Johnson syndrome
- Fever
- Leukopenia
- Nausea
- Hyperkalemia
- Elevated liver function tests
Rash, fever, or leukopenia may occur in as many as 30–40% of patients.
Intravenous (IV) pentamidine:
- Progressive renal insufficiency
- Pancreatitis

- Hypoglycemia or hyperglycemia
- Nausea
- Taste disturbances
- Cardiac arrhythmias
- Hypocalcemia

Atovaquone
- Rash (rare)
- Nausea

52. **List the indications for primary PCP prophylaxis.**
    - CD4+ count < 200/mm^3 or < 14% of total lymphocytes
    - Oral candidiasis
    - Immunosuppressive agents such as organ transplant agents
      The use of PCP prophylaxis after the initial episode of PCP is considered secondary prophylaxis.

53. **What drugs are used for PCP prophylaxis?**
    TMP-SMX (one double-strength daily) remains the drug of choice for prophylaxis but may be given as a single strength dose or three times a week. Alternatives include dapsone, atovaquone, and aerosolized pentamidine, but all efforts should be made, including desensitization, to allow use of TMP-SMX (Table 13-5).

TABLE 13-5. REGIMENS FOR *PNEUMOCYSTIS JIROVECI* PNEUMONIA PROPHYLAXIS

TMP-SMX
- TMP 160 mg, SMX 800 mg daily (one DS tablet)
- Side effects similar to but less common than with primary PCP treatment
- Decreasing dose by 50% (1 DS tablet three times/wk or single-strength daily) may limit side effects while preserving efficacy
- Also provides prophylaxis against CNS toxoplasmosis

Dapsone (+ Pyrimethamine)
- 50 mg twice-daily or 100 mg/day
- Provides prophylaxis against toxoplasmosis with addition of pyrimethamine

Aerosolized Pentamidine
- 300 mg once-monthly via nebulizer
- Transient taste alterations and coughing or wheezing (can be minimized by pretreatment with inhaled bronchodilators)
- Evaluate patients for active TB before starting therapy—administer in negative pressure room or booth

Atovaquone
- 1500 mg/day
- Gastrointestinal discomfort is main adverse event
- Also covers toxoplasmosis

CNS = central nervous system; DS = double-strength; PCP = *Pneumocystis carinii* (former name of *P. jiroveci*) pneumonia; TB = tuberculosis; TMP-SMX = trimethoprim-sulfamethoxazole.

Centers for Disease Control and Prevention: Guidelines for prevention and treatment of opportunistic infections in HIV-infected adults and adolescents. Recommended from CDC, the National Institutes of Health, and the HIV Medicine Association of the Infectious Diseases Society of America, *MMWR Morb Mortal Wkly Rep* 58:1–198, 2009. Available at: www.cdc.gov/mmwr/preview/mmwrhtml/rr5804a1.htm.

54. **Describe the relationship between HIV and tuberculosis (TB).**
    Until the mid-1980s, there had been a steady and rapid decline in the morbidity and mortality attributed to TB. In 1986, the number of new TB cases increased for the first time since nationwide reporting was initiated in 1953, concurrent with the beginning of widespread HIV infection. HIV patients are highly susceptible to primary TB, and there is a high rate of progression from latent to active TB in HIV patients with preexisting latent TB. In fact, ~30% of TB patients have HIV.

55. **How is this relationship explained?**
    Control of TB depends on cell-mediated immunity. In HIV infection, these immune cells are profoundly affected. The incidence of TB in an HIV-infected population can be expected to mirror that population's previous exposure to *Mycobacterium tuberculosis* (MTb). Immigrants, inner-city minorities, and IV drug users, groups with a high prevalence of both HIV and previous TB infection, will develop a high number of active TB cases unless prophylaxis is used. HIV strongly promotes the development of active TB from latent infection. With HIV infection, a person with latent TB is at a 5–9% risk per year of developing active disease compared with an HIV-negative person who carries a lifetime risk of 5%.

    Shafer RW, Edlin BR: Tuberculosis in patients infected with human immunodeficiency virus: Perspective on the past decade, *Clin Infect Dis* 22:683–704, 1996.

56. **Does TB differ in presentation in HIV-infected patients?**
    Yes. Although the common pulmonary symptoms of TB (cough, hemoptysis, fever, and weight loss) may be present in HIV patients, the incidence of extrapulmonary disease is much higher with frequent miliary and disseminated disease. Progressive fevers and wasting are common presenting symptoms. Cough for > 3 weeks or fever after antibiotic therapy for bronchitis in an HIV-infected patient should be considered TB until proven otherwise. Atypical or less common TB presentations are much more frequent in HIV, especially those with poor immunity CD4 < 200.

57. **How is the diagnosis of pulmonary TB made in an HIV-infected patient?**
    Four symptoms describe pulmonary TB:
    - Cough with or without hemoptysis
    - Fever
    - Night sweats
    - Weight loss

    Radiograph appearance is variable, but mediastinal adenopathy is highly suggestive of pulmonary TB. Clinical suspicion alone may warrant therapy while the sputum cultures are held in the microbiology laboratory for 8–12 weeks before final reporting. Induced sputum collection for acid-fast bacilli (AFB) smear and culture × 3 are suggested. Mycobacterial DNA probing (Mycobacterium Tuberculosis Direct [MTD] test) can be useful to detect organisms at a lower load.

58. **Describe the treatment of TB in an HIV-infected patient.**
    Multiple drugs given for 2 months, including:
    - Isoniazid (INH) 300 mg/day with vitamin B6 (to prevent neuropathy)
    - A rifamycin (such as rifabutin with less potential interaction with ARTs than rifampin)
    - Pyrazinamide (PZA) 20–30 mg/kg/day
    - Ethambutol 25 mg/kg/day.

This regimen is then followed by 4 months of INH and a rifamycin. Directly observed therapy (DOT, or observation of the patient actually swallowing pills) with a health-care provider or responsible person is preferred. Sometimes, medications can be given two or three times a week for DOT or DOT is provided only Monday through Friday. Treatment is extended beyond 6 months if cultures are still positive after the initial 2 months of therapy. TB is a curable infection in HIV patients. The recommended treatment is currently similar for both HIV-infected and non–HIV-infected patients.

Centers for Disease Control and Prevention: Guidelines for prevention and treatment of opportunistic infections in HIV-infected adults and adolescents. Recommended from CDC, the National Institutes of Health, and the HIV Medicine Association of the Infectious Diseases Society of America, *MMWR Morb Mortal Wkly Rep* 58, 2009. Available at: www.cdc.gov/mmwr/preview/mmwrhtml/rr5804.pdf.

KEY POINTS: TUBERCULOSIS AND HUMAN IMMUNODEFICIENCY VIRUS ✓

1. All TB patients need to be tested for HIV infection.

2. All HIV patients without prior history of TB need to have the tuberculin skin test (PPD) or a blood test measuring IFN-γ.

3. PPD induration of 5 mm in HIV is positive, and treatment for LTBI should be strongly considered.

4. Risk of TB reactivation from LTBI is higher than the risk of significant toxicity from treatment.

5. Rifamycins such as rifampin have drug interactions with many ARTs. Therefore, use of rifabutin, a less potent CYP450 inducer, is preferable.

6. IRIS is common in TB and can paradoxically present as a clinical worsening despite appropriate therapy.

ARTs = antiretroviral therapies; CYP450 = cytochrome P450; HIV = human immunodeficiency virus; IFN-γ = interferon-γ; IRIS = immune reconstitution inflammatory syndrome; LTBI = latent tuberculosis infection; PPD = purified protein derivative; TB = tuberculosis.

59. **Is tuberculin skin testing (TST) with purified protein derivative (PPD) of any use in HIV-infected patients?**
Yes. TST may be helpful, but a negative PPD TST does not rule out TB exposure or infection. The accuracy of TST depends on the prevalence of underlying TB infection in the screened population and the degree of immunosuppression present in the screened patient. About half of active TB cases are secondary to reactivation, and therefore, treatment of latent tuberculosis infection (LTBI) would significantly reduce new outbreaks of active tubercular disease. TST is recommended in all patients diagnosed with HIV infection. Patients with a reaction > 5 mm should receive INH prophylaxis for 9 months, regardless of age at the time of diagnosis. Anergy is common, so patients with a documented exposure to TB should be given INH prophylaxis even when the TST is negative. A newer technology available to screen for LTBI is interferon-releasing assays, which detect the release of interferon-γ (IFN-γ) in response to MTb peptides. Although commercially available, the clinical use of these assays is still under review, and it likely will be used in combination with TST to improve specificity and sensitivity. These assays also have high false-negative rates in immunodeficient patients.

Centers for Disease Control and Prevention: Guidelines for prevention and treatment of opportunistic infections in HIV-infected adults and adolescents. Recommended from CDC, the National Institutes of Health, and the HIV Medicine Association of the Infectious Diseases Society of America, *MMWR Morb Mortal Wkly Rep* 58:1–198, 2009. Available at: www.cdc.gov/mmwr/preview/mmwrhtml/rr5804a1.htm.

60. **Define "immune reconstitution inflammatory syndrome (IRIS)."**
Inflammation related to a "rebooted" immune system and commonly reported in patients with a poor immune status before initiating ART. Patients with TB may develop similar symptoms when antituberculous therapy is started. The IRIS results in symptomatic inflammatory responses to subclinical opportunistic infections present in the patient. The most common findings are lymphadenitis due to *Mycobacterium avium* complex (MAC), paradoxical reactions of TB (fever, malaise, weight loss, worsening of chest x-ray finding), and exacerbations of cryptococcal meningitis or cytomegalovirus (CMV) retinitis. In severe cases, steroid therapy is temporarily given to diminish the inflammation but is administered cautiously.

> Shelburne SA, Hamill RJ: The immune reconstitution inflammatory syndrome, *AIDS Rev* 5:67–79, 2003.

61. **What other mycobacterial infections in addition to MTb are seen in HIV-infected patients?**
MAC and *Mycobacterium kansasii*. MAC may have a prevalence of 50% in autopsy findings of death from AIDS, and clinical studies have shown an annual risk of ~20% in patients with AIDS.

> Nightingale SD, Bird TL, Southern PM, et al: Incidence of *M. Avium*–intracellulare complex bacteremia in human immunodeficiency virus-positive patients, *J Infect Dis* 165:1082–1085, 1992.

62. **What are the symptoms and laboratory findings of MAC infection?**
- Fever
- Night sweats
- Weight loss
- Fatigue
- Malaise
- Diarrhea (may be chronic with resulting malabsorption)
- Abdominal pain
- Anemia
- Elevated liver function tests
- CD4 cell count < 50

63. **Describe the standard therapy for MAC in patients with AIDS.**
At least two oral medications with good activity against MAC. One of these agents should be either azithromycin (500 mg/day) or clarithromycin (500 mg twice daily). The second drug is usually ethambutol (15 mg/kg/day). Other active agents include rifabutin (300 mg/day) and ciprofloxacin (750 mg twice daily). When AFB are initially seen in a specimen and not yet identified, therapy for both MTb and MAC is given with a regimen of RIPE (rifampin, INH, pyrazanimide, ethambutol) + azithromycin.

> Centers for Disease Control and Prevention: Guidelines for prevention and treatment of opportunistic infections in HIV-infected adults and adolescents. Recommended from CDC, the National Institutes of Health, and the HIV Medicine Association of the Infectious Diseases Society of America, *MMWR Morb Mortal Wkly Rep* 58:1–198, 2009. Available at: www.cdc.gov/mmwr/preview/mmwrhtml/rr5804a1.htm.

64. **Which drugs are used as prophylaxis against MAC?**
Rifabutin, clarithromycin, and azithromycin. Primary prophylaxis is initiated when the CD4 cell count < 50. Because of ease of dosing and lack of drug interactions, most practitioners use azithromycin (1200 mg once/wk). Rifabutin may cause cross-resistance to rifampin in a patient with MTb who is inadequately evaluated and then treated with this single drug inadvertently.

SYPHILIS

65. **Which HIV-infected patients should have a serologic test for syphilis (STS)?**
Every HIV-infected patient. In addition, a detailed history for all STDs and past treatments
should be obtained. Most literature in the pre-HAART era suggested an accelerated course
and unusual progression of syphilis in patients also infected with HIV. Transmission
routes for HIV and syphilis are similar and both infections are likely to be transmitted
simultaneously. Patients with a positive serology for one infection should be tested for
the other. If the initial HIV test is negative in a patient with primary syphilils, a second test
should be done in 3 months to evaluate for the possibility of early HIV infection with the
absence of antibodies at the initial visit.

66. **Which HIV-infected patients with syphilis need a lumbar puncture (LP)?**
Those with syphilis of >1 year's duration or with any clinical signs or symptoms of CNS
involvement. Although a few authorities recommend an LP in all HIV-infected patients with
syphilis, most agree that those with a clear episode of adequately treated primary or
secondary syphilis do not need an LP. Patients with early syphilis whose serologic titers
increase or fail to decrease fourfold in 6 months also should undergo an LP to evaluate for
CNS involvement with syphilis before retreatment.

67. **What is the treatment for neurosyphilis in HIV-infected patients?**
Aqueous crystalline penicillin G, 2.4 million units (mU) IV every 4 hours (12–24 mU/day) for
10–14 days. Patients with penicillin allergy should undergo desensitization in order to allow
appropriate treatment with penicillin.

68. **If a chancre is present, is initial therapy for syphilis changed?**
No. The recommended regimen remains one dose of benzathine penicillin G, 2.4 mU
intramuscularly (IM), but many authorities treat primary syphilis more aggressively
in patients co-infected with HIV and administer a total of 7.2 mU (2.4 mU benzathine
penicillin G IM weekly for 3 consecutive wk).

69. **How should patients with HIV infection and primary syphilis be followed?**
With repeat STS at 1, 3, 6, and 12 months. If at any time there is a fourfold increase in
titer, an LP should be done. If by 6 months, the titer has not decreased fourfold, an
LP should be done to evaluate the cerebrospinal fluid (CSF) for CNS syphilis.

CNS DISORDERS AND INFECTIONS

70. **What is the most common cause of meningitis in AIDS patients?**
Cryptococcus neoformans. Although only 5–10% of AIDS patients present with cryptococcal
infection, up to 15% are subsequently found to have infection.

71. **How does cryptococcal infection present?**
See Table 13-6.

72. **What findings in a patient with suspected cryptococcus suggests the need
for an urgent LP?**
- Undiagnosed fever and headache with CD4 count < 100
- Altered mental status, lethargy, psychosis, and vomiting (symptoms of increased
intracranial pressure) with CD4 count < 100
- Positive serum cryptococcal antigen (CrAg) or blood culture positive for cryptococcus

TABLE 13-6. FREQUENCY OF SIGNS AND SYMPTOMS OF CRYPTOCCCAL MENINGITIS

Sign or Symptom	Frequency (%)
Symptoms	
Malaise	76
Headache	73
Fever	65
Nausea or vomiting or both	42
Cough or dyspnea or both	31
Stiff neck	22
Diarrhea	21
Photophobia	18
Focal deficits (symptom of)	5
Seizures	4
Signs	
Fever	56
Meningeal signs	27
Altered mentation	17
Focal deficit on neurologic examination	15

Adapted from Chuck SL, Sande MA: Infections with *Cryptococcus neoformans* in acquired immunodeficiency syndrome. N Engl J Med 321:794–799, 1989.

Repeat LPs should be performed in patients in whom the initial opening pressure was elevated (>25 cmH$_2$O), sometimes as often as daily, to relieve increased intracranial pressure and prevent neurologic damage. LP should also be repeated after 2 weeks of therapy to help evaluate microbial response.

73. **What CSF findings are seen in cryptococcal meningitis?**
    - Elevated total protein
    - Mild white blood cell (WBC) elevation
    - Low glucose
    - Positive India ink preparation
    - Positive CrAg
    - Positive fungal culture
    CSF findings may also be relatively normal.

74. **What treatment is recommended for cryptococcosis in AIDS?**
    IV amphotericin B, or its liposomal preparations, and oral flucytosine for 14 days. Oral fluconazole is continued at a dose of 400 mg/day for 8 weeks for consolidation therapy and at a dose of 200 mg/day life-long for maintenance. In complicated disease or in the presence of high cryptococcal antigen titers, treatment with IV amphotericin B may be extended beyond 14 days and oral doses of fluconazole increased.

    Centers for Disease Control and Prevention: Guidelines for prevention and treatment of opportunistic infections in HIV-infected adults and adolescents. Recommended from CDC, the National Institutes of Health, and the HIV Medicine Association of the Infectious Diseases Society of America, *MMWR Morb Mortal Wkly Rep* 58:1–198, 2009. Available at: www.cdc.gov/mmwr/preview/mmwrhtml/rr5804a1.htm.

75. **Are serum CrAg levels good indicators of response to therapy?**
    No. Although the serum antigen test can be very helpful in the diagnosis of cryptococcal infection, it cannot be used to judge therapeutic response. In most cases of meningitis, the CSF antigen titer should be determined by repeat LP. If the serum titer does revert to very low titer or negative after therapy, an increasing titer in the future should raise concern about a relapse. High serum cryptococcal titers suggest a poorer prognosis.

76. **What is PML?**
    Progressive multifocal leukoencephalopathy, a CNS demyelinating disease resulting from infection with a prion, Jakob-Creutzfeldt (JC) virus. Although spread throughout the population, JC virus requires profound immunosuppression to cause disease; in HIV, the CD4 count is typically < 50. Any part of the CNS can be involved, and therefore, patients often present with cognitive decline, ataxia, aphasia, and other focal motor weaknesses. As the name implies, lesions are multifocal and result in focal neurologic defects. Diagnosis is based on clinical findings, classic findings on magnetic resonance imaging (MRI) of T2 flair, and positive CSF JC virus polymerase chain reaction (PCR). Although there is no specific treatment for PML, HAART is indicated.

77. **What is AIDS dementia complex?**
    Cognitive, behavioral, and motor dysfunction associated with AIDS. Although multiple opportunistic infections need to be ruled out (e.g., cryptococcosis, toxoplasmosis, and TB), direct CNS infection by HIV seems to cause this complex of signs and symptoms. Early in its course, neuropsychological testing may be needed to support a clinical suspicion of dementia, but the dementia can progress to a vegetative state. Patients may first complain of concentration difficulties, and family and friends may note personality changes. Treatment should focus on using HAART therapy with good CSF penetration.

78. **What are the most common causes of CNS mass lesions in AIDS?**
    Cerebral toxoplasmosis and primary CNS lymphoma. Other causes include PML, cryptococcoma, tuberculoma, bacterial and fungal abscesses, and metastatic disease such as lung and breast cancer.

79. **What computed tomography (CT) scan findings differentiate CNS toxoplasmosis from lymphoma?**
    See Table 13-7. Centers with access to single-photon emission computed tomography (SPECT) scanning can identify likely lymphoma when an increased signal ratio is demonstrated.

TABLE 13-7. BRAIN COMPUTED TOMOGRAPHY FINDINGS IN CENTRAL NERVOUS SYSTEM TOXOPLASMOSIS AND LYMPHOMA

CT Finding	Toxoplasmosis	Lymphoma
Area involved	Deep gray matter and basal ganglia	White matter, periventricular areas
Mass effect	Yes	Yes
Enhancement	Ring enhancement	Weakly, not ring-shaped
Number of lesions	Multiple	1–2

CT = computed tomography.

80. **How is CNS toxoplasmosis treated?**
Most clinicians recommend empirical treatment for toxoplasmosis (pyrimethamine, 100-mg loading dose, then 25 mg/day; sulfadiazine, 4–6 g/day in divided doses; and folinic acid, 10–20 mg/day). CNS toxoplasmosis usually readily responds to this treatment with rapid improvement on CT or MRI within 3–5 days. If no response is seen within 10–14 days, another etiology should be investigated.

81. **Should primary toxoplasmosis prophylaxis be given?**
Yes. Patients positive for toxoplasma antibodies who also have a CD4+ count < 100 but no symptoms of toxoplasmosis should receive primary prophylaxis. Oral TMP-SMX 160/800 mg is the preferred daily regimen, providing protection against both PCP and toxoplasmosis. If this regimen is not tolerated, oral dapsone-pyrimethamine or atovaquone can be given.

> Centers for Disease Control and Prevention: Guidelines for prevention and treatment of opportunistic infections in HIV-infected adults and adolescents. Recommended from CDC, the National Institutes of Health, and the HIV Medicine Association of the Infectious Diseases Society of America, *MMWR Morb Mortal Wkly Rep* 58:1–198, 2009. Available at: www.cdc.gov/mmwr/preview/mmwrhtml/rr5804a1.htm.

HBV AND HCV INFECTIONS

82. **What are the best treatment combinations for the treatment of HBV and HIV?**
A combination of tenofovir with emtricitabine or lamivudine. Much like treatment of HIV, monodrug therapy for the treatment of HBV has been associated with development of hepatitis B resistance including the YMDD mutation, occurring in ~13% of patients after 1 year. For this reason, HBV therapy should include more than one active agent. Another combination would be entecavir with one of the following: lamivudine or emtricitabine or tenofovir. If lamivudine is withdrawn from a HIV treatment regimen, hepatitis may flare if there is a co-infection with HBV. Successful therapy is often marked by immunoconversion with development of a surface antibody (HBsAb). The HBV DNA level is a prognostic marker for the risk for hepatocellular carcinoma and cirrhosis.

> Centers for Disease Control and Prevention: Guidelines for prevention and treatment of opportunistic infections in HIV-infected adults and adolescents. Recommended from CDC, the National Institutes of Health, and the HIV Medicine Association of the Infectious Diseases Society of America, *MMWR Morb Mortal Wkly Rep* 58:1–198, 2009. Available at: www.cdc.gov/mmwr/preview/mmwrhtml/rr5804a1.htm.

83. **Is there an interaction between HIV and HCV infection?**
Probably. Most studies have shown a more rapid course of HCV infection in the HIV-infected patient, but some studies have not. The positive studies have shown an increased percentage of patients developing cirrhosis and a shorter time from infection to cirrhosis. Patients co-infected with HIV and HCV have an increased risk for liver-related death.

84. **How common is HIV/HCV co-infection?**
Very common. Many HIV clinics have reported co-infection rates in the range of 15–30%.

85. **What are the best treatments currently available for the treatment of HCV in the presence of HIV?**
Combination peg-interferon and ribavirin therapy. HCV genotype 1 is less likely to respond to treatment as defined by a sustained viral response (SVR) compared with genotypes 2 and 3. Response is optimal when the weight-based ribavirin is maintained at > 13 mg/kg/day. Early viral response can be used to predict which patients are most likely to achieve success. Using HCV drop of 1 log 10 at week 4 as a point for evaluation, those who do not achieve this goal have only a 2–5% chance for success. HCV replicates rapidly at more

than a million copies per day and concerns for early development of resistance persist; but for the drugs currently available on the market, cross-resistance with HIV is not of concern.

Centers for Disease Control and Prevention: Guidelines for prevention and treatment of opportunistic infections in HIV-infected adults and adolescents. Recommended from CDC, the National Institutes of Health, and the HIV Medicine Association of the Infectious Diseases Society of America, *MMWR Morb Mortal Wkly Rep* 58:1–198, 2009. Available at: www.cdc.gov/mmwr/preview/mmwrhtml/rr5804a1.htm.

Torriani FJ, Rodriguez-Torres M, Rockstroh JK, et al: Peginterferon Alfa-2a plus ribavirin for chronic hepatitis C virus infection in HIV-infected patients, *N Engl J Med* 351:438–450, 2004.

86. **What factors are associated with poorer response to HCV therapy in patients co-infected with HIV?**
   - Low CD4 cell counts
   - HCV genotype 1
   - HCV viral load > 800,000 IU/mL
   - Presence of cirrhosis
   - Active alcohol use

87. **What is the major toxicity of ribavirin (RTV)?**
   Hemolytic anemia that is dose-dependent. In the AIDS Pegasys Ribavirin International Coinfection Trial (APRICOT) trial of pegylated IFN-α plus RTV and a Randomized Controlled Trial of Pegylated-Interferon-alfa-2b plus Ribavirin vs Interferon-alfa-2b plus Ribavirin for the Initial Treatment of Chronic Hepatitis C in HIV Co-infected Patients (RIBAVIC) trial, 10–16% of patients required dose reductions in RTV because of anemia. Decreasing the dose of RTV has been associated with higher rates of virologic failure.

   Chung RT, Andersen J, Volberding P, et al: Peginterferon alfa-2a plus ribavirin versus interferon alfa-2a plus ribavirin for chronic hepatitis C in HIV-coinfected persons, *N Engl J Med* 351:2340–2341, 2004.

   Torriani FJ, Rodriguez-Torres M, Rockstroh JK, et al: Peginterferon alfa-2a plus ribavirin for chronic hepatitis C virus infection in HIV-infected patients, *N Engl J Med* 351:438–450, 2004.

88. **What are the potential interactions between RTV and antiretroviral medications?**
   RTV interacts with didanosine, zidovudine, and abacavir. Didanosine is absolutely contraindicated for patient taking ribavirin. Ribavirin increases didanosine phosphorylation and increases risk for mitochondrial toxicity leading to lactic acidosis, hepatic decompensation, and death. RTV decreases zidovudine phosphorylation, leading to impaired HIV control. RTV and abacavir share common phosphorylation pathways (guanosine analogues), which can lead to decreased response to HCV therapy.

DERMATOLOGIC DISORDERS

89. **How would you describe Kaposi's sarcoma (KS)?**
   Thickened and edematous woody skin with erythematous purple nodules and plaques. Retention hyperkeratosis can look warty in appearance with surrounding purple color or erythema. Bacillary angiomatosis from *Bartonella henslae* can mimic KS. The human herpesvirus-8 (HHV-8) virus is the cause of KS, which occurs as a result of abnormal T-cell responses. ART is the backbone of treatment of limited infection. Biopsy-proven disease will usually be required in order to institute chemotherapy. Lymphedema is a sign of systemic involvement. In this instance, ART may not be adequate and liposomal doxorubicin will likely be required for treatment. Facial lesions may be treated with vincristine by injection or radiation therapy. Hemoptysis and hematochezia may indicate that patients will likely require chemotherapy.

90. **What skin conditions can be a marker of a low immune system?**
   - Prurigo nodularis (generally with CD4 count < 100)
   - Molluscum contagiosum
   - Cryptococcal infection.
   - KS

91. **What is the appearance of toxic epidermal necrolysis?**
   Triangular blisters that represent shearing of the skin due to the separation of the epidermis from the dermis. The disorder is usually drug-induced (trimethaprim, sulfa, and vancomycin). Dermatologic consultation and treatment with intravenous immunoglobulin (IVIG) are indicated. Toxic epidermal necrolysis is a life-threatening condition.

92. **What common ART has been described to cause skin eruptions?**
   NNRTI therapy such as efavirenz and nevirapine, and the integrase inhibitor, raltegravir. These medications can cause erythema multiforme. Once this has occurred, do not rechallenge the patient with the offending drug. Abacavir has also been described to have allergic reaction with rash in 5–8% of patients, and patients with human leukocyte antigen (HLA)-B*5701 are most likely to show hypersensitivity reactions. The U.S. Food and Drug Administration (FDA) now recommends that patients be screened with HLA typing before the initiation of therapy when abacavir is prescribed.

RENAL DISORDERS

93. **What is HIVAN?**
   HIV-associated nephropathy. Case reports of HIVAN were first described in 1984 as a rapidly progressive form of focal segmental glomerulosclerosis (FSGS). What differentiates HIVAN from other forms of FSGS is the hallmark finding of a collapsing glomerulonephropathy and the presence of microcystic tubular dilatation and interstitial inflammation. HIVAN primarily affects blacks of African descent, although other HIV-infected patients with low CD4 (<200 cells/mm^3) and high HIV viral load (>4000 copies/mL) are at risk for developing HIVAN.

94. **How does HIVAN present and how is it diagnosed?**
   HIVAN presents as proteinuria with either normal or abnormal glomerular filtration rate (GFR). There are recent reports of HIVAN presenting with microalbuminuria, but all of these reports are in uncontrolled HIV infection with low CD4 counts and high HIV viral load. HIVAN is diagnosed by renal biopsy. The following clinical findings are suggestive of HIVAN: nephrotic range proteinuria, abnormal renal function for > 3 months (estimated glomerular filtration rate [eGFR] < 60 mL/min), echogenic normal size or large unobstructed kidneys, and absence of diabetes mellitus, hypertension, pregnancy, collagen vascular disease, cirrhosis, or organ transplant.

95. **How is HIVAN managed?**
   With HAART. Since December 2007, the diagnosis of HIVAN by renal biopsy is an AIDS-defining illness; therefore, the initial treatment includes HAART. As in other proteinuric renal disease, angiotensin-converting enzyme (ACE) inhibitors and angiotensin receptor blockers may be beneficial. The adjunctive use of corticosteroids has not been proved, but small uncontrolled studies have suggested some benefit with regards to decreasing proteinuria and improving the clinical course of HIVAN. If chronic kidney disease stage 3 or worse has developed at the time of diagnosis, it is very likely that HIVAN will progress to end-stage renal disease (ESRD) rapidly. HIV-infected patients with ESRD will benefit from dialysis support. Renal transplant should be considered as long as the HIV infection is well

controlled. Although most reports show that acute rejection in the first year after renal transplant is higher in patients with HIV, the overall survival after the first year is almost equal to that in non–HIV-infected patients.

96. **Which HAART medications need to be adjusted based on eGFR?**
All NRTIs except abacavir.

97. **How does tenofovir nephrotoxicity present?**
With proximal tubular acidosis (renal tubular acidosis type 2) and global proximal tubular dysfunction, also known as "Fanconi's syndrome." Fanconi's syndrome can manifest as non–anion-gap metabolic acidosis, hypophosphatemia, hypokalemia, glucosuria, aminoaciduria, and proteinuria. Tenofovir has also been associated with acute tubular necrosis.

MISCELLANEOUS DISORDERS

98. **What is thrush?**
Oropharyngeal pseudomembranous candidiasis, which often presages AIDS. Thrush usually presents as white plaques called "pseudomembranes" on areas of less friction such as under the tongue and the posterior buccal wall. The lesions from *Candida albicans* easily rub off, leaving a red base. Fluconazole is the treatment of choice. Resistant forms of thrush (*Candida glabrata*) require non–azole-based therapy, such as echinocandins and amphotericin B. Thrush can be confused with oral hairy leukoplakia, a whitish corrugated growth along the margins of the tongue found in HIV-infected patients and caused by the Epstein-Barr virus (EBV).

99. **Explain the significance of thrush.**
Thrush often indicates significant immunosuppression and, if found during an initial examination, suggests the need for HIV-related medical interventions for prophylaxis of opportunistic infections regardless of CD4 count. If the patient is not known to be HIV-infected, the diagnosis of thrush warrants HIV testing.

100. **What is the most common cause of blindness in AIDS?**
CMV infection leading to chorioretinitis. Although formerly experienced by 5–10% of patients with AIDS during the course of their illness, the incidence of this AIDS-defining diagnosis has declined dramatically during the era of more effective ART.

101. **How is CMV retinitis diagnosed?**
By fundoscopic examination. Retinal examination usually reveals large white granular areas with hemorrhage (described as "cottage cheese in ketchup") with CMV retinitis. Symptoms may include blurred vision, decreased visual acuity, increasing "floaters," or a clear visual field cut. All patients with advanced HIV infection (CD4 counts < 100) should undergo routine retinal screening on a quarterly basis.

102. **In addition to chorioretinitis, what are the other manifestations of CMV infection in HIV infection?**
- Interstitial pneumonia
- Colitis
- Esophagitis
- Adrenal insufficiency
- Encephalitis

103. **Define HIV wasting syndrome.**
Weight loss > 10% of body weight with either chronic diarrhea or weakness and fever for > 30 days. HIV wasting syndrome is an AIDS-defining diagnosis. One should always evaluate a patient with suspected HIV wasting syndrome for other HIV-related causes of chronic diarrhea, weakness, and fever, but in the absence of other secondary causes, a diagnosis of HIV wasting syndrome can be made.

104. **In addition to KS and non-Hodgkin's lymphoma, what other malignancies are seen in HIV infection?**
See Table 13-8.

TABLE 13-8. MALIGNANCIES ASSOICATED WITH HUMAN IMMUNODEFICIENCY VIRUS AND CHANGES IN INCIDENCE SINCE 1998	
Malignancy	**Incidence Change**
Kaposi's sarcoma	↓
Central nervous system lymphoma	↓
Lymphoma (non-Hodgkin's)	↑
Lymphoma (Hodgkin's disease)	↑
Cervical cancer	↑
Anal cancer	↑
Lung cancer	↑
Prostate	↔
Breast	↔
Hepatoma	↔

From Patel P, Hanson DL, Sullivan PS, et al: Incidence of types of cancer among HIV-infected persons compared with the general population in the United States, 1992–2003. Ann Intern Med 148:728–736, 2008.

105. **How often does HIV infection result in anemia or thrombocytopenia?**
Frequently. Anemia occurs in up to 80%, neutropenia in 85%, and thrombocytopenia in 65% of cases. HIV-infected but asymptomatic patients are much less frequently cytopenic. Clinically significant thrombocytopenia indistinguishable from that seen in idiopathic thrombocytopenic purpura (ITP) may be a presentation of HIV infection. Typically, bone marrow is normal with adequate numbers of megakaryocytes. The disorder behaves much like classic ITP in that patients respond to steroids and splenectomy. An HIV antibody test is recommended in patients presenting with ITP. Of interest is the recent recognition of thrombotic thrombocytopenic purpura in association with HIV infection.

106. **What metabolic complications are associated with HIV treatments?**
- **Alterations in glucose metabolism:** insulin resistance, glucose intolerance, diabetes mellitus
- **Hyperlipidemia:** hypercholesterolemia, hypertriglyceridemia
- **Hyperlactatemia** and **lactic acidosis**
- **Fat redistribution:** visceral fat accumulation, subcutaneous fat atrophy
- **Osteoporosis**

107. **Describe the sensory neuropathy seen in HIV.**
Many patients with HIV experience a distal sensory polyneuropathy that may be due to HIV infection or HIV treatment with certain neurotoxic nucleoside analogues such as zalcitabine, didanosine, and stavudine. Patients present with paresthesias, numbness, or pain in the distal extremities. Symptoms are symmetrical and move proximally with progression. The temporal relationship of symptoms to initiation of medication is the only way to implicate a drug side effect as the etiology of the neuropathy. HIV-related neuropathy often responds to effective anti-HIV therapy, but this response is not uniform and can be delayed.

108. **How are rheumatologic studies affected by HIV infection?**
Patients with HIV make increased nonspecific antibodies, resulting in both an increased frequency of autoimmune disorders as well as an increased number of false-positive antibody based tests. Laboratory evaluations often reveal low titers of rheumatoid factor (RF), antinuclear antibodies (ANAs), and anticardiolipin antibodies. Generalized hypergammaglobulinemia is also seen, as are elevated creatine kinase (CK) levels of uncertain significance.

Mody GM, Parke FA, Reveille JD: Articular manifestations of human immunodeficiency virus infection, *Best Prac Res Clin Rheum* 17:580–591, 2003.

PRIMARY CARE OF HIV-INFECTED PATIENTS

109. **What vaccines are recommended in HIV-infected patients?**
- Hepatitis A, one complete series of two doses
- Hepatitis B, one complete series of three doses
- 23-valent pneumococcal polysaccharide vaccine every 5 years
- Inactivated influenza vaccine (intramuscular) annually
- For patients aged 19–64: Tetanus toxoid, reduced diphtheria toxoid, and acellular pertussis vaccine (Tdap) as a single dose followed by tetanus diphtheria toxoid (Td) every 10 years
- For patients aged > 64, Tetanus diphtheria toxoid every 10 years
- For women aged 13-26, Human papillomavirus (HPV) vaccine, one complete series of three doses

110. **What vaccines should be avoided in persons with HIV infection?**
- Combined measles-mumps-rubella vaccine (MMR) or any of its individual components
- Shingles vaccine (herpes zoster)
- Oral typhoid vaccine.
- Smallpox vaccine
These are all live vaccines and should not be given because of the risk for disseminated disease

111. **How well do HIV-infected patients respond to the influenza vaccine?**
Not as well as non–HIV-infected subjects, but administration of the influenza vaccine is indicated for all persons infected with HIV. CD4+ counts < 100 are associated with poor antibody responses. Studies showing increased HIV viral load and decreased CD4+ counts in study participants receiving influenza vaccine compared with placebo-injected controls have raised concerns, but no adverse clinical events have been demonstrated.

Tasker SA, O'Brien WA, Treanor JJ, et al: Effects of influenza vaccination in HIV-infected adults: A double-blind placebo-controlled trial, *Vaccine* 16:1039–1042, 1998.

112. **Do HIV-infected patients respond to the pneumococcal polysaccharide vaccine?**
    Partially. The response is impaired compared with normal control subjects. HIV-infected patients mount an adequate antibody response to fewer of the serotypes contained in the 23-valent vaccine, and this response rate decreases with decreasing CD4+ counts. As with influenza vaccination, there appears to be increased HIV viral activity after pneumococcal vaccination, but because morbidity due to pneumococcal disease is clearly and substantially increased in HIV-infected patients, the risk-to-benefit ratio supports vaccination.

    Moore D, Nelson M, Henderson D: Pneumococcal vaccination and HIV infection, *Int J STD AIDS* 9:1–7, 1999.

113. **Are there any travel restrictions for persons living with HIV?**
    Yes. In 1992, the International AIDS Conference moved outside of the United States because of visa restrictions for persons with HIV who enter the United States at that time. In January 2010, all restrictions for entering or migrating to the United States for people with HIV infection were lifted. Country-specific information can be obtained at www.hivtravel.org

ACKNOWLEDGMENT

The editor gratefully acknowledges contributions by Dr. Christopher J. Lahart that were retained from the previous edition of *Medical Secrets*.

WEBSITES

1. The AIDS Education and Training Center (AETC): http://www.aids-ed.org

2. AIDSInfo: http://www.aidsinfo.nih.gov/Guidelines

3. The American Academy of HIV Medicine (AAHIVM): http://aahivm.org

4. HIV Medicine Association (HIVMA): http://www.hivma.org

5. International AIDS Society (IAS-USA): http://www.iasusa.org

6. Stanford HIV RT and Protease Sequence Database: http://hivdb.stanford.edu/hiv

BIBLIOGRAPHY

1. Mandell GL, Bennett JE, Dolin R, editors. *Principles and Practice of Infectious Diseases*, ed 6, Philadelphia, 2005, Churchill Livingstone.
2. Sande MA, Volberding PA, editors: *The Medical Management of AIDS*, ed 6, Philadelphia, 1999, WB Saunders.

CHAPTER 14

HEMATOLOGY

Damian Silbermins, M.D., and Ara D. Metjian, M.D.

Blood is the originating cause of all men's diseases.

The Talmud, Baba Nathra, III.58a

The blood is the life.

The Bible, Deuteronomy 12:23

IRON METABOLISM AND IRON OVERLOAD

1. **Describe the major steps in iron absorption.**
   There are two sources of dietary iron: **heme** and **elemental iron.** Heme iron requires gastric acidity to release it from its apoprotein. In the duodenum (mostly), ferric iron (Fe^{3+}) is transformed into ferrous iron (Fe^{2+}) by the duodenal ferric reductase (Dcybt), which allows DMT1 (divalent metal transporter) to transfer the Fe^{2+} into the enterocyte. Ferritin is stored in the enterocyte. In order to be transported out of the cell into circulation, Fe^{2+} has to be converted back to Fe^{3+} (by hephaestin and other enzymes). Ferroprotein transports Fe^{3+} into the circulation, but only a limited amount of iron circulates. The remaining intracellular iron is lost with enterocyte shedding.

   Fleming RE, Bacon BR: Orchestration of iron homeostasis, *N Engl J Med* 352:1741–1744, 2005.

2. **Describe the mechanisms of iron utilization.**
   In the circulation, Fe^{3+} is bound to transferrin. The transferrin receptor in the hematopoietic precursors binds transferrin (iron bound) and creates an endosome to liberate the iron within the cell.

3. **What is hepcidin?**
   An acute-phase reactant that inhibits iron egress from the cells by binding to and inactivating the iron transport protein ferroprotein. Intestinal absorption of iron and iron release by macrophages is also negatively influenced by hepcidin. Hepcidin is produced by the liver and filtered by the kidney.

   Fleming MD: The regulation of hepcidin and its effects on systemic and cellular iron metabolism, *Hematology Am Soc Hematol Educ Program* 151–158, 2008.

4. **What causes iron overload?**
   - Chronic administration of iron to non–iron-deficient persons
   - Chronic transfusion therapy
   - Increased absorption of dietary iron (hemochromatosis, thalassemia intermedia or major, sideroblastic anemia)

5. **Summarize the consequences of iron overload.**
   - **Cardiac:** cardiomyopathy and arrhythmias
   - **Hepatic:** elevated liver enzymes (aspartate aminotransferase [AST] and alanine aminotransferase [ALT]), cirrhosis, and hepatocellular carcinoma
   - **Endocrine:** hypothyroidism, hypogonadotrophic hypogonadism, hyperpigmentation, and diabetes mellitus

- **Arthropathy:** chondrocalcinosis or pseudogout
- **Bone:** osteopenia and subcortical cysts
  If the transferrin saturation is > 75%, the percentage of labile iron (nontransferrin bound iron) increases significantly. This form of iron has a greater potential to cause end-organ damage.

6. **What test is frequently used to screen for hemochromatosis?**
   Ferritin. Levels > 300 ng/dL in males and > 200 ng/dL in females are suggestive of hemochromatosis. Ferritin is an acute-phase reactant and may be elevated in inflammatory conditions. The serum transferrin saturation (serum iron divided by the total iron-binding capacity) is also frequently used to screen for hemochromatosis. Because of the diurnal variation in serum iron, a fasting morning sample is best. A serum transferrin saturation > 50% for women and > 60% for men suggests the possibility of iron overload.

7. **What can cause increased ferritin other than iron overload?**
   - Chronic liver disease due to alcoholism, hepatitis, and nonalcoholic steatohepatitis
   - Inflammatory conditions such as rheumatoid arthritis
   - Malignancy
   - Hemophagocytic lymphohistiocytosis
   - Obesity
   - Ferritin/cataract syndrome

8. **Summarize the genetic link to hemochromatosis.**
   Mutations in the *HFE* gene may account for most cases in Caucasian patients, who appear to have genetic hemochromatosis. Homozygosity for C282Y or the combination of C282Y and another mutation, H63D in *HFE*, can be detected by the polymerase chain reaction (PCR) assay. Use of this genetic method in population studies shows that not all patients who appear to have the hemochromatosis genotype develop clinical iron overloading. If C282Y mutation is absent or the patient is not Caucasian and the patient is young (<30 yr), thinking about hemojuvelin or hepcidin mutation is appropriate. In older patients, ferroportin or transferrin receptor 2 mutation is possible. When iron overload is present in patients with normal or low transferrin saturation, a plasma ceruloplasmin should be drawn to exclude aceruloplasminemia. If normal, then genetic testing for ferroportin mutation (type 4A hemochromatosis) should be undertaken (V162del and A77D mutations)

   Brissot P, Troadec MB, Bardou-Jacquet E, et al: Current approach to hemochromatosis, *Blood Rev* 22:195–210, 2008.

9. **How is hemochromatosis treated?**
   Initially with weekly phlebotomy as long as the ferritin is > 300 for males and > 200 for females. Once this level is achieved, phlebotomy continues every other week until the ferritin is < 50. Phlebotomy is then continued every 2–4 months to maintain ferritin < 50. Transferrin saturation should be checked biannually. If the hemoglobin (Hb) is < 11, phlebotomy is contraindicated and iron chelators may be needed.

   Le Lan C, Loreal O, Cohen T, et al: Redox active plasma iron in C282Y/C282Y hemochromatosis, *Blood* 105:4527–4531, 2005.

HYPOPROLIFERATIVE ANEMIAS

10. **Define "anemia."**
    A reduction in the Hb or hematocrit (Hct). Different thresholds have been proposed:
    - The World Health Organization (WHO) defines anemia as Hb < 13 g/dL for men and < 12 g/dL for nonpregnant women.
    - National Comprehensive Cancer Network (NCCN) defines chemotherapy-induced anemia as Hb < 11 g/dL.

- Normal values may vary according to ethnicity. Regardless of age, anemia in African American females is defined as < 11.5 g/dL.
- Normal ranges may not apply to special populations such as athletes, smokers, and those who live at high altitude.

Beutler E, Waalen J: The definition of anemia: What is the lower limit of normal of the blood hemoglobin concentration? *Blood* 107:1747–1750, 2006.

11. **How are the anemias classified?**
By mechanism and duration. The mechanisms of anemia include underproduction, destruction (hemolysis), and blood loss. Anemia can be further classified as **acute** or **chronic.** Most anemias are chronic and allow the body to compensate to maintain sufficient Hb levels.

12. **How is anemia defined in pregnancy?**
Hb < 11 g/dL in the first and third trimesters and < 10.5 g/dL in second trimester. Severe anemia that requires immediate attention is Hb < 9 g/dL.

Milman N: Prepartum anemia: prevention and treatment, *Ann Hematol* 12:949–959, 2008.

13. **What is the mean cell volume (MCV)? Red cell distribution width (RDW)?**
The MCV is an average of the size of the red blood cell (RBC). The RDW is an index of the heterogeneity of cell size.

14. **How are MCV and RDW used in the evaluation of anemia?**
See Table 14-1.

TABLE 14-1.	CLASSIFICATION OF ANEMIAS BASED ON MEAN CELL VOLUME AND RED CELL DISTRIBUTION WIDTH*		
	MCV Low	**MCV Normal**	**MCV High**
RDW normal	Chronic disease	Normal	Aplastic anemia
	Nonanemic heterozygous thalassemia	Chronic disease	
		Nonanemic or enzyme abnormality	
	Children	Splenectomy	
		CLL (except extreme high-lymphocyte number)	
		Acute blood loss	
RDW high	Iron deficiency	Early or mixed nutritional deficiency	Folate or vitamin B_{12} deficiency
	HbS-α or β-thalassemia	Anemic abnormal hemoglobin	Sickle cell anemia (one third of cases)
		Myelofibrosis	Immune hemolytic anemia
		Sideroblastic anemia	Cold agglutinins
		Myelodysplasia	Preleukemia

CLL = chronic lymphocytic leukemia; HbS = hemoglobin S; MCV = mean cell volume; RDW = red cell distribution width.
*Chronic liver disease, chronic myelogenous leukemia, and cytotoxic chemotherapy may be associated with high or normal MCV and high or normal RDW.
From Bessman JD: Automated Blood Counts and Differentials: A Practical Guide. Baltimore, Johns Hopkins University Press, 1986, p 11.

15. **Summarize the symptoms and signs of iron deficiency.**
   ■ Fatigue
   ■ Exercise intolerance
   ■ Weakness
   ■ Headache
   ■ Pica (craving of nonfood items such as ice, starch, or dirt)
   ■ Restless leg syndrome
   ■ Symptoms of Plummer-Vinson syndrome
      ■ Dysphagia due to esophageal webs
      ■ Painless stomatis
      ■ Koilonychia (spooning of the fingernails)

   Moore DF Jr, Sears DA: Pica, iron deficiency, and the medical history, *Am J Med* 97:390–393, 1994.

16. **How is the diagnosis of iron-deficiency anemia (IDA) confirmed?**
   By bone marrow biopsy. The interpretation, though, can vary among pathologists, and this method is not useful for diagnosis after replacement with parenteral iron therapy.
   A ferritin < 30 µg/dL is diagnostic of iron deficiency, but relying only on this cutoff would miss milder forms of iron deficiency.

17. **In the treatment of IDA, how much iron should be administered, in what form, and for how long?**
   Usually oral ferrous sulfate, 325 mg three times/day until the anemia corrects and then continued for an additional several months. This regimen provides 60 mg of elemental iron per tablet, or 180 mg/day. Iron should not be taken with meals or within 2 hours of taking antacids. The major side effects are dyspepsia, constipation, and blackening of the stool. Patients usually need to start at once-daily dosing and gradually increase to three times/day to improve tolerance. Liquid iron preparations are sometimes better tolerated. Taking vitamin C (250 mg ascorbic acid) may improve iron absorption. Intravenous (IV) iron therapy has been used in patients undergoing renal dialysis to optimize the response to erythropoietin therapy, who have ongoing blood loss (e.g., inflammatory bowel disease or Osler-Weber-Rendu syndrome), who are intolerant of oral iron, or who are unable to absorb iron due to small intestinal disease (e.g., celiac disease).

18. **What are the common causes of iron deficiency?**
   ■ Dietary deficiency
   ■ Malabsorption (sprue and postgastrectomy patients)
   ■ Chronic blood loss
   ■ Menstrual blood loss (females)
   ■ Chronic intravascular hemolysis
   ■ Idiopathic pulmonary hemosiderosis
   ■ Repetitive phlebotomy

19. **When is it appropriate to order Hb electrophoresis to evaluate hypochromic microcytic anemia?**
   When iron stores are established as normal. The microcytic disorders that may be detected are β-thalassemia minor and the so-called thalassemic hemoglobinopathies (including hemoglobin E [HbE] in Asians). β-Thalassemia minor is marked by an increased HbA_2 and sometimes increased fetal Hb. Iron deficiency results in a decreased pool of alpha chains, for which the beta chain of HbA and the delta chain of HbA_2 must compete. Beta chains are more successful, resulting in diminished HbA_2 during iron deficiency. For this reason, a search for β-thalassemia may be thwarted when patients are also iron-deficient.

   Beutler E: The common anemias, *JAMA* 259:2433–2437, 1988.

20. **Which diseases are usually associated with the anemia of chronic disease (AOCD)?**
Inflammatory states, including malignancy, rheumatologic disease, and infection. AOCD is a subtype of underproduction anemia compounded by decreased RBC life span. Although it is typified by a low serum iron, low total iron-binding capacity, and low percent saturation but increased iron stores, as evidenced by an increased ferritin, these distinctive iron abnormalities are not central to its pathogenesis. A study of hospitalized patients showed that the laboratory pattern of AOCD occurs in a significant number of anemic patients who do not have inflammatory conditions. These patients were severely ill with complications of diabetes, renal failure, and hypertension.

   Spivak J: The blood in systemic disorders, *Lancet* 355:1707–1712, 2000.

21. **What causes macrocytosis?**
See Table 14-2.

TABLE 14-2. CAUSES OF MACROCYTOSIS

Megaloblastic anemia (macro-ovalocytosis)	Sideroblastic anemia*
	Chronic obstructive pulmonary disease
Alcoholism	Artifacts and idiopathic
Malignancy	Pregnancy
Hemolysis (usually poorly compensated)	Liver disease
	Drugs (zidovudine, hydroxyurea, azathioprine, anticonvulsants)
Aplastic anemia	
Hypothyroidism	Arsenic poisoning
Refractory anemias (myelodysplasia)	

RBCs = red blood cells.
*Often marked by dual populations of RBCs—one hypochromic microcytic and the other macrocytic.
From Colon-Otero G, et al: A practical approach to the differential diagnosis and evaluation of the adult patient with macrocytic anemia. Med Clin North Am 76:581–596, 1992; and Savage DG, et al: Etiology and diagnostic evaluation of macrocytosis. Am J Med Sci 319:343–352, 2000.

---

22. **How is cobalmin (vitamin B$_{12}$) deficiency diagnosed?**
By levels of vitamin B$_{12}$, methylmalonic acid (MMA), or homocysteine. The manifestations of clinical vitamin B$_{12}$ deficiency can vary in the individual patient, and may be mild. In 97% of the cases, vitamin B$_{12}$ level is low (<200 ng/L or <148 pmol/L) and often very low (<100 ng/L or 74 pmol/L). Subclinical vitamin B$_{12}$ deficiency can exist with levels of 250–350 ng/L (185–258 pmol/L). In clinical cobalamin deficiency, **MMA** is elevated in 98% of the cases and **homocysteine** is elevated in 96%. (See also Chapter 18, Geriatrics.)

   Carmel R, Green R, Rosenblatt DS, Watkins D: Update on cobalamine, folate, and homocysteine, *Hematology Am Soc Hematol Educ Program* 62–81, 2003.

23. **What disorders reduce vitamin B$_{12}$ absorption?**
   - Pernicious anemia associated with gastric atrophy and loss of intrinsic factor due to an autoimmune-mediated attack on the gastric mucosa
   - Gastrectomy with development of megaloblastic anemia within 5–6 years
   - Disorders of the small intestine such as ileal resection, Crohn's disease, and celiac sprue

- Competition with intestinal flora associated with blind-loop syndrome and fish tapeworm (*Diphyllobothrium latum*)
- Pancreatic disease
- Diet of strict vegetarians (no meat, eggs, or milk) and breast-fed infants of strict vegetarians
- Drugs such as aspirin, neomycin, colchicines, slow-release potassium chloride, cholestyramine, and proton pump inhibitors

24. **Describe the pattern of neurologic disease associated with vitamin B_{12} deficiency.**
    - **Posterior column:** paresthesia, disturbed vibratory sense, and loss of proprioception
    - **Pyramidal:** spastic weakness and hyperactive reflexes
    - **Cerebral:** dementia, psychosis (megaloblastic madness), and optic atrophy

KEY POINTS: HYPOPROLIFERATIVE ANEMIA ✔

1. The approach to anemia requires a thorough history and physician examination, careful examination of the peripheral blood smear, and reticulocyte count.

2. In evaluation of microcytic anemia, the first tests should include serum iron, total iron-binding capacity, and ferritin to look for iron-deficiency anemia.

3. Thalassemia is best evaluated after iron deficiency is ruled out or corrected.

4. Vitamin B_{12} and folate deficiencies should be initially considered in evaluation of macrocytic anemias.

5. Anemia of chronic disease is the first consideration for a patient with a normochromic normocytic anemia.

6. Renal insufficiency and diabetes mellitus are common chronic diseases contributing to anemia.

25. **Is the severity of anemia a good predictor of neurologic involvement?**
    No. A significant minority of patients with peripheral neuropathy or other neurologic manifestations of vitamin B_{12} deficiency have a normal Hct and MCV, but low or low-normal vitamin B_{12} levels. Serum MMA and homocystine can detect vitamin B_{12} deficiency at an earlier stage than RBC indices and vitamin B_{12} levels.

    Lindenbaum J, Healton EB, Savage DG, et al: Neuropsychiatric disorders caused by cobalamin deficiency in the absence of anemia or macrocytosis, *N Engl J Med* 318:1720–1728, 1988.

26. **What blood cell disorders are diagnosed by bone marrow biopsy and aspiration?**
    - **Pancytopenia:** myelodysplasia, aplastic anemia, myelophthisic states, hypersplenism, and megaloblastic anemia
    - **Anemia:** sideroblastic anemia, refractory anemia, and pure RBC aplasia
    - **Staging of malignancy:** Hodgkin's disease, leukemias, non-Hodgkin's lymphoma (NHL), and multiple myeloma
    - **Thrombocytopenia:** evaluation of idiopathic thrombocytopenic purpura (ITP)
    - **Neutropenia**

- **Infectious diseases:** typhoid, tuberculosis, pancytopenia seen in acquired immunodeficiency syndrome (AIDS), brucellosis, and fever of unknown origin
- **Lipid-storage diseases** (such as Gaucher's disease)

27. **Why is bone marrow biopsy essential to the diagnosis of sideroblastic anemia?**
To detect ringed sideroblasts.

28. **Define "aplastic anemia."**
As peripheral pancytopenia. Bone marrow examination shows a hypocellular bone marrow with the absence of an infiltrative process and no increase in bone marrow reticulin. Commonly used criteria for severe aplastic anemia include:
- Marrow biopsy cellularity < 25% or 25–50% with < 30% residual hematopoietic cells
- Two of the following:
  - Neutrophil count < 0.5×10^9/L
  - Platelet count < 20×10^9/L
  - Reticulocyte count< 20×10^9/L
  Very severe aplastic anemia is as above and with absolute neutrophil count (ANC) < 200.

29. **What tests should be ordered in the work-up of aplastic anemia?**
- Complete blood count (CBC) with differential, reticulocyte count, peripheral blood smear, and HbF
- Bone marrow biopsy and aspirate
- Blood chromosomal breakage analysis to exclude Fanconi's anemia if < 50 years old
- Flow cytometry to rule out paroxysmal nocturnal hemoglobinuria
- Vitamin B_{12} and folate
- Viral studies (hepatitis A, B [HBV], and C [HCV] viruses; Epstein-Barr virus [EBV], human immunodeficiency virus [HIV], and cytomegalovirus [CMV])
- Antinuclear antibody (ANA) and anti-double-stranded DNA (anti-dsDNA) antibodies
- Chest x-ray to evaluate for the presence of a thymoma
- Abdominal scan
- Echocardiogram
- Peripheral blood gene mutation analysis for dyskeratosis congenital (*DKC1, TERC, TERT*) if there are clinical features or lack of response to immunotherapy

    Marsh JC, Ball SE, Cavenagh J, et al: Guidelines for the diagnosis and management of aplastic anaemia, *Br J Haematol* 147:43–70, 2009.

30. **What is the differential diagnosis for pancytopenia and a hypocellular marrow?**
- Hypocellular myelodysplastic syndrome (MDS)/acute myelogenous leukemia (AML)
- Hypocellular acute lymphocytic leukemia (ALL)
- Hairy cell leukemia
- Lymphomas
- Mycobacterial infections
- Anorexia nervosa or prolonged starvation

31. **What supportive measures should be taken in the care of patients with aplastic anemias?**
1. Prophylactic platelet transfusion (if <10,000 or <20,000 if the patient is febrile)
2. *Irradiated* blood products for any transfusions
3. Prophylactic antibiotics and antifungals if ANC < 200
4. Human leukocyte antigen (HLA) typing as soon as possible to permit for bone marrow donor search as well as platelet transfusion if there is refractoriness
5. Iron chelation if serum ferritin >1000 ng/dL

32. **What is the best therapy for aplastic anemia in a young person?**
For patients who are younger than 40 years, bone marrow transplantation (BMT) from a HLA-identical sibling is the current standard of care. If there is not an HLA-identical sibling, cyclosporine and antithymocyte should be started, but response may take months. High-resolution HLA-identical but nonrelated donors may be used for such patients.

33. **What are the most important causes of death in patients undergoing BMT?**
Infection. After conditioning, patients become pancytopenic during the 3 weeks or so required for engraftment. The objective of the myeloablative preparation is to both eradicate the cancer and induce immunosuppression to allow engraftment. During that time, these patients are prone to **infectious complications** similar to those experienced by patients undergoing remission-induction chemotherapy for AML. These patients are treated prophylactically with antibiotics and transfusions of RBCs and platelets. Blood products must be irradiated to prevent **GVHD** (graft-versus-host disease) from donor lymphocytes. After engraftment, **interstitial pneumonitis** is a frequent complication, with a high mortality rate. Some of these deaths are due to infectious agents such as CMV. Recently, a severe form of **veno-occlusive disease** of the liver has emerged as a cause of morbidity and mortality after BMT. Owing to the high mortality rate of conditioning regimens, some patients may benefit from reduced-intensity conditioning (RIC), although it can be offset by a higher rate of relapse. RIC has been most effective in slow-growing cancers (chronic lymphocytic leukemia [CLL], low-grade NHL). If transplantation is urgent and a match cannot be found, cord blood can be safely used. The transplantation of cord blood requires less stringent HLA matching but is complicated by a longer time to engraftment.

   Copelan EA: Hematopoietic stem cell transplantation, *N Engl J Med* 354:1813–1826, 2006.

34. **What are the characteristics of acute GVHD?**
Acute GVHD arises during the first 100 days after transplant, with donor T cells targeting the host's skin, liver, and gastrointestinal tract. Patients may have mild skin rashes or more severe disease resulting in toxic epidermal necrolysis. Diarrhea and transient elevation of liver enzymes may occur and, in some patients, are more severe, resulting in massive diarrhea and liver failure. Immunologic competence is also delayed by GVHD, so that patients are susceptible to new infections, including those mediated by encapsulated organisms such as pneumococci. A regimen of total lymphoid irradiation and an antithymocyte regimen (i.e., T-cell depletion) has been shown to reduce acute GVHD.

   Lowsky R, Takahashi T, Lui YP, et al: Protective conditioning for acute graft versus host disease, *N Engl J Med* 353:1321–1331, 2005.

35. **Characterize chronic GVHD.**
Forty to 60% of survivors of allogenic BMT will develop chronic GVHD. This affects the same organs as acute GVHD, with the additional features of a scleroderma-like illness. Dry eyes, dry mouth, myasthenia, bronchiolitis, and infections are also observed. Three variables have been associated with shortened survival: extensive skin involvement (>50% of the body surface), platelet count < 100,000/µL and progressive onset. The main treatment is immunosuppression, although patients are best treated under investigational protocols.

   Vogelsang GB, Lee L, Bensen-Kennedy DM: Pathogenesis and treatment of graft-versus-host disease after bone marrow transplant, *Annu Rev Med* 54:29–52, 2003.

36. **What is the principal indication for erythropoietin-stimulating agents (ESAs) therapy in the treatment of anemia?**
   - Chronic kidney disease (CKD)
   - HIV infection and AIDS if treated with zidovudine (AZT)
   - Cancer with chemotherapy for palliative care
   - MDS

37. **What concomitant studies should be checked before initiation of ESAs?**
Iron studies including ferritin and percent saturation (calculated from the iron and total iron-binding capacity [TIBC]). ESAs require sufficient iron stores to be effective. In practice, a ferritin level > 100 ng/dL and an iron saturation > 20% are necessary. For patients with MDS, the pretreatment erythropoietin (EPO) level should be < 500.

38. **What are the potential adverse events of ESAs?**
Hypertension, fever, and local reactions. Less common but serious adverse events include vascular thrombotic events, increase in certain cancers, splenic rupture, and pure RBC aplasia. Diabetic patients treated with ESAs for CKD have a higher risk of stroke. A rapid raise in the Hb (>1 g/dL/wk) is an adverse prognostic factor.

39. **What are the current indications for ESA use in chemotherapy-induced anemia?**
An Hb concentration that is approaching or falling below 10 g/dL. In patients with a higher risk of vascular events (elderly; those with uncontrolled hypertension, limited cardiopulmonary reserve, or underlying coronary artery disease; frail patients), watchful waiting is recommended until the Hb < 10 g/dL. ESAs should be used cautiously in patients at a high risk for venous thromboembolism such as those with pancreatic and stomach cancer, thrombocytosis, leukocytosis, and morbid obesity. ESAs should only be used in patients receiving **palliative chemotherapy** and not in **adjuvant chemotherapy.**

Rizzo JD, Somerfield MR, Hagerty KL, et al: Use of epoetin and darbopoetin in patients with cancer: 2007 American Society of Hematology/American Society of Clinical Oncology clinical practice guideline update, *Blood* 111:25–41, 2008.

Khorana AA, Kuderer NM, Culakova E, et al: Development and validation of a predictive model for chemotherapy associated thrombosis, *Blood* 111:4902–4907, 2008.

HEMOLYTIC ANEMIAS

40. **List some of the causes of hemolytic anemia (HA).**
Disorders of:
- Immune system
- RBC membrane
- RBC enzymes
- Globin synthesis
- External causes

41. **List the complications of chronic HA.**
- Aplastic crises (associated with parvovirus B19)
- Hemolytic crises
- Megaloblastic crises (increased demand for folate)
- Pigment gallstones
- Splenomegaly
- Stasis ulcers
- Pulmonary artery hypertension
- Thrombosis, arterial or venous

42. **What supplement is mandatory for all patients with HA?**
Folate 1 mg by mouth daily.

43. **What are the immunologic causes of HA?**
- **Alloimmune:** result from the receipt of incompatible blood
- **Autoimmune:**

- Autoimmune hemolytic anemia (AIHA) due to warm antibodies
- AIHA due to cold antibodies
- Drug-induced

44. **Explain the mechanism of immediate and delayed hemolytic transfusion reactions.**
An immediate reaction can be mediated by preformed immunoglobulin M (IgM) antibodies owing to inappropriately cross-matched blood (e.g., type A receiving type B blood). Delayed hemolytic transfusion reactions occur when the patient has been sensitized to a foreign RBC antigen, which can be from pregnancy or a prior transfusion. Eventually, the alloantibody decreases in titer and is no longer detected on a typical type and cross. However, if blood containing that same RBC epitope is transfused again, the patient develops a rapid immune response against the transfused RBCs.

> Gehrs BC, Friedberg RC: Autoimmune hemolytic anemia, *Am J Hematol* 69:258–271, 2002.

45. **Describe the characteristics of AIHA due to warm antibodies.**
The warm antibody of AIHA is usually IgG, which is able to bind to the RBCs at 37°C, hence the "warm" designation. Warm autoimmune AIHA can be seen in a variety of conditions, including autoimmune disease such as systemic lupus erythematosus (SLE); lymphoproliferative disorders (chronic lymphocytic leukemia, Hodgkin's disease, and NHLs); postinfections that are usually viral; or idiopathic.

46. **Describe the characteristics of AIHA due to cold-reactive antibodies.**
Cold-reactive AIHA is typically induced by IgM antibodies that bind to RBCs at much lower temperatures. Cold agglutinin disease may be a self-limited disorder brought on by mycoplasmal infection (usually anti-I) or infectious mononucleosis (usually anti-i). Chronic cold agglutination disease may be an idiopathic syndrome or associated with a lymphoproliferative disorder.

47. **What is paroxysmal cold hemoglobinuria (PCH)?**
A cold-reactive HA in which antibodies to the P antigen are formed. The autoantibody is termed the **Donath-Landsteiner** antibody and binds to the P-glycoprotein on RBCs. The reaction shows "biphasic hemolysin" properties, meaning that the autoantibody will bind to RBCs, without lysing them at 0°C; however, when the sample is warmed to 37°C, hemolysis will occur. Although PCH is historically associated with syphilis, it is now more common in children after infections, particularly parvovirus. (The P antigen is the binding site for the virus.)

48. **Explain the direct Coombs' test used to evaluate AIHA.**
The direct Coombs' test detects antibodies on RBCs (direct Coombs' or direct antiglobulin test [DAT] positive) or in plasma. In the direct test, the RBCs are washed and incubated with an antiglobulin serum (rabbit or other species) and then examined for agglutination.

49. **Explain the indirect Coombs' test.**
In the indirect test, the serum is reacted with a panel of RBCs bearing antigens of interest. Antibodies, if present in the sera, bind to the RBCs bearing the relevant antigen. The panel cells are washed to reduce nonspecific binding and then incubated with an antiglobulin serum to detect agglutination. The antiglobulin reagent is necessary because antibodies attached to RBCs are usually IgG in low numbers and cannot ordinarily cross-link to agglutinate. The antiglobulin serum bridges these antibodies, favoring agglutination.

50. **How is the Coombs' test used to evaluate AIHA?**
In AIHA, the direct test is usually positive, indicating the presence of an autoantibody on the RBCs. The indirect test, indicating the presence of the same antibody in serum, also may

be positive. Persons who have been exposed to blood or have had pregnancy losses may develop antibodies to certain antigens on the transfused RBCs that do not exist on native RBCs. Later, they have a positive indirect Coombs' test and negative direct Coombs' test.

51. **What are some of the disorders of RBC membranes that lead to anemia?**
    - Hereditary spherocytosis (HS)
    - Hereditary elliptocytosis (HE)
    - Hereditary pyropokilocytosis
    - Rh deficiency
    - Dehydrated hereditary stomatocytosis (formerly known as "xerocytosis")
    - Overhydrated hereditary stomatocytosis

52. **Describe the underlying protein deficiency associated with HS.**
    Spectrin, the principal membrane protein found in erythrocytes. Spectrin has self-associative properties and forms a lattice with other RBC membrane proteins and actin. This supportive lattice on the inner aspect of the lipid bilayer gives the RBC its unique properties of strength and suppleness. The extent of spectrin deficiency correlates with the degree of hemolysis, changes in osmotic fragility, and response to splenectomy. The most common genetic defect in HS is in the ankyrin gene. Spectrin deficiency is often present with other genetic mutations as alterations in their products affect the assembly of spectrin into the cytoskeleton.

    An X, Mohandas N: Disorders of the red cell membrane, *Br J Haematol* 141:367–375, 2008.

53. **What is the differential diagnosis of spherocytosis in the peripheral blood film?**
    - ABO incompatibility
    - Phospholipase enzymes found in certain venoms or clostridial sepsis
    - Microangiopathic hemolytic anemias
    - AIHA

54. **What are the risks and benefits of splenectomy in patients with HS?**
    Splenectomy can markedly improve the anemia of HS, lower bilirubin levels that can contribute to gallstones, and improve skeletal growth. The risks include surgical complications (bleeding), postoperative thrombosis, pulmonary hypertension, and increased risk of infections, particularly from encapsulated organisms.

    Schilling RF: Risks and benefits of splenectomy versus no splenectomy for hereditary spherocytosis— a personal view, *Br J Haematol* 145:728–732, 2009.

55. **If a patient is scheduled for an elective splenectomy, what vaccines should be received before surgery?**
    - Pneumococcal polysaccharide
    - *Haemophilus influenzae* type B (HiB)
    - Meningococcal (aged 2–55 yr) or meningococcal polysaccharide (age > 55 yr)

56. **When should the patient receive these vaccines?**
    Preferably more than 14 days before surgery.

57. **What is HE?**
    A broad spectrum of disorders that result in an elliptical RBC shape and hemolysis. In general, HE results from genetic defects that arise in the horizontal interaction of the RBC membrane cytoskeleton that depends on alpha spectrin–beta spectrin association and interaction of spectrin with band 4.1 protein to form a high-molecular-weight oligomeric structure. Most patients with HE and its variants have a structural abnormality of the spectrin protein that results in failure of the protein to self-associate into higher-order tetramers and oligomers.

58. What are the most important subsets of HE?
- **Mild common HE:** normal Hct and mild reticulocytosis
- **Common HE with chronic hemolysis:** more striking degree of hemolysis, anemia, and more bizarre RBC morphology
- **Infantile poikilocytosis:** present at birth; later associated with striking hemolysis, bizarre RBCs, and jaundice
- **Homozygous HE:** rare subset accompanied by severe anemia
- **Hereditary pyropoikilocytosis:** rare subset in which the spectrin is abnormally sensitive to heat with a peripheral blood picture similar to that seen in hemolysis associated with severe burns
- **Spherocytic elliptocytosis:** unusual autosomal dominant disorder in which the elliptocytes are rounded with increased osmotic fragility
- **Southeast Asian ovalocytosis**

59. What are the RBC enzyme defects that lead to anemia?
- **Pyruvate kinase:** the most common cause of nonspherocytic chronic HA
- **Glucose 6-phosphate dehydrogenase (G6PD):** the most common disorder of the red blood cell
- **Glucose-6-phosphate isomerase**
- **Hexokinase:** rare, autosomal recessive
- **Phosphofructokinase:** rare, autosomal recessive
- **Aldolase:** extremely rare with only 6 reported cases
- **Triosephosphate isomerase:** very rare autosomal recessive disease
- **Phosphoglycerate kinase**

60. How is G6PD deficiency characterized?
As an X-linked disease that is one of the most common RBC enzyme deficiencies in the world, with an estimated 400 million affected individuals. The enzyme catalyzes the rate-limiting step in the generation of NADPH (nicotinamide adenine dinucleotide phosphate, reduced form) by converting glucose-6-PO_4 to 6-phosphoglucono-δ-lactose. NADPH is necessary for the reduction of glutathione-containing disulfides (GSSG [oxidized glutathione] to GSH [reduced glutathione]) in the reduction of oxidative species. Therefore, reduced or absent stores of NADPH in the RBC make it vulnerable to oxidative stress. In addition to hemolysis, oxidation results in precipitation of Hb, which can be detected as Heinz bodies by supravital staining with crystal violet. G6PD deficiency is categorized into five groups:
- **Class I:** severe deficiency in enzyme activity and is associated with a chronic non-spherocytic HA
- **Class II:** 1–10% of enzyme activity
- **Class III:** moderate deficiency with 10–60% of enzyme activity
- **Class IV:** normal activity 60–150% of enzyme activity
- **Class V:** elevated level of enzyme activity (>150%)

61. How do patients with G6PD present?
Typically with jaundice and HA early in life. However, many patients with G6PD deficiency may go through life without any symptoms. These patients typically present after some stress to their RBCs, whether by ingestion of medications, certain foods, or illness.

62. How is G6PD deficiency diagnosed?
By measurement of the enzymatic activity of G6PD by quantitative spectrophotometric analysis of the rate of NADPH production from NADP (nicotinamide adenine dinucleotide phosphate). This enzyme activity may be falsely negative during acute hemolysis or in the presence of reticulocytosis because the activity in young RBCs is higher than in more mature cells.

Cappellini MD, Fiorelli G: Glucose-6-phosphate dehydrogenase deficiency, *Lancet* 371:64–74, 2008.

63. **What is favism?**
An acute hemolytic crisis in patients with G6PD deficiency that occurs after eating fava beans. Compounds within the beans are thought to increase the activity of the erythrocytic hexose monophosphate shunt, leading to hemolysis.

64. **What else can cause hemolysis in G6PD deficiency?**
- Antimalarials (primaquine and possibly chloroquine)
- Sulfonamides
- Nitrofurantoin
- Acetanilide and possibly aspirin
- Naphtalene

65. **What are the laboratory features of intravascular hemolysis?**
- Increased reticulocyte count
- Indirect hyperbilirubinemia-acholuric jaundice (unconjugated bilirubin is not secreted in urine)
- Hemoglobinuria
- Fall of Hb > 1 g/7 days in the absence of bleeding or massive hematoma

KEY POINTS: HEMOLYSIS ✔

1. The peripheral blood smear should be reviewed to establish a diagnosis of hemolysis.

2. Reticulocyte counts will be elevated in patients without other complications.

3. The reticulocyte count may be low in patients with inflammation or renal failure. Hemolysis is suspected in these patients if the hemoglobin decreases 1 g/wk.

4. Acute blood loss or the presence of a large hematoma may be confused with hemolysis.

5. Ineffective erythropoiesis may have laboratory features resembling hemolysis including increased unconjugated bilirubin and LDH.

LDH = lactate dehydrogenase.

66. **Give examples of intravascular hemolytic disorders.**
- Hemolytic transfusion reactions
- Paroxysmal nocturnal hemoglobinuria
- March hemoglobinuria
- RBC fragmentation syndromes

67. **What are some other major acquired hemolytic disorders?**
- Malaria
- Hypersplenism
- Physical agents such as heat, copper, and certain oxidants

68. **What is fragmentation hemolysis?**
The appearance of schistocytes, helmet cells, burr cells (echinocytes), and spherocytes on a peripheral blood smear in a patient with HA. The hemolysis is intravascular and can be associated with a wide variety of conditions.

69. **What are some of the causes of microangiopathic HA?**
- Cavernous hemangiomas (Kasabach-Merritt syndrome)
- Thrombotic thrombocytopenic purpura (TTP)

- Hemolytic-uremic syndrome (HUS)
- Eclampsia and preeclampsia
- Malignant hypertension
- Scleroderma
- Valve hemolysis
- Disseminated carcinomatosis
- Disseminated intravascular coagulation (DIC)
  In addition to the anemia, thrombocytopenia may occur.

70. **What is the classic pentad of TTP?**
- Microangiopathic HA, with schistocytes on the peripheral smear
- Thrombocytopenia
- Renal insufficiency
- Fever
- Neurologic changes
  Most patients will not present with the classic pentad in the modern era. Currently, TTP is a diagnosis of exclusion and a platelet count of $< 100,000/\mu L$ and lactate dehydrogenase (LDH) levels > 1.5 times the upper limit of normal are necessary for diagnosis. TTP should not be diagnosed in patients with systolic blood pressure (BP) > 180 mmHg or diastolic BP > 120 mmHg until the BP has been controlled.

71. **How does HUS differ from TTP?**
In HUS, renal failure is the predominant organ syndrome associated with thrombocytopenia and fragmentation hemolysis. Metalloprotease activity, absent in TTP, is present in HUS, indicating a different pathogenesis. Ninety percent of HUS is associated with shiga-like toxin-producing bacteria. In some families, a deficiency in plasma factor H, a complement control factor, is associated with recurrent HUS. Another small population with atypical HUS may carry a mutation in thrombomodulin.

72. **What is ADAMTS13 and how is it implicated in TTP?**
A disintegrin **a**nd **m**etalloproteinase with **t**hrombo**s**pondin-1–like motif, member **13** that cleaves the ultralarge von Willebrand's factor (vWF) multimers produced by endothelial cells. Some patients with TTP have a deficiency in ADAMTS13 and, therefore, have a high concentration of the ultralarge VWF multimers. This leads to extensive microvascular platelet deposition with thrombocytopenia and blockade of small vessels. Activity of ADAMTS13 but not antibodies against ADAMTS13 has been associated with relapse of TTP. Although the effectiveness of plasma exchange had been attributed to removal of antibodies against ADAMTS13 and replacement of this critical enzyme, it has also been demonstrated to be useful in patients without a severe deficiency.

Jin M, Casper TC, Cataland SR, et al: Relationship between ADAMTS13 activity in clinical remission and the risk of TTP relapse, *Br J Haematol* 141:651–658, 2008.

Vesely SJ, George JN, Lammle E, et al: ADAMTS13 activity in thrombotic thrombocytopenic purpura–hemolytic-uremic syndrome: Relation to presenting features and clinical outcomes in a prospective cohort of 142 patients, *Blood* 102:60–68, 2003.

73. **How is TTP treated?**
With plasma exchange. Patients are typically exposed to 11–22 units of plasma/day for 1–3 weeks with a high number of expected allergic reactions (~66%). Prednisone 1 mg/kg/day is often added as adjuvant, and rituximab has been used in refractory cases.

Reutter JC, Sanders KF, Brecher ME, et al: Incidence of allergic reactions with fresh frozen plasma or cryo-supernatant plasma in the treatment of thrombotic thrombocytopenic purpura, *J Clin Apheresis* 16:134–138, 2001.

Rock GA, Shumak KH, Buskard NA, et al: Comparison of plasma exchange with plasma infusion in the treatment of thrombotic thrombocytopenic purpura, *N Engl J Med* 325:393–397, 1991.

74. **What are the disorders of globin synthesis?**
    - Hemoglobinopathies, including the thalassemias
    - Sickle cell syndromes
    - Unstable Hbs

75. **What is thalassemia?**
    Any disorder in which the synthesis of a globin chain required for the production of Hb is disrupted. In adults, RBCs contain mostly HbA, typically $> 96\%$, with a minimal amount of HbA_2, and rare amounts of HbF. Whereas HbA is composed of 2 alpha and beta chains apiece ($\alpha_2\beta_2$), A_2 is $\alpha_2\delta_2$, and is HbF is $\alpha_2\gamma_2$. Normally, the ratio of alpha and beta chains in the RBC is tightly regulated to be 1:1.

76. **What is α-thalassemia?**
    The hemoglobinopathy resulting from a series of defects that lead to a decrease in the synthesis of α globin. Normal adults have two copies of the α globin gene on each copy of chromosome 16, denoted $\alpha\alpha/\alpha\alpha$. α-Thalassemia results from the deletion of one (-$\alpha/\alpha\alpha$), two (-$\alpha/$-α or --/$\alpha\alpha$), three (--/-α), or four (--/--) of the α-globin genes.

77. **What are the different α-thalassemias and how do they manifest?**
    Unfortunately, there are a variety of names in the literature, which often leads to confusion. These are the basic names/forms of the α-thalassemias:
    - α^+-Thalassemia or α-thalassemia trait (-$\alpha/\alpha\alpha$) occurs with the loss of one α globin, occurring frequently in African Americans. The majority of patients are "silent-carriers," meaning they are clinically normal. RBC morphology and indices can be normal, along with a normal HbEP.
    - α-Thalassemia-1, or α^0-thalassemia (--/$\alpha\alpha$) occurs with the loss of two α-globin genes on one chromosome alone. This is sometimes referred to as being in "*cis*-." This form is common in patients of Asian descent and is characterized by a mild, hypochromic, microcytic anemia. The HbEP can be normal and care must be taken not to mistake this for IDA. Of concern is that two parents can potentially have a child who may inherit no α-globin genes, leading to hydrops fetalis (see later).
    - One α-globin gene deleted from both chromosomes (-$\alpha/$-α) is α-thalassemia-2, α^+-thalassemia, or α-thalassemia minima. This deletion is said to be in "*trans*-." It is commonly seen in patients of African or Mediterranean descent. Like α-thalassemia-1, it is associated with a mild, hypochromic, microcytic anemia and a normal HbEP.
    - When a total of three α-globin genes are missing (--/-α), this leads to the production of HbH. Because very little α globin is made, β_4 tetramers form RBC inclusions, which can be visualized by staining with brilliant cresyl blue. The resulting HA is characterized by a marked anisopoikilocytosis, hypochromia, and reticulocytosis. HbEP shows the presence of HbH.
    - Deletion of all four α-globin genes (--/--) causes the total absence of alpha chains. Therefore, HbA, HbA_2, or HbF cannot be made, resulting in Hb-Bart (γ_4). The peripheral blood smear is remarkable for a marked anisopoikilocytosis, hypochromia, target cells, reticulocytosis, and nucleated red blood cells (NRBCs). The HbEP shows approximately 80% Hb-Bart and approximately 20% Hb-Portland ($\zeta_2\gamma_2$). These Hbs have a left-shifting oxygen dissociation, leading to significant fetal hypoxia, oftentimes causing death in utero or shortly thereafter. This is common in Asian populations, because the *cis*- mutations are needed for this to occur.

78. **What is β-thalassemia?**
A general term for a spectrum of diseases caused by the imbalance of available β-globin chains. Unlike α-thalassemia, β-thalassemia is characterized not by whole gene deletions, but by mutations within the β-globin genes on chromosome 11.

79. **What are the different types of β-thalassemia?**
- **β-thalassemia minor** or **β-thalassemia trait** refers to patients with a single defect in the β-globin gene, causing reduced expression of the beta chains. Patients are mildly anemic, hypochromic, and microcytic. The hallmark of β-thalassemia minor is an HbEP with an elevated HbA_2. As with the α-thalassemias, it is important to not inappropriately diagnose or treat these patients as iron-deficient.
- **β-thalassemia intermedia** refers to a broad spectrum of mutations and clinical symptoms caused by mutations in both β-globin genes. Those that are able to make some β globin are sometimes referred to as $β^+$-thalassemia. Symptoms range between that of β-thalassemia minor and β-thalassemia major. Patients are usually anemic, microcytic, and hypochromic. The HbEP will also show an increase in the HbA_2 levels.
- **$β^0$-thalassemia**, **β-thalassemia major**, and **Cooley's anemia** all refer to conditions in which no β-globin chains are made. This absence of β-globin causes the formation of $α_4$ tetramers that are highly toxic to the RBC membrane. Because no β-globin chains can be made, no HbA or HbA_2 will be seen on the HbEP. Developing RBCs perish in the marrow or limp out to live a short, withered existence in the circulation. Erythropoiesis is highly ineffective and patients have tremendous expansion of the bone marrow and extramedullary hematopoiesis, as evidenced by marked hepatosplenomegaly. Affected children are transfusion-dependent; if not transfused aggressively, they develop pathologic fractures and significant growth retardation.

    Oliveri N: The beta-thalassemias, *N Engl J Med* 341:99–109, 1999.

SICKLE CELL DISEASE

80. **What is sickle cell disease?**
The hematologic disorder resulting from mutations in the β-globin chain, which produces polymers that are poorly soluble when deoxygenated. Classically, "sickle cell disease" refers to HbS disease, which results from a substitution of a valine for glutamic acid at the sixth amino acid of the β-globin chain.

81. **Many abnormal Hbs with single amino acid changes are known. Of these, which sickle or participate in the sickling process during deoxygenation?**
- S-β-thalassemia
- SC
- SD-Punjab
- SO-Arab
- SLepore-Boston
- S-Antilles

82. **What is the incidence of sickle hemoglobinopathies in births among African Americans?**
- **AS:** 8%
- **AC:** 3%
- **SS:** 0.16%
- **SC:** 0.12%
- **$Sβ^0$:** 0.03%

Note that the incidence of $S\beta^0$ and SC is approximately that of SS. In adults, as many patients with sickle β-thalassemia or SC will be seen as homozygous S patients. Although $S\beta^0$ is clinically similar to SS disease, $S\beta^+$ and SC patients are more likely to have palpable spleens and may experience splenic sequestration and infarctive crises as adults rather than in early childhood, as is the case with SS disease. SC patients also tend to have higher Hbs. They may present with blindness due to retinopathy or aseptic necrosis of the hip.

83. **What morbidities are associated with sickle trait?**

Splenic infarction at high altitude	Medullary renal carcinoma	Sudden death after exertion
Hyposthenuria	Pulmonary embolism	Bacteremia in women
Hematuria	Glaucoma, anterior chamber bleeds	
Bacteriuria and pyelonephritis in pregnancy		

84. **What are sickle crises?**
Sudden, unheralded, vaso-occlusive events that can have multiple symptoms but most commonly present as a pain crisis affecting the limbs, low back, chest, or abdomen. Sometimes specific organs are affected by definite infarcts, including the bone and spleen (if splenic tissue has been preserved).

85. **What is acute chest syndrome?**
Dyspnea, fever, pain, and sudden appearance of an infiltrate on chest x-ray consistent with pneumonia in patients in sickle crisis. Although an overt pneumonia may not exist, a number of patients may have atypical infections, notably *Chlamydophila pneumoniae*. Recent studies of chest syndrome have emphasized the role of fat embolism from bone marrow infarcts and infections. Splinting while the patient is suffering a rib infarct may lead to hypoventilation and pulmonary vaso-occlusion. Incentive spirometry has been advocated to reduce the risk of chest syndrome in patients hospitalized with sickle crises and chest pain. Among older patients and those with neurologic dysfunction, the symptoms can progress to respiratory failure. In a large multicenter trial, neurologic events occurred in 11% of patients. Acute chest syndrome progressed to respiratory failure in 13% of the patients and 3% of the cohort died.

Vichinsky EP, Neumayr LD, Earles AN, et al: Causes and outcomes of the acute chest syndrome in sickle cell disease, *N Engl J Med* 342:1855–1865, 2000.

86. **How are patients in a sickle crisis managed?**
Patients with chest syndrome often receive antibiotics and require oxygen. When hypoxemia continues despite oxygen therapy, exchange transfusions are helpful. The pathophysiology of the pain crisis is not well understood. Strict adherence to National Institutes of Health (NIH) guidelines in the treatment of vaso-occlusive episodes is recommended. Careful history and review of prior hospitalizations is necessary for prompt pain relief and to recognize subtle changes that may require more aggressive therapy.

National Institutes of Health: *National Heart, Blood, and Lung Institute: The Management of Sickle Disease*, ed 4, 2002. Available at: www.nhlbi.nih.gov/health/prof/blood/sickle/sc_mngt.pdf.

87. **How often do crises occur?**
Once every year or 2. About 20% of patients, however, are troubled by more frequent crises and may visit the emergency department or hospital monthly. Why some patients with sickle

cell disease do poorly while others do relatively well is one of the mysteries of sickle cell disease. Similarly, it is not known what initiates crises or what mechanisms of spontaneous recovery terminate crises while patients are receiving only supportive care. The severity and duration of crises are variable. Stays for patients requiring hospitalization vary from 3–10 days.

Platt OS, Thorington BD, Brambilla DJ, et al: Pain in sickle cell disease: Rates and risk factors, *N Engl J Med* 325:11–16, 1991.

88. **Summarize routine health maintenance for adults with sickle cell anemia.**
    - Preventive services as recommended for specific age group
    - Genetic counseling about the risk of sickle cell disease in relatives or children
    - Folic acid supplementation
    - Periodic ophthalmoscopic examinations
    - Pneumococcal polysaccharide 23-valent vaccine (PPSV23). A second dose of PPSV23 is recommended 5 years after the first dose of PPSV23
    - Annual (or more often as indicated) renal function evaluation
    - Iron studies to evaluate for iron overload if multiple transfusions received

89. **What are the main complications of sickle cell disease?**
    - Painful episodes
    - Ischemic strokes (can be silent and lead to cognitive impairment)
    - Acute chest syndrome
    - Priapism
    - Liver disease (from iron overload and HBV and HCV infection)
    - Splenic sequestration
    - Miscarriages
    - Leg ulcers
    - Osteonecrosis
    - Proliferative retinopathy
    - Renal insufficiency
    - Pulmonary hypertension
    - Cholelithiasis
    - Acute aplastic episodes
    - Osteomyelitis
    - Alloimmunization
    - Functional asplenia

90. **How often does pulmonary arterial hypertension (PAH) occur in sickle cell disease?**
    In about 30% of adult patients homozygous for Hb SS and confers an increased risk of death (~20% mortality at 2 yr). (See also Chapter 6, Pulmonary Medicine.)

    Gladwin MT, Sachdev V, Jison ML, et al: Pulmonary hypertension as a risk factor for death in patients with sickle cell disease, *N Engl J Med* 350:886–895, 2004.

91. **What is the average life span of patients with SS disease?**
    Rarely beyond 50 years of age. Because of the extent of complications and despite high mortality and morbidity, BMT is becoming an attractive option for patients with severe disease.

92. **Is RBC transfusion routinely recommended for the treatment of typical pain crises?**
    No.

93. **Under what circumstances should RBC transfusion be considered in the treatment of sickle cell disease?**

STRONG INDICATIONS	RELATIVE INDICATIONS
Aplastic crises	Before general anesthesia
Hypoxemia and chest syndrome	During pregnancy
Heart failure	Baseline anemia
Central nervous system (CNS) events and stroke	Simple surgery
Sequestration crises	Priapism
Intractable pain	Before arteriography

Wanko SO, Telen MJ: Transfusion management in sickle cell disease, *Hematol Oncol Clin N Am* 19:803–826, 2005.

94. **What protocol is recommended for RBC transfusion in sickle cell disease?**
A national cooperative study found that simple transfusions to an arbitrary level of Hb seemed to enable patients to undergo general anesthesia with no worse outcome than patients who had exchange transfusions. Because less blood was used, the conservative transfusion protocol was complicated less often by alloimmunization.

Claster S, Vichinsky EP: Managing sickle cell disease, *BMJ* 327:1151–1155, 2003.

95. **A patient with sickle cell disease presents with a history of a viral syndrome, followed by dramatic worsening of the anemia. What entity needs to be strongly considered?**
Aplastic crisis. Typically, patients have a flulike illness, with or without an evanescent rash, fever, and myalgias, followed 5–10 days later by weakness and dyspnea. The patient presents with a sharply reduced Hct. A key finding is the nearly absolute absence of reticulocytes. This disorder is in fact a transient pure RBC aplasia. The platelet and white blood cell (WBC) counts are usually unaffected. Bone marrow shows the absence of erythroid progenitors, except for a few "giant pronormoblasts."

96. **What is the most common cause of aplastic syndrome?**
Infection with parvovirus B19, which has a unique tropism for erythroid progenitors.

97. **Explain the physiologic and clinical significance of parvovirus-induced aplasia.**
In patients with a compensated chronic hemolytic disorder, parvovirus-induced aplasia is significant because the duration of aplasia (5–10 days) coincides with the half-life of RBCs. Thus, cessation of RBC production for 10 days in a patient with an Hct of 22% and RBC life span of 9 days spells trouble. Transfusions of packed RBCs are life-saving. The 10-day cessation of erythropoiesis caused by the parvovirus goes unnoticed in a normal person with an Hct of 40% and an RBC life span of 120 days. The parvovirus may be the cause of fifth disease, arthritis, and spontaneous abortions.

Saarinen UM, Chorba TL, Chattersall P, et al: Human parvovirus B19–induced epidemic acute red cell aplasia in patients with hereditary hemolytic anemia, *Blood* 67:1411–1417, 1986.

98. **What is the role of hydroxyurea (HU) in the treatment of patients with severe and frequent (>3 crises/yr) sickle cell anemia?**
Perhaps the greatest therapeutic advance in sickle hemoglobinopathy was the recognition that certain chemotherapeutic agents can reverse the developmental "switch" from fetal to adult Hb synthesis. The rise in HbF in each RBC suppresses sickling and offers the promise

of reduced hemolysis and vaso-occlusive phenomena. A double-blinded trial of HU was halted early when it was shown to reduce the rate of crises by ~40% and also to reduce the incidence of chest syndrome and frequency of transfusions and, in a follow-up study, prolonged survival.

Charache S, Terrin ML, Moore RD, et al: Effect of hydroxyurea on the frequency of painful crises in sickle cell anemia, *N Engl J Med* 332:317–322, 1995.

KEY POINTS: SICKLE CELL DISEASE ✓

1. Patients should have hemoglobin electrophoresis or HPLC or both to determine the exact sickling disorder.

2. All patients with sickle hemoglobinopathies should receive pneumococcal, HiB, and meningococcal vaccines.

3. Adult patients with SS Hb and more than three severe pain crises/yr should be considered for hydroxyurea treatment.

4. Transfusions in sickle cell patients have significant risk and should be avoided unless the patient has a severe complication (acute chest syndrome, stroke, or aplastic crisis).

5. Acute chest syndrome is a frequent cause of death in hospitalized patients with sickle cell disease. Treatment with RBC transfusions or exchange transfusions, antibiotics, and oxygen is essential.

Hb = hemoglobin; HiB = *Haemophilus influenzae* type B; HPLC = high performance liquid chromatography; RBC = red blood cell.

99. **Is HU leukemogenic?**
Uncertain. Reports of leukemia and other cancers have been described in patients who have received HU; however, this was observed in patients with other blood conditions (e.g., polycythemia vera [PCV] or essential thrombocytosis), which can progress to leukemia on their own. Therefore, it is difficult to confirm or refute the role of HU in this regard. Although cases of leukemia and other cancers have been described in sickle cell patients treated with HU, they are rare and are no more common than seen in the regular population. At this point, there are no data to support the theory of leukemogenicity of HU in practice.

Brawley OW, Cornelius LJ, Edwards LR, et al: National Institutes of Health Consensus Development Conference Statement: Hydroxyurea treatment for sickle cell disease, *Ann Intern Med* 148:932–938, 2008.

LEUKOCYTE DISORDERS

100. **What is the lower limit for the ANC?**
Usually 1.8×10^9/L (1800/mm^3). When the neutrophil count $< 0.5 \times 10^9$/L (500/mm^3), neutropenia is severe with a greater risk of infection. African Americans have a lower mean neutrophil count, without increased incidence or severity of infections. Recent data suggest that lower neutrophils in the African American population could be tied to CC genotype of the Duffy (Fy) because in these individuals, the Duffy antigen receptor for chemokines (DARC) is not expressed.

Grann VR, Ziv E, Joseph CK, et al: Duffy (Fy), DARC, and neutropenia among women from the United States, Europe and the Caribbean, *Br J Haematol* 143:288–293, 2008.

101. **What disorders cause decreased production of neutrophils?**
   - Drug-induced disorders (see later)
   - Hematologic diseases (idiopathic disease, cyclic neutropenia, Chediak-Higashi syndrome, aplastic anemia, and infantile genetic disorders)
   - Tumor invasion and myelofibrosis
   - Nutritional deficiencies (vitamin B_{12}, folate, and alcoholism)
   - Infections (tuberculosis, typhoid fever, brucellosis, tularemia, measles, dengue fever, mononucleosis, malaria, viral hepatitis, leishmaniasis, and AIDS)

102. **Which drugs commonly cause neutropenia?**
   See Table 14-3.

TABLE 14-3. DRUGS THAT CAUSE NEUTROPENIA

Antiarrhythmics: tocainide, procainamide, propranolol, quinidine

Antibiotics: chloramphenicol, penicillins, sulfonamides, *para*-aminosalicylic acid, rifampin, vancomycin, isoniazid, nitrofurantoin, ganciclovir

Antimalarials: dapsone, quinine, pyrimethamine

Anticonvulsants: phenytoin, mephenytoin, trimethadione, ethosuximide, carbamazepine

Hypoglycemic agents: tolbutamide, chlorpropamide

Antihistamines: cimetidine, brompheniramine, tripelennamine

Antihypertensives: methyldopa, captopril

Anti-inflammatory agents: aminopyrine, phenylbutazone, gold salts, ibuprofen, indomethacin

Antithyroid agents: propylthiouracil, methimazole, thiouracil

Diuretics: acetazolamide, hydrochlorothiazide, chlorthalidone

Phenothiazines: chlorpromazine, promazine, prochlorperazine

Immunosuppressive agents: antimetabolites

Cytotoxic agents: alkylating agents, antimetabolites, anthracyclines, vinca alkaloids, cisplatin, hydroxyurea, dactinomycin

Other agents: recombinant interferons, allopurinol, ethanol, levamisole, penicillamine, zidovudine, streptokinase, carbamazepine, clozapine

From Bagby JC Jr: Leukopenia and leucocytosis. In Goldman L, Ausiello D (eds): In Cecil Textbook of Medicine, 23rd ed. Philadelphia, Saunders Elsevier, 2008.

103. **Describe the features of lymphocytosis caused by viral infections.**
   Usually unusual or atypical lymphocyte morphology. Infection with EBV or CMV can cause an infectious mononucleosis syndrome of fever, sore throat, lymphadenopathy, hepatosplenomegaly, and in the case of EBV, an increased titer of the heterophile antibody. In EBV infection, B cells are penetrated by the virus, eliciting a polyclonal T-cell response manifested in the peripheral blood as atypical lymphocytosis. Cold agglutinin disease also may occur in EBV disease. The IgM antibodies are usually directed against the i antigen. An acute lymphocytosis may be associated with primary infection with HIV-1, adenovirus, rubella, or herpes simplex II.

104. **What is Felty's syndrome?**
An extra-articular manifestation of longstanding rheumatoid arthritis in which neutropenia often develops in conjunction with splenomegaly. Careful examination of the peripheral blood film should be undertaken because it can overlap with T subtype large granular lymphocyte (T-LGL) leukemia.

MYELOPROLIFERATIVE DISORDERS

105. **Polycythemia is frequently encountered by internists. Before you embark on a long and expensive work-up, how is the presence of polycythemia established?**
Patients must meet these criteria:
- Hct > 48 in females or 52 in males or Hb > 16.5 g/dL in females or 18.5 g/dL in males
- Normal oxygen saturation ($SaO_2 > 92\%$)
- Not elevated erythropoietin level

   Tefferi A, Thiele J, Orazi A, et al: Proposals and rationale for revision of the World Health Organization diagnostic criteria for polycythemia vera, essential thrombocythemia, and primary myelofibrosis: Recommendations for an ad hoc international expert panel, *Blood* 110:1092–1097, 2007.

106. **What are the 2008 criteria for PCV?**
Major criteria:
1. Hb >18.5 g/dL in men or 16.5 g/dL in women or other evidence of increased RBC volume
2. JAK 2 mutation (either 617V>F or exon 12)
Minor criteria:
1. Bone marrow biopsy showing hypercellularity for age with trilineage growth (panmyelosis) with prominent erythroid, granulocytic, and megakaryocytic proliferation
2. Serum EPO level lower than normal
3. Endogenous erythroid colony formation in vitro
   PCV requires the presence of both major criteria plus one minor criteria or one major criteria and two minor criteria.

107. **What secondary causes of polycythemia must be considered?**
- Elevated carboxyhemoglobin levels (found in heavy smokers)
- Inherited high-affinity Hb
- Alteration of the gene for the EPO receptor resulting in familial erythrocytosis
- Chuvash polycythemia (mutation in hypoxia-inducing factor-α)
- Neoplasm-produced ectopic EPO

108. **What particular situation warrants the thorough search for an occult MPD?**
Abdominal vein thrombosis including Budd-Chiari syndrome involving the hepatic and intrahepatic veins and portal, mesenteric, or splenic veins.

109. **How are patients with PCV risk-stratified?**
Patients who are > 60 years old or have had prior thromboembolic events should be considered high risk and may warrant cytoreductive therapy. Although leukocytosis has recently been found to be a potential adverse prognostic factor, similar findings have yet to be confirmed in other studies. Thrombocytosis is **not** a risk factor in PCV.

   Marchioli R, Finazzi G, Landolfi R, et al: Vascular and neoplastic risk in a large cohort of patients with polycythemia vera, *J Clin Oncol* 23:2224–2232, 2005.

110. **Once the diagnosis of PCV is established, how are patients treated?**
With phlebotomy of 500 mL of blood every other day as tolerated until the Hct is reduced to a normal range. In the elderly or those with cardiovascular disease, phlebotomies of 200–300 mL twice a week might be preferred. Once the target has been reached, maintenance phlebotomies can be scheduled in order to keep the Hb in the desired range. Phlebotomy alone usually suffices for younger patients, but some conditions are not well-controlled and require myelosuppressive therapy with HU.

111. **How does the treatment of high-risk patients differ from low-risk patients?**
High-risk patients should be offered cytoreductive therapy. Although there are no HU placebo-controlled, randomized trials in PCV, extrapolating from studies in patients with high-risk essential thrombocythemia, HU has been shown to be effective in the prevention of thrombosis and should be considered the drug of choice in high-risk patients. The starting dose of HU is 15–20 mg/kg/day until response is obtained without reducing WBC to $< 3 \times 10^6$/dL.

Cortelazzo S, Finazzi G, Ruggieri M, et al: Hydroxyurea in the treatment of patients with essential thrombocythemia at high risk of thrombosis: A prospective randomized trial, *N Engl J Med* 332: 1132–1136, 1995.

112. **Should HU be used during pregnancy?**
No. HU is teratogenic and embryotoxic. If PCV patients desire to become pregnant, HU should be stopped for a sufficient time before attempting conception. In low-risk pregnancies, the target Hct should be kept $< 45\%$ and low-dose aspirin should be given throughout the pregnancy. Low-molecular-weight heparin (LMWH) prophylaxis to prevent thrombosis should be offered in the postpartum period for at least 6 weeks. In high-risk pregnancies (either previous thrombotic complications or pregnancy complications), LMWH prophylaxis similar to the regimen used for antiphospholipid syndrome patients should be offered throughout the pregnancy. Furthermore, if myelosuppression is desired and there are no contraindications, interferon should be considered.

113. **Is aspirin effective for reducing complications in PCV?**
Yes. The ECLAP (European Collaboration on Low-dose Aspirin in Polycythemia Vera) study randomized patients to low-dose aspirin or placebo. Aspirin use reduced the combined end-point of cardiovascular death, nonfatal myocardial infarction, nonfatal stroke, and major venous thromboembolism. Overall mortality was also decreased, and therefore, low-dose aspirin is recommended in all PCV patients without history of gastrointestinal bleeding or gastric intolerance. This is recommended in **both** low-risk and high-risk patients.

Landolfi R, Marchioli R, Kutti J, et al: Efficacy and safety of low-dose aspirin in polycythemia vera, *N Engl J Med* 351:114–124, 2004.

114. **How is pruritus from PCV managed?**
Antihistamines initially, then paroxetine (20 mg/day) or photochemotherapy with psoralen and ultraviolet A light (UVA) if needed. Interferon has been reported to be successful as well.

Tefferi A, Fonseca R: Selective serotonin reuptake inhibitors are effective in the treatment of polycythemia vera–associated pruritus, *Blood* 99:2627, 2002.

115. **Is a bone marrow biopsy needed for diagnosis of chronic myelogenous leukemia (CML)?**
Yes. Although it might be tempting to diagnose CML only through peripheral blood testing, a bone marrow biopsy is needed for a thorough work-up to identify other potential cytogenetic defects.

116. **Describe the clinical features of accelerated CML and CML blast phase.**
WHO defines accelerated phase as 10–19% blasts in the peripheral blood or bone marrow, peripheral basophilia > 20%, persistent thrombocytopenia (<100 × 10⁶/dL) unrelated to therapy or persistent thrombocytosis (>1000 × 10⁶/dL) unresponsive to therapy, increasing spleen size or WBC count unresponsive to therapy, or cytogenetic evidence of clonal evolution. The clinical criteria for blast crisis or blast phase are defined as the presence of ≥ 20% blasts in the peripheral blood or bone marrow or by the presence of extramedullary blast cell disease. It should be noted that in most chemotherapy studies the criteria was ≥ 30% blasts.

Swerdlow SH, Campo E, Harris NL, et al: *World Health Organization Classification of Tumours of Haematopoietic and Lymphoid Tissues,* Lyon, France, 2008, IARC Press.

117. **Patients presenting with large spleens, fibrotic marrows, and teardrop-shaped erythrocytes on the peripheral blood film have what myeloproliferative disorder?**
Primary myelofibrosis (PMF), or agnogenic myeloid metaplasia. Extramedullary hematopoiesis is usually present in the liver and spleen. Patients may have neutrophilia, thrombocytosis, and anemia, but other patients, typically with massively enlarged spleens, may be cytopenic instead. Patients with enlarged spleens and neutrophilia resemble patients with CML. Determination of the presence of Ph[1] chromosome may distinguish the two.

118. **How is myelofibrosis treated?**
Currently, the only treatment that might offer the potential for cure is an allogeneic BMT. Other treatment modalities are palliative and include splenectomy, thalidomide, lenalidomide, pomalidomide, androgens, and HU.

119. **What are the causes of platelet counts > 1,000,000/mL?**
Severe iron deficiency with concurrent hemorrhage or inflammatory disease and essential thrombocythemia.

120. **What are the signs and symptoms of essential thrombocythemia?**
- Splenic enlargement
- Purpura
- Epistaxis
- Gingival bleeding (due to acquired von Willebrand's deficiency)
- Erythromelalgia (localized pain and warmth of the distal extremities relieved by small doses of aspirin)
- Neurologic manifestations (dizziness, seizures, and transient ischemic attacks)

121. **List the causes of thrombocytosis.**

Reactive disease	Infection	Essential thrombo-
Malignancy	Collagen-vascular	cythemia
Iron deficiency	diseases	PCV
Splenectomy	Myeloproliferative	CML (Ph[1]+)
Inflammatory bowel	disorders	Myelofibrosis
disease		MDS

122. **What is the long-term outcome of patients with essential thrombocythemia?**
Although it is generally safe to observe low-risk patients, long-term follow-up suggests that even after an uneventful first decade, the mortality is worse when compared with their normal counterparts. In higher-risk patients, despite cytoreductive therapy and

appropriate management, there is a small but very important potential of transformation into an acute leukemia, and an approximate 10% risk of venous thromboembolic events at 10 years.

Palandri F, Catani L, Testoni N, et al: Long-term follow-up of 386 consecutive patients with essential thrombocythemia: Safety of cytoreductive therapy, *Am J Hematol* 84:215–220, 2009.

123. **What is the most likely complication in a patient with a myeloproliferative disease who presents with a swollen, hot ankle?**
Gout. Patients with myeloproliferative syndromes (PCV, CML, myelofibrosis, and essential thrombocythemia) may develop hyperuricemia. Arthritis in such patients should be investigated thoroughly, including arthrocentesis and examination for intracellular, negatively birefringent crystals under polarized light.

ACUTE MYELOGENOUS LEUKEMIA

124. **What are the symptoms of leukostasis?**

Dyspnea	Dizziness	Cardiac ischemia
Limitation in activity	Visual disturbances	Ischemic necrosis
Tinnitus	Confusion	Strokes
Headache	Priapism	

Patients with AML and WBC > 100,000/dL or > 50,000/dL and symptoms of leukostasis should undergo leukapheresis.

125. **How is AML diagnosed?**
With a cellular bone marrow aspirate showing blasts representing > 20% of all nucleated WBCs. If erythroblasts comprise > 50% of the nucleated bone marrow cells, erythroleukemia (M6) is present. If the marrow is cellular but blasts account for < 20% of the NRBCs, myelodysplasia is present. For acute megakaryoblastic leukemia (M7), at least 50% of the blasts should be of megarkaryocytic lineage (CD41, CD61).

126. **What are the subgroups of AML and how has this changed?**
The original French-American-British (FAB) classification has been replaced by the newer WHO schema. The WHO classification takes into account cytogenetics, in addition to therapy related or leukemia arising from MDS (Table 14-4).

127. **What characteristic suggests a poorer prognosis for patients with AML?**
- Age > 55–60 years
- Prior myelodysplastic or myeloproliferative disorders
- Presence of specific karyotypes

Ferrara F, Palmieri S, Leoni F: Clinically useful prognostic factors in acute myeloid leukemia, *Crit Rev Oncol Hematol* 66:181–193, 2008.

128. **How can patients with AML and normal karyotype be further subdivided?**
With additional identification of genomic abnormalities. Mutant NPM1 (nucleophosmin) without FLT3-ITD and mutant CEBPA confer the best prognosis within this subgroup. Other genotypes (FLT3-ITD; MLL-PTD) confer a worse prognosis.

Akagi T, Ogawa S, Dugas M, et al: Frequent genomic abnormalities in acute myeloid leukemia/myelodysplatic syndrome with normal karyotype, *Haematologica* 94:213–223, 2009.

TABLE 14-4. WORLD HEALTH ORGANIZATION (WHO) CLASSIFICATION OF ACUTE MYELOGENOUS LEUKEMIA

Type	Description	Criteria
M1	Myeloblastic leukemia without maturation	>3% of blasts are peroxidase-positive. A few granules, Auer rods, or both; one or more distinct nucleoli; no further maturation.
M2	Myeloblastic leukemia with maturation	>50% of marrow cells are myeloblasts and promyelocytes. Myelocytes, metamyelocytes, and mature granulocytes are seen; eosinophilia may predominate in some cases.
M3	Hypergranular promyelocytic leukemia	Majority of cells are abnormal promyelocytes, reniform (kidney-shaped) nuclei, bundles of Auer rods; also some have closely packed bright pink or purple granules.
M4	Myelomonocytic leukemia	>20% of bone marrow, peripheral blood nucleated cells, or both are promonocytes and monocytes; an eosinophilic variant is also recognized.
M5	Monocytic leukemia (M5a = poorly differentiated) (M5b = differentiated)	Granulocyte component, 10% of marrow cells, monocytoid cells have a fluoride-sensitive esterase reaction cytochemically.
M6	Erythroleukemia	>50% of cells are erythroblasts; myeloblasts represent > 30% of nonerythroid nucleated cells.
M7	Megakaryoblastic	>30% of marrow cells are blasts; platelets peroxidase-positive on electron microscopy, or blasts react with antiplatelet monoclonal antibodies; marrow fibrosis is prominent; cytoplasmic budding is also a feature.

From Vardiman JW, Harris NL, Brunning RD: The World Health Organization (WHO) classification of the myeloid neoplasms. Blood 100:2292–2302, 2002.

129. **How does the presentation of acute promyelocytic leukemia (APL) differ from other AML subtypes?**
With lower or normal WBC counts when the patient is first seen. Careful attention to the morphology of the circulating WBCs discloses the presence of the hypergranular blasts or blasts with multiple Auer rods. Less frequently, the blasts are hypogranular. A significant hemorrhagic diathesis may complicate either the presentation or the treatment of APL with standard AML chemotherapy. A picture resembling DIC is characteristic and may be accompanied by CNS bleeding, which is sometimes fatal. Patients may require intensive support with platelets, fresh frozen plasma, and cryoprecipitate.

130. **What is the differentiation syndrome?**
Dyspnea, unexplained fever, weight gain, peripheral edema, hypotension, acute renal failure, or congestive heart failure occurring in patients with APL treated with either ATRA (tretinoin) or ATO (arsenic trioxide). Should a patient develop these symptoms, prompt treatment with dexamethasone 10 mg IV twice-daily should be started. ATRA or ATO should be discontinued only in severe cases.

131. **What antibiotics are selected for treatment of neutropenic infections?**
The selection of initial antibiotic therapy must take into account the type, frequency of occurrence, and antibiotic susceptibility of the local hospital-acquired infections. Although patients with low-risk neutropenic infections can be managed with oral antibiotics, this requires vigilant observation and prompt access to appropriate medical care 24 hr/day, 7 days/wk. In practice, unless strict criteria can be met, patients are treated as in-patients with broad-spectrum antibiotic coverage as per Infectious Diseases Society of America (IDSA) guidelines. Vancomycin is not generally recommended initially unless the hospital has a local flora of drug resistant *Streptococcus viridians* or the patient has clinically suspected serious catheter-related infection, known colonization with methicillin-resistant *Staphylococcus aureus* (MRSA), blood cultures with gram-positive cocci, or hemodynamic instability. Patients with severe mucositis, fever > 40°C, or who have had quinolone prophylaxis should also be considered for initial treatment with vancomycin. If the patient remains febrile after 5 days of broad-spectrum antibiotics, antifungal agents should be added.

Hughes WT, Armstrong D, Bodey GP, et al: 2002 Guidelines for the use of antimicrobial agents in neutropenic patients with cancer, *Clin Infect Dis* 34:730–751, 2002.

132. **What are the indications of removal of an indwelling cathether in patients with neutropenic fever?**
Evidence of a subcutaneous infection, septic emboli, hypotension associated with the cathether, or a nonfunctioning catheter. Prompt catheter removal should also be strongly considered if there is documented bacteremia with *Bacillus* spp., *Pseudomonas aeruginosa*, *Stenotrophomonas maltophila*, *Cornyebacterium jeikeium*, vancomycin-resistant *Enterococci* (VRE), or fungemia due to *Candida* spp.

Mermel LA, Farr BM, Sheretz RJ, et al: Guidelines for the management of intravascular cathether-related infection, *Clin Infect Dis* 32:1249–1272, 2001.

ACUTE LYMPHOBLASTIC LEUKEMIA

133. **What are the three main categories of ALL?**
- T cell
- Mature B cell
- B-cell precursor

134. **Define "molecular remission."**
As disease below the detection of PCR techniques (generally 1×10^4 cells or 1 blast in 10,000 normal cells)

135. **What are the indicators of a poor prognosis in adults with ALL?**
- WBC > 50,000 in B cell and > 100,000 in T cell
- Extreme leukocytosis (>400,000)
- Age > 35 years

- T-cell or mature B-cell phenotype
- Delayed time to complete response
- High-risk cytogenetics:
  - t(9;22): Philadelphia chromosome
  - t (4;11) MLL translocation or other 11q23 translocation
  - hypodiploidy (<45 chromosomes)
  - Balanced t(1;19)

136. **What test should be sent if a patient has hematologic toxicity out of proportion to the expected side effects?**
Measurement of thiopurine methyltransferase (TPMT) enzyme activity or determination of TPMT phenotype or both. This enzyme catalyzes S-methylation of thiopurines (mercaptopurine and thioguanine). Ten percent of the population has one functioning and one nonfunctioning allele (intermediate activity), 1/300 will inherit two nonfunctioning alleles with no enzyme activity (which can lead to fatal toxicity).

Relling MV, Pui CH, Cheng C, et al: Thiopurine methyltransferase in acute lymphoblastic leukemia, *Blood* 107:843–844, 2006.

LYMPHOPROLIFERATIVE DISEASE

137. **What is the most common leukemia of adults?**
CLL. Patients are often elderly (median age 70 for males and 74 for females). Lymphadenopathy and splenomegaly are also relatively common. Some patients present only with an elevated WBC count, composed of lymphocytes with a normal morphology.

138. **List the diagnostic criteria for CLL.**
- Sustained lymphocyte count $> 5 \times 10^9$/L for at least 3 months. Morphology should be "typical." The presence of cytopenias caused by a typical lymphoproliferative bone marrow infiltration makes the diagnosis regardless of the lymphocyte count.
- B-cell immunophenotypes (typically weak expression of membrane immunoglobulin, CD 20, expression of the T-cell antigen CD5).

Hallek M, Cheson B, Catovsky D, et al: Guidelines for the diagnosis and treatment of chronic lymphocytic leukemia: A report from the International Workshop on Chronic Lymphocytic Leukemia updating the National Cancer Institute-Working Group 1996 guidelines, *Blood* 111: 5446–5456, 2008.

139. **What is monoclonal B-cell lymphocytosis (MBL)?**
The presence of a monoclonal B-cell population in numbers < 5000/mL with no other features of a lymphoproliferative disorder. Akin to MGUS (monoclonal gammopathy of undetermined significance) and its relationship with multiple myeloma, CLL that requires treatment develops in patients with MBL at a rate of 1.1%/yr.

Rawson AC, Bennett FL, O'Connor SJM, et al: Monoclonal B cell lymphocytosis and chronic lymphocytic leukemia, *N Engl J Med* 359:575–583, 2008.

140. **What are the two currently used staging systems for CLL?**
The Rai Staging System (Table 14-5) and the Binet Staging System (Table 14-6).

141. **How are cytogenetics incorporated into the work-up for CLL?**
Chromosome abnormalities are well documented in CLL. From worst to best prognosis, the cytogenetics are:
- 17p deletion has the worse prognosis and is usually refractory to standard treatment.
- 11q deletions.

TABLE 14-5. RAI'S STAGING SYSTEM FOR CHRONIC LYMPHOCYTIC LEUKEMIA

Stage	Clinical Features	Survival (YR)
0	Lymphocytosis in blood and bone marrow only	>10
I	Lymphocytosis and enlarged lymph nodes	8
II	Lymphocytosis plus hepatomegaly, splenomegaly, or both	6
III	Lymphocytosis and anemia (hemoglobin < 110 g/L)	1.5–4
IV	Lymphocytosis and thrombocytopenia (platelets < 100×10^9/L)	1.5–4

From Rai KR, Sawitsky A, Cronkite EP, et al: Clinical staging of chronic lymphocytic leukemia. Blood 46:219–234, 1975.

TABLE 14-6. BINET'S STAGING SYSTEM FOR CHRONIC LYMPHOCYTIC LEUKEMIA

Stage	Clinical Features	Survival (YR)*
A	Hemoglobin > 100 g/L; platelets > 100×10^9/L and < three areas involved	12
B	Hemoglobin > 100 g/L; platelets > 100×10^9/L and > three areas involved	7
C	Hemoglobin < 100 g/L or platelets < 100×10^9/L or both (independent of the areas involved)	2–4

*Derived from 2 series (295 patients).
From Binet JL, Auquier A, Dighiero G, et al: A new prognostic classification of chronic lymphocytic leukemia derived from a multivariate survival analysis. Cancer 48:198–206, 1981.

- Normal karyotype, trisomy 12.
- 13q deletion has the best prognosis, contrary to its effect in multiple myeloma.

  Dohner H, Stilgenbauer S, Benner A, et al: Genomic aberrations and survival in chronic lymphocytic leukemia, *N Engl J Med* 343:1910–1916, 2000.

142. **What are the complications of CLL?**
- Autoimmune phenomena (warm antibody AIHA, ITP, neutropenia) that can be detected by DAT
- Pure RBC aplasia
- Hypogammaglobulinemia
- Transformation into a large cell lymphoma with poor prognosis (Richer's syndrome)

  Rozman C, Montserrat E: Chronic lymphocytic leukemia, *N Engl J Med* 333:1052–1057, 1995.

143. **When is treatment started in CLL?**
According to the International Workshop on Chronic Lymphocytic Leukemia (IWCLL), treatment is indicated when one of the following is present:

- Evidence of marrow failure (worsening anemia or thrombocytopenia)
- Massive splenomegaly (>6 cm below costal margin) or progressive and symptomatic splenomegaly
- Massive lymphadenopathy (>10 cm) or progressive and symptomatic lymphadenopathy
- Progressive lymphocytosis with > 50% increase in 2 months or a lymphocyte doubling time of < 6 months
- Autoimmune anemia or thrombocytopenia that is poorly responsive to standard treatment (note that autoimmune HA or ITP is **not** an indication of treatment for CLL)

Furthermore, at least one of the following must be present before initiating treatment:

- Unintentional weight loss (10% in previous 6 mo)
- Fatigue
- Fevers > 100.5°F or 38°C
- Night sweats of > 1 month in duration without signs of infection.

144. **Which lymphoproliferative disorder is associated with pancytopenia, splenomegaly, absence of lymphadenopathy, and circulating lymphoid cells with multiple projections?**
Hairy cell leukemia (HCL). Although an uncommon malignancy (2% of all leukemias), HCL receives a great deal of attention because of advances in treatment and the unusual infections observed in the course of the disease. HCL is an important consideration in the work-up of patients who present with pancytopenia. Some patients have presented with aplasia.

145. **How is HCL diagnosed?**
Through bone marrow biopsy. Although the bone marrow aspirate is often scanty, characteristic "hairy" lymphs may be observed. The biopsy may show a diffusely involved marrow with mononuclear cells situated in a network of fibrosis. Although hairy cells may be present in the marrow, the biopsy picture is one of profound hypocellularity. The hairy cell is a B lymphocyte with an immunophenotype consistent with a cell between a CLL-lymphocyte and a plasma cell. Hairy cells also possess the Tac antigen (CD25), a receptor for interleukin-2, usually seen on activated T cells. The distinctive cytochemical feature of the hairy cell is a tartrate-resistant acid phosphatase activity (TRAP). Monocytopenia is frequent.

Wanko SO, De Castro C: Hairy cell leukemia: An elusive but treatable disease, *Oncologist* 11:780–789, 2006.

146. **How does the HCL variant differ from classic HCL?**
Patients are older, splenomegaly is less common, and the bone marrow is usually hypercellular with mild myelofibrosis. Circulating hairy cells resemble prolymphocytes and respond poorly to standard therapy. Instead of being strongly positive, CD103 is mildly positive or negative.

147. **Describe the manifestations of large granular lymphocyte leukemia (LGLL).**
The presentation of LGLL is highly variable. LGLLs can be divided into either T cells (CD3-positive and T-cell receptor rearrangement positive) or natural killer (NK) cells (CD3-negative, CD16-positive, and CD56-positive). The leukemias can be indolent or aggressive. The aggressive variants are treated with ALL regimens, whereas the indolent disease can be watched and treated with oral immunosuppressants after patients become symptomatic (methotrexate, cyclophosphamide, and cyclosporine).

Sokol L, Loughran TP: Large granular lymphocyte leukemia, *Oncologist* 11:263–273, 2006.

HODGKIN'S AND NON-HODGKIN'S LYMPHOMAS

148. **What are the common presentations of Hodgkin's lymphoma (HL)?**
Lymphadenopathy in the neck or axilla. Lymph nodes are nontender, rubbery, and discrete.
Sometimes the nodes wax and wane in size until attention is sought. Important symptoms in
the staging of HL are fever, weight loss (>10% of body weight), and night sweats. Some
patients are troubled by pruritus or flushing after drinking alcohol. HL tends to originate in
central lymph nodes, so that some patients present with mediastinal lymphadenopathy.

149. **How is HL staged?**
See Table 14-7.

TABLE 14-7. STAGES OF HODGKIN'S LYMPHOMA

Stage	Substage	Involvement
I	I	Single lymph node
	IE	Single extralymphatic organ
II	II	Lymph nodes on same side of diaphragm
	IIE	With localized extralymphatic site
III	III	Lymph nodes above and below diaphragm
	IIIE	With localized extralymphatic site
	IIIS	With isolated splenic site
	IIISE	With both extralymphatic and splenic sites
IV	IV	Disseminated or diffuse involvement of one or more extralymphatic sites
	IVA	Asymptomatic
	IVB	Fever, sweats, weight loss > 10% body weight

From Aisenberg A: The staging and treatment of Hodgkin's disease. N Engl J Med 299:1228–1232, 1978.

150. **What features suggest a poor prognosis for advanced HL?**
- Age > 45 years
- Male gender
- Stage IV
- Hb < 10.5
- Albumin 4
- WBC > 15
- Absolute lymphocyte count < 600 or < 8% in the differential count

Hasenclaver D, Diehl V, for the International Prognostic Factors Project on Advanced Hodgkin's Disease: A prognostic score to predict tumor control in advanced Hodgkin's Disease, *N Engl J Med* 339:1506–1514, 1998.

151. **What is the initial work-up recommended for HL?**
- CBC, albumin, serum LDH, erythrocyte sedimentation rate (ESR), HBV, HCV, and HIV.
- Computed tomography (CT) of the neck, thorax, abdomen, and pelvis.
- Echocardiogram to assess ejection fraction.
- Pregnancy test in women of childbearing potential.

- Bone marrow biopsy (unilateral) for patients with B symptoms or stage III/IV disease or blood count abnormalities.
- Positron-emission tomography (PET) scan at baseline is strongly recommended.
- Thyroid function tests for patients who are candidates for neck radiation therapy.

Brusamolino E, Bacigalupo A, Barosi G, et al: Classical Hodgkin's lymphoma in adults: Guidelines of the Italian Society of Hematology, the Italian Society of Experimental Hematology and the Italian Bone Marrow Transplantation on initial work-up, management and follow-up, *Haematologica* 94:550–565, 2009.

152. **What are the histologic subtypes of HL?**
   - Nodular lymphocyte predominant classic HL
   - Classic HL which is subdivided into nodular sclerosis, mixed cellularity, lymphocyte-rich and lymphocyte-depleted HL

153. **What is the immunophenotype of HL?**
   CD15 is expressed in the Hodgkin/Reed Sternberg (H/RS) cells in 70–85%. CD30 and fascin are positive in almost all cases. CD20 can be expressed in H/RS cells in 30–40% of cases with variable intensity.

154. **Which subtypes carry the worst prognosis?**
   Although staging generally determines the outlook, histologic subtype is also important. Nodular-sclerosing and lymphocyte-predominant subtypes tend to present with limited disease. Lymphocyte depletion is associated with more advanced disease, retroperitoneal involvement, and presentation in older adults.

   Dann EJ, Bar-Shalom R, Tamir A, et al: Risk-adapted BEACOPP regimen can reduce the cumulative dose of chemotherapy for standard and high-risk Hodgkin lymphoma with no impairment on outcome, *Blood* 109:905–909, 2007.

155. **In patients cured of HL, what are the late sequelae of therapy?**
   Myelodysplasia, leukemia, and NHL (3–10 yr after therapy). Certain complications of the high-dose irradiation are also evident, which include acute radiation pneumonitis with fever, cough, and shortness of breath. Cardiac effects of irradiation include pericarditis, pericardial effusions, and pericardial fibrosis. Coronary artery disease may be accelerated. Neurologic effects of irradiation include Lhermitte's sign (paresthesia produced by flexion of the neck). Hypothyroidism is also a frequent sequela of radiation therapy.

   Bookman MA, Longo DI: Concomitant illness in patients treated for Hodgkin's disease, *Cancer Treat Rev* 13:77–111, 1986.

156. **How are NHLS subdivided?**
   NHL can arise from either B or T cells. B-cell NHLs can be further subdivided into aggressive and indolent. Within the aggressive forms, the most common ones are Burkitt's lymphoma (BL), diffuse large B-cell lymphoma (DLBCL), and mantle cell lymphoma (MCL). Within the indolent categories, the most common disorders are follicular lymphoma, MALT (mucosal-associated lymphoid tissue), and marginal zone lymphomas. Within the non–B-cell lymphomas, the most common ones are peripheral T-cell lymphomas, cutaneous T-cell lymphomas, angioimmunoblastic T-cell lymphomas, and NK-cell lymphomas.

   Tomita N, Tokunaka M, Nakamura N, et al: Clinicopathological features of lymphoma/leukemia patients carrying both BCL2 and MYC translocations, *Haematologica* 94:935–943, 2009.

157. **In Africa, Denis P. Burkitt described an aggressive neoplasm that bears his name. What are the clinical features of this lymphoma?**
   BL results from a proliferation of B lymphocytes with a striking appearance. They present as round or oval cells with abundant basophilic cytoplasm-containing vacuoles that stain

positively for fat. The tissue is replaced with a monotonous infiltrate of cells with interspersed macrophages, giving a "starry sky" appearance. When it presents as leukemia, it is classified as L3 in the FAB scheme. These cells proliferate rapidly and have a potential doubling time of 24 hours; this is one of the few hematologic emergencies.

The WHO classification describes two variants: classical and with plasmacytoid differentiation. Both express surface IgM, pan B-cell antigens (CD19, CD20, CD22, and CD79a). The plasmacytoid variant has monotypic cytoplasmic immunoglobulin. A defining feature of BL is the presence of a translocation between *c-myc* and the *IgH* gene (t[8;14]) in 80% or *IgL* gene (t[2;8] or t[8;22]) in the other 20% of cases.

158. **Distinguish the African and American forms of BL.**
In African BL, patients present with large extranodal tumors of the jaws, abdominal viscera (including kidney), ovaries, and retroperitoneum. In the American form of BL, patients present with intra-abdominal tumors arising from the ileocecal region or mesenteric lymph nodes. Bilateral involvement of the breast can be seen in puberty or associated with lactation. In Africa, the disease is associated with EBV, but this association is less common in American cases. Immunodeficiency-associated BL occurs mainly in patients with HIV, although it can also be seen in allograft recipients.

   Ferry J: Burkitt's lymphoma: Clinicopathological features and differential diagnosis, *Oncologist* 11:375–383, 2006.

159. **In which patients with DLBCL should a lumbar puncture be performed?**
Those presenting with testicular, epidural, or sinus involvement.

160. **What are the typical characteristics of MCL?**
There are four cytologic variants of MCL: small cell, marginal zone, blastoid, and pleomorphic. Both blastoid (typically with skin involvement) and pleomorphic have a worse prognosis.

   MCL cells are usually CD10-negative, CD5-positive, and CD23-negative. They express IgM or IgD surface immunoglobulins and cyclin D1 expression (t(11;14)) can be shown in almost all cases. Gastrointestinal involvement is very frequent and endoscopies are recommended at diagnosis (80% involvement when a biopsy from normal-appearing mucosa is taken).

161. **How are follicular lymphomas (FLs) graded?**
Morphologically, FL is graded depending on the proportion of centroblasts per high-power field into grades I, II, and III. FL expresses CD19, CD20, CD22, and surface immunoglobulin. Translocation 14;18 leading to overexpression of the antiapoptotic protein BCL2 is a hallmark of this lymphoma. The correct diagnosis of FL requires a complete excisional biopsy. A fine-needle aspiration is **not** adequate.

162. **When is treatment initiated in FL?**
According to the Groupe pour l'Etude de Lymphome Folliculaire (GELF, French) criteria, patients ought to be followed if **all** of the following are present: maximum diameter of disease < 7 cm, <3 nodal sites, no systemic symptoms, spleen < 16 cm on CT, no significant effusions, no risk of local compressive symptoms, no circulating lymphoma cells, and no bone marrow compromise (Hb > 10, WBC > 1.5, and platelet count > 100). Conversely, the British National Lymphoma Investigation (BNLI, British) group recommends prompt treatment if any of the following are present: B symptoms or pruritus, rapid disease progression, bone marrow compromise (Hb < 10, WBC < 3 as opposed to 1.5, PLT < 100), life-threatening organ involvement, renal infiltration or bone lesions.

163. **How can FL be risk-stratified?**
Traditionally, the Follicular Lymphoma International Prognostic Index 1 (FLIPI1) was used for risk stratification. Five adverse prognostic factors were identified: age > 60, Ann

Arbor stage III or IV, Hb < 12 g/dL, >4 involved nodal areas, and serum LDH greater than the upper limit of normal. There has been an update with a new Follicular Lymphoma International Prognostic Index 2 (FLIPI2) (Table 14-8).

TABLE 14-8. RISK STRATIFICATION OF FOLLICULAR LYMPHOMA		
Risk Stratification	Number of Risk Factors*	5 Year (%)
Low	0–1	80
Intermediate	1–2	51
High	3–5	19

Hb = hemoglobin.
*Elevated β_2-microglobulin; largest lymph node > 6 cm; Hb < 12 g/dL,; bone marrow involvement; and age > 60.
From Federico M, Bellei M, Marcheselli L, et al: Follicular Lymphoma International Prognostic Index 2: A new prognostic index for follicular lymphoma developed by the international follicular lymphoma prognostic factor project. J Clin Oncol 27:4555–4562, 2009.

PLASMA CELL DYSCRASIAS

164. **How should the discovery of a monoclonal protein (M-protein) be evaluated?**
With CBC, urinalysis for protein, calcium and renal function measurement, and bone survey for lytic lesions. The discovery of an M-protein on serum protein electrophoresis should be followed by a careful work-up for multiple myeloma (MM). Patients who have a small serum spike (<1.5 g/dL), normal CBC, no proteinuria, and no lytic lesions, hypercalcemia, or renal dysfunction are usually followed with periodic serum protein electrophoresis. Patients meeting some of the criteria for MM but showing no progression with follow-up are described as having "indolent" or "smoldering" MM. Up to 5% of patients in their eighth decade have MGUS.

165. **What is the differential diagnosis of an M-protein?**
- MGUS
- MM
- Solitary plasmacytoma
- Amyloid light-chain (AC) amyloidosis
- Waldenstrom macroglobulinemia (IgM)
- Low-grade lymphoproliferative disorder
- Cryoglobulinemia

166. **How is the diagnosis of smoldering multiple myeloma (SMM) made?**
MGUS can be differentiated from SMM by the lack of an M-spike > 3 g/dL **and** bone marrow plasma cells > 10%. The lack of myeloma-related organ or tissue impairment differentiates SMM from MM.

International Myeloma Working Group: Criteria for the classification of monoclonal gammopathies, multiple myeloma and related disorders: A report of the International Myeloma Working Group, Br J Haematol 121:749–757, 2003.

167. **What are the myeloma-related organ or tissue impairments (ROTIs)?**
Hypercalcemia, renal insufficiency attributable to MM, anemia (Hb < 10 g/dL), lytic lesions, **or** osteoporosis with compression fractures, symptomatic hyperviscocity, amyloidosis, and recurrent bacterial infections (>2 in 12 mo).

168. **What is the prognosis of MGUS and what are the predictors of malignant transformation?**
The overall risk of malignant transformation in patients with MGUS is approximately 1%/yr. A non-IgG monoclonal protein, serum M-spike > 1.5 g/dL, and an abnormal serum free light chain denote a higher risk of transformation. Patients with none of these risk factors have a 5% chance of transformation at 20% whereas patients with one, two, and three risk factors have a 21%, 37%, and 58% chance of transformation at 20 years, respectively.

Rajkumar SV, Kyle RA, Thernau TM, et al: Serum free light chain is an independent risk factor for progression in monoclonal gammopathy of unknown significance, *Blood* 106:812–817, 2005.

169. **Which patients with MGUS should be referred to hematology?**
Those with symptoms or physical signs of myeloma, lymphoproliferative disorders, or AL amyloidosis. Furthermore, patients with significant Bence-Jones proteinuria (>500 mg/L) or non-IgG M-spike should also be considered for referral.

Bird J, Behrens J, Westin J, et al: U.K. Myeloma Forum (UKMF) and Nordic Myeloma Study Group (NMSG): Guidelines for the investigation of newly detected M-proteins and the management of monoclonal gammopathy of undetermined significance (MGUS), *Br J Haematol* 147:22–42, 2009.

170. **What are the prognostic factors in multiple myeloma?**
See Table 14-9. Furthermore, t(4;14), t(14;16), t(14;20), deletion 17p13, and deletion 13 have poor prognosis, whereas t(11;14), t(6;14), and hyperdiploidy denote a good prognosis.

TABLE 14-9. PROGNOSTIC FACTORS IN MULTIPLE MYELOMA		
Stage	Findings	Median survival (MO)
I	β_2-microglobulin < 3.5 mg/L Serum albumin > 3.5 g/dL	62
II	Neither stage I nor III	44
III	β_2-microglobulin > 5.5 mg/L	209

171. **Is MM curable?**
No. To date, MM is not curable short of an allogeneic stem cell transplant, which is not an early option owing to its high mortality and morbidity. With current therapies, the survival of myeloma patients is measured in years.

172. **Describe the clinical manifestations of Waldenström's macroglobulinemia (WM).**
A B-cell disorder of proliferating plasmacytoid lymphocytes that produce an IgM monoclonal protein, most often seen in the elderly. Patients frequently have hepatosplenomegaly, lymphadenopathy, bone marrow involvement, and neurologic disease (including peripheral neuropathy and cerebellar dysfunction). Other features include retinopathy with large sausage-shaped, dilated retinal veins, bleeding, purpura, and hyperviscosity syndrome.

Alexanian R: Waldenstrom's macroglobulinemia, *Blood* 83:1452–1459, 1994.

173. **List the manifestations of the hyperviscosity syndrome.**

Global CNS dysfunction and stupor	Papilledema	Headache, vertigo, ataxia
Retinopathy	Hypervolemia, congestive heart failure	Stroke
Retinal hemorrhages		Coagulopathy

174. **How is WM treated?**
    The choice of treatment varies according to the severity of the disease and the comorbidities of the patient. Asymptomatic WM should be observed and alkylators should be avoided in patients who are candidates for autologous stem cell transplantation (ASCT). Symptomatic hyperviscosity should be promptly treated with plasmapheresis and once the symptoms have resolved, treatment should be instituted. Careful monitoring for hyperviscosity flare (IgM flare) during the initial phase of treatment is needed and prompt pheresis should be readily available.

175. **What gammopathies are associated with AL amyloidosis?**
    - WM
    - IgM MGUS
    - NHL

176. **How do patients with AL amyloidosis present?**
    With purpura from skin involvement, hepatosplenomegaly, macroglossia, orthostatic hypotension, congestive heart failure, malabsorption, nephrotic syndrome, peripheral neuropathy, and carpal tunnel syndrome. Of interest, the consequences of amyloid include an acquired Factor X deficiency, resulting in a prolonged prothrombin time and partial thromboplastin time and functional hyposplenism. The latter results in the presence of Howell-Jolly bodies, even though the spleen is present.

HEMOSTASIS

177. **What are the four basic contributors to effective hemostasis?**
    - Platelets
    - Coagulation
    - Antithrombotic/fibrinolytic system
    - Endothelium

178. **How are disorders of platelets categorized?**
    As quantitative or qualitative defects.

179. **What is the definition of thrombocytopenia?**
    A decrease in platelet number, usually < 150,000.

180. **What are the causes of quantitative defects of platelets?**
    - Pseudothrombocytopenia
    - Sequestration, usually due to splenomegaly
    - Increased consumption
    - Increased destruction
    - Bone marrow hypoproliferation

181. **What is pseudothrombocytopenia?**
    A falsely low platelet count usually associated with blood drawing errors, platelet satellites, or clumping. Platelet satellites occur when WBCs become coated with platelets. The in vitro clumping of platelets is usually caused by agglutination of the platelets by an autoantibody that reacts with the anticoagulant ethylenediaminetetracetic acid (EDTA). Examination of the peripheral smear and redrawing the CBC in a citrated or heparinized tube will reveal the clumping and the true platelet count, respectively.

KEY POINTS: THROMBOCYTOPENIA ✓

1. A thorough history includes questions about prescription and nonprescription medications and herbal supplements.

2. A thorough history also includes questions about risk factors for human immunodeficiency virus infection.

3. A thorough physical examination includes temperature, blood pressure, assessment for bleeding sites, lymphadenopathy, and hepatosplenomegaly.

4. The peripheral blood smear must be reviewed carefully to look for platelet clumping (spurious thrombocytopenia), schizocytes and other fragmented RBCs, macro-ovalocytes (megaloblastic anemia), and atypical WBCs (viral syndrome, leukemia, and lymphoma).

RBCs = red blood cells; WBCs = white blood cells.

182. **What is ITP?**
Immune thrombocytopenic purpura, an autoimmune-mediated disorder in which platelets and megakaryocytes are targeted by platelet-specific antibodies and cleared through the reticuloendothelial system.

183. **How is ITP diagnosed?**
By excluding all other mechanisms of thrombocytopenia. The recommended initial work-up should include patient history, family history, physical examination, CBC, reticulocyte count, peripheral blood film review, bone marrow examination in selected patients, blood group (Rh), DAT, and *Helicobacter pylori*, HIV, and HCV testing. Additional tests that can have potential utility include glycoprotein-specific antibody, antiphospholipid antibodies, antithyroid antibodies and thyroid function, pregnancy test, antinuclear antibodies, and viral PCR for parvovirus and CMV.

> Provan D, Stasi R, Newland AC, et al: International consensus report on the investigation and management of primary immune thrombocytopenia, *Blood* 115:168–186, 2010.

184. **How is ITP treated?**
Until recently, the main method of treating ITP focused on immunosuppression (steroids) or immunomodulation (splenectomy, intravenous immunoglobulin [IVIG], rituximab). In 2008, the U.S. Food and Drug Administration (FDA) granted approval to the use of thrombopoietin (TPO) mimetics to treat chronic ITP.

185. **What is TPO and how would this affect ITP treatment?**
A substance that binds to the thrombopoietin receptor, inducing proliferation and differentiation of megakaryocytes with increase in the platelet count. Originally, the thrombocytopenia observed in ITP was thought to result from the peripheral destruction of platelets that outpaced the ability of the bone marrow to produce platelets. However, subsequent studies showed a relative deficiency in TPO levels in patients with ITP.

186. **What are some of the congenital causes of thrombocytopenia?**
- MYH9-associated disorders
- Bernard-Soulier syndrome
- Wiskott-Aldrich syndrome

- Congenital amegakaryocytic thrombocytopenia
- Thrombocytopenia and absent radii

Drachman JG: Inherited thrombocytopenia: When a low platelet count does not mean ITP, *Blood* 103:390–398, 2004.

187. **What are the MYH9-associated disorders?**
Although previously known by a number of eponyms (May-Hegglin anomaly, Fechtner's syndrome, Sebastian's syndrome, or Epstein's syndrome), these disorders are all linked by mutations in the *MYH9* gene, which codes for nonmuscle myosin heavy chain IIA (NMMHC-IIA). They are characterized by the presence of giant platelets on the peripheral blood smear, Döhle-like inclusions within neutrophils, an autosomal dominant pedigree, and a variable degree of sensorineural hearing loss. It is important to recognize the presence of giant platelets and the familial mode of transmission so that patients are not inappropriately diagnosed and/or treated for ITP.

188. **List the coagulation factors.**
- **I:** fibrinogen
- **II:** prothrombin
- **III:** tissue factor
- **IV:** calcium
- **V:** proaccelerin or labile factor
- **VI:** original name for activated Factor V, but no longer used, currently there is no Factor VI designation.
- **VII:** stable factor, proconvertin, co-thromboplastin, serum prothrombin conversion accelerator
- **VIII:** antihemophilic factor (AHF), thromboplastinogen
- **IX:** Christmas factor, plasma thromboplastin component
- **X:** Stuart-Prower factor
- **XI:** plasma thromboplastin antecedent
- **XII:** Hageman factor
- **XIII:** fibrin-stabilizing factor, Laki-Lorand factor

189. **What is the PT and which factors are involved in its measurement?**
Prothrombin time, which assesses activity of Factors II, III, V, VII, and X, and therefore, evaluates both the "extrinsic pathway" and the "common pathway." The extrinsic pathway includes Factors III and VII. The common pathway includes Factors II, V, and X.

190. **How is the PT performed?**
Blood is placed into a citrated tube, which chelates calcium, inhibiting clot formation. The tube is then spun down and the platelet-poor plasma extracted. When ready for testing, calcium is added back in excess to the sample. A "thromboplastin" (i.e., tissue factor) is added, commonly from cow or rabbit brains or a recombinant source. The time to clot formation is then measured, most commonly spectrophotometrically: unclotted plasma is turbid and clot formation increases the lucency of the sample, which is measured as an increase in light transmission. The time to peak light transmission is the PT.

191. **What is the International Normalized Ratio (INR)?**
The INR is a calculated value used **only** for patients on warfarin therapy. Whereas the PT may have different values across laboratories, the INR is standardized to give a reproducible value from different laboratories. The INR is the ratio of the PT of the patient to a control, raised to the ISI (International Sensitivity Index). The ISI is different for each batch of thromboplastin and each manufacturer compares their thromboplastin against a standardized sample.

$$INR = (PT_{patient}/PT_{control})^{ISI}$$

192. **Which factors are measured by the activated partial thromboplastin time (aPTT)?**

Factors XII, XI, IX, and VIII, which are part of the "intrinsic pathway," and Factors II, V, and X, part of the "common pathway."

193. **How do you work up an abnormal PT or aPTT?**

Initially with a thorough history and physical examination. In the **history,** attention must be paid to medications (including over-the-counter medications and known anticoagulants), concomitant medical conditions, surgical outcomes and associated bleeding complications, use of alcohol, and any family history of bleeding disorders. For female patients, a detailed gynecologic history is crucial, with attention paid to the menstrual cycle. If the patient is hospitalized, the "history" of the blood sample should be investigated to determine whether the blood was drawn from an IV line that contains an anticoagulant.

During the **physical examination**, the location of hemorrhagic stigmata can give a clue to the underlying defect: mucocutaneous bleeding with von Willebrand's disease (vWD) or platelet disorders; hemarthrosis with hemophilia. Finally, the abnormal test result must be compared with a previous known value to establish whether this is a new or an old laboratory finding.

194. **Which laboratory test should be performed next?**

A mixing study.

195. **What is a mixing study?**

A test in which an aliquot of the patient's plasma is mixed 1:1 with normal plasma, and the PT or aPTT is repeated. If the repeat test gives a "normal" value, then the sample is said to have "corrected," implying a factor deficiency. However, if the result remains abnormal, even if the time has improved by a significant amount, then the test is said to have "not corrected," which indicates the presence of an inhibitor. For a Factor VIII inhibitor, the aPTT may correct initially, but then on prolonged incubation, prolong again.

196. **What are the causes of an abnormal aPTT?**

- Congenital deficiencies of Factors VIII, IX, XI, XII, high-molecular-weight kininogen (HMWK, which circulates with Factor XI), or prekallikrein (PK, associated with Factor XI)
- Acquired Factor VIII inhibitor (associated with malignancy, postpartum state, and autoimmune disorders)
- Lupus anticoagulant (LA)

A shortened aPTT is usually due to an increase in an intrinsic pathway factor, most commonly Factor VIII.

197. **What are the causes of *only* an abnormal PT?**

- Congenital Factor VII deficiency
- Liver dysfunction (decreasing vitamin K–dependent factors)
- Use of vitamin K antagonists

198. **What are the diseases caused by coagulation factor deficiencies?**

See Table 14-10.

199. **What is the most common inherited hemorrhagic condition?**

VWD. In 1926, Erik von Willebrand first described a family with a severe bleeding phenotype that was eventually found to have a severe deficiency of vWF. The index patient, a 14-year-old girl, bled to death after her fourth menses.

TABLE 14-10. COAGULATION DEFICIENCIES

Factor Deficiency	Prevalence	Inheritance	Treatment	Notes
Fibrinogen	1:1,000,000	Recessive	Fibrinogen concentrates to obtain a level > 100 mg/dL	Higher incidence in consanguineous families
Factor II (Prothrombin)	1:2,000,000	Recessive	FFP or (PCC)	Complete deficiency (<1%) has not been described
Factor V	1:1,000,000	Recessive	FFP	Check FVIII levels to make sure not combined deficiency
Factor VII	1:300,000	Recessive	PCC or rFVIIa	Need to evaluate for dietary or environmental variables
Factor VIII	1:5,000 live male births	X-linked	FVIII concentrates	In women with low FVIII levels, need to exclude vWD or combined FV deficiency
Factor IX	1:30,000 live male births	X-linked	FIX concentrates	"Christmas disease." Has marked heterogeneity
Factor X	1:1,000,000	Recessive	PCC	Heterozygous FX deficiency estimated at 1:500, but generally asymptomatic
Factor XI	Variable	Recessive	FFP	Although found in all racial groups, predominantly seen in Ashkenazi Jews
Factor XII	~1%	Recessive	None	Need to exclude LA as cause of deficiency. Not considered to be a hemorrhagic state
Factor XIII	1:1,000,000	Recessive	FFP, cryoprecipitate, or FXIII	Characterized by umbilical bleeding after birth

FFP = fresh frozen plasma; LA = lupus anticoagulant; PCC = prothrombin complex concentrates; vWD = von Willebrand's disease.

200. **What does vWF do?**

It functions as a carrier for Factor VIII that prolongs its half-life and a binder to a platelet receptor, GPIb, to initiate adhesion of platelets to the damaged endothelium (primary hemostasis).

201. **How is vWD diagnosed?**
- **History:** family history, menstrual history for females, history of mucocutaneous bleeding (epistaxis, gum bleeding, and menorrhagia)
- **Physical examination:** signs of mucocutaneous bleeding
- **Laboratory tests:** von Willebrand's factor antigen (vWF-Ag), and activity, von WIllebrand's factor ristocetin cofactor assay (VWF-RCo), multimer analysis, ristocetin titration, and collagen or Factor VIII binding assays

  Nichols WL, Rick ME, Ortel TL, et al: Clinical and laboratory diagnosis of von Willebrand disease: A synopsis of the 2008 NHLBI/NIH guidelines, *Am J Hematol* 284:366–370, 2009.

202. **What are the different types of vWD?**
- **Type 1:** vWF deficiency of at least 50% of normal that must be distinguished from "very low vWF levels"
- **Type 2:** characterized by qualitative defects
  - **2A:** loss of high-molecular-weight multimers of vWF
  - **2B:** mutation leads to inappropriate binding of vWF
  - **2M:** mutations in GPIb or collagen-binding domain
  - **2N:** mutations in the Factor VIII–binding domain abolishes its carrier capacity, decreasing Factor VIII levels
- **Type 3:** complete absence of vWF levels and activity
  vWF levels vary depending on the subtype of patient's blood group. Patients with type O blood have lower levels.

203. **What are the hemophilias?**
- **Hemophilia A:** Factor VIII deficiency
- **Hemophilia B:** Factor IX deficiency
- **Factor XI deficiency:** used to be called "Hemophilia C"

204. **What is an LA?**

An autoantibody that binds plasma proteins such as β_2-glycoprotein 1, cardiolipin, or annexin V that are bound to anionic phospholipids. Although the LA was originally described in 1952 in two patients with SLE who were noted to have a prolonged PT and bleeding symptoms, it was eventually observed that other lupus patients had prolonged aPTTs, and instead of bleeding, this prolonged aPTT was associated with thrombosis.

205. **What is the antiphospholipid syndrome (aPS)?**

The constellation of a prolonged aPTT or the presence of other antiphospholipid antibodies (anticardiolipin antibodies and anti-β_2-glycoprotein) occurring with vascular events, whether thrombosis or recurrent miscarriages. In order to correctly diagnose aPS, both the clinical and the laboratory components must be present. The clinical requirements are documented thrombotic events or recurrent pregnancy losses. The laboratory investigation requires a number of important components:
- Prolongation of a phospholipid dependent clotting assay (i.e., aPTT)
- No correction with mixing studies
- Addition of excess exogenous phospholipids (e.g., platelet neutralization or hexagonal-phase phospholipids) overcomes inhibition

- No specific clotting factor found for the inhibitor
- Persistent abnormality $\geq$ 12 weeks

Giannakopoulos B, Passam F, Ioannou Y, et al: How we diagnose the antiphospholipid syndrome, *Blood* 113:985–994, 2009.

206. **What is an acquired Factor VIII inhibitor?**
A rare development of an autoantibody against a patient's Factor VIII seen in pregnancy, malignancy, autoimmune disorders, and the elderly. Patients present with minor or even life-threatening hemorrhage, a newly prolonged aPTT that does not correct with mixing, and a low level of Factor VIII. The syndrome is also called "acquired hemophilia."

207. **What is a Bethesda titer and why is it important?**
The reciprocal of the dilution required to get 50% Factor VIII activity. In other words, when the mixing study is performed, serial dilutions are made of the patient's sample (e.g., 1:2, 1:5, 1:10, 1:100, or even greater) in order to overcome the inhibitor. Therefore, if the patient's sample was diluted 1:64 and a Factor VIII level of 50% was obtained, the Bethesda titer would be the reciprocal of this dilution (i.e., 64). The absolute value of the Bethesda titer is important, because levels $<$ 5 can be overcome with increased doses of Factor VIII. However, a Bethesda titer $\geq$ 5 will not respond to Factor VIII infusions and will require a bypassing agent.

208. **What are bypassing agents?**
Therapeutic agents used to overcome or "bypass" the block in the intrinsic pathway caused by the Factor VIII inhibitor. Currently, two agents available are: (1) recombinant Factor VIIa (rFVIIa) and (2) Factor VIII inhibitor bypassing activity (FEIBA). rFVIIa given in pharmacologic doses leads to thrombin generation on the surface of activated platelets. FEIBA is a factor concentrate that is enriched in activated vitamin K–dependent factors.

Kempton CL, White GC II: How we treat a hemophilia A patient with a factor VIII inhibitor, *Blood* 113:11–17, 2009.

209. **What are the vitamin K–dependent clotting factors (VKDCFs)?**
Factors II, VII, IX, and X.

210. **Which clotting factors are decreased in vitamin K deficiency, liver disease, and DIC?**
- **Vitamin K deficiency:** VKDCF and anticoagulants protein C and S
- **Liver disease:** VKDCF, fibrinogen, antithrombin, and Factors V and XI
- **DIC:** all factors including Factor VIII, which is not vitamin K–dependent or manufactured in the liver

211. **What is DIC?**
A syndrome in which the coagulation factors are all consumed and described as "... the circulating plasma is transformed into circulating *serum*." Findings include a microangiopathic HA (as evidenced by the presence of RBC fragments, or schistocytes, on the peripheral blood smear), thrombocytopenia, a prolongation initially of the PT and then the aPTT, and signs of hemorrhage.

Rodriquez-Erdmann F: Bleeding due to increased intravascular blood coagulation—Hemorrhagic syndromes caused by consumption of blood-clotting factors (consumption-coagulopathies). *N Engl J Med* 273:1370–1378, 1965.

212. **How is DIC scored?**
See Table 14-11.

TABLE 14-11. SCORING SYSTEM FOR ASSESSMENT OF MORTALITY RISK IN DISSEMINATED INTRAVASCULAR COAGULATION

Laboratory Test	Value	Points*
Platelet count	$>100 \times 10^9$/L	0
	$<100 \times 10^9$/L	1
	$<50 \times 10^9$/L	2
Elevated fibrin markers	No increase	0
	Moderate increase	2
	Strong increase	3
Prolonged PT	<3 sec	0
	>3 but <6 sec	1
	>6 sec	2
Fibrinogen level	>1 g/L	0
	<1 g/L	1

DIC = disseminated intravascular coagulation.
*A score ≥ 5 is compatible with overt DIC. For each point in the score, the odds ratio for mortality was 1.29.
From Levi M, Toh CH, Thachil J, et al: Guidelines for the diagnosis and management of disseminated intravascular coagulation. Br J Haematol 145:24–33, 2009.

213. **What are the naturally occurring anticoagulants?**
- Antithrombin
- Protein C
- Protein S

214. **What is their mechanism of action?**
    Antithrombin, particularly when combined with unfractionated heparin, is stimulated to inactivate thrombin and Factor Xa. The low-molecular-weight anticoagulants activate only antithrombin's anti-Factor Xa activity. **Protein C** circulates in an inactive form. However, when thrombin combines with thrombomodulin on the intact endothelium, it activates protein C (APC). APC then combines with its cofactor, **Protein S**, to inactive Factors Va and VIIIa.

215. **Is there a risk of increased thrombosis when starting warfarin for treatment or prevention of thrombotic events?**
    Yes, in select patients, treatment with warfarin alone can increase the risk for thrombosis. Because protein C and protein S are vitamin K–dependent, any deficiency in these anticoagulants, whether congenital or acquired, can be exacerbated with warfarin treatment. Complications include warfarin-induced skin necrosis or gangrene of the limbs. These risks can be avoided by initially or simultaneously treating with an alternative anticoagulant, such as unfractionated heparin, low-molecular-weight heparins, fondaparinux, or direct thrombin inhibitors. (See also Chapter 6, Pulmonary Medicine.)

216. **What thrombotic risk is associated with heparin use?**
The occurrence of heparin-induced thrombocytopenia (HIT). In HIT, the unfractionated heparin combines with platelet factor 4 (PF4) and induces a conformational change, which in some people is immunogenic. The resultant IgG combines with the heparin/PF4 complex. This IgG/heparin/PF4 complex can then bind to the FcγRIIa on platelets, leading to platelet activation, thrombocytopenia, and thrombin generation. Despite treatment with an anticoagulant (heparin) that results in thrombocytopenia, the risks of HIT are not of hemorrhage, but of thrombosis. In fact, the risk for thrombosis is increased so greatly, that it must be treated.

Arepally GM, Ortel TL: Heparin-induced thrombocytopenia, *N Engl J Med* 355:809–817, 2006.

217. **How is HIT treated?**
First, it must be recognized. Next, all heparin-containing products, *including heparin-containing flushes for IV lines,* must be discontinued immediately. Subsequent use of low-molecular-weight heparin is also contraindicated. A direct thrombin inhibitor is administered until the platelet count normalizes, at which point warfarin is initiated.

Warkentin TE, Greinacher A, Koster A, et al: Treatment and prevention of heparin-induced thrombocytopenia: American College of Chest Physicians Evidence-Based Clinical Practice Guidelines (8th ed.), *Chest* 133:340–380, 2008.

KEY POINTS: HEMOSTASIS ✔

1. A thorough history included previous history of aspirin use, bleeding episodes, and liver or kidney disease.

2. Disorders of primary hemostasis (thrombocytopenia and von Willebrand's disease) demonstrate purpura and mucosal bleeding.

3. Disorders of secondary hemostasis (hemophilia) demonstrate deep tissue bleeding and hemarthroses.

4. The initial laboratory evaluation of a bleeding disorder includes PT and aPTT with mixing study if prolonged and CBC with platelet count.

5. Hereditary thrombophilia is more likely in patients with thrombosis who are young or who have a thrombosis in an unusual site. The most common disorder in European patients is Factor V Leiden.

6. Increased homocysteine, lupus anticoagulants, and the related antiphospholipid antibody syndrome are important causes of acquired thrombophilia.

aPTT = activated partial thromboplastin time; CBC = complete blood count; PT = prothrombin time.

218. **What is activated protein C resistance (APCR)?**
Most commonly, an inherited mutation in the Factor V gene, wherein a G→A substitution at nucleotide 1,691 renders Factor Va resistant to inactivation by the activated protein C/S complex. This mutation is known as "Factor V Leiden (FVL)," after Leiden, Netherlands, where it was discovered. Whereas approximately 95% of APCR is due to FVL resistance, acquired cases of APCR can be due to elevated Factor VIII levels, use of oral contraceptive therapy, lupus, or malignancy.

ACKNOWLEDGMENT

The editor gratefully acknowledges contributions by Drs. Mark M. Udden and Martha P. Mims that were retained from the previous edition of *Medical Secrets*.

WESTES

1. www.hematology.com

2. www.bloodline.net

3. National Comprehensive Cancer Network: www.nccn.org. Provides risk stratification and treatment guidelines for hematology malignancies.

BIBLIOGRAPHY

1. Greer JP, Goerster J, Rodgers GM, et al, editors: *Wintrobe's Clinical Hematology*, ed 12, Philadelphia, 2008, Lippincott Williams & Wilkins.

2. Loscalzo J, Achaefer AI, editors. *Thrombosis and Hemorrhage*, ed 3, Philadelphia, 2002, Lippincott Williams & Wilkins.

CHAPTER 15

ONCOLOGY

Teresa G. Hayes, M.D., Ph.D.

> *While there are several chronic diseases more destructive to life than cancer, none is more feared.*
> Charles H. Mayo (1865–1939)
> *Annals of Surgery* 83:357, 1926

GENERAL ISSUES

1. **Define "carcinogenesis."**
   The alteration of normal cells into malignant cells. Through a multistage evolution of genetic and epigenetic alterations, cells can escape the normal growth constraints of their host.

2. **What are the known gene categories that influence the mechanisms of neoplasia?**
   - Oncogenes
   - Tumor suppressor genes
   - Regulators of cell death
   - Mutation control genes (includes mismatch repair genes)

3. **Describe the effects of oncogenes.**
   Oncogenes in humans and other animals have the capacity to transform normal cells into malignant ones. These genes, acquired at conception or mutated during life, make the patient susceptible to cancer by altering or impairing several processes:
   - Production of nuclear transcription factors that control cell growth (e.g., *myc*)
   - Signal transduction within cells (e.g., *ras*)
   - Interaction of growth factors and their receptors (e.g., *her/neu*)

   More than 100 different oncogenes have been identified, but only some have been associated exclusively with human cancers. Mutations convert proto-oncogenes to oncogenes by amplification, translocation, and point mutation.

4. **How do tumor suppressor genes affect carcinogenesis?**
   When functioning normally, tumor suppressor genes regulate the growth and division of cells. When mutations occur in both alleles of these genes, cellular regulatory function is lost and tumor growth can occur. Multiple tumor suppressor genes have been identified (e.g., *p53* and *rb*) and are found in many different types of cancers. These mutations are the basis of the inherited predispositions to cancers, when they are often inherited in the heterozygous state.

5. **How is cell death regulated?**
   Cell death genes are involved in the programmed death (**apoptosis**) of cells no longer needed by the body. Mutation in one of these genes (e.g., *bcl-2*) allows cells to live that should have died, causing excessive accumulation of cells. Activation of the **telomerase** gene, which controls cell senescence, is thought to cause cells to become immortal by turning off the normal aging process.

6. **What are mutation control genes?**
   Mismatch repair genes such as *hMSH2* and *hMLH1* that are responsible for ensuring the fidelity of the DNA duplication process. Microsatellite instability results from the faulty DNA editing process. Subsequently, the mutation rate increases and cancers occur.

7. **List common environmental causes of cancer.**
   - **Social agents:** tobacco and alcohol
   - **Occupational exposure:** arsenic, benzene, CCl_4, chromium, combustion byproducts (engine exhaust), and polycyclic hydrocarbons (coal byproducts)
   - **Ionizing radiation:** ultraviolet B light (UVB; sunlight), mining, and others
   - **Dietary factors:** aflatoxin B, high-fat diet, nitrates/nitrites (converted endogenously to nitrosamines), smoked foods, and diet low in fresh fruits and vegetables
   - **Foreign body reactants:** asbestos fiber
   - **Chronic inflammation:** ulcerative colitis
   - **Infectious agents:** Epstein-Barr virus (EBV), hepatitis B and C viruses, human papillomavirus (HPV), human T-lymphotropic virus, and *Helicobacter pylori*
   - **Iatrogenic agents:** cancer chemotherapeutic drugs, estrogens, and immune suppressants

8. **Summarize dietary "protective" factors.**
   Diets high in antioxidants and lycopene that include many fruits and vegetables (e.g., tomatoes and broccoli) are thought to protect against cancer development by scavenging for free radicals. Some vitamins may modify the effect of chemical carcinogenesis such as vitamin A (which promotes the differentiation of epithelial tissues), vitamin C (which blocks the formation of *N*-nitrosocarcinogens from nitrites and secondary amines), and vitamin E (which is a free radical scavenger). In general, these agents are more effective for cancer prevention when consumed in the diet rather than being taken in supplement form.

9. **Which cancers tend to cluster in families?**
   Breast, endometrial, colon, prostate, lung, melanoma, and stomach have an increased risk of development in first-degree relatives. This cluster may be due to hereditary factors, shared exposures to environmental carcinogens, chance associations, or a combination of all three.

10. **Summarize the familial clustering of breast cancer.**
    Mutation in a genetic locus (*BRCA1, BRCA2,* and several others) predisposes to the development of familial breast or ovarian cancer or both and occurs in approximately 10–15% of breast cancer cases.

KEY POINTS: FAMILIAL CANCER ✔

1. Up to 15% of cancers are familial, due to inherited chromosomal alterations.

2. A careful family history is essential.

3. Screening of family members is indicated in autosomal dominant conditions.

4. Chemoprevention (e.g., tamoxifen for breast cancer) or prophylactic removal of the tissue at risk may be considered in very high-risk families.

11. **Describe the Lynch cancer family syndrome.**

    Nonpolyposis colorectal cancer with an increased incidence of other cancers, including endometrial, ovarian, breast, stomach, small intestine, pancreatic, urinary tract, and biliary tract that is associated with an autosomal dominant pattern of predisposition. Mutations in the mismatch repair genes *hMLH1*, *hMSH2*, *hMSH6*, and *hPMS2* cause microsatellite instability and are associated with this syndrome.

12. **What is Li-Fraumeni syndrome?**

    A familial cancer syndrome with an autosomal dominant pattern of inheritance leading to a varied spectrum of mesenchymal and epithelial tumors, and multiple primary neoplasms in children and young adults. The gene for this cancer (*p53*) is located on the short arm of chromosome 17. *P53*, sometimes called "guardian of the genome," is a gene that is very important in preventing damaged cells from duplicating themselves.

13. **Describe the MEN I syndrome.**

    Multiple endocrine neoplasia type I (MEN I), associated with a defect in the *MEN1* gene on chromosome 11, is associated with tumors of the parathyroid, pituitary (most commonly prolactinoma), and islet cells of the pancreas.

14. **Summarize the two phenotypes of the MEN II syndrome.**

    - **Type A:** medullary thyroid carcinoma, pheochromocytoma, and parathyroid hyperplasia
    - **Type B:** medullary thyroid carcinoma, pheochromocytoma, marfanoid habitus, and mucosal neuromas

      Germ-line point mutations of the *RET* proto-oncogene on chromosome 10 are responsible for both types of MEN II.

15. **What are tumor markers?**

    Enzymes, hormones, and oncofetal antigens that are associated with particular tumors. These markers are sometimes present on the cell surface or secreted by the malignant cells and can be detected in the bloodstream or by staining tissue samples. The markers reflect the presence of the tumor and sometimes also the quantity of the tumor or tumor burden. Many cancers do not produce tumor markers, and tumors known to produce markers may sometimes fail to do so, particularly if they are very poorly differentiated.

16. **How are tumor markers used?**

    To follow the effects of therapy on tumor burden and in detecting recurrent disease after initial therapy. Some of the tumor markers, such as prostate-specific antigen (PSA) and alpha-fetoprotein (AFP), are highly sensitive and specific, strongly correlating with the presence of a particular type of cancer. Others, such as carcinoembryonic antigen (CEA), are nonspecific and may be elevated in many conditions besides malignancies.

17. **Summarize the significance of CEA.**

    High CEA can be found in a variety of cancers including lung cancer, colon cancer, breast cancer, and other adenocarcinomas. CEA is a glycoprotein of 200,000 Da that is found in gastrointestinal (GI) mucosal cells and pancreaticobiliary secretions. Elevations of CEA occur with breaks in the mucosal basement membrane by a tumor but can also occur in smokers and persons with cirrhosis, pancreatitis, inflammatory bowel disease, and rectal polyps. CEA is most useful in colorectal cancer and is used to monitor the activity of disease if the CEA level was elevated before treatment.

18. **Why is PSA important?**

    The serum level of PSA may be elevated in benign prostate disease, including benign prostatic hypertrophy and prostatitis, as well as in prostate cancer. PSA is a serine protease found only in the prostate that normally liquefies seminal gel. High levels of PSA, especially in patients with small-volume prostates, are a strong indicator of probable prostate cancer. Very elevated PSA levels (>100 ng/mL) correlate well with the presence of metastatic disease. The rate of rise of the PSA and the percentage of free PSA also can help to determine whether an elevated PSA level is due to benign or malignant causes. (See also Chapter 2, General Medicine and Ambulatory Care.)

19. **Discuss the role of AFP as a tumor marker.**
    AFP is a 70,000 Da α-globulin protein that is made by the yolk sac and liver of the human fetus. AFP is elevated in hepatocellular carcinoma and certain germ cell neoplasms and is a highly sensitive marker for disease activity. Very high levels of AFP (>400 ng/mL) correlate with the presence of these malignancies, although the marker is also elevated in acute and chronic hepatitis.

20. **What is β-human chorionic gonadotropin (β-hCG)?**
    A glycoprotein normally secreted by the trophoblastic epithelium of the placenta that is used as a sensitive and specific marker for germ cell tumors of the testes and ovary and extragonadal presentations of these tumors.

KEY POINTS: TUMOR MARKERS ✓

1. Tumor markers are generally nonspecific and can be elevated in a variety of conditions.

2. Other than PSA, most tumor markers are not useful in screening for malignancies in the general population.

3. Tumor markers are used to assist in diagnosis and therapy in patients suspected to have malignancy by clinical parameters.

4. CEA and CA-125 have clinical utility in patients diagnosed with colorectal and ovarian cancer, respectively, but only if the level was elevated before treatment of the cancer.

5. CA 19-9 can be highly elevated in cases of benign biliary tract obstruction.

6. PSA levels > 10 ng/mL have a 60% probability of prostate cancer; levels > 100 ng/mL correlate strongly with metastatic disease.

CEA = carcinoembryonic antigen; PSA = prostate-specific antigen.

21. **List the principles used in formulating combination chemotherapy regimens.**
    - Drugs used should have activity against the tumor.
    - Drugs should be selected with dissimilar toxicities.
    - Drugs with different mechanisms of action should be used.
    - Several cycles of therapy, with adequate biologic effect, should be used before determining efficacy.
    - Recovery of normal tissues should be allowed before starting the next cycle.

22. **What are the mechanisms of tumor resistance to chemotherapeutic agents?**
    - Intrinsic cellular or biochemical resistance
    - Impaired transport of the drug into the cell or active extrusion from the cell
    - Altered drug affinity for the target enzyme
    - Amplification of genes
    - Membrane alterations from overproduction of high-weight glycoproteins

23. **Summarize the toxic effects of chemotherapy.**
See Table 15-1. Nausea and vomiting are the most common immediate effects and may vary in presence and degree with the type of drug. Some medications, such as cisplatin, are very emetogenic, whereas others, like fludarabine, are less likely to cause emesis. Many chemotherapy drugs cause myelosuppression. When myelosuppression occurs, leukopenia predisposes to acute and serious infections; thrombocytopenia predisposes to bleeding; and anemia may worsen symptoms from other problems, such as chronic obstructive pulmonary disease and atherosclerotic cardiovascular disease. Many, but not all, chemotherapy agents cause hair loss (alopecia).

TABLE 15-1. TOXICITIES OF CHEMOTHERAPEUTIC AGENTS

Drug	Acute Toxicity	Delayed Toxicity
Bleomycin (Blenoxane)	Nausea/vomiting, fever, hypersensitivity reactions	**Pneumonitis, pulmonary fibrosis,*** rash and hyperpigmentation, stomatitis, alopecia, Raynaud's phenomenon, cavitating granulomas
Carboplatin (Paraplatin)	Nausea/vomiting	**Myelosuppression,*** peripheral neuropathy (uncommon), hearing loss, hemolytic anemia, transient cortical blindness
Capecitabine (Xeloda)	Nausea, diarrhea, stomatitis	**Hand-foot syndrome*** (palmar-plantar erythrodysesthesia), hyperbilirubinemia
Chlorambucil (Leukeran)	Seizures, nausea/vomiting	**Myelosuppression,*** pulmonary infiltrates and fibrosis, leukemia, hepatic toxicity, sterility
Cisplatin (Platinol)	Nausea/vomiting, anaphylactic reaction	**Renal damage,*** ototoxicity, myelosuppression, hemolysis, ↓ $Mg^{2+}/Ca^{2+}/K^+$, peripheral neuropathy, Raynaud phenomenom
Cytarabine (ara-C)	Nausea/vomiting, diarrhea, anaphylaxis	**Myelosuppression,*** oral ulceration, conjunctivitis, hepatic damage, fever, pulmonary edema, neurotoxicity (high dose), rhabdomyolysis, pancreatitis with asparaginase

(continued)

TABLE 15-1. TOXICITIES OF CHEMOTHERAPEUTIC AGENTS—*(continued)*

Drug	Acute Toxicity	Delayed Toxicity
Dacarbazine (DTIC)	Nausea/vomiting, diarrhea, anaphylaxis, pain on administration	**Myelosuppression,*** cardiotoxicity,* alopecia, flulike syndrome, renal impairment, hepatic necrosis, facial flushing, paresthesias, photosensitivity, urticarial rash
Daunorubicin (Cerubidine)	Nausea/vomiting, diarrhea, red urine, severe local tissue necrosis on extravasation, transient ECG changes, anaphylactoid reaction	**Myelosuppression,*** cardiotoxicity,* alopecia, stomatitis, anorexia, diarrhea, fever and chills, dermatitis in previously irradiated areas, skin and nail pigmentation
Doxorubicin (Adriamycin)	Nausea/vomiting, red urine, severe local tissue necrosis on extravasation, diarrhea, fever, transient ECG changes, ventricular arrhythmia, anaphylactoid reaction	**Myelosuppression,*** cardiotoxicity,* alopecia, stomatitis, anorexia, conjunctivitis, acral pigmentation, dermatitis in previously irradiated areas, acral erythrodysesthesia, mucositis
Etoposide (VP16)	Nausea/vomiting, diarrhea, fever, hypotension, allergic reaction	**Myelosuppression,*** alopecia, peripheral neuropathy, mucositis and hepatic damage with high doses, leukemia
Floxuridine (FUDR)	Nausea/vomiting, diarrhea	**Oral and GI ulceration,*** **myelosuppression,*** alopecia, dermatitis, hepatic dysfunction with infusion
Fluorouracil (5-FU)	Nausea/vomiting, diarrhea, hypersensitivity, photosensitivity	**Oral and GI ulcers, myelosuppression,*** diarrhea, ataxia, arrhythmias, angina, hyperpigmentation, hand-foot syndrome, conjunctivitis
Gemcitabine (Gemzar)	Fatigue, nausea and vomiting	**Bone marrow depression,** especially thrombocytopenia; edema; pulmonary toxicity; anal pruritus
Ifosfamide (Ifex)	Nausea/vomiting, confusion, nephrotoxicity, metabolic acidosis, **cardiac toxicity with higher doses***	**Myelosuppression,*** **hemorrhagic cystitis**, alopecia, SIADH, neurotoxicity

(continued)

TABLE 15-1. TOXICITIES OF CHEMOTHERAPEUTIC AGENTS—*(continued)*

Drug	Acute Toxicity	Delayed Toxicity
Irinotecan (Camptosar)	Nausea and vomiting, diarrhea, fever	**Diarrhea, anorexia,** stomatitis, bone marrow depression, alopecia, abdominal cramping
Mechlorethamine (nitrogen mustard)	Nausea/vomiting, local reaction and phlebitis	**Myelosuppression,*** alopecia, diarrhea, oral ulcers, leukemia, amenorrhea, sterility
Methotrexate	Nausea/vomiting, diarrhea, fever, anaphylaxis, hepatic necrosis	**Oral/GI ulceration,*** **myelosuppression,*** hepatic toxicity, renal toxicity, **pulmonary infiltrates and fibrosis,*** osteoporosis, conjunctivitis, alopecia, depigmentation
Mitoxantrone (Novantrone)	Blue-green sclera and pigment in urine, nausea/vomiting, stomatitis	**Myelosuppression,*** cardiotoxicity, alopecia, white hair, skin lesions, hepatic damage, renal failure
Paclitaxel (Taxol), docetaxel (Taxotere)	Hypersensitivity, hypotension, nausea, pain on extravasation	**Myelosuppression,*** alopecia, peripheral neuropathy, rash and edema (docetaxel)
Topotecan (Hycamtin)	Nausea/vomiting, diarrhea, headache	**Myelosuppression,*** alopecia, transient elevations in hepatic enzymes
Vinblastine (Velban)	Nausea/vomiting, local reaction and phlebitis with extravasation	**Myelosuppression,*** alopecia, stomatitis, loss of DTRs, jaw pain, muscle pain, paralytic ileus
Vincristine (Oncovin)	Local reaction with extravasation	**Peripheral neuropathy,*** alopecia, mild myelosuppression, constipation, paralytic ileus, jaw pain, SIADH
Vinorelbine (Navelbine)	Local reaction with extravasation	**Granulocytopenia,*** anemia, fatigue

CHF = chronic heart failure; DTRs = deep tendon reflexes; ECG = electrocardiographic; GI = gastrointestinal; SIADH = syndrome of inappropriate antidiuretic hormone.
*Dose-limiting effects.
Modified from Drugs of choice for cancer chemotherapy. Med Lett 42:83–92, 2000.

24. **Which chemotherapeutic drugs are associated with cardiotoxicity?**
Doxorubicin (Adriamycin) and other drugs of the anthracycline class, which cause a progressive loss of cardiac muscle cells. In previously normal hearts, toxicity is dose-related and does not become clinically important until a total dose of approximately 450 mg/m^2 of doxorubicin is administered. In patients with already compromised cardiac function, toxicity may occur at lower dosages.

25. **How is doxorubicin-related cardiotoxicity monitored?**
With cardiac radionuclide gated wall motion studies (multiple-gated acquisition scans) or echocardiograms measuring ejection fraction.

26. **Distinguish between neoadjuvant therapy and adjuvant therapy.**
Neoadjuvant therapy means treatment such as chemotherapy or hormones before definitive surgery or radiotherapy. Patients given neoadjuvant therapy often have large or fixed tumors, and the goal is to shrink these tumors to make subsequent surgical removal or radiation therapy easier and more complete. **Adjuvant therapy** is given after surgery. Adjuvant chemotherapy and/or radiotherapy are administered after an operation to eradicate possible micrometastatic disease and, therefore, prevent recurrence.

27. **What are radiation sensitizers?**
Chemical agents that increase the sensitivity of cells to radiation. This class of compounds includes drugs such as 5-fluorouracil (5-FU), platinum analogues, gemcitabine, and cetuximab. Radiosensitization by these compounds may be mediated by a variety of poorly understood mechanisms. Radiation sensitizers likely have effects on the induction and/or repair of radiation-induced damage.

28. **Define "tumor doubling time."**
The time required for the tumor to double in volume. The doubling time varies greatly among types of cancer and, in a single cancer type, may vary among different individuals. Cancers with a slow doubling time include prostate cancer and colon cancer. Cancers with more rapid doubling times include lung cancer, cancers of the pancreas and esophagus, and certain types of lymphomas.

29. **How is the doubling time of tumors calculated from x-rays?**
By measuring the diameter of the lesion (assuming that it is approximately spherical) and calculating its volume with the formula:

$$\text{volume} = 4/3\pi r^3$$

where π is the constant pi and r is the radius of the lesion. After the volume is calculated on two separate occasions, doubling time can be derived from a plot of volume versus time.

30. **What is the Gompertz equation?**
A calculation that describes the effect of size and other factors on slowing of tumor growth. Doubling time calculation is a rough estimate because it assumes simple growth kinetics and the absence of other factors that affect tumor growth. However, tumor cell populations exhibit a reduction in growth rate with increasing size because they receive less blood supply to the center of the tumor as the mass grows, and the Gompertz equation accounts for this effect.

31. **What is the most common cause of cancer death in the United States today?**
Lung cancer, for both men and women (Table 15-2).

TABLE 15-2. LEADING SITES OF NEW CANCER CASES AND DEATHS IN THE UNITED STATES

Male			Female		
Estimated New Cases					
Prostate	217,730	25%	Breast	207,090	28%
Lung and bronchus	116,750	15%	Lung and bronchus	105,770	14%
Colon and rectum	72,090	9%	Colon and rectum	70,480	10%
Urinary bladder	52,760	7%	Uterine corpus	43,470	6%
Melanoma of the skin	38,870	5%	Thyroid	33,930	5%
Non-Hodgkin's lymphoma	35,380	5%	Non-Hodgkin's lymphoma	30,160	4%
Kidney and renal pelvis	35,370	5%	Melanoma of the skin	29,260	4%
Oral cavity and pharynx	25,420	3%	Kidney and renal pelvis	22,870	3%
Leukemia	24,690	3%	Ovary	21,880	3%
Pancreas	21,370	3%	Pancreas	21,770	3%
All sites	**789,620**	**100%**	**All sites**	**739,940**	**100%**
Estimated Deaths					
Lung and bronchus	86,220	29%	Lung and bronchus	71,080	26%
Prostate	32,050	11%	Breast	39,840	15%
Colon and rectum	26,580	9%	Colon and rectum	24,790	9%
Pancreas	18,770	6%	Pancreas	18,030	7%
Liver and intrahepatic bile duct	12,720	4%	Ovary	13,850	5%
Leukemia	12,660	4%	Non-Hodgkin's lymphoma	9,500	4%
Esophagus	11,650	4%	Leukemia	9,180	3%
Non-Hodgkin's lymphoma	10,710	4%	Uterine corpus	7,950	3%
Urinary bladder	10,410	3%	Liver and intrahepatic bile duct	6,190	2%
Kidney and renal pelvis	8,210	3%	Brain and other nervous system	5,720	2%
All sites	**299,200**	**100%**	**All sites**	**270,290**	**100%**

Excludes basal and squamous cell skin cancers and in situ carcinoma except urinary bladder. Estimates are rounded to the nearest 10.
Modified from Jemal A, Siegal R, Xu J, Ward R: Cancer Statistics, 2010. CA Cancer J Clin 60:277–300, 2010.

COMPLICATIONS OF CANCER

32. **What are the causes of anemia in patients with cancer?**
    - Anemia of chronic disease
    - Bone marrow suppression by chemotherapy
    - Marrow involvement by tumor
    - Hemolysis secondary to tumor-associated antibodies
    - Certain chemotherapeutic agents
    - Sepsis
    - Disseminated intravascular coagulation (DIC)
    - Paraneoplastic syndrome
    - Gastritis and GI bleeding from medications for pain control (such as nonsteroidal anti-inflammatory agents [NSAIDs])
    - Decreased erythropoietin owing to renal effects due to chemotherapeutic agents such as cisplatin

33. **What are the predisposing factors for infection in patients with cancer?**
    - Defects in cellular and humoral immunity
    - Organ compromise due to tumor-related obstruction
    - Chemotherapy-related granulocytopenia
    - Disruption of mucosal (e.g., respiratory and alimentary tract) and integumental surfaces
    - Iatrogenic procedures or indwelling prosthetic devices
    - Hyposplenic or postsplenectomy states

34. **Discuss the sources of infection in patients with cancer.**
    The vast majority of infections originate from the patient's own endogenous flora. Sources of infection in neutropenic patients include the lungs, urinary tract, skin, upper aerodigestive tract (mouth, skin, teeth), central nervous system, rectum, perirectum, biopsy sites, and GI tract (appendicitis, cholecystitis, perforations). In investigating the cause of an infection, cultures should include blood, urine, sputum, and if appropriate to the patient's clinical status, stool, pleural fluid, or peritoneal fluid.

35. **Which malignancies commonly spread to bone?**

Lung	Prostate	Malignant
Breast	Thyroid	melanoma
Kidney	Multiple myeloma	

36. **Are metastatic bone lesions osteoblastic or osteolytic?**
    Both. Renal cell carcinoma and multiple myeloma tend to be purely lytic, prostate carcinoma tends to be mostly blastic, and other bone lesions are mixed. Lytic bone lesions are often associated with hypercalcemia, unlike blastic metastases.

37. **To which bones does cancer most often metastasize?**
    - Spine
    - Ribs
    - Pelvis
    - Long bones

38. **Characterize the pain associated with bone metastases.**
    A dull, aching discomfort that is worse at night and may improve with physical activity.

39. **Which tumors metastasize to the lungs?**
    Most types of tumors can metastasize to the lungs; therefore, the more common the tumor, the more common the lung metastases. GI cancers tend to metastasize locally first and to the

liver before pulmonary involvement is seen. Tumors that spread via the bloodstream, such as sarcomas, renal cell carcinoma, and colon cancer, tend to produce nodular lung lesions. Those that spread via lymphatic routes, such as cancers of the breast, lung, pancreas, stomach, and liver, may manifest a pattern of lymphangitic spread.

40. **Discuss the symptoms of intracranial metastases.**
Headache occurs in up to 50% of patients with intracranial metastases and is classically described as occurring early in the morning, disappearing or decreasing after arising, and associated with nausea and/or projectile vomiting. Other symptoms include focal signs such as unilateral weakness, numbness, seizures, or cranial nerve abnormalities. Nonfocal complaints such as mental status changes or ataxia may occur.

41. **How are intracranial metastases diagnosed?**
By contrast-enhanced computed tomography (CT) or magnetic resonance imaging (MRI) of the brain.

42. **How are intracranial metastases treated?**
By decreasing intracranial pressure with steroids, followed by definitive therapy. Surgery is recommended for patients with single intracranial lesions if technically possible, whereas radiation therapy is generally administered for multiple lesions. Chemotherapy may also be used, but the results are not as reliable as the other modalities owing to the difficulty of chemotherapy agents penetrating the blood-brain barrier.

43. **What are the signs and symptoms of malignant pericardial effusion?**
Frequently similar to the symptoms of heart failure with dyspnea, peripheral edema, and an enlarged heart on chest x-ray. However, the dyspnea is often out of proportion to the degree of pulmonary congestion seen on the x-ray. Kussmaul's sign, or jugulovenous distention with inspiration, and pulsus paradoxus of > 10 mmHg with distant heart sounds are clues to the presence of a pericardial effusion. See also Chapter 4, Cardiology.

44. **How is the diagnosis of malignant pericardial effusion confirmed?**
By echocardiogram or CT scan and by taking a sample of the pericardial fluid. Malignant effusions are usually exudates and are often hemorrhagic. Cytology is helpful if positive but does not exclude cancer if negative.

45. **Discuss the treatment of malignant pericardial effusion.**
Treatment depends on the patient's condition but should include drainage of the fluid for diagnostic as well as therapeutic reasons. A nonsurgical approach is preferred, with catheter drainage followed by sclerosis of the pericardium, sometimes with a sclerosing agent such as doxycycline. Other approaches include subxiphoid pericardiectomy, balloon pericardiectomy, pericardial window, and pericardial stripping for patients with prolonged life expectancy.

46. **What are the presenting symptoms and signs of spinal cord compression?**
Back pain in 95% of cancer patients. Other symptoms include lower extremity weakness, bowel or bladder incontinence, or increased deep tendon reflexes in the lower extremities. Once neurologic symptoms appear, the nerve damage may be irreversible; therefore, early diagnosis of cord compression is essential.

47. **How is spinal cord compression diagnosed?**
By MRI or myelography with CT, which will demonstrate blockage or pressure on the spinal canal or nerve roots.

48. **How is spinal cord compression treated?**
Initially by decreasing spinal cord swelling and pain with high-dose steroids and adequate pain medication. Definitive treatment with surgery or radiation therapy must be carried out emergently to prevent irreversible neurologic deterioration. Preservation of neurologic function is generally better with surgery. Radiation treatment is given to patients not eligible for surgical decompression.

49. **Which malignancies most commonly cause spinal cord compression?**
   - Lung
   - Breast
   - Prostate
   - Carcinoma of unknown primary
   - Lymphoma
   - Multiple myeloma

   The most common site of cord compression is the thoracic spine, followed by the lumbosacral spine and the cervical spine.

50. **Which tumors are associated with nonbacterial thrombotic endocarditis?**
Mucinous adenocarcinomas, most commonly of the lung, pancreas, stomach, or ovary. This paraneoplastic syndrome is also known as "marantic endocarditis" and has also been described in other types of cancers.

51. **How does nonbacterial thrombotic endocarditis present?**
Usually the appearance of embolic peripheral or cerebral vascular events causing arterial insufficiency, encephalopathy, or focal neurologic defects. The emboli originate from sterile, verrucous, fibrin-platelet vegetations that accumulate on the heart valves, likely due to a hypercoagulable state from malignancy. Heart murmurs are not always present.

52. **How is nonbacterial thrombotic endocarditis diagnosed and treated?**
By transesophageal echocardiogram (TEE). However, echocardiograms may be negative, and the diagnosis is usually made postmortem. Treatment with anticoagulants or antiplatelet drugs has been tried with little success.

53. **What are the tumor-related causes of hypercalcemia?**
   - **Lytic bone metastases:** release calcium into the bloodstream and are the most common cause of hypercalcemia in solid tumors with bony metastases.
   - **Humoral hypercalcemia of malignancy (HHM):** occurs in patients without bony metastases. Cancers associated with this syndrome secrete a non-PTH (parathyroid hormone) substance with activity similar to PTH. HHM is associated most commonly with squamous cell cancers of the lung, esophagus, or head and neck but can also be found in renal cell carcinoma, transitional cell carcinoma of the bladder, and ovarian carcinoma.
   - **Osteoclast-activating factors:** includes interleukin-1 (IL-1), IL-6, and tumor necrosis factor-α (TNF-α; lymphotoxin) that may cause hypercalcemia in plasma cell dyscrasias.
   - **Vitamin D metabolites:** produced by some lymphomas and promote intestinal calcium absorption.

54. **What is tumor lysis syndrome?**
Electrolyte and metabolic disturbances such as hyperuricemia, hyperkalemia, hyperphosphatemia, and hypocalcemia that can result in renal failure, arrhythmias, and seizures. These disturbances occur when rapidly growing tumors are effectively treated with chemotherapy and breakdown products of dying tumor cells are released in large amounts into the bloodstream. The complication is seen within hours to days after treatment of malignancies such as acute leukemia and high-grade lymphomas such as Burkitt's lymphoma. Although rarely seen with solid tumors, tumor lysis syndrome has been described in stage IV neuroblastoma and hepatoblastoma.

55. **How is tumor lysis syndrome treated?**
With allopurinol and supportive measures for renal failure such as vigorous hydration, dialysis if necessary, and appropriate treatment of electrolyte disorders. Rasburicase (recombinant urate oxidase) can be administered when uric acid levels are not lowered by standard approaches. Prophylactic treatment with aggressive hydration and allopurinol can prevent this serious complication and should always be given before chemotherapy in malignancies with high proliferative index.

56. **Which medications are commonly used for cancer pain?**
Pain medications are to be administered in a stepped approach according to the intensity and pathophysiology of symptoms and individual requirements. For mild pain, the recommended baseline drugs are NSAIDs. Patients with moderate-to-severe pain generally require an opioid agent such as codeine or oxycodone; severe pain requires a stronger opioid such as morphine. See also Chapter 19, Palliative Care.

57. **What are the neuromuscular complications of cancer?**
See Table 15-3.

TABLE 15-3. NEUROMUSCULAR COMPLICATIONS OF CANCER*

Site	Paraneoplastic Syndrome	Autoantibodies (Associated Cancer)
Brain and cranial nerves	Paraneoplastic cerebellar degeneration	Anti-Yo (gyn, breast cancer)
		Anti-Hu, CV 2 (SCLC)
		Anti-Tr (HD)
		Anti-Ma (others)
	Opsoclonus-myoclonus	Anti-Hu (neuroblastoma)
		Anti-Ri (breast cancer)
	Carcinoma-associated retinopathy	Anti-recoverin, CV2 (SCLC)
		Anti-rod-bipolar cell (melanoma)
	Limbic encephalitis	Anti-Hu, CV2, amphiphysin (SCLC)
		Anti-Ma2 (testicular)
		Anti-VGKC (thymoma, SCLC)
	Encephalomyelitis	Anti-Hu, CV2, amphiphysin (SCLC)
Spinal cord	Myelitis	Anti-Hu (SCLC)
	Subacute motor neuronopathy	Anti-Hu (SCLC)
	Motor neuron disease/ALS	Anti-Hu (rarely)
	Stiff-man syndrome	Anti-amphiphysin (breast, SCLC)
Peripheral nerves and dorsal root ganglia	Subacute or chronic sensorimotor neuropathy	Anti-Hu, CV2 (SCLC)
	Acute polyradiculopathy (GBS)	
	Neuropathy associated with plasma cell dyscrasias	Anti-MAG
	Brachial neuritis	
	Mononeuritis multiplex	
	Sensory neuronopathy	
	Autonomic neuronopathy	

(continued)

TABLE 15-3. NEUROMUSCULAR COMPLICATIONS OF CANCER*—*(continued)*		
Site	Paraneoplastic Syndrome	Autoantibodies (Associated Cancer)
Neuromuscular junction	Lambert-Eaton myasthenic syndrome	Anti-VGCC, anti-Sox1 (SCLC)
	Myasthenia gravis	Acetylcholine receptor Ab
Muscle	Dermatomyositis/polymyositis	
	Acute necrotizing myopathy	
	Carcinoid myopathy	
	Neuromyopathy	
	Neuromyotonia	Ab to potassium channels

Ab = antibody; ALS = amyotrophic lateral sclerosis; GBS = Guillain-Barré syndrome; gyn = gynecologic; HD = Hodgkin's disease; MAG = myelin-associated glycoprotein, SCLC = small cell lung cancer; VGCC = voltage-gated calcium channel.
*These syndromes frequently occur together as part of paraneoplastic encephalomyelitis/sensory neuronopathy with anti-Hu antibody.
Data from Schiff D, Batchelor T, Wyn PY, et al: Neurologic emergencies in cancer patients. Neurol Clin 16:449–481, 1998; and Didelot A, Honnorat J: Update on paraneoplastic neurological syndromes. Curr Opin Oncol 21:566–572, 2009.

GASTROINTESTINAL AND LIVER CANCERS

58. **Who gets squamous cell carcinoma of the esophagus?**
Usually men aged 40–60 years. The incidence is increased and nearly equal in men and women, in China, Africa, Russia, Japan, Scotland, and the Caspian region of Iran. In the United States, African American men living in urban areas are at increased risk.

59. **List the risk factors for squamous cell carcinoma of the esophagus.**
   - Excessive alcohol and/or tobacco use.
   - Native Bantu beer (southern Africa).
   - Betel nut chewing (Asia).
   - Chronic hot beverage ingestion.
   - Caustic strictures (due to accidental or intentional ingestion): >30% of cases develop esophageal cancer.
   - Tylosis (inherited disease with hyperkeratosis of palms and soles): >40% of cases develop esophageal cancer.
   - Achalasia.
   - Plummer-Vinson syndrome (presence of esophageal webs due to chronic iron-deficiency anemia).
   - Nontropical sprue.
   - Prior oral and pharyngeal cancer.
   - Occupational exposure to asbestos, combustion products, and ionizing radiation.
   - Decreased dietary intake of fruits and vegetables throughout adulthood.

60. **Discuss the incidence of adenocarcinoma of the esophagus.**
The incidence of esophageal adenocarcinoma has greatly increased since the 1970s. Adenocarcinoma of the esophagus is now more prevalent than squamous cell carcinoma in the United States and Western Europe, with most tumors located in the distal esophagus and esophagogastric junction.

61. **What are the risk factors for adenocarcinoma of the esophagus?**
   - Obesity
   - Chronic esophagitis
   - Gastroesophageal reflux disease (GERD)
   - Barrett's esophagus

62. **How does esophageal cancer present?**

Dysphagia: first with solids, then with liquids	Aspiration pneumonia	Chest pain on swallowing
	Hoarseness	
	Weight loss	Regurgitation
Occult GI bleeding	Cough	Fever
Choking		GERD

63. **How should esophageal cancer be treated?**
   By surgical resection. Fewer than half of patients appear to be operable at the time of presentation, and of these, only one half to two thirds have tumors that are completely resectable. Nonsurgical patients are treated with combined chemoradiotherapy or palliative measures if their performance status is too poor for active therapy.
   Some evidence indicates that survival in patients with adenocarcinoma of the esophagus is improved with preoperative combined chemotherapy and radiotherapy. Ongoing trials are investigating whether the outcome with chemoradiotherapy is equivalent to that of surgery.

64. **List the risk factors for gastric cancer.**

PRECURSOR CONDITIONS	GENETIC AND ENVIRONMENTAL FACTORS
Chronic atrophic gastritis and intestinal metaplasia	Family history of gastric cancer
Pernicious anemia	Blood type A
Partial gastrectomy for benign disease	Hereditary nonpolyposis colon cancer (HNPCC) syndrome
H. pylori infection	Low socioeconomic status
Ménétrier's disease	Low consumption of fruits and vegetables
Gastric adenomatous polyps	Consumption of salted, smoked, or poorly preserved foods
Barrett's esophagus	Cigarette smoking

65. **Discuss the role of gene mutations in gastric cancer.**
   Allelic deletions of the *APC*, *E-cadherin* (*CDH1*, *p53*), and microsatellite instability genes have been reported in a significant proportion of gastric cancers, and the exact role of oncogenes and tumor suppressor genes is currently being elucidated. Differences between mutations associated with the intestinal and diffuse types of gastric cancers may account for their different natural histories.

66. **List the symptoms of gastric cancer at the time of diagnosis.**

Weight loss: 61.6%	**Anorexia:** 32.0%	**Ulcer-type pain:** 17.1%
Abdominal pain: 51.6%	**Dysphagia:** 26.1%	**Lower extremity edema:** 5.9%
Nausea: 34.3%	**Melena:** 20.2%	
	Early satiety: 17.5%	

Fuchs CS, Mayer RJ: Gastric carcinoma, *N Engl J Med* 333:32–41, 1995.

67. **List the risk factors for pancreatic cancer.**
    - Smoking (2–3 times increased risk)
    - Diet high in calories, fat, and protein, low in fruits and vegetables
    - Diabetes mellitus
    - Chronic pancreatitis
    - Surgery for peptic ulcer disease
    - Occupational exposure to 2-naphthylamine and petroleum products (>10 yr increases risk to 5:1), dichlorodiphenyltrichloroethane (DDT)

68. **What hereditary syndromes increase the risk for pancreatic cancer?**
    - Familial pancreatic cancer
    - Hereditary pancreatitis
    - Familial adenomatous polyposis (FAP) syndrome
    - Familial atypical multiple mole melanoma syndrome (hereditary dysplastic nevus syndrome)
    - *BRCA2* gene
    - Peutz-Jeghers syndrome

69. **Do gender and ethnicity affect the risk for pancreatic cancer?**
    Yes. Males are affected more than females, and African Americans more than whites.

70. **List the symptoms and signs of pancreatic cancer based on tumor location.**
    See Table 15-4.

TABLE 15-4. SIGNS AND SYMPTOMS OF CANCER OF THE PANCREATIC HEAD AND BODY OR TAIL

Signs and Symptoms	Frequency of Occurrence by Pancreatic Site (%)	
	Head	Body/Tail
Weight loss	92	100
Jaundice	82	7
Pain	72	87
Anorexia	64	33
Nausea	45	43
Vomiting	37	37
Weakness	35	43
Palpable liver	83	–
Palpable gallbladder	29	–
Tenderness	26	27
Ascites	19	20

Adapted from Moossa AR, et al: Tumors of the pancreas. In Moossa AR, et al (eds): Comprehensive Textbook of Oncology, 2nd ed. Baltimore, Williams & Wilkins, 1991, p 964.

71. **Describe the diagnostic and staging evaluation for patients suspected of having pancreatic cancer.**

Endoscopic ultrasound (EUS) and helical CT are useful diagnostic modalities for suspected carcinoma of the pancreas that allow accurate depiction of local tumor extent, involvement of adjacent vascular structures, and distant metastases. Gadolinium-enhanced MRI is available, but is not commonly used to assess pancreatic cancer. Endoscopic retrograde cholangiopancreatography (ERCP) has a higher complication rate and should be reserved for patients in need of endoscopic stenting, nondiagnostic findings on standard evaluation, or those in whom tissue diagnosis is needed and cannot be obtained by EUS.

A high level of CA 19-9 is specific for pancreatic cancer only if the bilirubin is not elevated, because biliary tract obstruction can cause extremely high levels of CA 19-9 (Table 15-5).

TABLE 15-5. DIAGNOSTIC EVALUATION FOR PANCREATIC CANCER	
Test	Diagnostic Yield in Various Series (%)
CA 19-9 level > 200 U/mL	97
CT scan of abdomen	74–94
ERCP	91–94
EUS	94
Angiography	88–90
Ultrasound of abdomen	69–90
MRI of abdomen	Not applicable

CT = computed tomography; ERCP = endoscopic retrograde cholangiopancreatography; EUS = endoscopic ultrasound; MRI = magnetic resonance imaging.

72. **How is the diagnosis of pancreatic cancer confirmed and the extent of metastatic disease evaluated?**

By CT or EUS-guided fine-needle aspirate. Additional staging includes routine laboratory studies, chest x-ray, and other tests as directed by the history and physical. If there is bone pain or elevated alkaline phosphatase, bone scan should be done.

73. **What is the most important risk factor for hepatocellular carcinoma (HCC)?**

Cirrhosis. Macronodular cirrhosis is found in 85% of patients with HCC. In the United States, alcohol use is an important cause of cirrhosis. Chronic infection with hepatitis B or C viruses leading to cirrhosis is the major etiologic agent for HCC worldwide. Nonalcoholic steatohepatitis can also lead to cirrhosis and possible increased risk of HCC. See also Chapter 7, Gastroenterology.

74. **List the common presenting features of primary tumors of the liver.**
- **Asthenia**: 85–90%
- **Hepatomegaly**: 50–100%
- **Abdominal pain**: 50–70%
- **Jaundice**: 45–80%
- **Fever**: 10%

75. **List the unusual ways in which hepatomas may present.**
- Hemoptysis secondary to pulmonary metastases
- Rib mass secondary to bony metastasis

- Encephalitis-like picture secondary to brain metastasis or liver failure
- Heart failure secondary to cardiac metastasis and thrombosis of the inferior vena cava
- Priapism secondary to soft tissue metastasis
- Bone pain and pathologic fractures secondary to bony metastases

76. **What are the systemic manifestations of hepatocellular carcinoma?**
    - **Endocrine:** erythrocytosis and hypercalcemia
    - **Nonendocrine:** hypoglycemia, porphyria cutanea tarda, cryofibrinogenemia, osteoporosis, hyperlipidemia, dysfibrinogenemia, and alpha fetoprotein synthesis

    Margolis S, Horncy C: Systemic manifestations of hepatoma, *Medicine* 51:381–390, 1972.

77. **Which environmental factors are thought to be related to the development of colon cancer?**
    Increased risk:
    - Diet high in fat and red meat
    - Physical inactivity and central obesity
    Decreased risk:
    - Diet high in fresh fruits and vegetables
    - Regular use of NSAIDs, especially aspirin
      Nevertheless, as with all epidemiologic data, confounding factors not yet identified may be significant.

78. **What genetic syndromes are associated with colon cancer?**
    - FAP
    - Gardner's syndrome
    - Lynch syndrome (HNPCC)
      These all are autosomal dominant syndromes. The first two account for < 1% of all colorectal cancers, and the last for 6–15%.

79. **What is FAP?**
    A syndrome characterized by the occurrence of thousands of adenomatous polyps throughout the large bowel. If left untreated, cancer will develop in all patients with this syndrome, usually before the age of 40. If FAP syndrome is confirmed, total proctocolectomy should be done, because cancer surveillance is not possible among the thousands of polyps present. FAP is associated with mutations of the adenomatous polyposis coli (APC) tumor suppressor gene.

80. **What is Gardner's syndrome?**
    A syndrome related to mutations of the APC gene leading to colonic polyps and associated with other extraintestinal disorders such as osteomas, dental abnormalities, desmoid tumors, retinal pigment epithelial abnormalities, adrenal adenomas, and nasal angiofibromas.

81. **What is Lynch's syndrome?**
    The most common hereditary colon cancer syndrome that is also associated with extracolonic cancers such as endometrial, ovarian, pancreatic, gastric, renal, hepatic, and small bowel.

82. **What are the presenting signs and symptoms of colon cancer?**
    Ascending colon
    - Fatigue, lethargy, dyspnea (due to anemia related to chronic blood loss)
    - Positive fecal occult blood testing (FOBT)

Transverse colon
- Abdominal cramping and pain
- Bowel perforation

Rectosigmoid colon
- Tenesmus
- Decreased stool caliber
- Hematochezia

83. **What are the uses and limitations for CEA level testing?**
CEA is an antigen produced by many colorectal cancers and should not be used for cancer screening because it is nonspecific and not sensitive enough to pick up early cancers. CEA is often normal in patients with stage I disease, who are most amenable to curative surgery. CEA has also been found to be elevated in cancers of the stomach, pancreas, breast, ovary, and lung and with various nonmalignant conditions such as alcoholic liver disease, inflammatory bowel disease, heavy cigarette smoking, chronic bronchitis, and pancreatitis. If elevated before cancer surgery, CEA should return to normal within 1 month after surgery. A subsequent rise in CEA will be strongly indicative of recurrent cancer. CEA can also be used as a marker for response to chemotherapy.

84. **When should CEA testing be done?**
Preoperatively in patients undergoing resection for colon cancer. If elevated, it should be retested 30–45 days after complete resection of the cancer. National Comprehensive Cancer Network (NCCN) guidelines recommend obtaining a postoperative CEA every 3–6 months for 2 years, then every 6 months for a total of 5 years.

   NCCN Clinical Practice Guidelines in Oncology, Colon Cancer, version 2.2011, p COL-3. Available at: www.nccn.org.

85. **List the two roles of chemotherapy in the treatment of colon cancer.**
Treatment of metastatic disease and adjuvant treatment.

86. **Which agents are commonly used for treatment of metastatic disease?**
5-FU, leucovorin, capecitabine, irinotecan (CPT-11), and oxaliplatin, alone or in combination, plus targeted agents such as bevacizumab, cetuximab, and panitumumab. Use of these chemotherapy regimens has significantly prolonged survival in patients with metastatic colorectal cancer.

87. **How is chemotherapy used as an adjuvant treatment for colon cancer?**
As standard postoperative therapy for stage III patients. In stage II disease, adjuvant treatment is sometimes given to patients at high risk for recurrence, as judged by pathologic features of the resected specimens. In clinical studies, patients who were treated with adjuvant chemotherapy after curative-intent resections of stage III colon cancer were found to have reduced recurrence rate and death rate compared with untreated controls.

   Sargent D, Sobrero A, Grothey A, et al: Evidence for cure by adjuvant therapy in colon cancer: Observations based on individual patient data from 20,898 patients on 18 randomized trials, *J Clin Oncol* 27:872–877, 2009.

GENITOURINARY CANCERS

88. **What tests are available for the diagnosis and staging of prostate cancer? How do their results correlate with the stage?**
See Table 15-6.

TABLE 15-6. DIAGNOSTIC EVALUATION AND STAGING OF PROSTATE CANCER

Prostate Stage	Histology of Biopsy Specimen	Urinary Symptoms	Noninvasive Assessment of Metastatic Disease				Surgical LN Sampling
			SAP	PSA	Bone Scan	Pelvic CT Scan	
I	Incidental histologic finding in ≤5% of resected tissue, well differentiated	Compatible with BPH	N	Often ↑	—	—	Usually not performed
II	Incidental histologic finding in > 5% of resected tissue, or tumor not well differentiated, or palpable nodule confined to prostate	Compatible with BPH	N	Often ↑	—	—	+ in 8–25% (indicating stage IV disease)
III	Extends through prostate capsule	Present	N	Usually ↑	—	—	+ in 40–50% (indicating stage IV disease)
IV	Invades other organs or metastatic	Present	Often ↑	Usually ↑	±	±	+ in 95% of patients with elevated SAP

↑ = elevated; − = negative; + = positive; BPH = benign prostatic hypertrophy; CT = computed tomography; LN = lymph node; PSA = prostate-specific antigen; SAP = serum alkaline phosphatase.

89. What is the long-term survival of patients with prostate cancer?
100% disease-specific survival at 5 years for patients with a localized or regionally advanced stage of prostate cancer. Thirty-one percent of patients with distant metastases at the time of diagnosis will be alive after 5 years.

Surveillance, End Results and Survival Program, SEER Cancer Statistics Review 1975–2006: Available at: http://seer.cancer.gov/csr/1975_2006/browse_csr.php?section=23&page=sect_23_table.07.html. Accessed August 31, 2009.

90. Summarize the effects and mechanisms of the various androgen-deprivation therapies for prostate cancer.
See Figure 15-1.

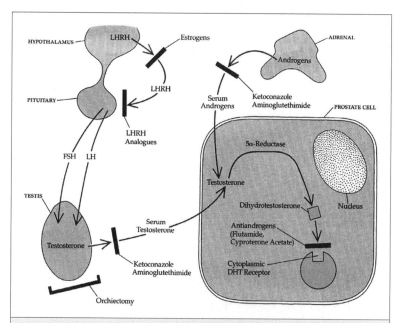

Figure 15-1. Androgen deprivation, which prevents the trophic influence of testosterone on the prostate in advanced prostate carcinoma, can be affected in a variety of ways. Estrogens such as diethylstilbestrol inhibit the release of luteinizing hormone–releasing hormone (LHRH) from the hypothalamus, thus diminishing the release of follicle-stimulating hormone (FSH) and luteinizing hormone (LH) from the anterior pituitary and reducing the signal that stimulates testosterone production by the testes. LHRH analogues such as leuprolide initially stimulate but ultimately inhibit the release of FSH and LH from the anterior pituitary and thus have an estrogen-like effect. The testes, which produce most of the testosterone, can be removed by orchiectomy. Ketoconazole and aminoglutethimide inhibit a variety of steroid synthetic pathways, including those that produce androgens in the testes and adrenal glands. In the prostate cells, testosterone is converted into dihydrotestosterone (DHT) by the enzyme 5α-reductase. Antiandrogens such as bicalutamide, cyproterone acetate, and certain progestational agents block the binding of DHT to its cytoplasmic receptor. (From Rubenstein E, Federman DD [eds]: Scientific American Medicine. New York, Scientific American, 1993, p 12[IXA]:8, with permission.)

91. What does Gleason's score predict about a prostate cancer?
How aggressive a prostate cancer is likely to be, based on its appearance on light microscopy. The pathologist assigns a number from 1 to 5 to the two most common

patterns of differentiation in the specimen. A score of 1 represents the most well differentiated and 5 the most poorly differentiated pattern. The sum of the two numbers is Gleason's score. Values of 2–4 represent the least aggressive cancers and 8–10 the most aggressive. Cancers with Gleason's scores of 5–7 are intermediate in their behavior.

92. **What is appropriate therapy for stage I prostate cancer?**
    - Watchful waiting for patients who would not benefit from definitive treatment but receive symptom relief through palliative care.
    - Active surveillance including close monitoring of serum PSA, digital rectal examination, and prostate biopsy with subsequent treatment if indicated.
    (Note that some physicians use the terms "watchful waiting" and "active surveillance" interchangeably.)
    - Radical prostatectomy
    - External-beam radiation therapy
    - Brachytherapy
    - Transurethral prostatectomy (TURP) if needed for symptoms of benign prostatic hypertrophy (BPH)

93. **List the appropriate therapy options for stage II prostate cancer.**
    - Radical prostatectomy
    - External-beam radiation therapy
    - Brachytherapy
    - Watchful waiting for selected patients
    - Active surveillance for selected patients

94. **List the appropriate therapy options for stage III prostate cancer.**
    - Radiation therapy ± hormonal therapy
    - Radical prostatectomy with pelvic lymphadenectomy ± hormonal therapy
    - Watchful waiting for selected patients.

95. **What is appropriate therapy for stage IV prostate cancer?**
    - TURP or radiation therapy for urinary obstruction
    - Endocrine manipulation or close observation for asymptomatic patients
    - Hormonal therapy for symptomatic disease
    - Palliative radiation therapy for localized symptoms
    - Chemotherapy for disease refractory to hormonal therapy

96. **List the environmental risk factors for the development of bladder cancer.**
    - Occupational hazards (workers in dye industry, hairdressers, painters, and leather workers)
    - Geographic factors causing chronic bladder irritation (endemic schistosomiasis)
    - Self-ingested toxins (tobacco, phenacetin, and possibly artificial sweeteners)
    - Alkylating agents (cyclophosphamide)
    - Previous cancers, especially those of the urothelial tract

97. **What is the classic triad of symptoms of renal cell cancer and the frequency of occurrence?**
    - **Gross hematuria:** 59%
    - **Abdominal mass:** 45%
    - **Pain:** 41%
    All three symptoms, however, are present in only 9% of patients with renal cell cancer.

98. List other symptoms of renal cell cancer and their frequency.
- **Weight loss:** 28%
- **Anemia:** 21%
- **Tumor calcification on x-ray:** 13%
- **Symptoms from metastases:** 10%
- **Fever:** 7%
- **Asymptomatic when diagnosed:** 7%
- **Hypercalcemia:** 3%
- **Acute varicocoele:** 2%

> Skinner DG, Colvin RB, Vermillion CD, et al: Diagnosis and management of renal cell carcinoma: A clinical and pathologic study of 309 cases, *Cancer* 28:1165–1177, 1971.

99. Why is renal cell cancer called "the internist's tumor"?
Because of the varied and unusual presentations that may obscure the true diagnosis. Many of these signs and symptoms are the result of paraneoplastic syndromes and include hypercalcemia, hypertension, hepatopathy without liver metastases, enteropathy, heart failure, cachexia, erythrocytosis, immune complex glomerulonephritis, amyloidosis, and a polymyalgia rheumatica (PMR) type syndrome.

100. What determines the prognosis for renal cell cancer?
The stage and grade of the tumor.

101. What are the molecular alterations associated with the different histologic types of renal cell carcinoma?
- **Clear cell:** von Hippel–Lindau gene (VHL)
- **Papillary type 1:** hereditary papillary renal carcinoma (HPRC): *Met* oncogene
- **Papillary type 2:** hereditary leiomyomatosis renal cell cancer (HLRCC): *FH* (fumarate hydratase gene)
- **Chromophobe RCC/oncocytoma:** Birt Hogg Dubé (BHD) syndrome: *BHD* (folliculin gene)

102. Give the 5-year survival rates for the four stages of renal cell cancer.
- **Stage I** (confined to the renal parenchyma, ≤ 7 cm in greatest dimension): 88–95%
- **Stage II** (confined to the renal parenchyma, >7 cm in greatest dimension): 67–88%
- **Stage III** (involves the renal vein, inferior vena cava, or regional lymph nodes): 40–59%
- **Stage IV** (invades beyond Gerota's fascia or distant metastases): 2–20%

103. Give the 5-year survival rates for the various grades of renal cell cancer.
- **Grade I** (highly differentiated tumors, sharply demarcated from surrounding tissue): 100%
- **Grade IIA** (moderately differentiated tumors, locally well circumscribed but not necessarily provided with capsule): 59%
- **Grade IIB** (moderately differentiated tumors, poorly circumscribed but not diffusely infiltrating or markedly polymorphous and mitotic): 36%
- **Grade III** (poorly differentiated, markedly polymorphous tumors that are diffusely infiltrating; tumors with abundant growth in capillary vessels): 0%

> American Joint Committee on Cancer: *Cancer Staging Manual*, ed 5, Philadelphia, 1997, Lippincott.

104. What treatments are available for advanced stage renal cell cancer? How effective are they?
Once renal cell carcinoma is widespread, there are few curative therapies, but there are several agents that can delay progression or induce partial remissions. Biologic response modifiers such as interferon and IL-2 induce long-term remissions in a minority of patients. Targeted agents such as sunitinib, sorafenib, temsirolimus, everolimus, and bevacizumab can significantly prolong progression-free survival in many patients.

105. **How often does testicular cancer occur in the United States?**
Approximately 1% of all cancers in U.S. males. The majority of these are men 29–35 years of age, with 8400 new cases annually. The incidence of testicular cancer is higher in patients with cryptorchidism, Klinefelter's syndrome, and testicular feminization syndrome.

   Jemal A, Siegal R, Xu J, Ward R: Cancer Statistics, 2010. *CA Cancer J Clin* 60:277–300, 2010.

106. **What causes testicular cancer?**
The cause is unknown, but age, genetic influences, repeated infection, radiation, and possible endocrine abnormalities have been suggested. Almost all tumors show an increased copy number of the short arm of chromosome 12 (12p), either as an isochromosome (an abnormal chromosome with two identical arms) or as tandem duplications. When 12p is present in multiple copies, the prognosis is poor.

107. **What are the presenting features of testicular cancer?**
Frequently as a painless scrotal mass, although pain is noted in ~25% of reported cases. When the tumor has already spread (5–15%), symptoms of metastases to the lungs and liver are demonstrated.

108. **Which pathologic types are most commonly seen among testicular cancers?**
Tumors of one histologic type
- Seminoma (germinoma)
  - Typical (35%)
  - Anaplastic (4%)
  - Spermatocytic (1%)
- Embryonal carcinoma (20%)
- Teratoma (10%)
- Choriocarcinoma (1%)
Tumors of mixed histologic type
- Embryonal carcinoma and teratoma (teratocarcinoma) (24%)
- Other combinations (5%)

109. **What are the stages of testicular cancer?**
- **Stage I:** no lymph node involvement or distant metastases, normal tumor markers
- **Stage II:** regional lymph node metastasis, with or without elevated tumor markers
- **Stage III:** distant metastasis to nonregional lymph nodes, lungs, or other sites, with or without elevated tumor markers.

110. **What tumor markers are associated with testicular cancer?**
- Serum lactic dehydrogenase (LDH)
- AFP
- β-hCG

111. **What determines survival rate in testicular cancer?**
The response to therapy. Survival is not determined on the basis of stage. In patients who respond to therapy, the survival curves plateau at ~90%.

112. **How should stage I testicular cancer be treated?**
With transinguinal orchiectomy.

113. **How is pure seminoma treated?**
Limited-stage cases are treated with radiation to the retroperitoneal nodes or close observation followed by radiation if there is relapse. Disseminated disease is treated with combination chemotherapy.

114. **How are nonseminomatous tumors treated?**
With retroperitoneal lymphadenectomy. If nodes are positive, patients may be treated with two to four cycles of adjuvant chemotherapy.

115. **Describe the treatment for stage III disease.**
With bulky mediastinal or retroperitoneal masses, three to four courses of chemotherapy are given, followed by resection of any residual disease.

116. **How are patients followed for recurrent disease?**
With tumor markers. Many patients with germ cell tumors will have elevated levels of the tumor markers AFP or β-hCG or both. AFP is not elevated in pure seminoma. AFP and β-hCG should return to normal levels after treatment and can be monitored subsequently for evidence of recurrent disease. These markers are very sensitive for the presence of disease, although normal values do not rule out malignancy.

117. **Describe the extragonadal germ cell syndrome.**
The occurrence of germ cell tumors in the mediastinum, retroperitoneum, or pineal gland in relatively young males, with elevated β-hCG or AFP and marked elevation of LDH. Patients often respond to treatment with chemotherapy developed for testicular cancer. A careful search for an occult testicular primary tumor must be carried out, because the testis is a relative sanctuary from the effects of chemotherapy. Ultrasound evaluation is useful in this setting.

LUNG CANCER

118. **Describe the extent of lung cancer spread that can influence the presenting signs and symptoms.**
   - Central or endobronchial growth of the primary tumor
   - Peripheral growth of the primary tumor
   - Regional spread of the tumor in the thorax by contiguity or by metastasis to regional lymph nodes
   - Distant metastases or systemic effects

119. **List symptoms secondary to central or endobronchial growth of the primary tumor.**
   - Cough
   - Dyspnea from obstruction
   - Wheezing and stridor
   - Pneumonitis from obstruction with fever and productive cough
   - Hemoptysis

120. **Which symptoms may be secondary to peripheral growth of the primary tumor?**
   - Pain from pleural or chest wall involvement
   - Dyspnea from restriction
   - Lung abscess syndrome from tumor cavitation
   - Cough

121. **List symptoms related to regional spread of the tumor in the thorax by contiguity or by metastasis to regional lymph nodes.**

Tracheal obstruction

Recurrent laryngeal nerve paralysis with hoarseness

Sympathetic nerve paralysis with Horner's syndrome

Superior vena cava (SVC) syndrome from vascular obstruction

Lymphatic obstruction with pleural effusion

Esophageal compression with dysphagia

Phrenic nerve paralysis with elevation of the hemidiaphragm and dyspnea

C8 and T1 nerve compression with ulnar pain and Pancoast's syndrome

Pericardial and cardiac extension with resultant tamponade, arrhythmia, or cardiac failure

Lymphangitic spread through the lungs with hypoxemia and dyspnea

122. **Which symptoms may be due to distant metastases or systemic effects?**

Bone pain

Painful lympha-denopathy

Hypercalcemia

Hemiparesis

Weight loss

Fatigue, malaise

Cohen MH: Signs and symptoms of bronchogenic carcinoma. In Straus MJ, editor: *Lung Cancer: Clinical Diagnosis and Treatment*, ed 2, New York, 1983, Grune & Stratton, pp 97–111.

123. **What are the accepted and proposed risk factors for lung cancer?**
   - **Cigarette smoking:** Causes 85% of lung cancers in men. In women, lung cancer has surpassed breast cancer as the leading cause of cancer death. Passive smoking also increases the risk of lung cancer, causing 25% of the lung cancers in nonsmokers.
   - **Radon exposure:** Increases the risk of lung cancer, especially in smokers, who have a 10-fold higher risk. An estimated 25% of lung cancer in nonsmokers and 5% in smokers is attributed to radon daughter exposure in the home.
   - **Marijuana smoking:** Increases the risk of lung cancer in smokers.
   - **Other agents:** Bis-chloromethyl ether, arsenic, nickel, ionizing radiation, asbestos, and chromates.
   - **Radiation therapy**
   - **Pulmonary fibrosis**
   - **Human immunodeficiency virus (HIV) infection and/or acquired immunodeficiency syndrome (AIDS):** Increases the risk of multiple cancers, including lung cancer.

   Patel P, Hanson DL, Sullivan PS, et al: Incidence of types of cancer among HIV-infected persons compared with the general population in the United States, 1992–2003, *Ann Intern Med* 148:728–736, 2008.

124. **Which chromosomal defects are associated with lung cancer?**
   Deletion of 3p (usually 3p14–23) occurring in virtually all cases (93%) of small cell lung cancer (SCLC), in 100% of bronchial carcinoids, and 25% of non–small cell lung cancer (NSCLC). Also seen are absent or reduced expression of the *rb* gene at 13q14, increased production of the c-*jun* oncogene product, and constitutive expression of c-*raf*-1 gene on 3p25. More than 50% of all lung cancers contain a mutation of the *p53* tumor suppressor gene. A *ras* family oncogene is mutated in ~20% of NSCLC, but not in SCLC. A mutation of the epidermal growth factor receptor (EGFR) is frequently found in Asian female nonsmokers with bronchoalveolar lung cancer.

125. **Which tests are used for the evaluation of suspected lung cancer?**
Chest x-ray and sputum cytology. If the expectorated sputum cytology is negative, bronchoscopy with biopsy, percutaneous biopsy, or thoracoscopy may be done. Preoperative evaluation includes CT scanning of the chest and upper abdomen to evaluate for mediastinal and hilar nodes and for liver and/or adrenal metastases. Pulmonary function tests, mediastinoscopy, and positron-emission tomography (PET) scan should be performed if surgical resection of NSCLC is considered. (SCLC is treated with radiation and chemotherapy, not surgery.) In SCLC and advanced-stage NSCLC, screening for the presence of brain metastases is recommended, using CT or MRI with contrast. Elevated alkaline phosphatase with normal liver CT suggests bony metastasis, which can be demonstrated by bone scan or PET scan.

126. **Which paraneoplastic syndromes are associated with lung cancer?**
See Table 15-7.

TABLE 15-7. PARANEOPLASTIC SYNDROMES IN LUNG CANCER

1. Systemic Symptoms	**5. Neurologic-Myopathic Symptoms**
Anorexia-cachexia (31%)	Lambert-Eaton syndrome (SCLC)
Fever (21%)	Peripheral neuropathy
Suppressed immunity	Subacute cerebellar
2. Endocrine Symptoms (12%)	degeneration
Ectopic PTH: hypercalcemia (NSCLC)	Cortical degeneration
SIADH (SCLC)	Polymyositis
Ectopic secretion of ACTH: Cushing's	Retinal blindness
syndrome	**6. Cutaneous Symptoms**
3. Skeletal Symptoms	Dermatomyositis
Clubbing (29%)	Acanthosis nigricans
Hypertrophic pulmonary	**7. Hematologic Symptoms (8%)**
osteoarthropathy: periostitis (1–10%)	Anemia
(adenocarcinoma)	Granulocytosis
4. Coagulation-Thrombosis	Leukoerythroblastosis
Migratory thrombophlebitis, Trousseau's	**8. Renal Symptoms (1%)**
syndrome: venous thrombosis,	Nephrotic syndrome
nonbacterial thrombotic	Glomerulonephritis
endocarditis: arterial emboli; DIC:	
hemorrhage	

ACTH = adrenocorticotropic hormone; DIC = disseminated intravascular coagulation; NSCLC = non–small cell lung cancer; PTH = parathyroid hormone; SCLC = small cell lung cancer; SIADH = syndrome of inappropriate antidiuretic hormone.,
Data from Cohen MH: Signs and symptoms of bronchogenic carcinoma. In Straus MJ (ed): Lung Cancer: Clinical Diagnosis and Treatment. New York, Grune & Stratton, 1977, pp 85–94.

KEY POINTS: LUNG CANCER ✓

1. The most common cause of cancer death in the United States for both men and women is lung cancer.

2. Eighty-five percent of lung cancer is caused by smoking; these deaths are entirely preventable.

3. Lung cancer is rarely curable unless it is diagnosed in a very early stage.

4. Patients should be counseled at every physician's visit to quit all forms of tobacco use.

127. **Which treatment modalities are used to manage SCLC?**
Chemotherapy (using combinations of drugs such as etoposide, cisplatin, carboplatin, or CPT-11) and radiotherapy are used concurrently or sequentially. These therapies in limited-stage disease have resulted in complete remission rates of 40–60%, median survival of 16–24 months, and 5-year survivals of 5–10%. Prophylactic radiotherapy to the brain is recommended for patients with limited-stage disease who achieve a complete response to therapy. Because of early hematogenous spread, surgery is not generally an option for patients with SCLC.

128. **How effective is the treatment of advanced stage (IV) SCLC?**
Generally fairly good for short-term survival. Patients with advanced-stage SCLC often have good partial responses to chemotherapy, but the responses are not durable. Median survival for patients with extensive disease who respond to treatment is 6–12 months. However, this is a significant improvement compared with the survival of untreated patients, which is measured in weeks.

129. **What is the SVC syndrome? What is its significance in lung cancer?**
Symptoms resulting from blood flow obstruction in the SVC due to thrombosis within the vessel or external compression of the vein by tumor (Fig. 15-2). The obstruction generally occurs when there is a lesion in the right upper lobe. Lung cancer, especially SCLC, accounts for up to 80% of cases. Lymphoma and other mediastinal malignancies account for the remaining 20% of SVC syndrome caused by neoplastic disease. Other causes of SVC syndrome include catheter thrombosis and sclerosis of the mediastinum.

130. **What are the presenting signs and symptoms of SVC syndrome?**
   - Dyspnea
   - Face and arm edema
   - Sense of fullness in the head
   - Cough
   - Prominent veins over the neck and chest
   - Failure of hand veins to collapse when the arms are lifted above the head

131. **Why are the symptoms of SVC syndrome not more significant?**
Because collateral circulation develops around the obstruction. Although obstruction of the vena cava has been considered a life-threatening oncologic emergency, only rarely does it progress to cause laryngeal edema, seizures, coma, and death.

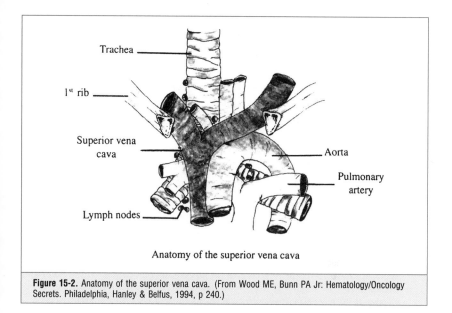

Anatomy of the superior vena cava

Figure 15-2. Anatomy of the superior vena cava. (From Wood ME, Bunn PA Jr: Hematology/Oncology Secrets. Philadelphia, Hanley & Belfus, 1994, p 240.)

132. **How is SVC syndrome treated?**
With radiotherapy or stent placement. Patients with SVC syndrome should not be given intravenous medications in the upper extremities owing to obstruction of the venous circulation.

133. **How is NSCLC treated?**
With surgery as a potential cure if the patient is a candidate for resection. Resection should be performed if the patient is medically fit and there is no evidence of the following:
- Distant metastases
- Malignant pleural effusion
- SVC obstruction
- Involvement of supraclavicular, cervical, or contralateral mediastinal nodes
- Recurrent laryngeal nerve paralysis
- Involvement of the mediastinum, tracheal wall, or mainstem bronchus < 2 cm from the carina
- Small cell carcinoma histology

134. **How is stage IIIA (large tumor or mediastinal node involvement) NSCLC treated?**
Neoadjuvant chemotherapy (given before surgery) may improve survival. If patients are unable to undergo surgery or the tumor is locally advanced but inoperable, combined chemotherapy and radiotherapy are indicated. In higher-stage disease, systemic chemotherapy or palliative care are options, depending on the performance status of the patient.

HEAD AND NECK CANCER

135. **What are the presenting symptoms of head and neck cancer?**
See Table 15-8.

TABLE 15-8. PRESENTING SYMPTOMS OF HEAD AND NECK CANCER	
Site	Symptoms
Oral cavity: lips, buccal mucosa, alveolar ridge, retromolar trigone, floor of mouth, hard palate, anterior two thirds of tongue	Mass, ulcer, leukoplakia, erythroplasia, bleeding, pain, loose teeth, earache, trismus, halitosis
Larynx: supraglottic (false cords, arytenoid), glottic (true vocal cords), subglottic	Hoarseness, bleeding, sore throat, thyroid cartilage pain
Pharynx: nasopharynx, oropharynx, soft palate, uvula, tonsil, base of tongue, hypopharynx, pyriform sinus	Sore throat, earache, epistaxis, nasal voice, dysphagia, masses, hearing loss, blood-streaked saliva
Maxillary sinus	Sinusitis, epistaxis, headache
All sites	Bleeding (oral or nasal), neck nodes, pain at site of tumor or referred pain

136. **What are the two major risk factors for squamous cell cancer of the head and neck area?**
   Tobacco is the most significant contributing factor to the development of head and neck cancers. Nine of 10 patients with cancer in this area are smokers. Snuff dipping and tobacco chewing are important causes of oral cancer. Smokers have an increased mortality related to head and neck cancer once it has been diagnosed, showing a twofold increase in mortality over nonsmokers.
   Alcohol is also strongly correlated with the development of head and neck cancer. About half of patients with head and neck cancer have cirrhosis, and three quarters drink alcohol excessively.

137. **What other risk factors have been identified?**
   - **Viral exposure:** HPV, EBV, and herpes simplex (HSV) type I
   - **Occupation:** woodworkers and nickel compound exposure
   - **Syphilis:** glossitis
   - **Other:** poor dental hygiene

138. **Describe the evaluation and initial staging of patients with head and neck cancer.**
   Triple endoscopy of upper and lower airway and upper aerodigestive tract, with biopsy of any suspicious lesions. Measurement and biopsy, if indicated, of any cervical or supraclavicular nodes should be performed. A **CT scan** of the head/neck and chest and/or a **PET scan** help to determine the extent of disease.

139. **What are the most common sites of metastases of head and neck cancer?**
   Local lymph nodes in the neck, followed by lung metastases. Bone metastases occur in up to 15% of patients. Brain metastases are rare and are seen mainly in patients with nasopharyngeal cancer. Depending on tobacco and alcohol history, a second cancer of the head and neck, esophagus, or lung may occur in up to 20% of patients at some time in the course of their disease, especially if they continue to smoke and drink.

140. **What is the most appropriate treatment of head and neck cancer?**
   Primarily surgery for early-stage cancer, sometimes involving radical neck node dissection and/or postoperative radiotherapy. Radiation therapy is used for locations not amenable

to surgery or if surgery would be too disfiguring. In more advanced stages, head and neck cancers are treated with **multimodality therapy,** using chemotherapy or targeted agents in combination with radiotherapy. For cancer of the larynx, vocal cord preservation with chemotherapy and radiotherapy is preferred whenever possible. Cessation of smoking and alcohol consumption is essential to decrease the occurrence of second primary cancers in the head and neck region.

141. **Which chemotherapeutic agents are used in the treatment of squamous cell cancers of the head and neck? How effective are they?**
    5-FU infusions with cisplatin or carboplatin, taxanes, and methotrexate, singly and in combination. Tumors may also respond to treatment with cetuximab, a monoclonal antibody against EGFR. Response rates for these agents vary depending on the agent, schedule, tumor type/location, previous treatment, and patient performance status. Combination chemotherapy regimens usually show higher initial response rates but have yet to show an increase in survival rates.

BREAST CANCER

See also Chapter 2, General Medicine and Ambulatory Care, for screening guidelines.

142. **How do you identify women at high risk for breast cancer?**
    Initially by family history of breast or ovarian cancer. These patients have a high incidence of mutations in the *BRCA1* and *BRCA2* genes on chromosome 17 and 13, respectively. In families with these mutations, generally over half of the female relatives have breast or ovarian cancer that is usually multifocal and has early age of onset. Patients with these gene mutations have a cumulative lifetime risk of developing breast cancer ranging up to 87%.

143. **What factors other that *BRCA* mutations significantly increase a woman's risk of breast cancer?**
    - Age > 40 years
    - Previous cancer in one breast
    - Breast cancer in a first- or second-degree family member
    - History of multiple breast biopsies
    - Parity: nulliparous, or first pregnancy after age 31 years
    - Lobular carcinoma in situ
    - Gene mutations: *BRCA1*, *BRCA2*, *p53*, Peutz-Jeghers syndrome, others
    - Radiation exposure to chest wall during childhood or adolescence

144. **What factors also increase a woman's risk for breast cancer?**
    - Early menarche or late menopause
    - Hormone replacement therapy (HRT) with estrogen and progesterone
    - Long-term use of estrogen therapy
    - History of cancer of the ovary, uterus, or colon
    - Alcohol use
    - Obesity
    - Lack of physical activity
    - Diethystilbesterol (DES) exposure in utero

    A computer model breast cancer risk assessment tool is available at: www.cancer.gov/bcrisktool/.

145. **What can women do to reduce their risk of breast cancer?**
    Prophylactic tamoxifen or raloxifene may reduce the occurrence of new breast cancers in women at high risk owing to a previous personal history of breast cancer, first-degree family

members with breast cancer, and other factors, but there is an increased risk of thromboembolism and uterine cancer. Prophylactic mastectomy may also be selected by women who are known to carry the *BRCA1* or *BRCA2* gene mutations, which may reduce the incidence of breast cancer by about 90%.

Visyanathan K, Chlebowski RT, Hurley P, et al: American Society of Clinical Oncology Clinical Practice Guideline update on the use of pharmacologic interventions including tamoxifen, raloxifene, and aromatase inhibition for breast cancer risk reduction, *J Clin Oncol* 24:3235–3258, 2009.

146. **What are the poor prognostic factors in primary breast cancer?**

Estrogen or progesterone receptors negative	Distant metastasis	Positive axillary nodes
	Premenopausal patient	High S-phase fraction
	Aneuploidy and high cathepsin D	Local skin involvement
Fixed axillary nodes	Large tumor size	
Positive *HER-2/neu* status	Nuclear grade 3 (poor)	

147. **Summarize the surgical options for treatment of localized breast cancer.**
The two surgical options are modified radical mastectomy or breast conservation surgery (lumpectomy) followed by radiation therapy. In both types of surgery, axillary node staging with sentinel node biopsy or axillary node dissection is performed. Lumpectomy followed by radiotherapy is used if complete excision is possible and radiation therapy can be delivered to the tumor bed. Modified radical mastectomy is performed if tumor mass is large relative to breast size, the cancer is multifocal, or radiation therapy is not technically feasible.

148. **What are the overall treatment guidelines for localized breast cancer?**
If the tumor is large or has unfavorable prognostic characteristics on the preliminary biopsy, preoperative (neoadjuvant) chemotherapy may be administered, followed by surgery. After the operation, adjuvant therapy with chemotherapy, hormone therapy, and/or trastuzumab, or combination therapy may be given to help eradicate any possible micrometastases in the circulation. The types of agents chosen will depend on tumor characteristics that include estrogen and progesterone receptor status and *Her2/neu* status. Patient-specific factors such as menopausal category, age, and comorbidities are also important in the choice of adjuvant therapy. Local radiation therapy is administered to patients whose tumors are at high risk for local recurrence.

149. **When is radiation therapy given to the chest wall and regional lymph nodes after breast cancer surgery?**
For high-risk patients for recurrence identified by:
- Lumpectomy as procedure for initial treatment
- Four or more axillary nodes positive for cancer
- Extracapsular nodal extension
- Large (>5 cm) primary tumor
- Positive or very close tumor resection margin

150. **How is adjuvant therapy used in the management of breast cancer?**
See Table 15-9.

151. **How is stage IV breast cancer treated?**
With either systemic chemotherapy or hormone therapy, depending on hormone receptor status, location of metastases, and patient characteristics, reserving surgery and radiotherapy for local control. Trastuzumab, an antibody against the *Her2/neu* receptor, may be added for patients whose tumors are *Her2/neu*-positive.

TABLE 15-9. CURRENT RECOMMENDATIONS FOR THE USE OF ADJUVANT SYSTEMIC THERAPY IN BREAST CANCER

	Premenopausal	Postmenopausal
Node Negative*†‡		
ER and PR negative	Chemotherapy	Chemotherapy
ER or PR positive	Chemotherapy + TAM, ± ovarian ablation or LHRH agonist	Endocrine therapy§ ± chemotherapy
Node Positive‡‖		
ER and PR negative	Chemotherapy	Chemotherapy
ER or PR positive	Chemotherapy + TAM, ± ovarian ablation or LHRH agonist	Endocrine therapy§ ± chemotherapy

ER = estrogen receptor; LHRH = luteinizing hormone–releasing hormone; PR = progesterone receptor; TAM = tamoxifen.
*Adjuvant therapy is not recommended for tumors < 0.5 cm or well-differentiated tumors < 1 cm.
†Adjuvant therapy is recommended for all tumors > 1 cm and for tumors 0.5–1.0 cm with poor prognosis features: poorly differentiated, high nuclear grade, lymphovascular invasion, high S-phase fraction.
‡Patients with Her2/neu-positive tumors require ≤ 1 year of adjuvant trastuzumab in addition to chemotherapy and/or endocrine therapy.
§Endocrine therapy may consist of an aromatase inhibitor for 5 years or tamoxifen for 2–3 years followed by an aromatase inhibitor for a total of ≥ 5 years.
‖Adjuvant therapy is recommended for all patients.

152. Discuss the role of aromatase inhibitors in adjuvant therapy for breast cancer.
In postmenopausal women with hormone-positive breast cancers, aromatase inhibitors such as anastrozole may be more effective than tamoxifen, and the addition of letrozole after 5 years of adjuvant tamoxifen may offer additional benefit.

153. Which chemotherapy agents are used in the treatment of metastatic breast cancer?
Paclitaxel, docetaxel, doxorubicin, epirubicin, vinorelbine, cyclophosphamide, methotrexate, fluorouracil, and capecitabine. These agents are used singly or in combination in the treatment of advanced or metastatic breast cancer. If the tumor overexpresses the Her2/neu oncogene, trastuzumab or lapatinib may be added to improve the effectiveness of chemotherapy.

154. How effective are chemotherapy agents in the treatment of metastatic breast cancer?
Overall induction response rates range from 55–65%. Median survival times are 14–18 months. The survival rates depend more on the site of the metastatic disease than on the treatment, with visceral disease faring more poorly than bony or soft tissue metastases. Most patients receive more than one treatment regimen, because the median time to failure of most programs is about 6 months.

155. What other drugs may be used to treat metastatic breast cancer?
Hormonal agents such as tamoxifen, anastrozole, letrozole, exemestane, or luteinizing hormone–releasing hormone (LHRH) agonists (in premenopausal women) can be used for bony or soft tissue metastases in patients with estrogen or progesterone receptor–positive breast cancer and can be effective palliation lasting many months. Newer drugs that target growth factor pathways in breast cancer are currently in development.

GYNECOLOGIC CANCERS

See Chapter 2, General Medicine and Ambulatory Care, for screening guidelines.

156. **What should be done if invasive cancer is found on cervical biopsy?**
Metastatic work-up to determine the extent of disease. For early-stage disease, treatment options include radiation therapy or surgery with postoperative radiation therapy plus chemotherapy. For locally advanced disease, the treatment is radiation therapy combined with chemotherapy. Once the cancer is metastatic, it is treated with chemotherapy. Radiation therapy may be used to palliate local symptoms or distant metastases.

157. **Which studies are used in the staging of carcinoma of the cervix?**
- Pelvic examination.
- Biochemical profile.
- Chest x-ray.
- CT scan or MRI (MRI is preferred).
- Lymphangiograms may be useful in selected cases.
- Cystoscopy and proctosigmoidoscopy for advanced disease.

158. **What are the 5-year survival rates, relative to stage, for carcinoma of the cervix?**
See Table 15-10.

TABLE 15-10.	FIVE-YEAR SURVIVAL RATES FOR CERVICAL CANCER RELATIVE TO STAGE	
Stage	Description	5-Year Survival Rate (%)
I	Tumor strictly confined to the cervix.	89–100
II	Tumor extends beyond the uterus but not to the pelvic wall. The tumor involves the vagina but not the lower third.	67
III	Tumor extends to the pelvic wall, and/or involves the lower third of the vagina, and/or causes hydronephrosis or nonfunctioning kidney.	53
IV	Tumor extends beyond the true pelvis, or has involved the bladder or rectal mucosa, or has distant metastases.	5–24

159. **How is stage I carcinoma of the cervix treated?**
- **IA:** total or modified radical hysterectomy, conization, or intracavitary radiation.
- **IB:** external-beam pelvic irradiation combined with two or more intracavitary radiation applications; radical hysterectomy with bilateral pelvic lymphadenectomy ± postoperative total pelvic irradiation plus chemotherapy; or radiation therapy plus chemotherapy with cisplatin or cisplatin/5-FU for patients with bulky tumors.

160. **Summarize the treatment of stage II carcinoma of the cervix.**
- **IIA:** same as stage IB.
- **IIB:** radiation therapy plus chemotherapy: intracavitary radiation and external-beam pelvic irradiation combined with cisplatin or cisplatin/fluorouracil.

161. **How is stage III carcinoma of the cervix treated?**
The same as stage IIB.

162. **Summarize the treatment of stage IV carcinoma of the cervix.**
- **IVA:** same as stage IIB and stage III.
- **IVB:** chemotherapy with agents such as cisplatin, paclitaxel, ifosfamide-cisplatin, or irinotecan. Radiotherapy may be used for palliation.

   Cervical Cancer Treatment (PDQ), National Cancer Institute: Available at: www.cancer.gov/cancertopics/pdq/treatment/cervical/HealthProfessional/.

163. **Name the risk factors for carcinoma of the endometrium.**
1. Infertility
2. Obesity
3. Failure of ovulation
4. Dysfunctional bleeding
5. Prolonged estrogen use
6. Diabetes mellitus
7. Hypertension
8. Polycystic ovaries
9. Familial cancer syndrome (Lynch)
10. Tamoxifen use

164. **What are the 5-year survival rates for the various grades and stages of endometrial cancer?**
See Table 15-11.

TABLE 15-11. FIVE-YEAR SURVIVAL RATES FOR GRADES AND STAGES OF ENDOMETRIAL CANCER	
Description	5-Year Survival Rate (%)
Grade	
I Differentiated.	81
II Intermediate.	74
III Undifferentiated.	50
Stage	
I Tumor confined to the corpus.	92
II Tumor involves the corpus and cervix.	78
III Tumor extends outside the corpus, but not outside the true pelvis (may involve the vaginal wall or parametrium but not the bladder or rectum).	42
IV Tumor involves the bladder or rectum, extends outside the pelvis, or has distant metastases.	14

165. **List the risk factors for ovarian cancer.**
- Nulliparity or low parity
- Presence of basal cell nevus syndrome
- Family history of ovarian cancer or ovarian cancer syndromes, including *BRCA1* and *BRCA2* mutations
- Gonadal dysgenesis (46XY type)
- History of breast, endometrial, or colon cancer
- Asbestos exposure
- Presence of Peutz-Jeghers syndrome

166. **Discuss the appropriate use of the CA-125 antigen.**
CA-125 serum tumor marker, an antigenic determinant detected by radioimmunoassay, is elevated in 80% of epithelial ovarian cancers. Because it is high in only half of patients with stage I cancers and is increased in a significant proportion of healthy women and women with benign disease, it is not a sensitive or specific test and should not be used for screening in women with average risk for ovarian cancer. In high-risk patients or in patients suspected of having an ovarian cancer, it can be used in conjunction with bimanual rectovaginal pelvic examination and transvaginal ultrasonography. When the CA-125 value is elevated before treatment in a patient with an established diagnosis of ovarian cancer, it is useful as a marker of disease recurrence after surgical resection.

167. **List the neurologic paraneoplastic syndromes associated with ovarian cancer.**
- Peripheral neuropathy
- Organic brain syndrome
- Acute myelogenous leukemia–like syndrome
- Cerebellar ataxia (anti-Yo paraneoplastic cerebellar degeneration)
- Cancer-associated retinopathy
- Opsoclonus-myoclonus

168. **What other paraneoplastic syndromes may be associated with ovarian cancer?**
- Cross-matching of blood antigens
- Cushing's syndrome
- Hypercalcemia
- Thrombophlebitis
- Dermatomyositis
- Palmar fasciitis and polyarthritis

169. **What are the 5-year survival rates for the various stages of carcinoma of the ovary?**
- **I:** growth limited to the ovaries: 84%
- **II:** growth involving one or both ovaries with pelvic extension: 63%
- **III:** tumor involving ovaries with peritoneal implants outside the pelvis and/or positive retroperitoneal or inguinal nodes: 29%
- **IV:** distant metastases: 17%

170. **Describe the treatment for advanced-stage ovarian cancer.**
Patients with stage III epithelial ovarian cancers are first treated with surgery, consisting of total abdominal hysterectomy and bilateral salpingo-oophorectomy with omentectomy and debulking of as much gross tumor as possible. This is followed by intravenous chemotherapy with cisplatin or carboplatin combined with paclitaxel or cyclophosphamide. Patients with stage IV disease are given combination chemotherapy. The survival benefit of surgical debulking in patients with stage IV extra-abdominal disease is not yet known.

MISCELLANEOUS TOPICS

171. **Which cancers are associated with AIDS and are AIDS-defining conditions?**
- Kaposi's sarcoma (decreasing incidence)
- Non-Hodgkin's lymphoma including primary central nervous system lymphoma (most frequent)
- Cervical cancer

172. **What are other AIDS-related cancers?**
Hodgkin's disease and cancers of the lung, oral cavity, cervix, and anus.

173. **What phenotype is most highly associated with the development of melanoma?**
Fair skin, reddish hair, and freckles. Melanoma families have been described in which > 25% of the kindred are affected, with a vertical distribution of disease. There is an early age of onset, from the third to fourth decades. The incidence of multiple primary melanomas is increased, as is the presence of atypical nevi (B-K moles or familial atypical multiple melanoma with melanocyte dysplasia). However, there is a superior overall survival, possibly related to earlier detection. Ocular melanoma is also seen in this group of patients. The gene for the dysplastic nevus syndrome/familial melanoma is located on chromosome 1.

174. **Where does melanoma metastasize?**
To anywhere in the body, including lungs, liver, bowels, and bones. Melanoma is one of the few cancers that can cross the placenta and spread to a developing fetus. Bowel metastases can cause obstruction and bleeding, and lesions appear on barium dye studies as ulcerated with a central crater and a surrounding heaped-up border, causing the barium to pool in a "target" configuration.

WEXSITES

1. National Cancer Database: www.facs.org/cancer/ncdb/index.html

2. National Guideline Clearinghouse: www.guideline.gov/

3. PDQ Cancer Information Summaries: www.cancer.gov/

4. SEER Cancer Statistics Review, 1975–2006: http://seer.cancer.gov/csr/1975_2006/index.html

BIBLIOGRAPHY

1. American Joint Committee on Cancer: *Cancer Staging Manual*, ed 7, New York, 2010, Springer-Verlag.
2. Casciato DA, Territo MC, editors: *Manual of Clinical Oncology*, ed 6, Boston, 2009, Little, Brown.
3. DeVita T Jr, Lawrence T, Rosenberg SA, editors: *Cancer Principles and Practice of Oncology*, ed 8, Philadelphia, 2008, Lippincott Williams & Wilkins.
4. Jemal A, Siegel R, Ward E, et al, Cancer Statistics, 2009. *CA Cancer J Clin* 59:225–249, 2009.
5. Kufe DW, Frei E, Holland JF, et al, editors: *Holland-Frei Cancer Medicine*, ed 8, Shelton, CT, 2010, People's Medical Publishing House.

CHAPTER 16

ENDOCRINOLOGY

Susan E. Spratt, M.D., and Whitney W. Woodmansee, M.D.

In diabetes the thirst is greater for the fluid dries the body.... For the thirst there is need of a powerful remedy, for in kind it is the greatest of all sufferings, and when a fluid is drunk, it stimulates the discharge of urine.

Aretaeus of Cappadocia
2nd-Century Greek Physician
From *Therapeutics of Chronic Diseases* II, Chapter II, pp 485–486

DIABETES MELLITUS AND GLYCEMIC DISORDERS

1. List the three main categories of diabetes mellitus (DM).
   - **Type 1** (previously called "insulin-dependent DM" or "juvenile-onset DM")
   - **Type 2** (previously called "non–insulin-dependent DM" or "adult-onset DM")
   - **Gestational diabetes mellitus** (GDM; diabetes diagnosed in pregnancy)

2. Describe type 1 DM.
   Type 1 DM accounts for approximately 5–10% of patients and is generally due to autoimmune destruction of the pancreatic beta cells, leading to absolute insulin deficiency. Although typically diagnosed in patients before age 30, it can present at any age due to variability in the rate of beta-cell destruction.

3. What autoimmune diseases are associated with type 1 DM?
   - Adrenal insufficiency
   - Hyperthyroidism
   - Hypothyroidism
   - Celiac sprue
   - Pernicious anemia

4. What autoimmune diseases should be considered when a patient with type 1 DM presents with iron deficiency?
   Celiac sprue and pernicious anemia.

5. What are the major characteristics of type 2 DM?
   Insulin resistance and relative insulin deficiency. Most patients are obese with predominantly abdominal accumulation of fat. Type 2 DM is usually diagnosed in adults, but increasing numbers of children and adolescents are now diagnosed with type 2 DM as childhood obesity rates increase. These patients are not prone to developing ketoacidosis except in association with the stress from another illness.

6. Compare and contrast the general features of type 1 and type 2 DM.
   See Table 16-1.

TABLE 16-1. CHARACTERISTICS OF DIABETES MELLITUS

Type 1 Diabetes Mellitus	Type 2 Diabetes Mellitus
Usually presents at a younger age	Typically presents age > 40 yr
Normal weight or thin	Obese
Usually no family history	Strong family history
Autoimmune markers may be positive (anti-GAD and anti-islet cell antibodies)	Not autoimmune in nature
Insulin-sensitive	Insulin-resistant
Requires insulin for treatment	Often managed with diet or oral agents
	Usually eventually requires insulin

GAD = glutamic acid decarboxylase.

7. **Which pregnant women should be screened for GDM?**
Those who are obese or have a prior history of GDM, polycystic ovarian syndrome (PCOS), glycosuria, or family history of type 2 DM should be screened for GDM at the first prenatal visit using standard diagnostic criteria. (See Question 12.) All other women can be screened for GDM between weeks 24 and 28 of gestation with a 75-g OGTT. (See Question 9.)

8. **What is GDM?**
Diabetes diagnosed during pregnancy that is not clearly overt diabetes. New criteria for GDM will likely lead to an increased prevalence. Glucose tolerance usually returns to normal after delivery, but women with GDM should be screened for diabetes 6–12 weeks postpartum and routinely approximately every 3 years.

Bellamy L, Casas JP, Hingorani AD, et al: Type 2 diabetes mellitus after gestational diabetes: A systematic review and meta-analysis, *Lancet* 373:1773–1779, 2009.

9. **What are the diagnostic criteria for GDM?**
During a 75-g OGTT, a glucose value exceeding one of the following values:
- Fasting ≥ 92 mg/dL
- 1 hour ≥ 180 mg/dL
- 2 hour ≥ 153 mg/dL

10. **What are the complications of GDM?**
- Preeclampasia
- Polyhydramnios
- Fetal macrosomia
- Birth trauma
- Cesarean section
- Perinatal mortality and morbidity

11. **Summarize other specific types of DM.**
Other specific types of DM include genetic defects in beta-cell function, also known as "maturity-onset diabetes of the young," genetic defects in insulin action (i.e., mutations in the insulin receptor), diseases of the exocrine pancreas (e.g., hemochromatosis, neoplasm, cystic fibrosis), endocrinopathies (e.g., Cushing's syndrome, acromegaly, somatostatinoma,

glucagonoma), drug-induced DM (e.g., pentamidine, glucocorticoids, interferon-α), infections, and other rare genetic disorders.

12. **What criteria are used to diagnose DM?**
    One of the following:
    - Symptoms of diabetes (polyuria, polydipsia, and unexplained weight loss) plus casual plasma glucose (PG) concentration $\geq$ 200 mg/dL (11.1 mmol/L). "Casual" is defined as any time of day without regard to last meal.
    - Fasting plasma glucose $\geq$ 126 mg/dL (7.0 mmol/L). "Fasting" is defined as no caloric intake for at least 8 hours.
    - Two-hour PG > 200 mg/dL with OGTT using a 75-g glucose challenge.
    - Hemoglobin A$_1$C (A$_1$C) $\geq$ 6.5%

13. **Is a single reading of any of these values sufficient to diagnose DM?**
    No. In the absence of unequivocal hyperglycemia with acute metabolic decompensation, these criteria should be confirmed by repeat testing on a different day.

14. **What is the OGTT?**
    A specialized test for the diagnosis of DM that should be performed as described by the World Health Organization (WHO), using a glucose load containing the equivalent of 75 g of anhydrous glucose dissolved in water. A positive test is defined as 2-hour PG $\geq$ 200 mg/dL (11.1 mmol/L). The OGTT is an accepted method for diagnosing DM; however, it is not used routinely because it is more cumbersome than PG or A$_1$C.

15. **What is the role of A$_1$C in the diagnosis of DM?**
    Estimating blood glucose control in patients with diagnosed DM and, more recently, for initial diagnosis of DM with confirmatory testing.

16. **What is prediabetes?**
    A condition in which the glucose values are too high to be considered normal but do not fit the criteria for the diagnosis of DM. It includes the syndromes of impaired glucose tolerance (IGT) and impaired fasting glucose (IFG).

17. **Define IGT and IFG.**
    - **IGT:** A 2-hour postload glucose of 140–199 mg/dL (7.8–11.1 mmol/L), using the OGTT
    - **IFG:** A fasting PG of 100–125 mg/dL (5.6–6.9 mmol/L)

    IGT and IFG are associated with the metabolic syndrome and a high risk of developing DM and cardiovascular disease.

18. **List the diagnostic criteria for the metabolic syndrome.**
    - Prediabetes or diabetes (hyperinsulinemia)
    - Abdominal (central) obesity
    - Hypertension
    - Atherosclerosis
    - Polycystic ovarian syndrome
    - Waist circumference $\geq$ 102 cm in men and $\geq$ 88 cm in women
    - Triglycerides (TG) $\geq$ 150 mg/dL*
    - Systolic BP $\geq$ 130 mmHg or diastolic BP $\geq$ 85 mmHg*
    - High-density lipoprotein (HDL) cholesterol <40 mg/dL in men and <50 mg/dL in women*
    - Fasting glucose $\geq$ 100 mg/dL

    Metabolic syndrome is diagnosed if three of the above criteria are present.

---

*or history of drug treatment for the condition.

Grundy SM, Cleerman JI, Daniels SR, et al: Diagnosis and management of the metabolic syndrome: An American Heart Association/National Heart, and Blood Institute Scientific Statement, *Circulation* 112:2735–2752, 2005.

KEY POINTS: CRITERIA FOR CONDITIONS ASSOCIATED ✔️ WITH METABOLIC SYNDROME

1. Atherogenic dyslipidemia (elevated TG, apolipoprotein B, small density LDL, and low HDL)

2. Prothrombotic state (impaired fibrinolysis, elevated plasminogen activator inhibitor-1)

3. Proinflammatory state (elevated high-sensitivity C-reactive protein and inflammatory cytokines)

4. Polycystic ovarian syndrome

5. Vascular dysregulation (microalbuminuria and chronic kidney disease)

6. Insulin resistance

7. Abnormal body fat distribution

HDL = high-density liproprotein; LDL = low-density lipoprotein.

19. **Describe the pathophysiology of diabetic ketoacidosis (DKA).**
An increase in counterregulatory hormones (catecholamines, cortisol, glucagon, and growth hormone) accompanied by insulin deficiency. All of these hormonal factors contribute to increased hepatic and renal glucose production and decreased peripheral glucose utilization. These hormonal changes also serve to enhance lipolysis and ketogenesis as well as glycogenolysis and gluconeogenesis and serve to worsen hyperglycemia and acidosis. Insulin is required to block glycogenolysis and gluconeogenesis. Lipolysis leads to increased free fatty acid synthesis for ultimate conversion by the liver to ketones. This state is associated with increased production and decreased utilization of glucose and ketones. Glucosuria leads to osmotic diuresis and dehydration that is associated with reduced renal function and worsening acidosis.

20. **List the clinical features of DKA.**
    - Polydipsia
    - Polyphagia
    - Polyuria
    - Severe dehydration
    - Altered mental status (including coma)
    - Gastrointestinal (GI) distress (nausea, vomiting, abdominal pain)
    - Weight loss
    - Hyperventilation
    - Weakness

21. **What physical examination findings are associated with DKA?**
    - Dehydration
    - Poor skin turgor
    - Rapid shallow breathing (initially) followed in late DKA by Kussmaul breathing (deep, gasping breath)

- Mental status changes (wide range)
- Hypotension
- Tachycardia
- Musty (fruity) breath
- Hyporeflexia
- Hypothermia

Findings will vary with the severity of DKA. Untreated DKA can progress to coma, shock, and death.

22. **Summarize the laboratory data associated with DKA.**
Laboratory data, which varies with the severity of DKA, includes PG > 250 mg/dL, arterial pH < 7.3, serum bicarbonate < 18 mEq/L, positive serum and urine ketones, and elevated anion gap (>10–12). Although these laboratory results are diagnostic for DKA, one may see other abnormalities, including elevated blood urea nitrogen and creatinine with dehydration, leukocytosis, low serum sodium, and elevated serum potassium due to extracellular shifting caused by insulin deficiency.

23. **How is DKA managed?**
With fluid resuscitation, insulin therapy, and careful monitoring and correction of electrolyte imbalances. Any precipitating factors should be identified when possible. The most common precipitating factor is infection. The hospitalized patient should have appropriate bacterial cultures (e.g., blood, urine) and antibiotic therapy if infection is suspected.

24. **What factors other than infection may precipitate DKA?**
Other precipitating factors include myocardial infarction, stroke, pancreatitis, trauma, alcohol abuse, or medications (particularly inadequate insulin therapy).

25. **Should patients with DKA be hospitalized?**
Possibly. Hospitalization depends on the severity of DKA, and very mild DKA in experienced patients with type 1 DM can be managed in the outpatient setting. Most patients, however, require hospitalization for intravenous (IV) fluid management, insulin (IV insulin infusion is the treatment of choice), and correction of electrolytes (sodium, potassium, phosphate, bicarbonate).

26. **What principle should be kept in mind when patients are transitioned from IV to subcutaneous (SC) insulin?**
That SC insulin must be given before discontinuing IV insulin (usually 1–2 hr to allow for adequate plasma insulin levels) to avoid return of hyperglycemia and/or DKA.

27. **What is hyperglycemic hyperosmolar nonketotic syndrome (HHNS)?**
Severe hyperglycemia with profound dehydration and some degree of alteration in mental status (50%). Typically, patients have type 2 DM and mild renal impairment. The plasma glucose is frequently very elevated (>600 mg/dL). Ketosis is usually only very mild or absent. Plasma hyperosmolarity (>340 mOsm/L) is one hallmark of this condition.

28. **How is HHNS treated?**
With aggressive fluid replacement, insulin, and correction of electrolyte disturbances. As with DKA, a search for the precipitating factor is warranted.

29. **What is A_1C?**
Glycosylated hemoglobin or glycohemoglobin and is used as a measure of average serum glucose concentrations over the prior 2–3 months.

30. **How is A_1C used clinically?**
As an overall indicator of glycemic control. A_1C should be measured biannually in patients who meet treatment goals (typically $A_1C < 7\%$) or quarterly in patients whose therapy is actively changing. Although an ideal goal for $A_1C < 7\%$, this goal must be individualized. Less intensive goals may be indicated in patients with frequent hypoglycemia, cardiovascular disease, the elderly, and limited life expectancy. More intensive goals are desired in pregnant patients, those who need to further reduce diabetes complications, and those who can easily obtain better glycemic control without hypoglycemia.

31. **What are the currently recommended goals for glycemic control in patients with DM?**
$A_1C < 7\%$.

32. **What diseases or conditions reduce the accuracy of A_1C?**
- Hemolysis (from artificial cardiac valves and transjugular intrahepatic portosystemic shunts [TIPS])
- Transfusion
- Dialysis
- Hemoglobinopathies such as sickle cell disease and thalassemia

33. **How should one screen for diabetic nephropathy?**
With an annual urine spot albumin-to-creatinine ratio to detect microalbuminuria. Microalbuminuria is defined as 30–299 µg albumin/mg creatinine and must be confirmed on repeated examinations. Clinical albuminuria is defined as ≥ 300 µg albumin/mg creatinine. Any abnormal results should be repeated over a several-month period. Patients with type 1 DM should begin microalbuminuria screening when they have had DM for longer than 5 years; patients with type 2 DM should begin screening at the time of diagnosis.

34. **Summarize the screening recommendations for diabetic retinopathy.**
Patients with type 1 DM should receive a comprehensive dilated eye examination within 3–5 years of diagnosis and annually thereafter. Patients with type 2 DM should receive a comprehensive dilated examination at the time of diagnosis and annually. The eye-care specialist may determine altered timing of follow-up examinations.

35. **How are patients screened for diabetic neuropathy?**
With monofilament sensory testing of the foot in addition to a detailed foot examination and patient education about foot care.

36. **Identify the oral agents available for the treatment of type 2 DM.**
See Table 16-2.

37. **What vitamin deficiency is associated with the use of metformin?**
Vitamin B_{12}.

38. **Describe the different types of insulin.**
See Table 16-3.

39. **Where is insulin cleared?**
Mainly in the liver. Approximately 50% of insulin is cleared via first pass through the liver. Once insulin is in the periphery, 30% is cleared by the kidney. IV insulin has an extremely short half-life regardless of the type of insulin used (e.g., regular or lispro). As soon as the insulin IV infusion is discontinued, it is generally cleared quickly (i.e., within 5 min) from the circulation.

TABLE 16-2. AVAILABLE NON-INSULIN AGENTS FOR THE TREATMENT OF TYPE 2 DM

Class	Generic Name (Brand Name)	Common Side Effects
Augment Insulin Release		
Sulfonylureas	Glyburide (Micronase, DiaBeta, Glynase) Glipizide (Glucotrol, Glucotrol XL) Glimepiride (Amaryl)	Hypoglycemia, dizziness, GI upset.
Meglitinides	Repaglinide (Prandin) Nateglinide (Starlix)	Hypoglycemia, GI upset.
Insulin Sensitizers		
Biguanides	Metformin (Glucophage) Metformin XL (Glucophage XL)	Anorexia, diarrhea, GI upset, lactic acidosis (rare). Do not use in renal disease (Cr > 1.4 women, 1.5 men) or CHF.
Thiazolidinediones	Pioglitazone (Actos) Rosiglitazone (Avandia)*	Weight gain, fluid retention (do not use in CHF), hepatotoxicity, hypoglycemia when used with insulin.
α-Glucosidase inhibitor	Acarbose (Precose) Miglitol (Glyset)	Flatulence, diarrhea, GI distress.
DPP-IV Inhibitors	Sitagliptin (Januvia) Saxiglitpin (Onyglyza)	
Mixtures	Glyburide/metformin (Glucovance) Glypizide/metformin (Metaglip) Metformin/rosiglitazone (Avandamet)	Same as single agents.
GLP-1 Agonists	Exenatide (Byetta)	Nausea, weight loss, GI upset, possibly pancreatitis.
GLP-1 Agonist	Liraglutide (Victoza)	C-Cell hyperplasia.

CHF = congestive heart failure; Cr = creatinine; DPP = dipeptidyl peptidase; GI = gastrointestinal; GLP = glucagon-like peptide.
*Only for use in patients whose glucose is uncontrolled with any other medicine.

TABLE 16-3. TYPES OF INSULIN*

Insulin Type	Time of Onset	Peak	Duration of Onset
Rapid-Acting			
Lispro (Humalog)	<30 min	30–90 min	3–5 hr
Aspart (Novolog)	<15 min	1–3 hr	3–5 hr
Glulisine (Apidra)	12–30 min	1.6–1.8 hr	3–4 hr
Short-Acting			
Regular	0.5–1 hr	2–4 hr	6–12 hr
Intermediate-Acting			
NPH	1–2 hr	4–14 hr	10–24 hr
Lente	1–3 hr	6–16 hr	12–24 hr
Long-acting			
Glargine (Lantus)	3 hr	No real peak	20–24 hr
Detemir (Levemir)	1–3 hr	Small peak at 6–8 hr	12–24 hr
Ultralente	4–8 hr	10–30 hr	18–36 hr
Mixtures			
70% NPH/30% regular	30 min	4–8 hr	16–24 hr
50% NPH/50% regular	30 min	7–12 hr	16–24 hr
75% NPL/25% lispro	<30 min	Lispro 30–90 min Protamine 2–4 hr	6–12 hr
70% NPA/25% aspart	<15 min	1–4 hr	12–24 hr

NPA = neutral protamine aspart; NPH = neutral protamine hagedorn; NPL = neutral protamine lispro.
*These values are highly variable among individual patients. Even in a given person, these values vary depending on the site and depth of injection, skin temperature, and exercise. *Note:* Insulin glargine cannot be mixed with other insulins owing to the low pH of its diluent. Rapid-acting insulins can be mixed with NPH, Lente, and Ultralente.

40. **What are the indications for an insulin pump?**
Motivated patients who require flexibility in insulin dosing and meal timing. Although both continuous subcutaneous insulin infusion (CSII) and multiple daily insulin injections can effectively control blood glucose values, some patient and physician preferences may lead to the use of an insulin pump (CSIIP). CSIIP requires significant patient education, meticulous monitoring, and supervision by a health-care provider who is comfortable with this mode of insulin delivery.

41. **What are incretin hormones and which drugs are based on them?**
They are hormones produced in the GI tract when food is eaten that enhances the action of insulin. Their existence were postulated when it was noted that a glucose challenge given IV required more insulin to achieve glycemic control than a glucose challenge given orally. Incretin hormones include glucagon-like peptide-1 (GLP-1) and amylin. Drugs that have been manufactured to take advantage of these incretin hormones include Exenatide (GLP-1 agonist), Symlin (amylin agonist), and dipeptidyl peptidase (DPP) IV inhibitors, which block the degradation of GLP-1.

42. List the chronic complications of DM.
Microvascular
- Neuropathy (painful paresthesias, autonomic neuropathy)
- Retinopathy (nonproliferative and proliferative retinopathy, blindness)
- Nephropathy (spectrum of disease from microalbuminuria to end-stage renal disease)

Macrovascular (cardiovascular and peripheral vascular disease)
- Nonhealing ulcers, amputations
- Peripheral artery disease
- Hypertension
- Dyslipidemia
- Coronary artery disease
- Stroke

43. What is important to know about diabetes in pregnancy?
Patients with diabetes should plan all pregnancies. A₁C should be < 7% before pregnancy is attempted. Medications such as angiotensin-converting enzyme (ACE) inhibitors, angiotensin receptor blockers, statins, fibrates, and certain antidepressant medications should be discontinued. Diabetes health-care maintenance screening, including thyroid, urine albumin, and retinal examination should be up to date. Women should take 1000 μg of folate daily before conception and during pregnancy. Once pregnant, glucose levels are much more stringent. Fasting glucose should be < 90 mg/dL and 2-hour postmeal blood glucose should be < 120 mg/dL. Patients should check fingerstick glucose six times per day.

44. What are the symptoms of hypoglycemia?
See Table 16-4. Symptoms can be divided into two categories: **adrenergic** (due to excess secretion of epinephrine) and **neuroglycopenic** (due to cerebral dysfunction). Patients with DM typically develop symptoms of hypoglycemia when blood glucose values fall below 50–60 mg/dL, but severity of symptoms can vary with the individual. In addition, some fasting individuals (particularly women) without DM can be completely asymptomatic with glucose values approximately 50 mg/dL.

TABLE 16-4. SYMPTOMS OF HYPOGLYCEMIA

Adrenergic	Neuroglycopenic
Sweating	Dizziness
Tachycardia	Headache
Tremor	Decreased cognition, confusion
Anxiety	Clouded vision
Hunger	Seizures
	Coma

45. How is hypoglycemia treated?
If profound hypoglycemia is likely and the patient is unable to speak or swallow, intramuscular (IM) glucagon and/or IV glucose should be administered. Patients who are unable to communicate or swallow on their own should not be force-fed juice or sugar. Patients who are awake and able to swallow can consume 15 g of rapid-acting carbohydrate in the form of 4 ounces of juice or soda, or glucose tablets. Ice cream, cake, or candy bars should not be used to treat hypoglycemia because fat delays absorption of glucose. Glucose should be rechecked in 15–30 minutes. Patients should not drive or operate heavy machinery until blood glucose is normal. Patients on insulin pumps should suspend insulin delivery for 15–30 minutes.

46. **Describe hypoglycemia-associated autonomic failure.**
A syndrome of inappropriate response to hypoglycemia that occurs in patients with DM. Under normal physiologic conditions, hypoglycemia induces a reduction in insulin levels and an enhancement of glucagon and epinephrine secretion, both of which serve to defend against continued hypoglycemia. Patients with type 1 DM and many patients with type 2 DM have defective glucose counterregulation. Because they cannot reduce exogenous insulin levels and have impaired glucagon and epinephrine responses to hypoglycemia, they become prone to severe iatrogenic hypoglycemia. In addition, they frequently have attenuated sympathoadrenal responses to hypoglycemia. Hypoglycemia-associated autonomic failure is induced by hypoglycemia and reversed by avoidance of hypoglycemia.

47. **What is hypoglycemic unawareness?**
Hypoglycemia that occurs unnoticed by the patient because it is not associated with any adrenergic symptoms. These patients may have exceedingly low glucose levels without symptoms and may rapidly progress to confusion, seizures, or coma without warning.

48. **What is the diagnostic approach to hypoglycemia in patients without diabetes?**
Confirmation of hypoglycemia through Whipple's triad: presence of symptoms consistent with hypoglycemia (e.g., sweating, hunger, palpitations, and weakness), documented low plasma glucose at the time of symptoms, and relief of symptoms when the plasma glucose concentration is raised to normal levels. Hypoglycemia in the fasting state is typically more clinically concerning than reactive (postprandial) hypoglycemia. Although the exact criteria are debated, glucose levels of < 50 mg/dL in men and < 40 mg/dL in women are generally accepted as indicative of hypoglycemia.

49. **Summarize the differential diagnosis of adult hypoglycemia not related to diabetes.**
   - Drug-induced or factitious hypoglycemia, particularly related to exposure to exogenous insulin and oral antidiabetic agents such as sulfonylureas. Other drugs associated with hypoglycemia include ethanol (inhibits gluconeogenesis), salicylates, sulfonamides, pentamidine, monoamine oxidase (MAO) inhibitors, and quinine.
   - Critical illness, including liver and renal failure.
   - Adrenal insufficiency due to lack of the counterregulatory hormone cortisol.
   - Insulinoma, a tumor of the pancreatic beta cells that produces too much insulin.
   - Non–beta-cell tumors, including mesenchymal tumors such as fibrosarcoma, mesothelioma, and leiomyosarcoma, that produce insulin-like growth factor-1 (IGF-1) or IGF-2.
   - Insulin or insulin receptor autoantibodies (rare).

50. **How do you distinguish between endogenous and exogenous hyperinsulinemia?**
By insulin and C-peptide levels. Insulin and its cleavage product C-peptide are secreted by the pancreatic beta cell in equimolar amounts. If a patient is getting exogenous insulin, insulin levels will be high and C-peptide levels low. Both values are elevated in patients with surreptitious sulfonylurea use because these drugs stimulate release of endogenous insulin and C-peptide. Sulfonylurea blood levels can also help rule out drug-induced hypoglycemia in this setting.

51. **List the most common pancreatic endocrine tumors and their clinical presentations.**
These tumors are derived from the islet cells of the pancreas and are named for the hormones that they secrete.

- **Insulinoma** (secretes insulin): hypoglycemia.
- **Gastrinoma** (secretes gastrin): Zollinger-Ellison syndrome, associated with excess gastric acid secretion and peptic ulcer disease.
- **Glucagonoma** (secretes glucagon): DM, weight loss, anemia, necrolytic migratory erythema.
- **Somatostatinoma** (secretes somatostatin): somatostatin inhibits secretion of insulin gastric acid and pancreatic enzymes, leading to diabetes, weight loss, hypochlorhydria, steatorrhea, and gallstones.
- **VIPoma** (secretes vasoactive intestinal peptide): watery diarrhea, hypokalemia, achlorhydria.
- **PPoma** (secretes pancreatic polypeptide alone or in combination with other pancreatic peptides): watery diarrhea.

52. **Identify the hereditary syndrome associated with pancreatic tumors.**
Multiple endocrine neoplasia syndrome type I (MEN I). MEN syndromes are characterized by neoplastic transformation in multiple endocrine glands. MEN I is now known to be caused by a mutation in the tumor suppressor *MEN I* gene, whose product is named "menin."

53. **What are the components of MEN I?**
- Pituitary tumors (most commonly prolactinoma)
- Primary hyperparathyroidism (typically due to parathyroid hyperplasia)
- Pancreatic tumors (most commonly gastrinoma, followed by insulinoma)

54. **What are MEN IIA and MEN IIB?**
MEN IIA includes neoplasms of the thyroid (medullary thyroid carcinoma), parathyroid (primary hyperparathyroidism), and adrenal gland (pheochromocytoma). MEN IIB includes medullary thyroid carcinoma, pheochromocytoma, and mucosal neuromas. MEN IIA and MEN IIB are due to activating mutations of the *RET* proto-oncogene

OBESITY

55. **How is obesity currently defined?**
Obesity is generally defined as excessive body fat and is determined by body mass index (BMI). The BMI is calculated by dividing weight in kilograms by height in meters squared (weight in kg)/(height in m)^2. BMI is defined as follows:
- **BMI < 25:** Normal
- **BMI 25–29.9:** Overweight
- **BMI > 30:** Obesity

56. **Is waist circumference significant for diagnosing obesity?**
Yes. Waist circumference can also be used to diagnose obesity. Health risks of obesity are correlated with visceral (abdominal) adiposity. People with larger waist sizes have increased risks of obesity-related disorders such as hypertension, cardiovascular disease, and diabetes. Waist circumference is determined by placing a tape measure horizontally around the abdomen at the level of the iliac crest. Measurements should be taken at the end of a normal expiration. The tape measure should be snug but not compress the skin. Increased risk of obesity-related disease occurs in men with a waist circumference $\geq$ 40 inches (102 cm) and women with a waist circumference $\geq$ 35 inches (88 cm).

57. **List the health risks associated with obesity.**
- Diabetes
- Hypertension
- Hyperlipidemia
- Coronary artery disease
- Cerebral vascular disease

- Degenerative arthritis
- Obstructive sleep apnea
- Gallbladder disease
- Cancers of endometrium, breast, colon, and prostate
- Psychological complications (depression, poor self-esteem, discrimination)

Stein CJ, Colditz GA: The epidemic of obesity, *J Clin Endocrinol Metab* 89:2522–2525, 2004.

58. **How common is obesity?**
Increasingly common. Obesity is now thought to be one of the leading health disorders in the United States. Its prevalence has increased dramatically and it is now estimated that approximately one third of the U.S. population is obese (BMI > 30). The prevalence is higher in ethnic minorities and is rapidly increasing in children and adolescents.

59. **What causes people to gain weight?**
Increased caloric intake or decreased energy expenditure relative to caloric intake. Weight gain occurs when a person is not in energy balance. Weight maintenance occurs when people consume as many calories as they expend per day.

60. **List the three components of total daily energy expenditure (EE).**
- Basal metabolic rate (~65% of total daily EE)
- Energy of physical activity (30% of average person's daily EE)
- Thermic effect of food (energy cost of digesting food, which accounts for 5% of daily EE)

61. **What factors control energy homeostasis?**
Complex interactions between the brain and neural factors that control appetite and satiety, nutrient metabolism, and hormonal systems. Much research is currently being conducted in the neural mechanisms that regulate feeding and energy balance. Most evidence suggests that obese people do not have major alterations in their basal metabolic rates. In fact, because total EE is linearly related to BMI, obese people actually require more calories for weight maintenance than lean people. It is much more likely that obesity develops as a multifactorial process involving genetic predisposition as well as environmental and behavioral factors.

62. **Who should be treated for obesity?**
All obese people should be instructed about proper diet and exercise to prevent obesity-related complications. People with more severe obesity or those who already have obesity-related complications should be treated more aggressively, including medications and surgery if indicated.

63. **Describe the general approach to treatment of obesity.**
Individualized treatment is important and the patient's goals must be discussed. Frequently, patients want a rapid, substantial weight loss. Unfortunately, this goal is usually not healthy or attainable in the patient's desired time frame. Because 1 lb of fat stores approximately 3500 kcal, in order to lose 1 lb of weight/wk, the person must decrease caloric intake by roughly 500 kcal/day. This regimen is often extremely difficult to follow. Consequently, a more moderate approach is to restrict caloric intake (250–500 kcal reduction from basal intake) and increase energy expenditure (30 min of moderate physical activity most days of the week).

64. **When should pharmacotherapy be considered for the treatment of obesity?**
In patients with a BMI > 30, a BMI > 27 with comorbidities, or minimal response after 6 months of lifestyle modifications. Typically, the first approach is diet and exercise with behavioral modifications followed by the addition of pharmacotherapy.

65. **What medications are U.S. Food and Drug Administration (FDA)–approved for the treatment of obesity?**
    - Phentermine, a norepinephrine agonist (15–30 mg/day)
    - Diethylpropion, a sympathomimetic (75 mg/day in multiple doses or as controlled release)
    - Benzphetamine, a sympathomimetic (up to 50 mg three times/day)
    - Orlistat, a pancreatic lipase inhibitor (120 mg three times/day before meals)

66. **How effective are medications in treating obesity?**
    In general, medications require chronic use for effectiveness and can be expected to produce a 5–10% weight loss in most people.

67. **What are the concerns about using phenteramine?**
    Phenteramine has a high potential for abuse.

68. **What medications are associated with weight loss in patients with type 2 diabetes?**
    Metformin, exenatide, and pramlitide.

69. **What other drugs used for treatment of depression or seizures may facilitate weight loss, although not FDA-approved for obesity treatment?**
    - Buproprion (not recommended owing to lack of long-term data)
    - Fluoxetine (high doses required preclude use)
    - Topimiramate and zonisamide (antiseizure medications that cause anorexia without enough data to justify use at this time)

70. **Summarize the role of surgery in the treatment of obesity.**
    Surgery is generally reserved for people with severe obesity (BMI > 40) who have failed other forms of therapy. The most frequently performed procedures are the vertical banded gastroplasty and gastric bypass.

PITUITARY GLAND

71. **Summarize the general functions of the pituitary gland.**
    The pituitary gland is the "master gland" of the endocrine system involved in many body functions, including growth and development, metabolism, and reproduction. These functions are regulated by the secretion of hormones that interact at specific target organ sites.

72. **Describe the anterior pituitary gland.**
    The anterior pituitary or adenohypophysis, which composes 80% of the entire gland, is derived embryologically from Rathke's pouch and is oral ectoderm in origin. Anterior pituitary hormones are synthesized in the pituitary by specific cell types and are regulated by hypothalamic and target organ factors.

73. **List the six major hormones secreted by the anterior pituitary.**
    - **Somatotropin** (growth hormone [GH])
    - **Prolactin**
    - **Corticotropin** (adrenocorticotropic hormone [ACTH])
    - **Thyrotropin** (thyroid-stimulating hormone [TSH])
    - **Luteinizing hormone** (LH)
    - **Follicle-stimulating hormone** (FSH)

74. **How is secretion of these hormones regulated?**
   By positive- and negative-feedback mechanisms. Most hormones are stimulated by a
   hypothalamic hormone and inhibited by a target organ hormone. The one exception
   is prolactin, which is under tonic inhibitory control by hypothalamic dopamine neurons.
   A schematic diagram is presented in Figure 16-1 (Table 16-5).

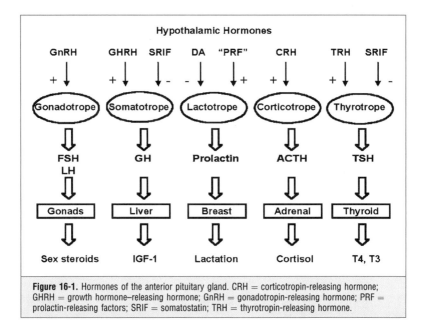

Figure 16-1. Hormones of the anterior pituitary gland. CRH = corticotropin-releasing hormone;
GHRH = growth hormone–releasing hormone; GnRH = gonadotropin-releasing hormone; PRF =
prolactin-releasing factors; SRIF = somatostatin; TRH = thyrotropin-releasing hormone.

TABLE 16-5. HORMONES OF THE ANTERIOR PITUITARY GLAND

Pituitary Cell Type	Hormone	Hypothalamic Factor
Corticotrope	Corticotropin (ACTH)	CRH stimulates
Thyrotrope	Thyrotropin (TSH)	TRH stimulates and SRIF inhibits
Gonadotrope	LH	GnRH
	FSH	
Somatotrope	GH	GHRH stimulates and SRIF inhibits
Lactotrope	Prolactin	Dopamine inhibits prolactin-releasing factors (e.g., TRH, suckling)

ACTH = adrenocorticotropic hormone; CRH = corticotropin-releasing hormone; FSH = follicle-
stimulating hormone; GH = growth hormone; GHRH = growth hormone–releasing hormone;
GnRH = gonadotropin-releasing hormone; LH = luteinizing hormone; SRIF = somatostatin;
TRH = thyrotropin-releasing hormone; TSH = thyroid-stimulating hormone.

75. **Describe the posterior pituitary. What hormones does it secrete?**
    The posterior pituitary or neurohypophysis is an extension of the floor of the third ventricle of the brain and originates from cells of the central nervous system. Posterior pituitary hormones include arginine vasopressin (AVP) or antidiuretic hormone (ADH), and oxytocin. These hormones are synthesized in the cell bodies of hypothalmic neurons and stored in the axons that terminate in the posterior pituitary.

76. **Describe the general approach to evaluating a patient with pituitary disease.**
    A detailed history regarding anterior and posterior pituitary function and hormonal hyper- or hypofunction will help identify the extent of the disease. Specific questions to assess hormone function related to a specific pituitary disorder include:
    - **Diabetes insipidus** (DI; deficient ADH): presence of polyuria, polydipsia, or nighttime polydipsia
    - **Hypothyroidism** (secondary): fatigue, constipation, cold intolerance, dry skin, weight gain
    - **Adrenal insufficiency** (secondary): fatigue, dizziness, nausea, weight loss
    - **Prolactinoma:** galactorrhea, amenorrhea or male hypogonadism, infertility, headache
    - **Acromegaly** (excessive GH): increased size of hands, head, and feet, hypertension, sweating, snoring, and fatigue (due to sleep apnea)
    - **Cushing's disease** (excessive ACTH): weight gain, purple striae, diabetes, osteoporosis, hypertension, depression

77. **In particular, what symptoms should be evaluated in patients with pituitary tumors?**
    Those suggestive of hormonal abnormalities and mass effects. Mass effects (symptoms) include neurologic findings and impaired anterior pituitary function.
    Posterior pituitary dysfunction is rarely a consequence of a pituitary tumor, but it can be seen in patients with pituitary trauma, surgery, or disorders of the pituitary stalk.

KEY POINTS: MECHANISMS BY WHICH PITUITARY TUMORS CAUSE PROBLEMS ✔

1. Mass effect: tumors apply pressure to surrounding structures causing functional disruption that may lead to:
    - Headaches (most common).
    - Visual loss or visual field defects (bitemporal hemianopsia).
    - Cranial nerve dysfunction (most commonly II, III, IV, and VI).
    - Anterior pituitary hormone deficiencies.
2. Endocrine hyperfunction: due to excessive secretion of a particular anterior pituitary hormone by the tumor.

78. **What physical examination findings suggest pituitary disease?**
    - Abnormal visual field testing by confrontation
    - Enlarged hands and feet, skin tags, and macroglossia (acromegaly)
    - Cranial nerve palsies
    - Purple striae, moon facies, proximal muscle wasting, hyperpigmentation, dorsocervical fat pad (Cushing's)

- Loss of body hair, gynecomastia (hypogonadism)
- Delayed deep tendon reflexes, coarse hair or hair loss, nonpitting edema (hypothyroidism)

79. **What causes acromegaly?**
An oversecretion of GH. Ninety-nine percent are caused by a GH-secreting pituitary adenoma, either a pure somatotrope (produces solely GH) or a mammosomatotrope (producing prolactin and GH). Rare causes of acromegaly include a pituitary or hypothalamic gangliocytoma, growth hormone–releasing hormone (GHRH)–secreting tumor found in a bronchial or GI carcinoid tumor, pancreatic islet cell tumor, adrenal adenoma, or small cell carcinoma.

80. **How does acromegaly present clinically?**
As gigantism if the tumor occurs in childhood before the closure of the epiphyses. Children with acromegaly can grow to heights much higher than genetic potential. When a GH-producing tumor is present in association with deficiency in gonadal hormones, epiphyses can remain open for even longer, allowing even higher growth heights to be obtained. GH and IGF-1 levels can be high during adolescence, but in patients without abnormal GH levels, GH suppresses with glucose challenge. Adult patients frequently present late in the disease with large tumors (macroadenomas in 85%) owing to the very slow development of the clinical features. Acromegaly often goes unrecognized by the patient, his or her family, and the physician because the physical changes occur so slowly. Such patients can present with soft tissue hypertrophy; headache; arthritis/carpal tunnel syndrome; increased size of hands, head, and feet; organomegaly, including cardiomegaly with congestive heart failure; and obstructive sleep apnea.

81. **What physical examination findings suggest acromegaly?**
Soft tissue changes (large doughy hands), frontal bossing, widening spaces in teeth, skin tags, organomegaly, large body size, signs of hyperprolactinemia (gynecomastia, galactorrhea), hypogonadism, and visual field deficits. Patients may also have diaphoresis and thick heel pads.

82. **How is acromegaly diagnosed?**
By clinical features, laboratory evaluation, and magnetic resonance imaging (MRI) of the pituitary. Diagnostic laboratory abnormalities include elevated GH with failure to suppress with oral glucose administration and an elevated IGF-1 (somatomedin-C). Patients may also have insulin resistance/DM, hyperprolactinemia due to stalk compression, hypogonadism, and hypercalciuria/nephrolithiasis. They are at higher risk of colon polyps/cancer and have increased mortality rates. Elevated phosphorous can also be seen.

83. **Explain the goal for treatment of acromegaly.**
To normalize anterior pituitary function and GH secretion. Mortality rates return to baseline levels if the GH is normalized (normal GH, normal IGF-1, and normal GH suppression [<1 μg/L or <0.4 if using ultrasensitive GH assay] following oral glucose).

84. **How can this goal be achieved?**
Through transsphenoidal surgical resection. Medical treatment postresection is often required because many tumors are too large at presentation to be completely excised by surgery. In such cases, somatostatin analogues are indicated for medical therapy to control GH secretion. GH cells have somatostatin receptors and treatment with somatostatin analogues (octreotide and lanreotide) has been shown to decrease GH levels and induce tumor shrinkage. GH receptor antagonist pegvisomant is also approved for medical therapy. Although less effective, dopamine agonists such as bromocriptine. Cabergoline may also

control GH levels, particularly in patients who also secrete prolactin. Finally, radiation therapy can be offered to patients who fail surgical and medical interventions. Radiation therapy can result in panhypopituitarism.

Melmed S, Colao A, Barkan A, et al: Guidelines for acromegaly management: an update, *J Clin Endocrinol Metab* 94:1509–1517, 2009.

85. **Prolactinomas are the most common type of pituitary tumor. In general, how do they present?**
Generally with hypogonadism, but the clinical picture of hyperprolactinemia is variable, depending on age, sex, duration of hyperprolactinemia, and tumor size. Hypogonadism is due to prolactin inhibition of gonadotropin-releasing hormone neurons and leads to suppression of the hypothalamic-pituitary-gonadal axis. Women of reproductive age present earlier with amenorrhea and galactorrhea. Men and postmenopausal women usually present later in the disease course with mass effect such as headache and visual deficits.

86. **List the clinical features of hyperprolactinemia.**
   - Galactorrhea
   - Amenorrhea/menstrual irregularities
   - Infertility
   - Hirsutism
   - Gynecomastia and erectile dysfunction in men
   - Growth arrest/delayed puberty
   - Mass lesions/visual field defects (primarily in men and postmenopausal women)
   - Osteopenia (due to hypogonadism)

87. **What is the differential diagnosis of hyperprolactinemia?**
If values > 200 ng/mL:
   - Prolactinoma
   - Renal failure
   - Pregnancy (normal physiologic cause of hyperprolactinemia)
If values < 100 ng/mL:
   - Prolactinoma
   - Pregnancy
   - Renal failure
   - Drugs (see Question 88)
   - Stalk effect from other pituitary tumors
   - Stalk effect from hypothalmic/sellar masses (craniopharyngioma, meningioma, metastatic disease)
   - Infiltrative disorders (sarcoidosis, tuberculosis)
   - Neurogenic disorder (chest wall lesion, suckling; do not measure prolactin after a breast examination)
   - Estrogen use
   - Primary hypothyroidism (thyrotropin-releasing hormone [TRH] also stimulates prolactin secretion)
   - Idiopathic disease

88. **What medications are associated with hyperprolactinemia?**
   - Antipsychotics (chlorpromazine, clomipramine, fluphenazine, prochlorperazine, thioridazine, haloperidol, respiradone, olanzapine)
   - Gastrointestinal agents (metoclopromide, cimetidine)
   - Selective serotonin reuptake inhibitors (SSRIs [fluoxetine])
   - Tricyclic antidepressants (TCAs [imipramine])

- Antihypertensive medication (reserpine, methyldopa, verapamil)
- Alcohol
- Morphine
- Cocaine

89. **What are the treatment options for hyperprolactinemia?**
Treatment depends on the etiology. When due to a medication, it is obviously best to stop the offending agent if possible. One may not be able to discontinue medical therapy, though, in patients with schizophrenia or severe mental illness; instead, replace sex hormone (estrogen or testosterone) if not contraindicated. Unlike other hyperfunctioning pituitary adenomas, medical therapy with dopamine agonists is the treatment of choice for prolactinomas. Oral contraceptives can be used to restore normal menstrual cycles and protect against bone loss in female patients who have mild elevations in prolactin in the absence of a visible pituitary tumor. Surgery is not typically the treatment of choice for prolactinomas owing to a high recurrence rate (especially for macroadenomas) but can be considered in invasive tumors or tumors resistant to medication. Radiation can always be considered in patients who fail other modalities.

90. **How do dopamine agonists work?**
By inhibiting prolactin secretion and causing tumor shrinkage. Examples include bromocriptine and cabergoline. All must be started at low doses and titrated upward very slowly to avoid side effects. The most common side effects include nausea, vomiting, and orthostatic hypotension. Cabergoline appears to be the best tolerated.

91. **What cardiac side effects are associated with dopamine agonists?**
Valvular heart disease and heart failure. Careful cardiac examination and screening echocardiogram are recommended periodically.

92. **What is the "stalk effect"?**
Compression of the pituitary stalk by large non–prolactin-secreting tumors, thus interrupting the tonic inhibitory effect of dopamine (or prolactin-inhibiting factor) on the pituitary. The result is elevation of prolactin levels ≤ 200 ng/mL.

93. **What is pituitary apoplexy?**
The syndrome of sudden headache, visual change, ophthalmoplegia, and altered mental status caused by the acute hemorrhage or infarction of the pituitary gland. Most cases are due to pituitary hemorrhage of a previously undiagnosed pituitary adenoma (65%), but can also be caused by Sheehan's syndrome, conditions that increase bleeding (such as anticoagulation), or intracranial pressure. Patient presentation may range from asymptomatic to symptoms of severe retro-orbital headache, visual defects, meningeal signs, altered sensorium, seizure, or coma depending on the extent of the lesion. Clinical symptoms and signs plus computed tomography (CT) scan or MRI of the pituitary aid in the diagnosis. This condition can be life-threatening if unrecognized.

94. **How is pituitary apoplexy treated?**
With stress doses of glucocorticoids (for cerebral edema and presumed adrenal insufficiency) and/or neurosurgical decompression. Hormonal deficiencies after apoplexy are the rule, and panhypopituitarism is common. Hypogonadism occurs in nearly 100%, GH deficiency in 88%, hyperprolactinemia in 67%, adrenal insufficiency in 66%, hypothyroidism in 42%, and DI in 3%.

95. **What is Sheehan's syndrome?**
Pituitary apoplexy after obstetric hemorrhage.

96. **What is a thyrotropinoma?**
A tumor of the TSH-producing cells. This rare tumor occurs in approximately one in a million people, producing a clinical syndrome of hyperthyroidism that is indistinguishable clinically from other more common causes (e.g., Graves' disease, toxic nodular goiter). Thyrotropinomas are differentiated from primary hyperthyroidism by an inappropriately normal or elevated TSH in the setting of elevated thyroid hormone levels, because TSH is secreted as a dimer peptide composed of the TSH beta and alpha subunits, alpha subunit levels are typically elevated. Patients have an elevated molar ratio of alpha-SU/TSH > 1.

97. **How is a thyrotropinoma diagnosed?**
By pituitary MRI and laboratory results. If not seen on MRI, octreotide scanning may be used for tumor localization, because these tumors display somatostatin receptors.

98. **What causes hypopituitarism?**
   - Mass lesions from tumors (pituitary adenoma, craniopharyngiomas, metastatic lesions)
   - Iatrogenic causes (pituitary surgery, radiation)
   - Infiltrative disease (hemochromatosis, lymphoma, sarcoid, histiocytosis X)
   - Pituitary infarction (Sheehan's syndrome, after coronary artery bypass grafting, trauma)
   - Pituitary apoplexy
   - Genetic disease (transcription factor mutations)
   - Empty sella syndrome (typically secondary)
   - Hypothalamic dysfunction (mass lesions, infiltrative diseases, radiation, trauma, infection)
   - Autoimmune lymphocytic hypophysitis
   - Miscellaneous (abscess/infection; aneurysm)
   Hypopituitarism can be partial or complete (panhypopituitarism).

99. **How do patients with hypopituitarism present?**
With signs and symptoms of hormonal deficiency. Evaluation is aimed at documenting deficiency and may include stimulation testing.

100. **How is hypopituitarism treated?**
With correction of the hormonal deficiency. Patients with adrenal insufficiency need to be educated about stress-dose steroids for acute illness, and all patients should wear medical alert jewelry.

101. **What are the goals of surgical management of pituitary adenomas?**
To correct hyperfunctioning/oversecretion of endocrine hormones (except in the case of prolactinoma in which medical treatment should be tried first), prevent or treat panhypopituitarism, prevent tumor recurrences, treat mass effect symptoms, and obtain definitive pathologic diagnosis. Emergency surgery is indicated in cases of pituitary apoplexy or other causes of mass effect.

102. **What is lymphocytic hypophysitis?**
A lymphocytic infiltration of the pituitary gland that often occurs after pregnancy and causes panhypopituitarism. Patients present with headache, visual field disturbances, weakness, and fatigue. Lymphocytic hypophysitis can be fatal if not recognized.

103. **What is DI? How is it treated?**
An inability to concentrate urine owing to insufficient AVP (ADH) release or activity. Large amounts of dilute urine are excreted inappropriately in the setting of hyperosmolality and hypernatremia.

104. **What are the two types of DI?**
Central (neurogenic) DI and nephrogenic DI. **Central DI** is due to impaired or inadequate secretion of AVP from the posterior pituitary. Central DI can be partial or complete and is typically an acquired condition related to trauma or infiltrative disease of the hypothalamus/ posterior pituitary. **Nephrogenic DI** is due to AVP resistance and can be acquired owing to hypercalcemia, hypokalemia, drug-induced (lithium), or congenital.

105. **How do patients with DI present?**
With polyuria (typically large volumes with osmolality < 200 mOsm/kg), polydipsia, and hypernatremia if the patients do not have an intact thirst mechanism or do not drink water. Diagnosis is confirmed by performing a water deprivation test.

106. **How is a water deprivation test performed?**
A patient suspected of having DI is asked to fast without drinking any liquids from a time point deemed safe by the physician. The patient is carefully monitored in the outpatient clinic or inpatient setting. Weight, urine output, blood pressure, and pulse are monitored hourly. Serum and urine osmolality and serum sodium are checked every 2 hours. Once serum osmolality or serum osmolality is over normal, desmopressin (DDAVP) is administered and serum and urine osmolality and serum sodium are monitored at 30 minutes and 1 hour postinjection of DDAVP. If serum osmolality is above normal and urine osmolality < 600, a diagnosis of DI is made. Patients who maintain normal serum osmolality and are able to concentrate urine osmolality over 600 and who have decreased urine output with time should be considered for primary polydipsia. Patients who are able to concentrate urine and decrease urine output after DDAVP have central DI and those who do not have nephrogenic DI.

107. **How is DI treated?**
Central DI is typically treated with AVP replacement in the form of DDAVP, a synthetic AVP agonist. There are no good therapies for nephrogenic DI, but treatment is usually aimed at volume contraction using thiazide diuretics, salt depletion, or prostaglandin synthesis inhibitors. These agents decrease renal blood flow by volume contraction and decrease urine output by reducing glomerular filtration rates.

ADRENAL GLANDS

108. **List the hormones secreted by the adrenal glands.**
See Table 16-6.

109. **Differentiate Cushing's syndrome from Cushing's disease.**
Cushing's syndrome refers to hypercortisolemia and its associated signs and symptoms due to any cause. **Cushing's disease** refers specifically to hypercortisolemia due to ACTH overproduction by a pituitary adenoma. The most common cause of Cushing's syndrome is iatrogenic owing to exogenous steroid treatment for a variety of conditions (rheumatologic, organ transplant, reactive airway disease). If one excludes iatrogenic hypercortisolemia, the most common cause of Cushing's syndrome is Cushing's disease, which accounts for approximately two thirds of all cases.

110. **What are the signs and symptoms of Cushing's disease?**
- Atrophic, thin skin; easy bruising and purple striae on abdomen, axilla, hips, and thighs
- Weight gain or central obesity
- Dorsocervical (buffalo hump) and supraclavicular fat accumulation
- Moon facies
- Menstrual irregularities

TABLE 16-6. ADRENAL HORMONES

Hormone	Synthesis	Syndromes
Cortisol	Synthesized from cholesterol in the adrenal cortex (zona fasciculata, zona reticularis)	Hyperfunction: Cushing's syndrome Hypofunction: adrenal insufficiency
Aldosterone	Synthesized from cholesterol in the adrenal cortex (zona glomerulosa)	Hyperfunction: hyperaldosteronism Hypofunction: adrenal insufficiency
Androgens/sex steroids	Synthesized from cholesterol in the adrenal cortex (zona fasciculata, zona reticularis)	Hyperfunction: hirsutism/virilization Hypofunction: no clear syndrome
Catecholamines (norepinephrine, epinephrine)	Synthesized in the adrenal medulla	Hyperfunction: pheochromocytoma Hypofunction: hypotension

- Hirsutism
- Diabetes or insulin resistance
- Muscle weakness
- Hypertension
- Increased susceptibility to infection
- Frequent fungal infections
- Osteoporosis or osteopenia
- Psychiatric symptom such as depression, mood changes, and even psychosis
- Hypercoagulable state

111. **List the four steps involved in evaluating a patient for Cushing's syndrome.**
   - **Step 1:** screen for and document hypercortisolemia with a 24-hour urine cortisol or dexamethasone suppression test (DST)
   - **Step 2:** differentiate between ACTH-dependent and ACTH-independent causes by measuring ACTH
   - **Step 3:** distinguish pituitary Cushing's disease from ectopic ACTH secretion with a pituitary MRI and/or inferior petrosal sinus sampling (IPSS)
   - **Step 4:** surgically resect the tumor once identified

112. **When should one screen for Cushing's syndrome?**
   In the presence of multiple clinical features of Cushing's syndrome or worsening symptoms suggestive of Cushing's syndrome. However, the symptoms that could be associated with Cushing's syndrome, such as weight gain, hypertension, diabetes, osteoporosis, and depression, are common. Consider screening adults with weight gain, an abnormal fat distribution, proximal muscle weakness, large ($>$1-cm-wide) purple striae, and new cognitive/depression complaints; young people with nontraumatic bone fractures, cutaneous atrophy, or hypertension; patients with incidental adrenal adenomas.

113. **How should one screen for Cushing's syndrome?**
With the low-dose (1-mg) overnight DST, 24-hour urine free cortisol levels, or late-evening salivary cortisol levels.

> Nieman LK, Biller BM, Findling JW, et al: The diagnosis of Cushing's syndrome: an Endocrine Society Clinical Practice Guideline, *J Clin Endocrinol Metab* 93:1526–1540, 2008.

114. **How is the low-dose DST performed?**
Give 1 mg of dexamethasone at 11 PM and measure cortisol at 8 AM the following morning. If the patient does not have Cushing's, the 8 AM cortisol is suppressed to < 1.8 μg/dL if a sensitive assay is used.

115. **How is the 24-hour urine free cortisol test done?**
By collecting urine over 24 hours to measure free cortisol. To ensure an accurate result, the urine collection should be confirmed with a complete and simultaneous urine creatinine excretion. Urinary cortisol should be normal in patients without Cushing's syndrome. This test should be repeated up to three times if the first tests are normal and there is a high index of suspicion.

116. **What is the late-evening salivary cortisol test?**
Measurement of cortisol levels in salivary samples collected late at night (11 PM). Some clinicians advocate this test because it is easy to perform and salivary and plasma cortisol levels are highly correlated. Normal cortisol levels should be low, confirming normal diurnal variation. Cushing's patients have abnormally high late-night levels. Normal ranges are assay-dependent and must be validated for each laboratory. Although helpful as an initial screening test, particularly in patients with episodic hypercortisolemia, many endocrinologists still use the DST or 24-hour urine free cortisol as first-line modalities.

117. **Once hypercortisolemia has been documented, what is the next step in evaluating a patient with Cushing's syndrome?**
Measurement of ACTH and cortisol. If the ACTH > 10 pg/mL, the patient most likely has an ACTH-dependent cause of Cushing's syndrome. In addition, an ACTH value > 10 pg/mL after peripheral corticotropin-releasing hormone (CRH) administration suggests ACTH dependency.
After ruling out ingestion of exogenous steroids, the next step is to differentiate between ACTH-dependent (80%) and ACTH-independent (20%) disease. ACTH-dependent disease is associated with pituitary adenoma (80%), ectopic ACTH (20%), and CRH hypersecretion (rare). ACTH-independent disease is associated with adrenal adenoma (40–50%), adrenal carcinoma (40–50%), nodular dysplasia (rare), and McCune-Albright syndrome (rare).

118. **Once ACTH-dependent Cushing's syndrome has been confirmed, what is the final step in making the biochemical diagnosis?**
A high-dose (8-mg) DST to differentiate between a corticotrope adenoma and an ectopic ACTH-secreting tumor. Patients with a pituitary source of ACTH retain suppressibility of cortisol to high-dose dexamethasone, whereas patients with ectopic ACTH tumors do not.

119. **How is the dexamethasone test confirmed?**
With IPSS. This test takes advantage of the concentration gradient between pituitary venous drainage via the inferior petrosal sinus (IPS—central) and peripheral venous values of ACTH to further determine whether an ACTH-producing corticotropic adenoma is present in the pituitary; the inclusion of CRH stimulation adds greater sensitivity to the test.

120. **Explain how the IPSS is done.**
Samples of ACTH and cortisol are obtained simultaneously from the IPS (central) and from a peripheral site (e.g., inferior vena cava [IVC]). In patients with Cushing's disease, the

central/peripheral ratio (C/P = IPS/IVC ratio) of ACTH > 2. In patients with ectopic ACTH, the ratio < 2 and selective venous sampling (e.g., of the pulmonary, pancreatic, or intestinal beds) may localize the ectopic tumor.

121. **How does the administration of CRH increase diagnostic accuracy during IPSS?**
By eliciting an ACTH response in the few patients with pituitary tumor who did not have a diagnostic C/P gradient in the basal samples. All patients with Cushing's disease have had a C/P ratio > 3 after CRH, whereas patients with ectopic ACTH or adrenal disease have had C/P ratios < 3 after CRH.

122. **What is the most significant limitation of IPSS with or without CRH?**
Because IPSS has not been extensively performed in normal subjects, correct interpretation of the results requires accurate catheter placement and that the patient be hypercortisolemic at the time of the study in order to suppress the response of normal corticotropes to CRH. See Figure 16-2. If results indicate an ectopic source, a CT or MRI of the chest is usually performed first because most are due to small cell carcinoma or bronchial or thymic carcinoid tumors. IPSS should be performed in tertiary-care centers that perform this invasive test often.

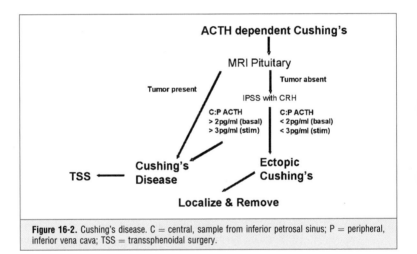

Figure 16-2. Cushing's disease. C = central, sample from inferior petrosal sinus; P = peripheral, inferior vena cava; TSS = transsphenoidal surgery.

123. **What is pseudo-Cushing's syndrome?**
A clinical state characterized by mild overactivity of the hypothalamic-pituitary-adrenal axis that is not associated with true Cushing's syndrome (hypercortisolemia) typically seen in a variety of psychiatric states (depression, anxiety), alcoholism, uncontrolled diabetes, and severe obesity. The dexamethasone-CRH stimulation test can be used to help distinguish this disorder from true Cushing's syndrome. Alternatively, an elevated midnight plasma cortisol level rules out pseudo-Cushing's because, unlike patients with true Cushing's syndrome, patients with pseudo-Cushing's retain the diurnal rhythm of cortisol secretion.

124. **Explain how the dexamethasone-CRH stimulation test is done.**
Patients take 0.5 mg of dexamethasone every 6 hours for 8 doses starting at noon. At 8 AM (after the eighth dose of dexamethasone), CRH (human recombinant CRH [Acthrel]) is given IV at a dose of 1 μg/kg, and cortisol is measured 15 minutes later. A cortisol value > 1.4 mg/dL indicates Cushing's syndrome.

125. **What is Nelson's syndrome?**
Symptoms of a mass effect of corticotrope hyperplasia or adenoma in patients after bilateral adrenalectomy. Nelson's syndrome occurs in up to 30% of patients after bilateral adrenalectomy and patients often present with headache, visual field deficits, ophthalmoplegia, and hyperpigmentation owing to high levels of ACTH (with resultant high levels of melanocyte-stimulating hormone). Pituitary tumor resection followed by pituitary radiation can prevent Nelson's in someone who has had bilateral adrenalectomy.

126. **Define "adrenal insufficiency."**
Insufficient release of adrenal hormone, typically from the adrenal cortex, including cortisol and aldosterone.

127. **What causes adrenal insufficiency?**
The causes can be divided into two categories: primary and central. **Primary adrenal insufficiency** (Addison's disease) is due to adrenal gland dysfunction. **Central adrenal insufficiency** includes both secondary (pituitary) and tertiary (hypothalamic) causes.

128. **List the causes of primary adrenal insufficiency.**
Autoimmune destruction (70–80%), tuberculosis (20%), adrenal destruction by bilateral hemorrhage or infarction, tumor, infections (other than tuberculosis), surgery, radiation, drugs, amyloidosis, sarcoidosis, hyporesponsiveness to ACTH, and congenital abnormalities.

129. **List the causes of central adrenal insufficiency.**
Withdrawal of exogenous steroids (common), treatment and cure of Cushing's syndrome, pituitary adenoma/infarction, other causes of panhypopituitarism, pituitary or brain irradiation, and hypothalamic abnormalities (rare).

130. **What are the major symptoms and signs of Addison's disease?**
See Table 16-7.

TABLE 16-7. CLINICAL PRESENTATION OF PRIMARY ADRENAL INSUFFICIENCY (ADDISON'S DISEASE)	
Symptoms	**Signs**
Weakness, fatigue	Hyperkalemia (mild)
Anorexia, weight loss	Hyponatremia
Dizziness	Orthostatic hypotension
GI upset: nausea, vomiting, diarrhea, abdominal pain	Hyperpigmentation (buccal mucosa, skinfolds, extensor surfaces, new scars)
Salt craving	Vitiligo
	Adrenal calcifications
GI = gastrointestinal.	

131. **How do Addison's disease and central adrenal insufficiency differ in their presentation?**
Primary adrenal insufficiency (Addison's disease) is caused by failure or destruction of the adrenal glands, leading to underproduction of glucocorticoids and mineralocorticoids and

an increase in ACTH production by the pituitary. **Central** adrenal insufficiency is caused by deficient production of ACTH, leading to underproduction of glucocorticoids. The manifestations are the same as those of Addison's disease with the following exceptions:

- Hyperpigmentation is not seen in central disease. Patients do not have hypersecretion of melanocyte-stimulating hormone (a product of the propiomelanocortin gene, like ACTH) that is responsible for the hyperpigmentation.
- Electrolyte abnormalities (hyponatremia, hyperkalemia) are not typically present in central disease because the aldosterone system is largely intact.
- Central disease may involve other manifestations of hypopituitarism.
- Hypoglycemia is more commonly seen with central disease owing to the presence of combined ACTH and GH deficiency.

132. **What test do most clinicians use to assess adrenal insufficiency?**
An ACTH stimulation test. In the classic test, a baseline cortisol is drawn and 250 μg of IV synthetic ACTH (Cortrosyn) is given. Blood samples for cortisol are collected at 30 and 60 minutes. A normal response is a stimulated cortisol value of > 18 μg/dL. A normal response rules out primary adrenal insufficiency. Patients with acute central adrenal insufficiency (i.e., pituitary apoplexy or head trauma) may respond to synthetic ACTH because the adrenal glands have not had sufficient time to become atrophic and unresponsive to ACTH. Lack of a normal response indicates decreased adrenal reserve but does not differentiate between primary and central adrenal insufficiency.

133. **How do you distinguish between primary and central adrenal insufficiency?**
By ACTH level. This level is high in primary adrenal insufficiency and low or normal in central. More recently, clinicians have considered the 250-μg ACTH test less accurate in detecting patients with mild secondary adrenal insufficiency (because it is a supraphysiologic dose) and have recommended a 1-μg ACTH stimulation test. The test is performed the same way as the higher-dose test but requires dilution of the ACTH. ACTH (Cortrosyn) is available only in a 250-μg vial and must be diluted for this low-dose test. Therefore, careful attention must be given to ensure proper administration of the drug to avoid a high false-positive rate.

134. **Summarize the differences in treatment of primary and central adrenal insufficiency.**
Patients with Addison's disease (primary adrenal insufficiency) typically require replacement of both glucocorticoid (prednisone or hydrocortisone) and mineralocorticoid (fludrocortisone) hormones, whereas patients with central adrenal insufficiency typically need only glucocorticoids. Patients with central disease do not usually require mineralocorticoids because aldosterone secretion is largely unaffected. All patients should be instructed to increase steroid replacement during times of illness and should wear medical alert jewelry. The goal of treatment is to ameliorate the signs and symptoms of adrenal insufficiency without causing Cushing's syndrome due to exogenous glucocorticoid replacement. Always use the lowest possible doses that control symptoms to avoid side effects.

135. **What is the gold standard test to assess adequacy of the hypothalamic-pituitary-adrenal axis?**
The insulin tolerance test (ITT). The principle of the test is to induce hypoglycemia (plasma glucose < 40 mg/dL) with IV insulin, which acts as a major stressor to stimulate production of ACTH, cortisol, and GH. The ITT can be dangerous and requires close monitoring.

136. **What are other tests that can be used to diagnose central adrenal insufficiency?**
Besides the ITT, metyrapone can be given at 11 pm to suppress cortisol synthesis. If the pituitary adrenal axis is intact, morning measurements of ACTH and 11-deoxycortisol,

the precursor to cortisol, will rise to > 75 pg/mL and 7 μg/dL, respectively, if there is no secondary adrenal insufficiency. Metyrapone is not commercially available but can be obtained by contacting the manufacturer, Novartis Pharmaceuticals.

137. **Why is it important to rule out adrenal insufficiency in pituitary patients with central hypothyroidism?**
Because patients with central hypothyroidism metabolize cortisol more slowly than euthyroid patients. Thyroid hormone replacement increases cortisol metabolism and can precipitate adrenal crisis in a patient with undiagnosed central adrenal insufficiency. Adrenal insufficiency should be detected and treated before starting thyroid hormone replacement.

138. **What is the "classic triad" of symptoms of pheochromocytoma?**
Episodic headache, diaphoresis, and tachycardia with or without hypertension. The hypertension may be paroxysmal. Other symptoms may include anxiety/psychiatric disturbances, tremor, pallor, visual changes (papilledema, blurred vision), weight loss, polyuria, polydipsia, hyperglycemia, dilated cardiomyopathy, and arrhythmias. Most patients have two of the three symptoms of the classic triad. If the patient is hypertensive and has the classic triad of symptoms, the sensitivity and specificity for pheochromocytoma are both $> 90\%$.

139. **What other diagnoses should be considered in the diagnosis of pheochromocytoma?**
Anxiety/panic attacks, alcoholism (or alcohol withdrawal), sympathomimetic drugs (cocaine, amphetamines, phencyclidine, epinephrine, phenylephrine, terbutaline, and phenylpropanolamine [a popular over-the-counter decongestant]), combined ingestion of MAO inhibitor and tyramine-containing food, hyperthyroidism, menopause, hypoglycemia, and abrupt discontinuation of short-acting sympathetic antagonists (e.g., clonidine).

140. **What is the "rule of 10" for pheochromocytomas?**
- 10% are extra-adrenal
- 10% are bilateral
- 10% are familial
- 10% are malignant

141. **How do you evaluate a patient with suspected pheochromocytoma?**
By making a biochemical diagnosis before embarking on radiographic imaging. Confirming the presence of excess catecholamines is crucial because people can have incidental adrenal tumors that do not hypersecrete catecholamines.

142. **Describe the main screening tests for pheochromocytoma.**
Although preferences may vary by institution, 24-hour urine catecholamines and metanephrines measurements are available in most laboratories. Plasma-free normetanephrine and metanephrine levels are also useful but not readily available. If these values are more than two- to fourfold higher than the upper limit of the normal reference range, proceed to abdominal CT scan or MRI to localize the tumor.

143. **What other tests may be helpful?**
Clonidine suppression test, chromagranin A, and neuropeptide Y.

144. **Under what conditions is the 24-hour urine test performed?**
Usually when the patient is symptomatic because catecholamine hypersecretion may be episodic. If possible, testing should be performed after discontinuing medications. TCAs and antipsychotics are most likely to interfere with the measurement. Caffeine, alcohol, acetaminophen, decongestants, and tobacco should be avoided during testing. Cocaine, appetite suppression drugs, and other sympathomimetics should also be discontinued.

145. **Describe the clonidine suppression test.**
Plasma catecholamines are measured before and 3 hours after oral administration of 0.3 mg of clonidine. Failure to suppress plasma catecholamines suggests the diagnosis of pheochromocytoma. This test must not be performed in hypovolemic patients or patients taking diuretics, beta blockers, or TCAs.

146. **After the biochemical diagnosis is made, how is the tumor localized?**
By using CT or MRI (first of the adrenals, then of the chest, abdomen, and pelvis). If the tumor cannot be localized with standard imaging, perform an ^{123}I metaiodobenzylguanidine (MIBG) scan to localize functional catecholamine-rich tissue.

Pacak K, Linehan WM, Eisenhofer G, et al: Recent advances in genetics, diagnosis, localization, and treatment of pheochromocytoma, *Ann Intern Med* 134:315–329, 2001.

147. **What is the treatment of choice for patients with pheochromocytomas?**
Surgery after the tumor is localized. All patients must be preoperatively treated with alpha adrenergic (phenoxybenzamine) and beta adrenergic (atenolol) blockade to avoid stress-induced catecholamine excess and hypertensive crisis during surgery. Dose should be titrated to cause orthostatic hypotension. If only beta adrenergic blockade is provided, the patient may develop peripheral vasoconstriction and an exacerbation of hypertension.

148. **What is an adrenal incidentaloma?**
Previously unsuspected adrenal mass that is detected in approximately 1% of all abdominal CT scans. These tumors fall into three categories: nonfunctioning mass, hyperfunctioning mass, and pseudoadrenal mass. Because approximately 10% are hormonally active and < 3% are adrenocortical carcinomas, it is important to assess hormonal hyperfunction and malignant potential.

149. **How do you evaluate an adrenal incidentaloma?**
Although there are numerous approaches, evaluations should be individualized. A careful history and physical examination may detect signs and symptoms of hormone excess. Screening for Cushing's syndrome (24-hr urine free cortisol and/or 1-mg overnight DST) and pheochromocytoma (24-hr urine metanephrines/catecholamines or plasma metanephrines) are helpful. If the patient is hypertensive, tests for hyperaldosteronism are indicated. Plasma aldosterone concentration (PAC) and plasma renin activity (PRA) may be used to test for an aldosterone-secreting tumor, looking for an PAC/PRA ratio > 20–25. Nonfunctioning tumors < 4 cm are typically observed for growth. Functional tumors or tumors > 4 cm (or growing) are typically removed by surgery. On unenhanced CT imaging, adrenal tumors with Hounsfield units < 10 and a smooth border are almost always benign. On delayed-contrast enhanced CT images, benign adenomas wash out contrast more than 50% compared with malignant adrenal tumors, metastases, or pheochromocytomas, which metabolize contrast more slowly and wash-out characteristics < 50%.

Young WF Jr: Clinical practice. The incidentally discovered adrenal mass, *N Engl J Med* 356:601–610, 2007.

150. **What is primary hyperaldosteronism?**
Excessive production of aldosterone independent of the renin-angiotensin system, found in approximately 0.5–2% of the population. The differential diagnosis includes solitary aldosterone-producing adenoma (65%), bilateral or unilateral adrenal hyperplasia, adrenal carcinoma, and glucocorticoid-remediable aldosteronism.

151. **How do patients with primary hyperaldosteronism present?**
With hypertension, hypokalemia (weakness, muscle cramping, paresthesias, headaches), low magnesium levels, and metabolic alkalosis.

152. **How should patients with primary hyperaldosteronism be evaluated initially?**
With a morning ambulatory plasma aldosterone level and PRA in the absence of drugs that alter the renin-aldosterone axis (spironolactone, eplerenone or high-dose amiloride). A ratio of plasma aldosterone concentration to plasma renin activity ratio of ≥ 20 and a plasma aldosterone concentration of ≥ 15 ng per deciliter makes the diagnosis of hyperaldosteronism likely.

153. **How is the diagnosis of primary hyperaldosteronism confirmed?**
With a high 24-hour urine aldosterone level in the presence of normokalemia and adequate volume status or inadequate suppression of aldosterone levels using the saline suppression or salt-loading test. As always, biochemical diagnosis should precede diagnostic imaging. Treatment depends on the etiology but usually includes surgery except in cases of adrenal hyperplasia or glucocorticoid-remediable hyperaldosteronism. Renal vein sampling can lateralize the aldosterone source before surgery.

154. **How should renal vein sampling be performed?**
By an experienced interventional radiologist. Cortisol and aldosterone should be sampled in the vena cava and right and left adrenal vein before and after cortrosyn stimulation. Cortisol concentration in the adrenal veins should be 10 times higher than peripheral (vena cava) measurements. Cortisol concentration should be slightly higher in the right over the left adrenal vein. Aldosterone measurements should be adjusted for this difference.

THYROID GLAND

155. **Diagram the hypothalamic-pituitary-thyroid axis.**
See Figure 16-3.

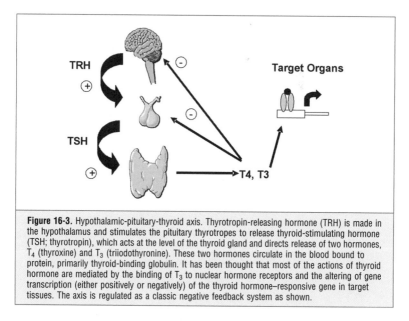

Figure 16-3. Hypothalamic-pituitary-thyroid axis. Thyrotropin-releasing hormone (TRH) is made in the hypothalamus and stimulates the pituitary thyrotropes to release thyroid-stimulating hormone (TSH; thyrotropin), which acts at the level of the thyroid gland and directs release of two hormones, T_4 (thyroxine) and T_3 (triiodothyronine). These two hormones circulate in the blood bound to protein, primarily thyroid-binding globulin. It has been thought that most of the actions of thyroid hormone are mediated by the binding of T_3 to nuclear hormone receptors and the altering of gene transcription (either positively or negatively) of the thyroid hormone-responsive gene in target tissues. The axis is regulated as a classic negative feedback system as shown.

156. **Describe the laboratory findings in hyperthyroidism and hypothyroidism.**
See Table 16-8.

TABLE 16-8.   LABORATORY TESTING IN THYROID DISEASE

Laboratory Test	Hyperthyroidism	Hypothyroidism
TSH	Low or undetectable	High
Free T_4	High	Low
Total T_4	High	Low
Free T_3 (not often accurate)	High	Low
Total T_3	High	Low
T_3 resin uptake*	Usually high if no TBG abnormality	Usually low if no TBG abnormality

T_3 = triiodothyronine; T_4 = thyroxine; TBG = thyroid-binding globulin; TSH = thyroid-stimulating hormone.
*Inverse measure of thyroid hormone binding sites on TBG.

---

157. **Distinguish between subclinical and overt thyroid disease.**
    Thyroid disease occurs along a continuum. At either end is hyperthyroidism or hypothyroidism. Milder forms of thyroid dysfunction are often referred to as **subclinical** disease, meaning below the limit of detection by clinical evaluation. **Overt** disease refers to hyperthyroidism or hypothyroidism with classic clinical signs and symptoms, abnormal TSH, and abnormal hormone levels.

158. **Discuss the significance of subclinical thyroid disease.**
    Subclinical disease was originally thought to be a laboratory diagnosis in which patients had an abnormal TSH and normal thyroid hormone levels and were "asymptomatic." We now know that subclinical disease is often associated with subtle clinical signs and symptoms and that it represents an early, mild form of thyroid disease. Although these milder forms of thyroid dysfunction have been shown to be associated with abnormal physiology (particularly subclinical hypothyroidism), treatment is currently quite controversial. Many thyroidologists believe that treatment should be initiated in patients with mild forms of the disease. However, a recent consensus panel concluded that the data regarding benefits of detection and treatment of subclinical cases were not well established. Therefore, clinical judgment should prevail. Women of childbearing age with subclinical hypothyroidism should be treated with thyroid hormone for several reasons. First, the effects of untreated maternal hypothyroidism can cause cognitive developmental delays in the fetus. Second, maternal thyroid hormone requirements increase by 30–50% during pregnancy owing to high estrogen effects to increase thyroid hormone–binding globulin and thus thyroid hormone–carrying capacity. Third, the fetus can not provide its own thyroid hormone until 12 weeks' gestation. Women with subclinical hypothyroidism who become pregnant may not be able to supply the 30–50% extra necessary. Treatment of patients with subclinical hyperthyroidism should also be considered when there is concomitant osteoporosis or atrial fibrillation present.

Col NF, Surks MI, Daniels GH: Subclinical thyroid disease: Clinical applications, *JAMA* 291:239–243, 2004.

Sirks MI, Ortiz E, Daniels GH, et al: Subclinical thyroid disease: Scientific review and guidelines for diagnosis and management, *JAMA* 291:228–238, 2004.

Helfand M: Screening for subclinical thyroid dysfunction in nonpregnant adults: A summary of the evidence for the U.S. Preventive Services Task Force, *Ann Intern Med* 140:128–141, 2004.

159. **How common is thyroid disease?**
Relatively common, affecting more women than men. Subclinical thyroid disease is more common than overt disease. The prevalence of hypothyroidism increases with age in both men and women. In fact, more than 20% of women older than 60 years have hypothyroidism. General overall prevalence rates are as follows.
- **Hyperthyroidism:** 1.2% (0.5% overt and 0.7% subclinical).
- **Hypothyroidism:** 4.6% (0.3% overt and 4.3% subclinical).

Hollowell JG, Staehling NW, Flanders WD, et al: Serum TSH, T(4), and thyroid antibodies in the United States population (1988–1994): National Health and Nutrition Examination Survey (NHANES III), *J Clin Endocrinol Metab* 87:489–499, 2002.

Canaris GJ, Manowitz MR, Mayor G, et al: The Colorado thyroid disease prevalence study, *Arch Intern Med* 160:526–534, 2000.

KEY POINTS: THYROID GLAND ✔

1. The best initial screening test for evaluation of thyroid status is the TSH level.

2. TSH is the most sensitive measure of thyroid function in the majority of patients.

3. The one exception is patients with pituitary/hypothalamic dysfunction, in whom TSH cannot be used to reliably to assess thyroid function.

TSH = thyroid-stimulating hormone.

160. **How do you evaluate a patient with hyperthyroidism?**
By history, physical examination, and thyroid function tests including TSH, thyroxine (T_4), and triiodothyronine (T_3). Thyroid function tests usually show a low or undetectable TSH, high or normal T_4, and high or normal T_3. Normal T_4 and T_3 in the presence of low or undetectable TSH typically suggest subclinical hyperthyroidism except in the patient with pituitary dysfunction. The TSH is not a reliable indicator of hyperthyroidism in patients with pituitary dysfunction.

161. **Describe the presentation of patients with hyperthyroidism.**
See Table 16-9.

162. **What is the differential diagnosis of hyperthyroidism?**
Thyroid gland hyperfunction as in Graves' disease and autonomously functioning nodule(s), inflammation and destruction of all or part of the gland with resultant release of stored hormone (thyroiditis), or an exogenous thyroid hormone source outside the thyroid.

163. **How does the thyroid ^{123}I scan help differentiate among the different causes of hyperthyroidism?**
By demonstrating the pattern and degree of ^{123}I uptake by the thyroid gland. See Table 16-10.

164. **What is Graves' disease?**
An autoimmune disease in which patients develop antibodies that mimic TSH by binding to its receptor on thyroid cells to stimulate thyroid hormone production. Graves' disease is the most common cause of endogenous hyperthyroidism.

165. **What is thyroid storm?**
A dramatic, life-threatening exacerbation of hyperthyroidism (thyrotoxicosis), associated with a 20% mortality rate if untreated. Thyroid storm is diagnosed clinically based on the severity of hyperthyroidism.

TABLE 16-9.   CLINICAL PRESENTATION OF HYPERTHYROIDISM

Symptoms	Signs
Lethargy, fatigue	Tremor
Anxiety/palpitations	Tachycardia/atrial arrhythmias/hypertension
Hyperactivity	Rarely congestive heart failure; often
Increased defecation	hyperdynamic precordium
Weight loss	Agitation (mental status alterations if severe or
Sleep disturbance/insomnia	in elderly patients)
Heat intolerance	Goiter
Menstrual irregularities in women	Increased deep tendon reflexes
Erectile dysfunction in men	Warm, moist, soft skin
Infertility	Proximal muscle weakness
Increased appetite	Ophthalmopathy: lid lag, stare (Graves' disease:
Poor exercise capacity, dyspnea	proptosis, diplopia, color vision changes,
	optic neuropathy, chemosis, eye irritation,
	extraocular muscle dysfunction)
	Brittle nails
	Edema (Graves' disease: pretibial myxedema)

TABLE 16-10.   CAUSES OF HYPERTHYROIDISM

Etiology	^{123}I Scan Pattern	RAIU (%)	Pathogenesis
Common Causes			
Graves' disease	Homogenous	High uptake (can be high normal)	Stimulating TSH receptor antibody
Multinodular goiter	Patchy	Moderate uptake	Autonomous thyroid function
Solitary toxic nodule	Suppressed gland with one area of high uptake	Normal gland with suppressed uptake, high nodule uptake	Autonomous thyroid function
Thyroiditis Silent Subacute Drug-induced Radiation-induced	Homogeneous	Low uptake	Release of preformed hormone
Exogenous thyroid hormone ingestion	Homogeneous	Low uptake	Excess thyroid hormone in drug or food

(continued)

TABLE 16-10.   CAUSES OF HYPERTHYROIDISM—*(continued)*

Etiology	¹²³I Scan Pattern	RAIU (%)	Pathogenesis
Less Common Causes			
Hashitoxicosis	Patchy	Moderate uptake	Release of preformed hormone
Iodine (Jod-Basedow)	Homogeneous	Low uptake	Iodine excess
Hyperemesis gravidarum	Do not scan due to pregnant state	Would expect high uptake	Circulating hCG
Lithium	Variable	High uptake	Variable
Rare Causes			
TSH-producing pituitary adenoma	Homogeneous	High uptake (can be normal)	Excess TSH production from tumor
Pituitary resistance to thyroid hormone	Homogeneous	High uptake (can be normal)	Excess TSH production from impaired feedback
Choriocarcinoma Trophoblastic disease	Homogeneous	High uptake	Circulating hCG cross-reacts with TSH receptor
Struma ovarii (teratoma)	Homogeneous	Low uptake	Ovarian teratoma
Metastatic thyroid cancer	Homogeneous	Low uptake	Foci of functional autonomous tissue
Thyroid adenoma infarction	Homogeneous	Low uptake	Release of preformed hormone

hCG = human choriogonadotropin; RAIU = radioactive iodine uptake; TSH = thyroid-stimulating hormone.

166. **Describe the presentation of thyroid storm.**
Severe signs and symptoms of hyperthyroidism including severe tachycardia, cardiac arrhythmias, heart failure, fever, GI disturbances (hepatitis, jaundice), and mental status changes.

167. **How is thyroid storm treated?**
With general supportive care (often in the intensive care unit) and initiation of the following medications:
- Antithyroid medication (propylthiouracil [PTU]) to block thyroid hormone synthesis and peripheral conversion of T_4 to T_3.
- Beta blockers (propranolol or IV esmolol) to inhibit the adrenergic system.
- Saturated solution of potassium iodide or other iodine-rich compounds (Gastrograffin, ipodate) to block the release of preformed thyroid hormones.

- Glucocorticoids may also be part of the initial management because thyroid hormones increase metabolism of endogenous cortisol and steroids can inhibit conversion of T_4 to T_3.

168. **Summarize the treatment approach to hyperthyroidism.**
Treatment is based on the etiology of the hyperthyroidism. The most common causes are overly zealous replacement of thyroid hormone, Graves' disease, hyperfunctioning nodular disease, and thyroiditis. Overreplacement is easily treated by titrating down the thyroid hormone dose. All hyperthyroid patients benefit from beta blockers to treat the hyperadrenergic state.

169. **How is Graves' disease treated?**
With ^{131}I radioiodine ablation or antithyroid drugs (ATDs). Surgery can be performed to remove the Graves' gland, but most patients prefer the nonsurgical options.

170. **How is solitary or multinodular disease treated?**
With ^{131}I ablation or surgery, particularly if the gland is large and the patient has compressive symptoms. ATDs can be used to render patients euthyroid, but typically not recommended for long-term use because they do not treat the underlying pathophysiology of the disease. The hyperthyroidism invariably returns if the ATD is discontinued.

171. **Describe the treatment of thyroiditis.**
With beta blockers until the usually transient thryoiditis resolves. Some patients with painful or subacute thyroiditis can be treated with steroids if the pain is particularly severe.

172. **How are ATDs used in Graves' patients?**
As primary treatment or short-term management in preparation for ^{131}I radioablation. If the second approach is chosen, the ATD must be discontinued 7–10 days prior to the ^{131}I ablation so that it will not inhibit iodine uptake into the gland. ATDs should be titrated to normalize the TSH and T_4 (total or free T_4). Because normalization of TSH lags behind normalization of the T_4 level (by $\sim$4–6 wk), both laboratory tests must be monitored initially to avoid induction of hypothyroidism. Patients are typically treated with an ATD for 12–18 months, then tapered off to determine whether they have remained in remission. Relapse rates are high (50–60%) within the first year and are highest in patients with large goiters and more severe hyperthyroidism.

173. **Compare the two available ATDs.**
Both ATDs, PTU and methimazole (Tapazole) inhibit T_4 and T_3 synthesis by the thyroid gland and are effective for treating hyperthyroidism. PTU has been associated with acute hepatic injury and should only be used in patients unable to tolerate other therapies or in pregnant women during or just before the first trimester. PTU is preferred for treating pregnant patients because methimazole has been associated with a rare congenital scalp defect known as "aplasia cutis." Methimazole is more convenient than PTU due to its once-daily dosing.

174. **Summarize the side effects of ATDs.**
   - Rash (most common)
   - Abnormal taste
   - Agranulocytosis (0.2–0.5%)
   - Mild elevated transaminases
   - Fulminant hepatitis (rare)
   - Vasculitis

Side effects can occur at any time and at any dose, although higher doses are associated with higher risk of adverse effects. Patients should be warned to stop the medication if they experience sore throat, fever, or joint pain.

175. **What is T_3 toxicosis?**
Hyperthyroidism that is due primarily to high T_3 levels. Such patients have a low or undetectable TSH, normal T_4, and elevated T_3. It is important to check the T_3 level in patients whom you suspect of having subclinical hyperthyroidism to rule out T_3 toxicosis. The differential diagnosis, evaluation, and treatment are otherwise the same as for patients with hyperthyroidism due to any cause.

176. **How do you confirm a diagnosis of hypothyroidism?**
By history, physical examination, and thyroid function tests that show elevated TSH, low or normal T_4, and low or normal T_3. Normal hormone levels in the presence of an elevated TSH suggest subclinical hypothyroidism. TSH is a more sensitive marker of thyroid disease than circulating hormone levels and even if the T_4 or T_3 laboratory measurement is normal, the thyroid hormone level may not be physiologically "normal" for that particular patient if the TSH is elevated. Measurement of thyroid antibodies is not routinely indicated in the evaluation of primary hypothyroidism, but can identify Hashimoto's thyroiditis.

177. **When should thyroid autoantibodies be measured?**
The presence of antithyroid peroxidase antibodies can be helpful in predicting which patients with subclinical hypothyroidism may progress over time to overt disease. Thyroid-stimulating immunoglobulins (TSIs) and thyrotropin receptor antibodies (TRAbs) should be monitored in pregnant women with a history of active or ablative Graves' in the second trimester to determine whether the fetus has a risk for fetal or neonatal Graves' or goiter.
Antithyroglobulin antibodies should be monitored in patients with well-differentiated thyroid cancer to assess the reliability of thyroglobulin as a tumor marker.

178. **How do hypothyroid patients present clinically?**
See Table 16-11.

179. **What are the pathologic types of hypothyroidism?**
Primary, secondary, tertiary, and peripheral (generalized) resistance to thyroid hormone

180. **Explain the mechanisms of primary hypothyroidism.**
Any pathologic process intrinsic to the thyroid gland, leading to defective production of thyroid hormone or destruction of the gland.

181. **What are the causes of primary hypothyroidism?**
- Thyroiditis (Hashimoto's, silent, painful/subacute, postpartum, and drug-induced)
- "Burnt-out" Graves' disease
- Thyroid ablation from any cause (radiation, radioactive iodine, surgical resection, and metastatic tumor/neoplasia)
- Thyroid hormone biosynthetic defects
- Iodine deficiency
- Thyroid agenesis or dysgenesis

182. **What is the most common cause of primary hypothyroidism?**
Hashimoto's thyroiditis

183. **How does secondary hypothyroidism develop?**
When there is a deficiency of TSH from the pituitary (central hypothyroidism), most frequently found in patients with pituitary tumors or pituitary damage (e.g., radiation, surgery).

TABLE 16-11. CLINICAL PRESENTATION OF HYPOTHYROIDISM

Symptoms	Signs
Lethargy, fatigue	Goiter
Dry skin	Dry skin (common in dry climates)
Hair loss, brittle hair, brittle nails	Coarse hair, alopecia, brittle nails
Decreased energy	Delayed relaxation phase of deep
Constipation	tendon reflexes
Weight gain (not usually > 50 lb)	Periorbital edema, edema
Hoarseness	Deepened voice
Cold intolerance	Hypothermia
Menstrual irregularities in women	Lipid abnormalities (elevated
Erectile dysfunction in men	cholesterol, LDL)
Infertility	Elevated transaminases, creatinine
Children: precocious or delayed puberty,	phosphokinase
abnormal growth/cognition	Reduced respiratory effort
Depression, cognitive dysfunction	Proximal muscle weakness
Poor exercise capacity, dyspnea	Bradycardia, hypertension,
Muscle pain, joint stiffness	cardiomegaly
Chest pain/angina	Neuropathy
Paresthesias	

LDL = low-density lipoprotein.

184. **Name the major cause of tertiary hypothyroidism.**
A deficiency of TRH from the hypothalamus (central hypothyroidism).

185. **What is peripheral (generalized) resistance to thyroid hormone?**
A rare genetic cause of hypothyroidism in which patients have generalized tissue resistance to thyroid hormone due to mutations in the thyroid hormone beta receptor gene. There is also a form that seems to cause primarily pituitary resistance to thyroid hormone. Unlike patients with generalized resistance, these patients present with symptoms of tissue hyperthyroidism and high T_4 and T_3 levels accompanied by an elevated or "inappropriately" normal TSH.

186. **How should hypothyroidism be treated?**
With levothyroxine (T_4). The goal is to reverse the clinical syndrome by restoring the TSH and hormone levels to the normal range. A typical replacement dose is 1.6 µg/kg/day in young healthy patients. Elderly patients often require lower doses. The best approach is to "start low, go slow." When initiating therapy, measure the TSH every 4–6 weeks with dose adjustments until the goal TSH is reached. More frequent measurements are not useful because the half-life of the drug is 7 days and the TSH should be measured in a state of equilibrium. Once the patient is on a stable dose, the TSH can be monitored annually unless there are changes in the patient's clinical status.

187. **How does iodide affect thyroid gland function?**
Through multiple inhibitory effects on thyroid function, including decreased iodide transport, decreased iodide organification, and decreased thyroid hormone secretion.

188. **Describe the Wolff-Chaikoff effect.**
The normal transient inhibitory effect of an iodide load on thyroid function causing hypothyroidism and/or decreased thyroid hormone production. Most patients "escape" from these inhibitory effects within 2–4 weeks after iodide exposure.

189. **What is the Jod-Basedow phenomenon?**
Iodide-induced thyrotoxicosis. This phenomenon typically occurs in elderly patients with underlying nodular thyroid disease after they receive an iodide load such as radiographic contrast. In iodide-deficient countries, the Jod-Basedow phenomenon can occur after reintroduction of iodide in patients with goiter.

190. **Describe postpartum thyroiditis.**
An inflammation of the thyroid that can cause both hyperthyroidism and hypothyroidism. This inflammation occurs in approximately 5–9% of women after pregnancy, with a higher frequency (25%) in women with type 1 DM. Pathology reveals an inflammatory process that is indistinguishable from lymphocytic thyroiditis (Hashimoto's disease). In fact, women with positive antithyroid antibodies are at much higher risk of developing postpartum thyroiditis and permanent thyroid dysfunction.

191. **What are the phases of postpartum thyroiditis?**
- **Hyperthyroidism** (lasting 1–3 mo)
- **Hypothyroidism** (lasting 4–8 mo)
- **Euthyroid state**
Only 25–30% of women develop permanent hypothyroidism, and the clinician should assess whether a woman has returned to a euthyroid phase before prescribing unnecessary life-long therapy with thyroid hormone.

192. **List the risk factors for malignancy in a thyroid nodule.**
- Family history of thyroid cancer
- Age < 20 or > 60 years
- Rapid growth of a preexisting nodule
- Large, painful, or firm nodule
- Invasive and compressive symptoms
- Lymphadenopathy
- Fixation of nodule to adjacent structures
- Vocal cord paresis
- History of head and neck irradiation
Any nodule $\geq$ 1–1.5 cm should be evaluated with fine-needle aspiration in a clinically euthyroid patient.

193. **What is the most cost-effective method for evaluating a thyroid nodule?**
TSH and fine-needle aspiration biopsy (FNAB). Radioiodide (RAI) thyroid scan is recommended only in patients with a low TSH to detect hyperthyroidism. FNAB is recommended for patients nodules detected on ultrasound and normal or high TSH.

Cooper DS, Doherty GM, Haugen BR, et al: Revised American Thyroid Association management guidelines for patients with thyroid nodules and differentiated thyroid cancer, *Thyroid* 19:1167–1214, 2009.

194. **What is the 5–10% rule for thyroid nodules?**
- 5–10% of people have palpable nodules (more common in women).
- 5–10% of nodules are cancerous (overall lifetime risk of thyroid cancer 1%).
- 5–10% of thyroid cancer is associated with high morbidity and mortality rates.

195. **List the types of thyroid cancer.**
  - **Thyroid epithelial cell cancers:** papillary (75%), follicular (10%), Hurthle cell, anaplastic. Papillary and follicular thyroid cancers are considered "differentiated" thyroid cancer.
  - **Thyroidal C-cell cancer** (calcitonin-secreting): medullary thyroid cancer.
  - **Primary thyroid lymphoma.**

196. **How should differentiated thyroid cancer be treated?**
  Usually with thyroidectomy. In higher risk patients, radioiodide (RAI) therapy can be used while TSH is elevated. Thyroid hormone withdrawal for four weeks can raise the TSH naturally or patients can receive synthetic recombinant human TSH (rhTSH [Thyrogen]). RAI has been shown to reduce the risk of cancer recurrence in selected patients. Some centers use RAI to facilitate monitoring, but other centers are moving away from this practice due to the risks of RAI, including the rare increase in secondary malignancy, siladenitis and tear duct dysfunction. Patients are treated with thyroid hormone to keep the TSH suppressed. The level of TSH suppression is determined by the aggressiveness of the disease (initial stage), risk of recurrence, and time elapsed from initial diagnosis. This therapy has been shown to decrease cancer recurrence and mortality and to facilitate monitoring for residual/recurrent cancer.

197. **Describe the typical follow-up for patients with differentiated thyroid cancer.**
  Serial physical examinations, thyroglobulin (tumor marker) measurements both on thyroid hormone suppression therapy and after TSH stimulation, diagnostic whole-body ^{131}I scans (WBSs), and thyroid ultrasound. Previously, TSH stimulation was achieved by induction of hypothyroidism after withdrawal of thyroid hormone. Because an elevated TSH is required to stimulate ^{131}I uptake into thyroid cells, patients typically discontinue thyroid hormone replacement a number of weeks before the WBS and thyroglobulin test. As expected, hypothyroidism is uncomfortable for most patients, and some patients experience very severe symptoms and refuse or delay these cancer-monitoring procedures. See Question 198 for a discussion of the use of rhTSH.

  Cooper DS, Doherty GM, Haugen BR, et al: Revised American Thyroid Association management guidelines for patients with thyroid nodules and differentiated thyroid cancer, *Thyroid* 19:1167–1214, 2009.

198. **What other option for monitoring is available?**
  Fortunately, the development of recombinant human thyroid-stimulating hormone (rhTSH) provides a tool whereby TSH levels can be elevated without the need for the patient to become hypothyroid. This discovery has revolutionized care of patients with thyroid cancer. Although rhTSH is currently approved by the FDA for diagnostic monitoring of differentiated thyroid cancer and remnant ablation, the overall goal is to have no evidence of disease based on negative imaging studies and undetectable thyroglobulin levels.

  Woodmansee WW, Haugen BR: A review of the potential uses for recombinant human TSH in patients with thyroid cancer and nodular goiter, *Clin Endocrinol* 61:163–173, 2004.

199. **What is thyroglobulin?**
  A normal protein produced by benign and malignant thyroid cells. Elevated levels of TSH can stimulate thyroglobulin production. Patients who have had thyroidectomy and ^{131}I remnant ablation should not have any residual cells to make thyroglobulin; thus, thyroglobulin can be used as a tumor marker to determine whether there are residual thyroid cells present.

200. **What are the limits of thyroglobulin measurement?**
  Thyroglobulin measurement in patients with thyroglobulin antibodies cannot be measured accurately. Patients who have been treated only with surgery and not ^{131}I therapy will have some residual thyroglobulin production. Dedifferentiated thyroid cancer may not produce thyroglobulin.

201. **How do you determine the initial degree of thyroid hormone suppression needed after thyroid cancer treatment?**
By the disease risk. Low-risk patients have no metastases, no residual tumor, no local tumor invasion, non-aggressive pathology, and no ^{131}I uptake outside the thyroid bed (if given). Low-risk patients should have TSH suppression to 0.1–0.5 mU/L. All other (intermediate and high-risk) patients should have TSH suppression to <0.1 mU/L. Patients with heart disease and elderly patients may also require a higher TSH goal. Long-term suppression goals will vary for the individual patient.

REPRODUCTIVE ENDOCRINOLOGY

202. **Define "erectile dysfunction (ED)."**
The inability to obtain and maintain an erection sufficient for sexual intercourse. ED is usually multifactorial in etiology, and most men have at least some psychogenic factors that contribute to the disorder (i.e., performance anxiety can exacerbate underlying organic etiology).

203. **List the six main categories of ED.**
- **Hormonal:** Hypogonadism (primary or secondary), hyperprolactinemia (with resultant hypogonadism), hyperthyroidism or hypothyroidism, diabetes, adrenal insufficiency, and Cushing's syndrome.
- **Pharmacologic:** Many causative medications such as antihypertensives (clonidine, beta blockers, vasodilators, thiazide diuretics, spironolactone); antidepressants (SSRIs, TCAs); antipsychotics; anxiolytics; cimetidine; phenytoin; carbamazepine; ketoconazole; metoclopramide; digoxin; alcohol; and, illicit drugs (marijuana, cocaine, and heroin).
- **Systemic disease:** Any severe illness that leads to hypogonadotrophic hypogonadism.
- **Vascular:** Diabetes, peripheral arterial disease.
- **Neurologic:** Diabetes, spinal cord injury, neuropathy.
- **Psychogenic:** Uncommon in isolation, but contributes to most cases owing to other etiologies and should be considered a diagnosis of exclusion.

204. **Describe the typical evaluation of a patient with ED.**
- Detailed history including alcohol and illicit drug use, timing of symptom onset (gradual vs. sudden), satisfaction with current sexual partner, occurrence of nocturnal erections, previous surgeries, and current medical illnesses
- Review of medications
- Physical examination with particular attention to lower extremity vasculature, genitals, and findings of hypogonadism
- Endocrine laboratory testing (TSH, prolactin, and testosterone)
- Systemic disease testing (urinalysis, complete chemisty panel, A_1C, and complete blood count)
- Nocturnal penile tumescence testing if assessment of erectile function is needed

205. **What are the most important steps in the management of ED?**
Identifying and treating organic etiologies and discontinuing any offending medications, if possible.

206. **What are the potential treatment options for men with ED?**
- Correction of any hormonal abnormality, such as testosterone replacement for hypogonadism, correction of thyroid dysfunction, maximal glycemic control in diabetes, and treatment of hyperprolactinemia with dopamine agonist.
- Treatment of any underlying systemic disorders, including depression, but note that, although SSRIs can cause ED, SSRIs may help to prevent premature ejaculation.

- Medical therapy (see Question 207).
- Mechanical devices including rings, vacuum pump device that may be cumbersome to some patients, but have minimal side effects.
- Surgical interventions, typically used as a last resort and include revascularization, removal of venous shunts, and penile implants.
- Supportive counseling and/or couples therapy.

207. **What medical therapies are available for ED?**
- Alpha$_2$ adrenergic receptor blocker: yohimbine (oral).
- Phosphodiesterase 5 inhibitors: sildenafil (Viagra), vardenafil (Levitra), and tadalafil (Cialis). All three are administered orally, but none should be used in combination with nitrates.
- Intracavernosal injections of vasodilating medications: alprostadil (Caverject), prostaglandin E$_1$, papaverine, and phentolamine.
- Transurethral alprostadil suppositories (Muse).

208. **List the three etiologic categories of gynecomastia.**
Idiopathic, physiologic, and pathologic.

209. **List the physiologic changes that occur throughout the life cycle that may lead to gynecomastia.**
- **Newborn:** Owing to fetal exposure to maternal estrogens during pregnancy.
- **Puberty:** Owing to increased estrogen-to-androgen ratio.
- **Older ages:** Likely due to combined effect of decreasing testosterone with age and increased estrogen owing to peripheral aromatization of androgens to estrogens in adipose tissue, but the exact mechanism is unclear.

210. **What causes pathologic gynecomastia?**
Usually, estrogen excess from either overproduction or peripheral aromatization including:
- Drugs that increase estrogen activity or production or reduce testosterone activity or production.
- Tumors that increase human chorionic gonadotropin (hCG) or estrogen production, such as testicular tumors (Leydig cell, Sertoli cell, germ cell, and granulosa cell), choriocarcinomas, and adrenal tumors. Male breast cancer is an uncommon cause.
- Decreased androgens or androgen resistance as found in hypogonadism due to any cause such as Klinefelter's syndrome (male with extra X chromosome) and Kallmann's syndrome (hypogonadotropic hypogonadism with absent sense of smell).
- Increased activity of enzyme that catalyzes estrogen production (aromatase) that is found in obesity, hyperthyroidism, and certain genetic mutations.
- Displacement of estrogens from sex hormone–binding globulin.
- Other illnesses such as end-stage liver disease, renal disease, human immunodeficiency virus (HIV) infection, familial syndromes, and starvation refeeding.

211. **How does one begin to evaluate the causes of amenorrhea?**
First, determine whether amenorrhea is primary (the patient has never had menses) or secondary (cessation of menses after she has started). Next, rule out pregnancy as a cause of amenorrhea. After pregnancy is ruled out, consider the following four broad categories of amenorrhea:
- Anatomic/outflow tract defect
- Ovarian failure
- Hypogonadotropic hypogonadism (pituitary or hypothalamic failure)
- Chronic anovulation

KEY POINTS: REPRODUCTIVE ENDOCRINOLOGY ✓

1. The most common presentation of hypogonadism in men is erectile dysfunction and decreased libido.

2. The most common presentation of hypogonadism in women is amenorrhea and infertility.

212. **Give examples of anatomic/outflow tract defects.**
   - Imperforate hymen
   - Asherman's syndrome (amenorrhea due to uterine adhesions)
   - Müllerian agenesis
   - Sexual differentiation disorders

213. **What are the causes of primary ovarian failure?**
   - Genetic alterations (Turner's syndrome with XO genotype)
   - Autoimmune destruction
   - LH or FSH receptor or postreceptor defects
   - Physical insults (radiation, chemotherapy, viral infection, oophorectomy)
   Levels of FSH and LH are generally high in these disorders (hypergonadotrophic hyogonadism).

214. **List the causes of hypogonadotropic hypogonadism.**
   - Hypothalmic dysfunction (induced by exercise or eating disorders)
   - Pituitary dysfunction (such as tumors and hypopituitarism)
   - Androgen excess (due to adrenal tumors, PCOS, tumors with high human choriogonadotropin, and congenital adrenal hyperplasia)
   - Thyroid dysfunction (hyperthyroidism and hypothyroidism)
   - Systemic illness (such as liver and renal disease)
   - Obesity
   - Adrenal dysfunction
   Levels of FSH and LH are generally low in these disorders.

215. **Describe PCOS.**
   Also known as "Stein-Leventhal syndrome," PCOS is characterized by (1) oligo- or anovulation, (2) hyperandrogenism, and (3) polycystic ovaries. Patients can be diagnosed with PCOS if they have at least two of the three classic features and other etiologies have been excluded.

216. **How do women with PCOS typically present?**
   With menstrual dysfunction, hirsutism, and insulin resistance. Long-term consequences of PCOS include increased risk of developing type 2 DM, hyperlipidemia, and endometrial cancer.

217. **Describe the management of PCOS.**
   Correction of the underlying metabolic disorder and addressing cosmetic concerns related to hirsutism. Weight loss and treatment of insulin resistance with thiozolidenediones or metformin are recommended. Oral contraceptives are used to regulate menstrual cycles and suppress hyperandrogenism. Because most patients have impaired ovulation, fertility must also be addressed. Most women can be treated with the ovulation-induction drug clomiphene citrate, either alone or in combination with insulin-sensitizing medication. Hirsutism is treated by suppressing androgen production with oral contraceptives, androgen receptor blockers, or 5-alpha-reductase inhibitors and appropriate cosmetic treatments.

218. **Summarize the traditional rationale behind hormonal treatment of menopausal women.**
Menopause represents the time in a woman's life that cyclic ovarian function ceases. Hormone replacement therapy (HRT), which consists of combined estrogen and progesterone in women with an intact uterus and estrogen only for women without a uterus, has become extremely controversial over the past few years. HRT was frequently given to women at the time of menopause and continued indefinitely because HRT was considered of clinical benefit to women by ameliorating vasomotor symptoms (hot flashes), improving lipids, and decreasing risk of cardiovascular disease, osteoporosis, and dementia.

219. **How have the recommendations of HRT changed in current practice?**
HRT is now mainly used for the short-term treatment of menopausal vasomotor symptoms, using the lowest effective dose based on the findings of the Women's Health Initiative (WHI). The WHI and subgroup studies showed that HRT was associated with an increased risk of breast cancer, thromboembolic diseases, and cardiovascular disease (coronary artery disease and stroke) and a reduced risk of colon cancer and osteoporosis. Although the absolute risk of these disorders is small, HRT is no longer recommended for disease prevention.

   U.S. Preventive Services Task Force: Hormone therapy for the prevention of chronic conditions in postmenopausal women: recommendations from the U.S. Preventive Services Task Force, *Ann Intern Med* 142:855–860, 2005.

220. **How does pregnancy affect thyroid disease?**
Pregnant women with hypothyroidism treated with thyroid hormone require approximately 30–50% more thyroid hormone than they did before pregnancy. Initially, thyroid hormone doses are increased by 30% at the time pregnancy test is positive. The thyroid hormone dose increase can by calculated by multiplying the current dose by 1.3 or by adding two extra pills per week. The dose would not be changed for women on thyroid hormone suppression therapy for thyroid cancer or who are already taking excessive thyroid hormone. Thyroid hormone levels should be measured at the diagnosis of pregnancy and every 4–6 weeks during pregnancy. Women can restart their prepregnancy dose the day of delivery.

221. **How does one manage pregnant patients previously treated for Graves' disease?**
TSIs and TRAbs should be monitored in the second trimester for patients who have been treated for Graves' disease and are now hypothyroid or euthyroid. If TSIs or TRAbs are positive, fetal Graves' disease may develop. Fetal thyroid ultrasound should be monitored for possible fetal goiter, which can contribute to respiratory distress at birth.

222. **How is hyperthyroidism treated during pregnancy?**
With PTU during the first trimester and methimazole starting in the second trimester. ^{131}I treatment should not be used in patients who are pregnant or nursing. Surgery can be attempted during the second trimester if necessary.

PARATHYROID HORMONE, CALCIUM, AND BONE DISORDERS

223. **Identify the principal organs responsible for maintaining serum calcium in the normal range.**
   - **Bone:** storage of calcium
   - **Kidney:** excretion of calcium
   - **Intestine:** absorption of calcium

   Marx SJ: Medical progress: Hyperparathyroid and hypoparathyroid disorders, *N Engl J Med* 343: 1863–1875, 2000.

224. **List the three main hormones involved in calcium regulation.**
   - Parathyroid hormone (PTH) increases serum calcium levels
   - Vitamin D increases serum calcium levels
   - Calcitonin decreases serum calcium levels

225. **List the mechanisms by which PTH increases serum calcium levels.**
   - Increases bone resorption
   - Increases $1,25\text{-}(OH)_2$ vitamin D production
   - Increases renal calcium retention
   - Increases renal phosphate excretion
     PTH is synthesized and secreted by the parathyroid gland in response to low calcium levels.

226. **Describe how vitamin D works to increase serum calcium levels.**
   - Increases bone resorption
   - Increases renal calcium and phosphate retention
   - Enhances intestinal calcium absorption
     The most active form is $1,25\text{-}(OH)_2$ vitamin D, which is synthesized in the kidney by conversion of $25\text{-}(OH)$ vitamin D by 1-alpha-hydroxylase.

227. **How does calcitonin work to decrease serum calcium levels?**
   By promoting calcium deposition in bone and inhibiting osteoclastic bone resorption. Calcitonin is synthesized by thyroidal C cells.

KEY POINTS: CALCIUM HOMEOSTASIS ✓

1. Calcium homeostasis is tightly regulated to keep calcium in a very narrow physiologic range.

2. The three organs involved in calcium homeostasis are the bone (storage), kidney (excretion), and intestine (absorption).

3. The three hormones involved in calcium homeostasis are parathyroid hormone, vitamin D, and calcitonin.

4. Parathyroid hormone and vitamin D work to increase calcium levels.

5. Calcitonin works to decrease calcium levels.

228. **List the signs and symptoms of hyper- and hypocalcemia.**
   See Table 16-12.

229. **Identify the two most common causes of hypercalcemia.**
   Primary hyperparathyroidism (55%) and hypercalcemia of malignancy (35%).

230. **Describe how you would distinguish between the two.**
   Hypercalcemia diagnosed on an outpatient basis is usually due to primary hyperparathyroidism, whereas malignancy is the most common cause in hospitalized patients. The PTH level distinguishes between hypercalcemia of malignancy (undetectable PTH with high levels of PTH-related peptide) and primary hyperparathyroidism (high PTH levels). When faced with an elevated calcium, always check PTH before embarking on an expensive evaluation. High or normal PTH levels confirm the diagnosis of hyperparathyroidism. PTH values < 20 suggest another cause of hypercalcemia.

TABLE 16-12. CLINICAL PRESENTATION OF CALCIUM DISORDERS*

Hypercalcemia		Hypocalcemia	
Symptoms	**Signs**	**Symptoms**	**Signs**
CNS: cognitive impairment (variable), weakness	Dehydration (patient may have hypotension if severe)	Perioral and peripheral paresthesias (initially)	Chvostek's sign Trousseau's sign Bradycardia/ arrhythmias,
GI symptoms (N/V), reflux, constipation	Hypertension	Carpal-pedal spasm	prolonged QT interval
Renal: impaired function, polyuria, polydipsia, nephrocalcinosis	Arrhythmias (shortened QT interval)	Irritability Tetany Seizures	Hypotension Laryngospasm Bronchospasm
Osteopenia		Congestive heart	
Pancreatitis		failure (rare)	

CNS = central nervous system; GI = gastrointestinal; N/V = nausea and vomiting.
*All signs and symptoms are a function of severity of calcium abnormality, acuteness of onset, and central patient's underlying medical status (often more severe in elderly patients).

231. **What are the uncommon causes of hypercalcemia?**
- Thyrotoxicosis
- Granulomatous disease (sarcoidosis, tuberculosis, histoplasmosis, coccidiomycosis)
- Drug-induced (thiazides, lithium, vitamins A and D intoxication, aluminum toxicity in renal failure)
- Immobilization
- Renal insufficiency with tertiary hyperparathyroidism
- Total parenteral nutrition

232. **List the rare causes of hypercalcemia.**
- Adrenal insufficiency
- Pheochromocytosis
- Pancreatic islet-cell tumors
- Familial hypocalciuric hypercalcemia (FHH)
- Milk alkali syndrome

233. **How does one diagnose primary hyperparathyroidism?**
By elevated levels of calcium and PTH. Primary hyperparathyroidism is usually due to a single parathyroid adenoma. FHH can be excluded with a 24-hour urine for calcium and family history.

234. **How is primary hyperparathyroidism treated?**
With surgery for patients <50 yr with identified complications of hypercalcemia. However, some patients do not present with classic signs and symptoms and are believed to have a mild form of the disease that has been termed **asymptomatic hyperparathyroidism**. Many of these patients have mild elevations in calcium and complain of mild cognitive symptoms or symptoms of depression that are not always clearly related to the disease. Because a large

number of patients are "asymptomatic" and may be observed, a list of indications for surgery has been developed. Table 16-13 lists the guidelines as revised in 2009.

Bilezkian JP, Khan AA, Potts JT Jr: Guidelines for the management of asymptomatic primary hyperparathyroidism: Summary statement from the Third International Workshop, *J Clin Endocrin Metab* 94:335–339, 2009.

TABLE 16-13.	INDICATIONS FOR SURGERY IN PRIMARY HYPERPARATHYROIDISM
Measurement	**Indication for Surgery**
Serum calcium	1 mg/dL above upper limit of normal
Creatinine clearance	<60 mL/min if hypercalcemia related to worsening renal function
Bone mineral density	T score: ≤ 2.5 at any site and/or previous fracture fragility
Age	<50 yr

235. **Identify the risk factors for low bone mineral density (BMD), fractures, and falls.**
See Table 16-14.

TABLE 16-14.	RISK FACTORS FOR LOW BONE MINERAL DENSITY, FRACTURES, AND FALLS	
Modifiable		**Nonmodifiable**
Nutrition: calcium/vitamin D intake		Age
Physical activity		Race/genetics
Habits: smoking, caffeine, alcohol		Body habitus (slender)
Medications		Family history
Secondary causes		Early menopause

236. **What is osteopenia?**
A bone density that is lower than normal, but not low enough for classification as osteoporosis.

237. **List the causes of secondary osteoporosis.**
   - **Endocrine:** DM, hyperthyroidism, hypogonadism, Cushing's syndrome, hyperparathyroidism, and osteomalacia
   - **GI:** gastrectomy/malabsorption syndromes, celiac disease, inflammatory bowel disease, malnutrition, liver disease, pancreatic insufficiency, and jejunoileal bypass
   - **Malignancy:** multiple myeloma, metastatic carcinoma, leukemia, and lymphoma
   - **Sarcoidosis**
   - **Renal disease:** idiopathic hypercalciuria
   - **Connective tissue disorders:** rheumatoid arthritis
   - **Medications:** steroids (most common), thyroid hormone when excessively replaced, anticonvulsants, heparin, isoniazid, loop diuretics, cyclosporine, and transplant antirejection medications
   - **Miscellaneous:** lifestyle factors such as poor nutrition, alcohol use, tobacco use, immobilization, anorexia nervosa, and amyloidosis

238. **List the treatment options for patients with osteoporosis. Which agents have been shown both to increase bone mineral density and to reduce fractures?**
See Table 16-15.

TABLE 16–15. MEDICATIONS CURRENTLY AVAILABLE FOR THE TREATMENT OF OSTEOPOROSIS

Drug	Mechanism of Action	Increases BMD Data Available	Reduces Fractures Data Available
Miscellaneous			
Calcitonin	Antiresorptive	Yes	Hip: not significant
			Spine: yes
Estrogen/HRT	Antiresorptive	Yes	Hip: yes
			Spine: yes
Raloxifene	Antiresorptive	Yes	Hip: not significant
			Spine: yes
Denosumab	Antiresorptive	Yes	Hip: yes
			Spine: yes
Bisphosphonates			
Alendronate	Antiresorptive	Yes	Hip: yes
			Spine: yes
Risedronate	Antiresorptive	Yes	Hip: yes
			Spine: yes
Zoledronate	Antiresorptive	Yes	Hip: yes
			Spine: yes
Ibandronate	Antiresorptive	Yes	Hip: not significant
			Spine: Yes
Recombinant PTH			
Teriparatide (human recombinant PTH 1–34)	Anabolic	Yes	Hip: uncertain (reduced nonvertebral fractures)
			Spine: yes

BMD = bone mineral density; FDA = U.S. Food and Drug Administration; HRT = hormone replacement therapy; PTH = parathyroid hormone.
Not significant: indicates effect on hip has been examined but no significant differences found. Trial may have been underpowered to detect differences. Hip data may have been combined in all nonvertebral fractures.
Uncertain: results variable or data insufficient to determine.
No data: has not been examined yet, or trial is under way.
FDA-approved drugs for prevention and treatment of osteoporosis: alendronate, risedronate, and raloxifene are approved for treatment and prevention. HRT is approved for prevention. Calcitonin and teriparatide are approved for treatment. Off-label use: drug has been used in this setting but is not FDA-approved for osteoporosis treatment.

239. **What is FRAX?**
A calculation that allows the practitioner to assess a patient's 10-year fracture risk by entering clinical data regarding fracture risk and femoral neck BMD measurement. Patients who have a

10-year fracture risk > 3% in the hip or 20% in other areas should be treated or considered for antiosteoporosis, anti-fracture medication. The calculation can be accessed at www.shef.ac.uk/FRAX

240. **What are the contraindications to teriparatide therapy?**
- Past or present history of radiation therapy
- Bone cancer
- Paget's disease
- Elevated PTH
- Vitamin D deficiency
- Past or present hypercalcemia

241. **What is FHH?**
A very rare autosomal dominant genetic disorder that has nearly 100% penetrance due to an inactivating germ-line mutation in the calcium-sensing receptor. In this disorder, parathyroid cells are insensitive to inhibition by calcium. Renal tubule cells are also insensitive to calcium.

242. **Summarize the clinical characteristics of FHH.**
FHH is generally a benign disorder that results in alteration of the calcium "set point." Patients have life-long moderately elevated calcium, normal–to–slightly elevated intact PTH, and normal-to-low calcium excretion. The fractional excretion of calcium (which normalizes calcium excretion for glomerular filtration rate) is usually low. Most patients have a ratio of calcium clearance (C_{Ca}) to creatinine clearance (C_{Cr}) < 0.01. This ratio is calculated by the following equation:

$$C_{Ca} : C_{Cr} = [U_{Ca} \times S_{Cr}]/[S_{Ca} \times U_{Cr}]$$

where U_{Ca} = urinary calcium, U_{Cr} = urinary creatinine, S_{Ca} = serum calcium, and S_{Cr} = serum creatinine. Owing to the abnormal calcium sensor, patients have "relative hypocalciuria" (unusually normal for the degree of hypercalcemia). An estimate of free serum calcium not bound by albumin should be used in this calculation by multiplying total calcium by 0.6.

243. **Why is it necessary to distinguish FHH from primary hyperparathyroidism?**
To avoid unnecessary parathyroidectomy.

244. **What is Paget's disease?**
A disorder of abnormal bone remodeling that can affect one or more skeletal sites. Initially, the disorder begins with abnormal bone resorption followed by compensatory bone formation, resulting in disorganized bone remodeling that predisposes the affected region to deformity and fracture. The exact etiology is unknown. Patients may be asymptomatic with elevated serum alkaline phosphatase levels noted on routine serum chemistries or present with bone pain and deformity.

245. **How is Paget's disease diagnosed?**
With bone scan and confirmatory plain radiographs of areas showing increased uptake.

246. **Summarize the management of Paget's disease.**
Biphosphonates are used for patients with progressive bone pain, planned surgery at an active bone site, and disease at bone sites that are at high risk for future complications such as skull, spine, weight-bearing bones, or bones near joints.

247. **How are the causes of hypocalcemia classified?**
As related to hypoparathyroidism or nonhypoparathyroidism. **Hypoparathyroidism** causes can be divided into PTH deficiency (e.g., surgical, autoimmune, congenital aplasia, radiation-induced, and infiltrative diseases) or PTH resistance (PTH antibodies, pseudohypoparathyroidism, and magnesium deficiency). **Nonhypoparathyroidism** causes include vitamin D deficiency or resistance (dietary deficiency, lack of sunlight, liver and renal disease), accelerated bone mineralization (hungry bone syndrome after parathyroidectomy), drugs (anticalcemic, antineoplastic), and acute complexing/ sequestration of calcium (rhabdomyolysis, tumor lysis syndrome, pancreatitis, phosphate infusions, blood transfusions).

248. **How should hypocalcemia be treated?**
Treatment depends on the severity and duration of symptoms. Patients with acute hypocalcemia should be hospitalized with telemetry monitoring and given IV calcium in addition to magnesium, if indicated. Patients with chronic hypocalcemic disorders are managed with oral calcium and vitamin D supplementation. *Note:* Never give calcium with phosphate.

LIPID DISORDERS

249. **What are the major classes of lipoprotein particles?**
See Table 16-16.

TABLE 16-16.	LIPOPROTEIN PARTICLES			
Lipoprotein Particle	Location of Origin	Composition	Apoproteins	Associated Disorders
Chylomicron	Intestine	80–95% TG 3–7% chol	Apo B48	Chylomicronemia
VLDL	Liver	50–65% TG 20–30% chol	Apo B100	Familial hypertriglyceridemia Familial combined hyperlipidemia
Remnants and IDL	Catabolism of VLDL & chylomicrons	30–40% TG 30–50% chol	Depends on particle of origin	Familial dysbeta lipoproteinemia (broad beta disease)
LDL	IDL, VLDL remnants	4–10% TG 45–55% chol	Apo B100	Familial hypercholesterolemia Familial combined hyperlipidemia
HDL	Liver, intestine	3–7% TG 25% chol	Apo A	Tangier's disease

Apo = apolipoprotein; chol = cholesterol; HDL = high-density lipoprotein; IDL = intermediate-density lipoprotein; LDL = low-density lipoprotein; TG = triglycerides; VLDL = very low density particle.

250. **What is familial hypercholesterolemia (FH)?**
An autosomal dominant disorder due to a mutation in the LDL receptor (causing a deficient or defective receptor) that leads to altered LDL catabolism and increased cholesterol synthesis. Approximately 1/500 people are heterozygous carriers of a mutation and 1/1,000,000 are homozygous for the disorder. Such people have higher rates of premature atherosclerosis and can have myocardial infarctions at a very young age. Physical examination often reveals tendinous xanthomas (cholesterol deposition in the extensor tendons) and corneal arcus. Management is aimed at aggressive LDL-lowering to reduce cardiovascular risk.

251. **What is the chylomicronemia syndrome?**
The hereditary occurrence of accumulation of chylomicrons in the serum due to severe triglyceride elevations resulting from dysfunction or absence of the enzyme lipoprotein lipase (LPL), which is responsible for triglyceride hydrolysis of chylomicrons. The chylomicronemia syndrome typically occurs when triglyceride levels > 1000 mg/dL, and the serum may appear lipemic.

252. **Describe the physical manifestations of chylomicronemia syndrome.**
Lipemia retinalis in which the retinal blood vessels appear creamy, eruptive xanthomas, and hepatomegaly. Patients are at increased risk of developing pancreatitis.

253. **How is chylomicronemia syndrome treated?**
By reducing triglyceride levels and may initially require fasting to lower the triglyceride levels into a safer range.

254. **List the genetic causes of lipid abnormalities.**
See Table 16-17.

TABLE 16-17. GENETIC DISORDERS OF LIPID METABOLISM

Disorder	Mechanism	Lipid Profile
Familial hypercholesterolemia (increased CHD risk)	Autosomal dominant mutation in LDL receptor	Elevated LDL
Familial defective Apo B-100 (increased CHD risk)	Autosomal dominant Impaired binding of LDL to receptor Mutant Apo B100 ligand	Elevated LDL
Familial combined hyperlipidemia (increased CHD risk)	Overproduction of VLDL Specific gene defect unknown High Apo B	Elevated LDL and TG
Polygenic hypercholesterolemia (increased CHD risk)	Genetics poorly understood Abnormal LDL metabolism Apo E4 phenotype	Elevated LDL
Familial hypertriglyceridemia	Autosomal dominant Overproduction and secretion of VLDL	Elevated TG

(continued)

TABLE 16-17. GENETIC DISORDERS OF LIPID METABOLISM—*(continued)*

Disorder	Mechanism	Lipid Profile
Familial dysbetalipoproteinemia (broad beta disease) (increased CHD risk)	Altered IDL and remnant metabolism Apo E2 phenotype	Elevated LDL and TG
Lipoprotein lipase deficiency	Mutation in LPL gene Decreased TG metabolism	Elevated TG, low HDL
Familial hypoalphalipoproteinemia (increased CHD risk)	Autosomal dominant Mutation in Apo A1 gene	Low HDL
Apo CII deficiency (cofactor for LPL)	Decreased TG metabolism	Elevated TG
Tangier's disease: cholesterol esters accumulate in tissues: tonsils (orange), peripheral nerves, liver, spleen, lymph nodes, cornea; unclear CHD risk Familial HDL deficiency like Tangier disease but no systemic finding	Autosomal recessive Mutation in the *ABC-A1* gene that allows cellular cholesterol efflux; abnormal intracellular cholesterol transport	Low HDL
LCAT deficiency (corneal opacities)	Mutation in the LCAT gene Abnormal cholesterol esterification	Low HDL
CETP excess	High CETP activity (allows cholesterol ester transfer from HDL to TG-rich lipoproteins); gene variants with altered activity	Low HDL

Apo = apolipoprotein; CETP = cholesterol ester transfer protein; CHD = coronary artery disease; HDL = high-density lipoprotein; IDL = intermediate-density lipoprotein; LCAT = lecithin-cholesterol acyltransferase; LDL = low-density lipoprotein; TG = triglycerides; VLDL = very low density lipoprotein.

255. **Identify some secondary/acquired causes of hyperlipidemia.**
See Table 16-18.

TABLE 16-18. SECONDARY AND ACQUIRED CAUSES OF HYPERLIPIDEMIA

Increased LDL, Cholesterol	Increased TG	Decreased HDL
Hypothyroidism	Hypothyroidism	Tobacco use
Poorly controlled diabetes	Poorly controlled diabetes	Poorly controlled diabetes
Obesity/metabolic syndrome	Obesity/metabolic syndrome	Obesity/metabolic syndrome
Drugs: anabolic steroids	Drugs: oral estrogens, alcohol, beta blockers, protease inhibitors, thiazides, glucocorticoids, retinoids	Drugs: androgens, progesterone, beta blockers
Nephrotic syndrome	Nephrotic syndrome	Sedentary lifestyle
Primary biliary cirrhosis		Diet restricted in fat
Diet high in saturated fat		

TG = triglycerides.

WEScreen WEBSITES

1. American Association of Clinical Endocrinologists: www.aace.com
2. American Diabetes Association: www.diabetes.org
3. American Heart Association: www.americanheart.org
4. American Society for Bone and Mineral Research: www.ASBMR.org
5. American Thyroid Association: www.thyroid.org
6. National Osteoporosis Foundation: www.nof.org
7. Pituitary Society: www.pituitarysociety.org
8. The Endocrine Society: www.endo-society.org

BIBLIOGRAPHY

1. American Diabetes Association: Clinical Practice Recommendations 2011, *Diabetes Care* 34(Suppl 1): S1–S100, 2011.
2. Basa ALP, Afsharkharaghan H: *Endocrinology in Medical Secrets*, (Zollo A, editor), ed 3, Philadelphia, 2001, Hanley and Belfus.
3. Braverman LE, Utiger RD, editors: *Werner and Ingbars' Thyroid. A Fundamental and Clinical Text*, Philadelphia, 2000, Lippincott Williams & Wilkins.
4. Casanueva FF, Molitch ME, Schlechte JA, et al: Guidelines of the Pituitary Society for the diagnosis and management of prolactinomas, *Clin Endocrinol* 65:265–273, 2006.

5. Dickey J: Diabetes, In *The Eye-Beaters, Blood, Victory, Madness, Buckhead, and Mercy*, Garden City, NY, 1970, Doubleday.

6. Favus MJ, editor: *Primer on the Metabolic Bone Diseases and Disorders of Mineral Metabolism*, ed 5, Washington, DC, 2003, American Society of Bone and Mineral Research.

7. Larson PR, et al: *Williams Textbook of Endocrinology*, ed 10, Philadelphia, 2003, WB Saunders.

8. Nieman LK, Biller BMK, Findling JW, et al: The diagnosis of Cushing's syndrome: An Endocrine Society clinical practice guideline, *J Clin Endocrinol Metab* 93:1526–1540, 2008.

9. Puxeddu E, Filetti S: The 2009 American Thyroid Association guidelines for management of thyroid nodules and differentiated thyroid cancer: Progress on the road from consensus to evidence-based practice, *Thyroid* 19:1145–1147, 2009.

10. Snow V, Barry P, Fitterman N, et al: Pharmacologic and surgical management of obesity in primary care: A clinical practice guideline from the American College of Physicians, *Ann Intern Med* 142:525–531, 2005.

11. The Guideline Development Group: Management of diabetes from preconception to the postnatal period: Summary of NICE guidance, *BMJ* 336:714–717, 2008.

12. Wierman ME, editor: *Diseases of the Pituitary: Diagnosis and Treatment*, Totowa, NJ, 1997, Humana Press.

NEUROLOGY

David B. Sommer, M.D., M.P.H.

> *My hand moves because certain forces—electric, magnetic, or whatever 'nerve-force' may prove to be—are impressed on it by my brain. This nerve-force, stored in the brain, would probably be traceable, if Science were complete, to chemical forces supplied to the brain by the blood, and ultimately derived from the food I eat and the air I breathe.*
>
> Lewis Carroll (1832–1898)
> from *Sylvie and Bruno, 1890*

OVERVIEW AND APPROACH TO THE PATIENT

1. **What is localization?**

   The process of determining which parts of the nervous system are malfunctioning in order to produce the patient's signs or symptoms. Localization is key to the neurologic evaluation and often plays an important role in teaching rounds. After the history and physical examination are presented, a discussion begins to "locate the lesion." A differential diagnosis of pathologic processes is discussed after localization—*where*, then *what!*

2. **How is the neurologic lesion localized?**

   Through the history and physical examination. Ancillary studies such as computed tomography (CT) or magnetic resonance imaging (MRI) results should not be cited during the initial localization evaluation because many laboratory or imaging results are coincidental and not causal of the patient's problem. Careful localization allows the examiner to tell the difference. Localization requires knowledge of functional neuroanatomy. Some of the first questions asked concern the distribution of the findings on the initial history and examination. One can ask:

   Is the process
   - **Focal:** explained by a single lesion?
   - **Diffuse:** affecting a specific level of the neuraxis symmetrically?
   - **Multifocal:** explained by multiple lesions?

   What level of the neuraxis is involved?
   - Muscle
   - Neuromuscular junction (NMJ)
   - Peripheral nerve
   - Nerve plexus
   - Nerve root
   - Spinal cord
   - Brainstem
   - Cerebellum
   - Subcortical brain
   - Cortex

3. **What are the components of the neurologic examination?**
See Table 17-1.

TABLE 17-1. THE NEUROLOGIC EXAMINATION		
Component Tested	Function Assessed	Maneuver or Observation
Mental status	Level of arousal	Alert, drowsy, stuporous, or comatose
	Attention and concentration	Attentive, neglectful, or easily distracted
	Language	Name objects, repeat sentences, comprehend directions
	Memory	Remember short lists of words
	Calculation, abstraction, and sequencing	Perform simple calculations
	Affect	Appropriate, shows full range
	Thought processes and content	Assess for presence of hallucinations and delusions, insight, judgment, and appropriateness
Cranial nerves	I	Identify scent (such as common spice)
	II	Visual acuity, visual fields by confrontation testing and pupillary responses
	III, IV, and VI	Extraocular movements
	V	Facial sensation to light touch
	VII	Facial movements (eyebrow raising, grimace, smiling)
	VIII	Hearing (whisper test), observe presence of nystagmus
	IX and X	Palatal movement
	XI	Trapezius and sternocleidomastoid strength (shoulder shrug)
	XII	Tongue movement or deviation
Motor	Bulk and appearance	Atrophy, hypertrophy, and fasciculation
	Tone	Increased with spasticity, rigidity, or geggenhalten* or decreased with flaccidity
	Strength	Graded as: 5—full strength 4—weak but can move against some resistance

(continued)

TABLE 17-1. THE NEUROLOGIC EXAMINATION—*(continued)*

Component Tested	Function Assessed	Maneuver or Observation
		3—can move against gravity but not resistance
		2—cannot move against gravity
		1—muscle contracts or twitches but limb does not move
	Pattern of abnormalities noted	Symmetrical vs. asymmetrical
		Proximal vs. distal
		Central or upper motor neuron pattern
Sensory	Sensations	Pinprick, temperature, vibration, proprioception
	Pattern of abnormalities noted	Proximal vs. distal
Reflexes	Deep tendon (biceps, brachioradialis, triceps, patellar, ankle)	Graded as:
		0—absent
		1—reduced
		2—normal
		3—hyperreflexic
		4—sustained clonus
	Plantar response	Babinski (positive with upgoing great toe and fanning of other toes)
Coordination		Finger to nose, heel to shin, rapid movement
Gait		Ability to get up without assistance or using arm support
		Posture (stooped, upright)
		Base width (between insides of feet)
		Stride length
		Arm swing present or absent
		Symmetry
		Weakness

*Geggenhalten: increased resistance to movement that is overcome when distracted.

4. **How is a neurologic examination performed if the patient is comatose?**
   Despite the apparent lack of responsiveness, several parts of the examination can be done in the comatose patient and assist in the localization of the pathology. The key parts of the examination for a comatose patient are:

TABLE 17-2. GLASCOW COMA SCALE

Points	Observed Response		
	Eye Opening	Vocal Response	Motor Response
1	None	None	None
2	To pain	Grunts	Extends to pain
3	To voice	Utters inappropriate words	Abnormal flexion to pain
4	Spontaneously	Confused or disoriented	Withdrawal from pain
5	—	Oriented and appropriate	Purposeful or localizes
6	—	—	Follows commands

Scoring: Add the points as indicated in the left column, based on the observed response.
- ≥13: Mild brain injury
- 9–12: Moderate brain injury
- ≤8: Severe brain injury

The minimum score is 3 and maximum score is 15.
Adapted from Teasdale G, Jennett B: Assessment of coma and impaired consciousness. A practical scale. Lancet 2:81–84, 1974.

- **Responsiveness,** with assessment of severity of brain injury by Glasgow Coma Scale (Table 17-2):
  - Response to painful stimuli in unrestrained limbs
  - Ability to track objects with eyes
  - Blink to threatening stimulus
  - Ability to follow commands ("look up," "blink")
  - Answer to yes/no questions.
- **Cranial nerves:**
  - Pupillary responses to light
  - Extraocular movements (EOMs)
  - Oculocephalic reflex ("doll's eyes") if EOMs absent or abnormal
  - Cold caloric testing if "doll's eyes" abnormal or not elicitable
- **Motor testing:**
  - Tone
  - Strength, even if able to assess only withdrawal and movement against gravity
- **Sensory testing:** although limited, can compare stimuli responses on right and left side of the body
- **Reflexes:**
  - Deep tendon
  - Plantar responses
- **Coordination and gait:** cannot be assessed

5. **What if the examiner thinks the patient is faking or imagining her or his symptoms?**
The term "functional" is used to describe neurologic phenomena or symptoms that occur when the basic structure and function of relevant neurologic symptoms are intact. Patients with functional symptoms are among the most challenging to care for and, consequently, often receive suboptimal care. Most patients with functional neurologic problems are not voluntarily producing their symptoms and may have concomitant or underlying organic neurologic problems (e.g., comorbid seizures and pseudoseizures). A careful neurologic examination is important, but the presence of a functional disorder

often makes this examination difficult. Many neurologic syndromes have subtle findings, though, that may be assumed to be functional. Honestly tell patients that their symptoms are difficult to explain given our understanding of neurology. Confrontation is generally not helpful, but suggesting that the symptoms will improve may be helpful.

NEUROLOGIC TESTS AND PROCEDURES

6. **When should the examiner order an electromyogram (EMG) or nerve conduction study (NCS) or both?**
   During the evaluation of neuropathies, myopathies, or NMJ disorders. Sometimes, an EMG laboratory may refer to both NCS and EMG as "EMG." Be sure to list the diagnoses being considered when submitting the request.

7. **How are EMG and NCS done?**
   - **Sensory NCS:** electrically stimulates a nerve and records a response at a distant point on the same nerve.
   - **Motor NCS:** electrically stimulates a nerve and records an electrical response over a target muscle belly.
   - **EMG:** places a needle electrode into various muscle bellies to observe electrical activity with rest and activation (no electrical stimulus is applied).

8. **List the uses of EMGs and NCSs for electrodiagnostic evaluation.**
   See Table 17-3.

TABLE 17-3. CLINICAL SYNDROMES IN WHICH ELECTROMYOGRAPHY AND NERVE CONDUCTION STUDIES ARE USED FOR DIAGNOSIS*

Myopathy	Differentiation between axonal and
Polyneuropathy	demyelinating neuropathies
Neuromuscular junction disease	Assessment of large sensory and motor fibers (may be normal in small fiber sensory neuropathy)
Focal compression neuropathies	Focal root, plexus, or nerve lesions

EMG = electromyography; NCS = nerve conduction studies.
*Both EMG and NCS are generally required for appropriate diagnosis.

9. **When is an electroencephalogram (EEG) helpful?**
   When trying to establish a diagnosis of epilepsy, evaluating coma, or confirming brain death. Prolonged EEG monitoring (over several days) can be helpful in determining whether transient alterations in behavior have an epileptic basis. Simultaneously recorded video and audio helps in correlating EEG findings to behavior change.

10. **How is an EEG done?**
    By placing multiple electrodes on a patient's scalp and recording electrical activity generated by the brain. From an electrician's standpoint, this is a fairly unsatisfactory way to record brain activity, given the significant amount of electrical insulation between cortex and

scalp. Nonetheless, it is impractical in most clinical circumstances to remove the skull, and surface (scalp) EEG can still be quite clinically useful.

11. **When should one order a polysomnogram (PSG; sleep study)?**
When evaluating sleep disorders such as sleep apnea and parasomnias (physical, sensory, or emotional disturbances during sleep). Although not necessary for the diagnosis of restless leg syndrome (RLS), PSG may be helpful in some instances.

12. **What is monitored during PSG?**
Respirations, cardiac rhythm, limb movement, and limited EMG are monitored overnight in a sleep laboratory. Video is typically recorded as well.

ALTERED MENTAL STATUS

13. **What is the most common cause of altered mental status in the hospitalized patient?**
Delirium, also called "toxic/metabolic encephalopathy." An encephalopathy is a diffuse higher-level brain dysfunction. Delirium in the hospitalized patient is most often due to an underlying medical process that reduces cerebral blood flow or "poisons" the blood with exogenous or endogenous toxins.

KEY POINTS: CAUSES OF DELIRIUM IN THE HOSPITALIZED PATIENT ✓

1. Infection
2. Fluid and electrolyte disturbances
3. Endocrine abnormalities
4. Medications or withdrawal from medications
5. Alcohol intoxication or withdrawal
6. Hypotension

14. **What is the appropriate initial evaluation for a patient with altered mental status?**
   - Review of current medications
   - If hospitalized, review of home medications that were not continued in the hospital, possibly resulting in a withdrawal syndrome
   - Review of current and past alcohol and nonprescription drug use
   - Laboratory tests: complete blood count (CBC), serum chemistries, hepatic enzymes, ammonia, thyroid function tests, urinalysis
   - Chest x-ray
   - Serum and urine drug screens (if indicated)
   - Urine and blood cultures
   - Oxygen saturation

15. **When is a brain CT scan or MRI indicated for evaluation of delirium?**
Whenever the cause of delirium is unclear after the initial evaluation or a structural process such as hemorrhage, mass lesion, ischemic stroke, or hydrocephalus is suspected.

Witnessed rapid onset of a focal neurologic deficit is a sure-fire indication for a CT scan. CT scans are usually done first in the acute setting because of easier availability, but MRI is more sensitive than CT for imaging cerebral ischemia and inflammation (especially with addition of gadolinium contrast) and posterior fossa lesions.

16. **When is a lumbar puncture (LP) indicated for evaluation of altered mental status?**
When the initial evaluation suggests infection, inflammation, or neoplasm involving the cerebrospinal fluid (CSF) or does not identify the etiology of the altered mental status. In the setting of encephalopathy, LP should be performed only **after** either CT or MRI, because the presence of a mass lesion (easily seen on imaging studies) could cause a significant intracranial mass effect with risk of cerebral herniation if the lumbar space is decompressed through an LP.

17. **What tests should be done on the CSF?**
- Cell counts on tubes 1 and 4
- Protein
- Glucose
- Gram stain
- India ink preparation and/or cryptococcal antigen testing if cryptococcal meningitis suspected
- Cytology if malignancy suspected
- Oligoclonal bands if multiple sclerosis (MS) suspected
- Immunoglobulin G (IgG) index which may be elevated in conditions such as neurosyphilis, MS, chronic infection, central nervous system (CNS) lupus erythematous
- CSF-VDRL (Venereal Disease Research Laboratory) and CSF-FTA-Abs (fluorescent treponemal antibody absorption) if syphilis suspected
- Viral polymerase chain reactions (PCR) if indicated

18. **How can an EEG aid in diagnosis of altered mental status?**
To identify seizure activity and help differentiate organic encephalopathy from psychiatric dysfunction. The EEG in organic encephalopathy shows diffuse slowing. Triphasic waves may be seen in hepatic encephalopathy. Patients with psychiatric disorders have normal EEGs. Rarely, altered mental status can be caused by ongoing seizure activity (complex partial status epilepticus) or a postictal state. In these cases, EEG may reveal epileptiform abnormalities.

DEMENTIA

See also Chapter 2, General Medicine and Ambulatory Care, Chapter 12, Infectious Diseases, and Chapter 18, Geriatrics.

19. **What is dementia?**
A chronic impairment in memory and at least one other cognitive domain (e.g., executive function, language, motor planning) of sufficient severity to impair performance of activities of daily living.

20. **What is the most common chronic dementia syndrome?**
Alzheimer's disease with a cortical pattern of symptoms, defined as:
- The development of multiple cognitive deficits manifested by both memory impairment and one or more of the following cognitive disturbances:
  - Aphasia.

- Apraxia.
- Agnosia.
- Disturbance in executive functioning.
- The cognitive deficits cause significant impairment in social or occupational functioning and represent a significant decline from a previous level of functioning.
- The course is characterized by gradual onset and continuing decline.
- The deficits are not due to another brain, systemic, or psychiatric condition.
- The deficits do not occur exclusively during the course of delirium.

American Psychiatric Association: *Diagnostic and Statistical Manual of Mental Disorders*, ed 4, text revised (DSM-IV-TR). Washington, DC, 2000, American Psychiatric Association.

21. **What are other causes of chronic dementia?**
   - Vascular dementia (VaD)
   - Frontotemporal dementias (FTDs)
   - Dementia with Lewy bodies (DLB)
   - Dementia associated with Parkinson's disease (PD)
   - Alcohol-related dementia (Korsikoff's)

22. **Describe the clinical features of FTD.**
   FTD typically presents with behavioral abnormalities and not an obvious impairment in memory. The most common presentation is a lack of insight and social awareness leading to inappropriate social interactions. Patients can appear apathetic or disinhibited. As the disease progresses, more global impairment becomes obvious. Initially, FTD is sometimes mistaken for primary psychiatric disease.

23. **Describe DLB.**
   DLB is characterized by the relatively simultaneous development of cognitive impairment and parkinsonian motor features. The cognitive impairment in DLB waxes and wanes and visual hallucinations appear early.

24. **Describe the characteristics of VaD?**
   Previously called "multi-infarct dementia," VaD can result from symptomatic strokes due to large vessel infarction or hemorrhage or small vessel cerebrovascular disease due to atherosclerosis or amyloid angiopathy. The latter patients usually do not have significant neurologic deficits other than memory impairment, psychomotor slowing, and extrapyramidal findings, indicating a subcortical pattern. VaD and Alzheimer's dementia may be present in the same patient.

25. **Is there a recommended work-up for dementia?**
   Yes. Some form of neuroimaging (CT or MRI) is recommended to evaluate for structural causes, including normal-pressure hydrocephalus (NPH). CBC, serum chemistries including liver function tests (LFTs), thyroid panel, vitamin B_{12} levels, and clinical screening for depression are indicated routinely. Specific testing for syphilis with FTA-Abs is not indicated unless there is suspicion of neurosyphilis. LP, genetic testing, EEG, and testing for Creutzfeld-Jakob disease are not routinely indicated but should be performed if clinical suspicion exists for a specific atypical etiology.

Knopman DS, DeKosky ST, Cummings JO, et al: Practice parameter: Diagnosis of dementia (an evidence-based review). Report of the Quality Standards Subcommittee of the American Academy of Neurology, *Neurology* 56:1143–1153, 2001. Available at: ww.aan.com/practice/guideline.

APHASIA

26. **What is aphasia?**
    A deficit in language function. Aphasia is important to recognize because of its localizing value as a focal deficit. Aphasia should be distinguished from global encephalopathy, but assessment becomes difficult when both are present. The aphasic patient will typically appear more frustrated than confused.

27. **What are the types of aphasia?**
    See Table 17-4.

TABLE 17-4.	TYPES OF APHASIAS AND THEIR CHARACTERISTICS				
Aphasia Type	Speech Function Affected				Localization
	Fluency	Naming	Repetition	Comprehension	
Broca's	+	+	+	−	Left posterior inferior frontal gyrus
Wernicke's	+	−	+	+	Left posterior superior temporal gyrus
Transcortical motor	+	+	−	−	Left frontal lobe
Transcortical sensory	−	+	−	+	Left temporal-parietal-occipital junction
Conductive	−	+	+	−	Arcuate fassiculus
Global	+	+	+	+	Large left hemispherical

+ = impaired; − = spared.

28. **How do you detect aphasia?**
    By assessing object naming. Patients with mild-to-moderate global encephalopathy will not have difficulty naming objects, but aphasic patients will. To detect mild deficits, have the patient name objects that are rarely named or subparts of objects (e.g., lenses of eyeglasses; stem of watch, second hand, minute hand; ring finger, or index finger) or both.

29. **What causes aphasia?**
    Any process that causes focal cerebral dysfunction (e.g., stroke, tumor, MS, or seizure) can cause aphasia. The most common cause of aphasia is stroke.

30. **Are reading and writing affected in aphasia?**
    Yes. Aphasia is a language problem, not a speech problem. Typically, reading and writing are affected in proportion to the ability to comprehend and produce spoken language.

31. **Is slurred speech aphasia?**
    No. Although some patients with aphasia may have slurred speech or dysarthria, slurred speech is usually not aphasia. Slurred speech can be produced by a focal process such as facial or bulbar weakness and can be a manifestation of a global encephalopathy. Many patients and families assume that slurred speech is a stroke or transient ischemic attack (TIA), but ischemia is not usually the etiology of the speech deficit.

VISUAL COMPLAINTS

32. **What questions should be asked to localize a visual disturbance?**
    - Is one (monocular) or are both (binocular) eyes affected?
    - Was the disturbance transient or fixed?
    - Was the disturbance gradual or abrupt?
    - If binocular, is one part of the visual field involved?
    - Are other phenomena present such as flashing lights and zigzag lines?

33. **What is the differential diagnosis for monocular vision loss?**
    - Glaucoma
    - Retinal detachment
    - Retinal artery occlusion
    - Ischemic optic neuropathy (e.g., giant cell arteritis or vasculitis)
    - Optic neuritis (ON)

34. **Where does a monocular visual disturbance localize?**
    Anterior to the optic chiasm, either within the eye itself or in the optic nerve.

35. **How does ON present?**
    As the relatively abrupt (hours to days) onset of vision loss or blurring. ON is usually monocular but can be binocular and sometimes is associated with pain, particularly with eye movement. Peripheral color perception, particularly for red, is reduced. An associated afferent pupillary defect may also be present and will appear on examination as greater constriction of both pupils when light is shone in the unaffected eye than when light is shone in the affected eye.

36. **What is the role of steroids in the treatment of ON?**
    The Optic Neuritis Treatment Trial randomized 457 patients with ON to receive low-dose oral prednisone (1 mg/kg/day for 14 days), high-dose intravenous (IV) methylprednisolone (250 mg every 6 hr for 3 days) followed by low-dose oral prednisone, or placebo. Low-dose oral prednisone was not effective. High-dose methylprednisolone led to faster visual recovery, but outcomes at 1 year were not significantly different.

    Beck RW, Cleary PA, Anderson MM Jr, et al: A randomized, controlled trial of corticosteroids in the treatment of acute optic neuritis. The Optic Neuritis Study Group, *N Engl J Med* 326:581–588, 1992.

37. **Do patients with ON have MS?**
    Possibly. ON can be the presenting symptom in MS. In the cohort from the Optic Neuritis Treatment Trial, the risk of subsequent diagnosis of MS depended heavily on whether there were MS-like abnormalities on initial MRI. Seventy-two percent of patients with one or more lesions on MRI went on to develop MS versus 25% of patients with no lesions.

    Optic Neuritis Study Group: Multiple sclerosis risk after optic neuritis: Final Optic Neuritis Treatment Trial follow-up, *Arch Neurol* 65:727–732, 2008.

38. **What is the localization of a homonymous field deficit?**
A left or right field cut localizes posterior to the optic chiasm. The farther posterior the defect is, the more congruent it will be in the two eyes. A lesion to the optic radiations in the temporal lobes (Meyer's loop) will produce a contralateral superior quadrantanopsia—a "pie in the sky" deficit.

39. **What is the significance of ischemic monocular vision loss?**
Significant risk of stroke. Although this symptom carries less subsequent risk of stroke than a TIA involving a cerebral hemisphere, these patients should undergo appropriate evaluation and treatment if significant stenoses are found (see Chapter 5, Vascular Medicine). The arterial supply for the eye derives from the internal carotid artery (ICA), which is a branch of the common carotid artery. A common cause for retinal artery occlusion is atheroembolism from plaques in the ICA. Sometimes, cholesterol emboli can be seen as bright yellow spots in the vessels on fundoscopic examination and are called "Hollenhorst's plaques."

Benavente O, Eliasziw M, Streifler JY, et al: Prognosis after transient monocular blindness associated with carotid-artery stenosis, *N Engl J Med* 345:1084–1090, 2001.

40. **What is the localization for binocular diplopia?**
Structures affecting eye alignment. Binocular diplopia (diplopia that resolves with closure of either eye) results from ocular misalignment. Asking historical questions about whether the double images are horizontally displaced, vertically displaced, or skewed and whether the diplopia consistently worsens in a particular direction of gaze can help localize which eye movement(s) are involved. A careful examination of eye movements to look for dysconjugate gaze is a must.

41. **What is the differential diagnosis of binocular diplopia?**
- Orbital abnormality that restricts eye movement
- NMJ disorder such as myasthenia gravis
- Cranial neuropathy of III, IV, or VI
- Brainstem lesion
  If the diplopia is inconsistent, then myasthenia gravis is likely.

HEADACHE

See also Chapter 2, General Medicine and Ambulatory Care.

42. **How are headaches classified?**
As primary or secondary. **Primary headaches** are *not* associated with any identifiable structural factor. **Secondary headaches** are associated with underlying disorders such as trauma, vasculitis, medications, infection, hypertension, and tumor.

The International Headache Society: The International Classification of Headache Disorders (2nd ed), *Cephalgia* 24(Suppl 1):1–160, 2004. Available at: www.ihs-headache.org.

43. **What is a migraine headache?**
Episodic primary headaches that can be preceded or accompanied by premonitory symptoms and auras. Migraines without aura are more common. Auras include specific neurologic deficits or disturbances such as visual, sensory, motor, or speech symptoms. When auras present as focal neurologic deficits, the headache can be mistaken for stroke. Premonitory symptoms include nausea, vomiting, photophobia (light sensitivity and avoidance), or phonophobia (sound sensitivity and avoidance). Patients typically feel better lying down in a quiet place. Migraines can occur with only neurologic symptoms without the headache.

44. **What drugs can be used to treat migraine acutely?**
    - Nonsteroidal anti-inflammatory drugs (NSAIDs)
    - 5-Hydroxytyramine (5-HT) agonists (triptans)
    - Ergotamine
    - Opiates
    - Magnesium
    - Dopamine antagonists (metoclopramide)

    In selecting a treatment for an individual patient with an acute headache, the most important guide is the determination of the treatment that was previously effective. Before use, the individual patient should be assessed for any contraindications to these medications.

KEY POINTS: CONTRAINDICATIONS TO TRIPTAN USE FOR MIGRAINE HEADACHE ✓

1. Uncontrolled hypertension
2. Pregnancy
3. Coronary artery disease
4. Variant or Prinzmetal's angina
5. Stroke
6. Familial hemiplegic migraine
7. Basilar migraine

45. **What drugs can be used to prevent migraine?**
    - Propranolol
    - Amitriptyline
    - Valproic acid
    - Gabapentin
    - Topirimate

    Generally a prophylactic medication is indicated if migraines occur more frequently than twice per month or if infrequent attacks are severe and disabling. Verapamil, angiotensin-converting enzyme (ACE) inhibitors, other tricyclic antidepressants, and other anticonvulsants have less robust evidence to support their use but may be effective.

46. **Describe a tension headache.**
    Tension headaches are the most common types of headache. The pathophysiology of tension headache is not understood nor is the role of cranial muscle tension (from which the headaches derive their name). Headaches are typically bilateral, have a pressing or tightening ("bandlike") quality, and are not associated with migranous features.

47. **What is a cluster headache?**
    A unilateral orbital, frontal, or temporal headache usually associated with ipsilateral conjunctival injection, lacrimation, rhinorrhea, facial sweating, miosis, or ptosis. Pain is severe and stabbing. Cluster headaches occur most commonly in men aged 20–40 years. High-flow oxygen can be an effective treatment.

48. **What is rebound headache?**

    A headache that occurs with withdrawal from many of the types of medications used to treat headaches including triptans, ergotamine, butalibital combinations, and other analgesics. Patients who use headache medications can get into a cycle of needing to treat headache with the same medication that is responsible for the headache. This type is also called "medication-overuse headache (MOH)." Treatment must include discontinuing the inciting medication.

DIZZINESS

49. **How does one differentiate vertigo, presyncope, and disequilibrium?**

    The most important step in taking the history from a dizzy patient is to figure out what is meant by "dizziness." **Vertigo** is the perception of translational or rotational movement in the absence of stimulus. A vertiginous patient should be able to identify the direction of movement (e.g., "the room is spinning from left to right" or "I feel like I'm falling backward"). If you've stepped off a rapidly spinning merry-go-round, you've experienced vertigo. **Presyncope** is a feeling of "lightheadedness" that is experienced in the setting of global cerebral hypoperfusion. The presyncopal patient, as implied by the term, often feels like "I was about to pass out." Others experience "blood rushing to the head," tinnitus, or "blacking out." **Disequilibrium** is an apt term for feelings of dizziness or unsteadiness that cannot be accurately described as vertiginous or presyncopal and can be used to describe ataxia, gait apraxia, postural instability, or anxiety. Disequilibrium can be either paroxysmal or constant. Patients will usually describe a feeling of the ground moving beneath them, being unsure of their footing, or "floating about" without a specific direction.

50. **What is the localization of vertigo?**

    The vestibular apparatus, the vestibulocochlear nerve (cranial nerve VIII), the brainstem, or the cerebellum. The key clinical differential localization of vertigo is whether it is peripheral (i.e., due to vestibular or nerve dysfunction) or central (i.e., localizing to the brainstem or cerebellum). **Peripheral vertigo** is typically accompanied by lateralized nystagmus (either spontaneous or elicited by head movement and either horizontal or rotatory in direction) and the absence of other brainstem or cerebellar findings. A positive Dix-Hallpike maneuver is relatively specific for benign positional vertigo. **Central vertigo** is often accompanied by other brainstem findings (cranial nerve deficits, crossed sensory or motor findings) or cerebellar findings. Vertical nystagmus is suggestive of a central etiology. (See also Chapter 18, Geriatrics.)

51. **What is benign (paroxysmal) positional vertigo (BPV/BPPV)?**

    A disorder in which brief intense periods of vertigo, often accompanied by nausea, are provoked by movement of the head. Classically, this is produced by extending the neck and twisting the head as if to look on a high shelf or rotating the head while supine (e.g., looking under a cabinet or rolling over in bed). The etiology of BPV is presumably precipitated crystals in the endolymph of the semicircular canals. Cannolith repositioning procedures can be remarkably effective at ameliorating symptoms.

    Fife TD, Iverson DJ, Lempert T, et al: Practice parameter: Therapies for benign paroxysmal positional vertigo (an evidence-based review): Report of the Quality Standards Subcommittee of the American Academy of Neurology, *Neurology* 70:2067–2074, 2008.

52. **What is the difference between vestibulitis and vestibular neuronitis?**

    Vestibulitis and vestibular neuronitis are idiopathic dysfunctions of vestibular function. In **vestibulitis,** the patient primarily experiences vertigo. In **vestibular neuronitis,** hearing loss or tinnitus or both are felt in addition to vertigo. Although the name implies an infectious or inflammatory etiology and a viral etiology is often suspected, an "-itis" has not been confirmed. Symptoms are not provoked by head movement and are less paroxysmal than in BPV.

53. **What is Ménière's disease?**
An inner ear disorder with symptoms of episodic vertigo, tinnitus, and sensorineural hearing loss. Hearing loss is typically progressive. Endolymphatic hydrops (excess hydrostatic pressure in the vestibular system) is associated with Ménière's, though the pathophysiology is incompletely understood. Diuretics are sometimes used for treatment.

54. **What are the causes of presyncope and syncope?**
Presyncope or syncope suggests global cerebral hypoperfusion or a toxic/metabolic derangement. Hypoperfusion usually results from a drop in blood pressure (BP). Although severe bilateral carotid stenoses or basilar artery stenosis could theoretically predispose to presyncope or syncope, there is seldom a focal vascular lesion responsible for these phenomena. The most common cause is activation of the parasympathetic autonomic nervous system leading to a bradycardia and vasodilation (i.e., vasovagal presyncope and syncope). The vasovagal response is the mechanism of presyncope and syncope induced by abdominal pain and cramping, defecation, micturition, cough, sexual activity, and fear. Intravascular volume depletion will predispose patients to vasovagal syncope. Hypoglycemia is the most common metabolic cause of presyncope or syncope and glucose should be checked while the patient is symptomatic, if possible. Cardiac dysrhythmias are much less common. Classically, cardiac syncope occurs without a presyncopal prodrome whereas vasovagal syncope is almost always preceded by a presyncopal prodrome. Orthostatic hypotension should always be considered in the setting of presyncope that comes on after standing from a sitting or supine position (see Chapter 18, Geriatrics). In the volume-depleted patient, falling BP is accompanied by an increase in pulse. In the patient with autonomic neuropathy or central autonomic dysfunction, falling BP is unaccompanied by an increase in pulse. (A lack of pulse increase is difficult to interpret if the patient is on a beta blocker.)

55. **What is the appropriate evaluation of disequilibrium?**
Nonspecific disequilibrium (which comprises a significant proportion of dizziness provoking neurologic consultation) is difficult to evaluate. Symptoms may be either continuous or paroxysmal. If symptoms are paroxysmal, a careful history for associated features or precipitants may give some clue to etiology. In either case, a careful neurologic examination including analysis of gait is imperative. Loss of proprioceptive function in the setting of a sensory neuropathy often leads to a mild gait ataxia and disequilibrium. Midline cerebellar dysfunction, whether toxic or degenerative, is another cause of disequilibrium. Postural responses should be assessed by observing the patient's ability to maintain posture when perturbed ("pull test"). To perform this test, the examiner first informs the patient what will happen, then stands behind the patient and gently pulls him or her backward by the shoulder. If the patient shuffles more than three steps, the response is abnormal.

MUSCLE WEAKNESS

56. **How can one distinguish peripheral from central facial weakness?**
In general, by determining the location of the involved muscles. The classic answer is that facial weakness caused by stroke or another central lesion should affect only the lower part of the face because the muscles of facial expression above the eye (corrugators and frontalis) have bilateral cerebral innervation. Thus, the patient with a Bell's palsy (peripheral) will have forehead weakness and eye closure weakness, whereas the patient with a hemispheric cerebrovascular accident (central) will not. A peripheral lesion affecting only the lower facial

nerve branches (V2 or V3 or both) could look like a central lesion, though, with lack of upper facial involvement. Taste sensation on the anterior two thirds of the tongue or tactile sense in the ear canal can be a clue to the location of the lesion. In addition, significant central facial weakness is often accompanied by subtle ipsilateral upper extremity weakness manifested by the presence of a pronator drift or decreased ipsilateral hand dexterity.

57. **What is the treatment for Bell's palsy?**
Oral corticosteroids and eye protection. In a randomized, controlled trial, oral steroids were shown to be effective, whereas acyclovir was not shown to be effective. Eye protection is needed because these patients frequently cannot close their eyes fully and can develop scleral damage. Applying a gel lubricant approved for eye use at night and taping the eye closed is cheap and effective. Ophthalmologic follow-up should be arranged.

Sullivan FM, Swan IR, Donnan PT, et al: Early treatment with prednisolone or acyclovir in Bell's palsy, *N Engl J Med* 357:1598–1607, 2007.

58. **How can one tell whether the patient has a neurologic disorder causing perceived weakness?**
By muscle strength testing (see Table 17-1). Focal or generalized weakness is a common complaint leading to neurologic evaluation. To the neurologist, true weakness is an inability to forcefully activate voluntary skeletal muscle despite maximal effort that can be due to a lesion in muscle, NMJ, lower motor neuron (anterior horn cell to NMJ), or upper motor neuron (motor cortex to anterior horn cell). True motor weakness has a characteristic feel on muscle strength testing with a steady but diminished resistance to movement of the limb. Functional or subjective weakness is characterized by inconsistent resistance that suddenly drops out or "gives way."

KEY POINTS: PATTERNS OF MUSCLE WEAKNESS AND LOCALIZATION ✔

1. Symmetrical suggests diffuse process.

2. Distal suggests neuropathy.

3. Proximal suggests myopathy.

4. Asymmetrical suggests focal structural problem.

5. Extensors weaker than flexors in upper extremities and flexors weaker than extensors in lower extremities suggest upper motor neuron lesion.

59. **Describe the settings in which a patient experiences subjective weakness without objective findings.**
For complaints of focal weakness, the most common cause of this discrepancy is pain. Patients will unconsciously guard against activating muscle groups that exacerbate pain from arthritis, fracture, or other structural problems. Pain elicited during confrontational testing is an obvious clue that this may be the case. In situations in which pain is the limiting factor, the best one can sometimes do is document "strength is at least 3 of 5 and examination is limited by pain." In the case of generalized fatigue or malaise, systemic illness may be the cause. However, fatigue and malaise also accompany other neurologic problems such as parkinsonism, spasticity, ataxia, or apraxia (inability to activate a complex coordinated movement). Thus, a careful examination of tone, coordination, and gait is a must in the patient with subjective weakness.

NUMBNESS

60. **Differentiate anesthesia, paresthesia, and dysesthesia.**
    - **Anesthesia:** lack of ability to detect sensory stimuli
    - **Paresthesia:** perception of sensory phenomena (e.g., tingling) in the absence of stimuli
    - **Dysesthesia:** experience of abnormal or unpleasant sensations with normal stimulus
      Patients may use the word "numbness" to describe any of these sensory abnormalities.

61. **Can an organic process cause subjective numbness without an objective sensory deficit?**
    Yes. The more central the lesion, the more likely there is to be a discrepancy between reported symptoms of numbness and ability to detect stimuli on a sensory examination. Infarcts to the thalamus can produce contralateral hemibody numbness with a normal sensory examination.

ATAXIA

62. **What is ataxia?**
    A deficit in coordination of voluntary movements leading to irregular deviations from the intended movement. Ataxia can affect the extremities, speech, or postural reflexes. During finger pointing tasks, intention tremor, which is a regular oscillation about the intended path, can be mistaken for ataxia.

63. **What is the location of lesions that cause ataxia?**
    The cerebellum. Strokes, degenerative diseases, and inflammatory or demyelinating diseases affecting the cerebellum or cerebellar outflow can cause ataxia. Disorders of the proprioceptive system or sensory nerves that lead to the cerebellum (either dorsal columns or peripheral nerves) also cause ataxia. In a number of genetically determined ataxias such as Friedrich's ataxia and spinocerebellar ataxia type 4, sensory deficits are prominent.

64. **Name some causes of ataxia that primarily affect the cerebellum.**
    - Intoxication with alcohol, medications, or other substances
    - Chronic alcohol use in the absence of intoxication
    - Cerebellar or brainstem hemorrhagic or ischemic stroke
    - Neurosyphilis
    - Vitamin B_{12} deficiency
    - Human immunodeficiency virus (HIV)–associated myelopathy
    - Paraneoplastic syndromes
    - Multiple system atrophy
    - MS
    - Postinfectious cerebellitis (usually in children)
    - Multiple genetic disorders

GAIT DYSFUNCTION

65. **Differentiate between an ataxic gait and an apraxic gait.**
    Both gait **ataxia** and **apraxia** are commonly associated with subjective balance difficulty and falls, though they look different clinically and have different localization. Gait ataxia is characterized by a wide-based gait and difficulty standing with the feet together. A Romberg sign is present if the patient can stand with feet together and eyes open but cannot maintain balance with eye closure. In marked gait or postural ataxia, patients cannot stand with the

feet together and the eyes open. Gait apraxia is a motor planning deficit and, thus, has a cerebral localization. Patients with gait apraxia have a hard time getting started with walking and may have a "magnetic" or shuffling gait. Gait apraxia is commonly seen in dementia (especially vascular dementia) and in NPH.

66. **When should one consider NPH?**
In any patient with gait apraxia. NPH is the classic triad of gait dysfunction, urinary incontinence, and memory difficulties. However, NPH produces a gait apraxia, and many patients with gait apraxia have memory difficulties, because this is frequently associated with dementia. Urinary incontinence is usually the last feature of NPH to appear and is not required in order to consider NPH.

KEY POINTS: CHARACTERISTICS OF NORMAL PRESSURE HYDROCEPHALUS ✔

1. Dementia.

2. Urinary incontinence.

3. Gait abnormalities.

4. Dementia may improve with ventricular shunting.

67. **How is NPH diagnosed?**
By brain imaging (CT or MRI). The radiologic hallmark of NPH is ventriculomegaly out of proportion to cerebral atrophy. Ventriculomegaly that results from cerebral atrophy is known as "ex vaccuo hydrocephalus." Whereas this distinction may sound simple, consensus about what is out of proportion to cerebral atrophy is elusive. In a patient with a gait apraxia and ventricles that are too big for her or his brain, the response to treatment with gait improvement is the ultimate diagnostic test.

68. **How is NPH treated?**
With drainage of CSF. However, there is little consensus about how to drain CSF and for how long. High-volume LP is frequently used as a first-line test. A positive response predicts a good response to ventriculoperitoneal (VP) or lumboperitoneal shunting. Temporary placement of a lumbar drain is another option. Empirical placement of a VP or lumboperitoneal shunt is sometimes performed on the basis of clinical suspicion.

69. **Do unsteady patients sway, rock, and swing their arms a lot to improve balance?**
Usually not. Exaggerated movements of the arms or swaying and rocking movements of the trunk (especially when superimposed on a narrow-based gait) should raise suspicion of a functional overlay to a gait problem.

STROKE AND CEREBROVASCULAR DISEASE

70. **What is a stroke?**
An acute, focal, cerebrovascular event leading to brain infarction or hemorrhage. Most strokes are ischemic (not getting blood to part of the brain). Hemorrhage within the cranial cavity, whether intraparencyhmal, subarachnoid, subdural, or epidural is also considered a stroke.

71. **What is a TIA?**
"A transient episode of neurological dysfunction caused by focal brain, spinal cord, or retinal ischemia without acute infarction." Although, historically, TIAs were defined as neurologic events that lasted < 24 hours, the advent of MRI that allows detection of stroke within this period has led to a new, tissue-based definition. If one can see infarction on an MRI, a stroke has occurred, even if the neurologic symptoms have resolved.

Easton JD, Saver JL, Albers GW, et al: Definition and evaluation of transient ischemic attack: A scientific statement for healthcare professionals from the American Heart Association/American Stroke Association Stroke Council; Council on Cardiovascular Surgery and Anesthesia; Council on Cardiovascular Radiology and Intervention; Council on Cardiovascular Nursing; and the Interdisciplinary Council on Peripheral Vascular Disease, *Stroke* 40:2276–2293, 2009.

72. **Name some possible mechanisms of ischemic stroke.**
- Thrombosis
- Embolism from carotid artery, aortic arch, or heart
- Hypoperfusion

73. **What cardiac conditions contribute to a cardiac source of the embolus or thrombosis?**
- Atrial fibrillation
- Ischemic or nonischemic cardiomyopathy with hypokinesis
- Atrial septal defect (venous thrombosis)
- Patent foramen ovale (venous thrombosis)
- Mechanical prosthetic valves
- Atrial myxoma
- Bacterial endocarditis

74. **What are the indications and contraindications for IV thrombolysis in acute ischemic stroke?**
See Table 17-5. Despite the expansion of eligibility to 4.5 hours, it is imperative to remember (and remind all those involved in acute stroke care) that the potential benefit from thrombolysis decreases with each passing minute. Therapy should be administered as soon as possible—time is brain!

TABLE 17-5. DETERMINANTS OF USE OF THROMBOLYTIC THERAPY IN ISCHEMIC STROKE

Presence of	Absence of
■ Persistent neurologic deficits that are not clearing ■ Neurologic deficits that are more than minor and isolated ■ Symptoms started < 3 hr before planned treatment* ■ Systolic BP < 185 mmHg and diastolic BP < 110 mmHg	■ Findings suggestive of SAH ■ History of head trauma in previous 3 mo ■ History of prior stroke in previous 3 mo ■ Myocardial infarction in previous 3 mo ■ Gastrointestinal or urinary tract hemorrhage in previous 21 days ■ Major surgery in previous 14 days

(continued)

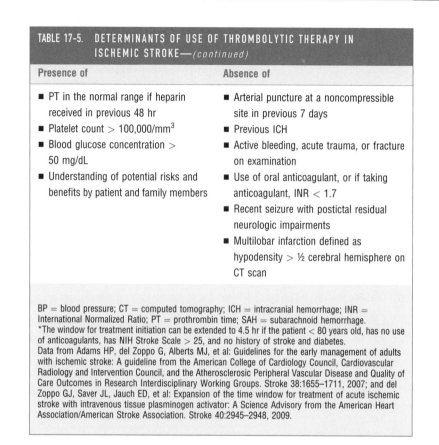

TABLE 17–5. DETERMINANTS OF USE OF THROMBOLYTIC THERAPY IN
ISCHEMIC STROKE—*(continued)*

Presence of	Absence of
▪ PT in the normal range if heparin received in previous 48 hr ▪ Platelet count > 100,000/mm³ ▪ Blood glucose concentration > 50 mg/dL ▪ Understanding of potential risks and benefits by patient and family members	▪ Arterial puncture at a noncompressible site in previous 7 days ▪ Previous ICH ▪ Active bleeding, acute trauma, or fracture on examination ▪ Use of oral anticoagulant, or if taking anticoagulant, INR < 1.7 ▪ Recent seizure with postictal residual neurologic impairments ▪ Multilobar infarction defined as hypodensity > ½ cerebral hemisphere on CT scan

BP = blood pressure; CT = computed tomography; ICH = intracranial hemorrhage; INR = International Normalized Ratio; PT = prothrombin time; SAH = subarachnoid hemorrhage.
*The window for treatment initiation can be extended to 4.5 hr if the patient < 80 years old, has no use of anticoagulants, has NIH Stroke Scale > 25, and no history of stroke and diabetes.
Data from Adams HP, del Zoppo G, Alberts MJ, et al: Guidelines for the early management of adults with ischemic stroke: A guideline from the American College of Cardiology Council, Cardiovascular Radiology and Intervention Council, and the Atherosclerosic Peripheral Vascular Disease and Quality of Care Outcomes in Research Interdisciplinary Working Groups. Stroke 38:1655–1711, 2007; and del Zoppo GJ, Saver JL, Jauch ED, et al: Expansion of the time window for treatment of acute ischemic stroke with intravenous tissue plasminogen activator: A Science Advisory from the American Heart Association/American Stroke Association. Stroke 40:2945–2948, 2009.

75. **Does IV thrombolysis in acute stroke improve outcomes? By how much?**
Yes. Various studies have shown an absolute increase in probability of a good functional recovery of approximately 15%. The number needed to treat (NNT) to prevent poor recovery is six acute strokes.

76. **When is intra-arterial thrombolysis, mechanical extraction of thrombus, or both considered for treatment of acute ischemic stroke?**
In many tertiary-care medical centers, there is a protocol for catheter-based intra-arterial thrombolysis or clot extraction or both in acute large vessel stroke that involve the middle cerebral artery or its branches and the basilar artery. Interventional procedures for acute stroke remain promising and are undergoing current evaluation through investigational protocols.

77. **Should BP be tightly controlled to normal levels for patients with acute ischemic stroke?**
No. For thrombolysis patients, systolic BP must be maintained < 180 mmHg, but excessive lowering of BP should be avoided. Reduction of BP to "normal" levels in the setting of acute stroke worsens functional recovery. Systemic hypertension is a physiologic response to cerebral ischemia and maximizes penumbral perfusion. In the first few days poststroke, antihypertensives should thus be used judiciously. Control of hypertension is, of course, an important part of secondary stroke prevention and should be achieved by the time of

hospital discharge. If patients have completely resolved deficits, then permissive hypertension is not necessary.

78. **What is the work-up of an acute ischemic stroke or TIA?**
Acute evaluation (should be focused to allow thrombolytic therapy if indicated):
- **CT scan** of the brain without contrast to evaluate for acute intracerebral hemorrhage
- **Laboratory data:** Glucose, CBC, platelet count, serum electrolytes, coagulation studies, lipid panel, cardiac enzymes, oxygen saturation
- **Electrocardiogram (ECG)** with continued telemetry monitoring

Etiology and risk factor evaluation:
- **Laboratory data in appropriate clinical setting:** erythrocyte sedimentation rate (ESR), antinuclear antibody (ANA), homocysteine
- **Carotid artery imaging** (duplex ultrasound or magnetic resonance angiography [MRA]) for anterior circulation symptoms
- **Transthoracic echocardiogram**
- **Echocardiogram** with "bubble study" to assess for intra-atrial shunt, if indicated
- **Evaluation of hypercoagulable state**, if indicated: protein C, protein S, Factor V Leiden, prothrombin gene mutation

79. **What is the role of antiplatelet therapy in secondary stroke prevention (or the occurrence of another stroke after the first event)?**
To reduce the risk of stroke. The relative risk reduction of stroke with aspirin is around 20–25% with both an acute and a long-term benefit. All patients with ischemic stroke should be on aspirin 81–325 mg daily or an alternative antiplatelet medication unless there is a compelling contraindication. Whereas there is broad agreement that stroke patients should be on some form of antiplatelet therapy, there is far less consensus about which agent (aspirin alone, aspirin + dipyridamole, clopidogrel alone, or aspirin + clopidogrel) is optimal. This can be, and often is, a subject of substantial debate about risks, benefits, and costs. See Figure 17-1 for detailed information regarding these multiple studies.

(Based on CAPRIE Steering Committee: A randomised, blinded, trial of clopidogrel versus aspirin in patients at risk of ischaemic events (CAPRIE). *Lancet* 348:1329–1339, 1996; Bhatt MD, Fox KA, Hacke W, et al: Clopidogrel and aspirin versus aspirin alone for the prevention of atherothrombotic events. *N Engl J Med* 354:1706–1717, 2006; ESPRIT Study Group, Halkes PH, van Gijn J, et al: Aspirin plus dipyridamole versus aspirin alone after cerebral ischaemia of arterial origin (ESPRIT): randomized

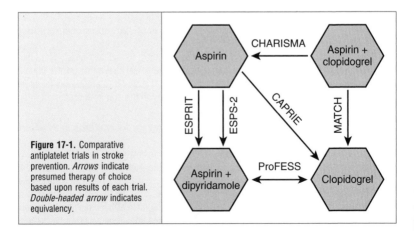

Figure 17-1. Comparative antiplatelet trials in stroke prevention. *Arrows* indicate presumed therapy of choice based upon results of each trial. *Double-headed arrow* indicates equivalency.

controlled trial. *Lancet* 367:1665–1673, 2006; Dippel DW, Maasland L, Halkes P, et al: Prevention with low-dose aspirin plus dipyridamole in patients with disabling stroke. *Stroke* 41:2684–2686, 2010; Diener HC, Bogousslavsky J, Brass LM, et al: Aspirin and clopidogrel compared with clopidogrel alone after recent ischaemic stroke or transient ischaemic attack in high-risk patients (MATCH): randomised, double-blind, placebo-controlled trial. *Lancet* 364:331–337, 2004; Bath PM, Cotton D, Martin RH, et al: Effect of combined aspirin and extended-release dipyridamole versus clopidogrel on functional outcome and recurrence in acute, mild ischemic stroke: PRoFESS subgroup analysis. *Stroke* 41:732–738, 2010.)

80. **What is the role of warfarin in secondary stroke prevention?**
    To reduce the risk of stroke in patients with persistent or paroxysmal atrial fibrillation. Relative risk is reduced by ≤ 68%. Warfarin should thus be strongly considered in all patients with stroke and atrial fibrillation or mechanical heart valves. In patients with noncardioembolic stroke, though, warfarin has not shown benefit over aspirin in multiple randomized trials. Warfarin has specifically not been shown to be superior to aspirin in preventing strokes in patients with intracranial stenosis.

81. **What is the role of statins in secondary stroke prevention?**
    To reduce recurrent stroke risk. In a randomized study, atorvastatin (80 mg daily) reduced absolute recurrent stroke risk by 2% over 5 years versus placebo in patients with low-density lipoprotein (LDL) between 100 and 190 mg/dL. Many experts feel that the benefit proved in this trial is generalizable across the statins and that statins are indicated in any patient with a history of ischemic stroke. The benefit in patients with LDL < 100 mg/dL is uncertain.

    Aggressive Reduction in Cholesterol Levels (SPARCL) Investigators: High-dose atorvastatin after stroke or transient ischemic attack, *N Engl J Med* 355:549–559, 2006.

82. **What are the etiologies and location of hemorrhagic stroke?**
    See Table 17-6.

TABLE 17-6. ETIOLOGIES AND LOCATIONS OF HEMORRHAGIC STROKE

Etiology	Stroke Location
Hypertension	Thalami, basal ganglia, pons, or cerebellum
Ruptured intracranial aneurysm	Subarachnoid
Amyloid angiopathy	Lobar
Neoplasm	Lobar
Vascular malformation	Lobar

83. **How does one work-up and treat nontraumatic subarachnoid hemorrhage (SAH)?**
    Initially, with CT angiography (CTA) or MRA to evaluate for a ruptured cerebral aneurysm. If an aneurysm is discovered, urgent intervention to secure the aneurysm via surgical clipping or intravascular coiling is typically indicated. Patients with aneurysmal SAH must be monitored closely for the development of delayed cerebral vasospasm 3–14 days post hemorrhage, which can cause delayed ischemic stroke. Nimodipine has been shown to improve outcomes and is typically given to SAH patients. SAH patients must also be monitored for the development of hydrocephalus.

84. **How do I work up and treat parenchymal hemorrhage (intracranial hemorrhage [ICH])?**
    Patients with ICH are typically diagnosed by CT scan without contrast. Unless the hemorrhage is in a classic location for hypertensive hemorrhage and the patient has a clear history of uncontrolled hypertension, both immediate and delayed (4–8 wk) contrasted imaging by CT or MRI is indicated to evaluate for the presence of underlying pathology that

may have caused the bleed. Any coagulopathy (iatrogenic or intrinsic) should be reversed promptly and anticoagulant and antiplatelet agents should be held. Trials of procoagulant administration have failed to show improvement in outcomes. BP should be managed typically to maintain a systolic pressure of 120–140 mmHg.

85. **When does one need to consult a neurosurgeon?**
A discussion of surgical triage and timing in subdural hemorrhage is beyond the scope of this chapter, but it is generally appropriate to consult a neurosurgeon in acute **subdural hematoma (SDH). Epidural hematoma** is typically another neurosurgical emergency, as is **posterior fossa hemorrhage** when there is a risk of brainstem compression. In cases of life-threatening mass effect from acute **supratentorial ICH,** surgical evacuation may be appropriate. If the patient has a normal level of consciousness, ICH can usually be managed nonsurgically. Urgent neurosurgical intervention, typically in the form of a ventriculostomy, is indicated in the development of acute obstructive hydrocephalus resulting from obstruction of ventricular outflow by **intraventricular hemorrhage.** Neurosurgery may be involved in securing aneurysms in aneurysmal SAH, but these are frequently handled by interventional radiologists. Surgical evacuation is not typically indicated in ICH.

SEIZURES AND EPILEPSY

86. **What is a seizure?**
An abnormal, rhythmic, synchronous firing of a group of neurons. Seizures can manifest as both positive (e.g., rhythmic shaking, hallucinations, or lip smacking) and negative (e.g., lack of responsiveness or inability to move) neurologic phenomena. A generalized tonic-clonic seizure has a typical appearance with generalized muscle contractions, followed by synchronous convulsions, followed by postictal period of slowly improving lethargy and confusion. Partial seizures, however, can look like just about anything in terms of neurologic symptoms depending on what area of brain is involved. The important thing to remember is that spells are typically stereotyped (i.e., the same from spell to spell) within a given patient.

87. **How are seizures and seizure disorders classified?**
   - **Generalized:** involves both cerebral hemispheres
   - **Partial: Focal**
     - **Complex partial:** impaired consciousness or responsiveness
     - **Simple partial:** unimpaired consciousness
   - **Partial with secondary generalization**
   The classification of seizures is a work in progress. The International League Against Epilepsy is tasked with being the official classifier.

   International League Against Epilepsy. Available at: www.ilae-epilepsy.org/.

88. **What is the most common seizure type in adults with new-onset seizures?**
Complex partial.

89. **What is the work-up for a first seizure in an adult?**
   - **History:** focusing on provocative factors such as substance use or withdrawal, recent infection, head trauma, strokes, or brain surgery.
   - **Laboratory data:** serum electrolytes, CBC.
   - **Neuroimaging:** preferably MRI.
   - **EEG:** preferably within 24 hours of the event. May be normal, which does not rule out the diagnosis of seizure disorder.

90. **When does driving need to be restricted?**
Whenever a patient has an unprovoked sudden impairment in consciousness or cognition that impairs operation of a motor vehicle. Seizure, syncope, and other unexplained alterations

in consciousness all fit this bill. Legal requirements about length of time event-free before returning to driving and physician reporting vary state by state.

www.epilepsy.com/epilepsy/rights_driving.

91. **When should one start a seizure medication?**
Most neurologists adhere to a "two-strikes-you're-out" policy for unprovoked seizures. If EEG findings are highly suggestive of a seizure disorder or there is a clear structural problem that correlates with localization of seizure onset, then it may be reasonable to start an antiepileptic drug (AED) after the first seizure.

92. **When should one add a second seizure medication or switch seizure medications?**
If a patient continues to have seizures on a given antiseizure regimen or cannot tolerate the initial medication. Common wisdom suggests that the dose and plasma level of each AED should be maximized before adding another AED or switching AEDs. If lack of efficacy rather than intolerability is the issue, then typically a second AED is added, and then, if the add-on AED provides good control, the first AED can be tapered to see whether control is maintained. For each subsequent AED regimen that fails to provide good seizure control, the odds of achieving good control with a subsequent change diminishes.

93. **Which AED should one start?**
Many AEDs are available and there is a paucity of conclusive head-to-head data to guide selection. Some childhood epilepsies have been found to respond well to specific AEDs (e.g., ethosuxamide for absence epilepsy). In adults, pragmatics often guide drug selection. Phenytoin is commonly used because it is inexpensive, available IV and orally, and levels can be easily followed. Lamotrigine is well tolerated but must be titrated up slowly to avoid severe rash. Levetiracetam has gained wide use as a first-line drug because of its wide therapeutic window (eliminating need for level monitoring), ability to start at full dose, lack of hepatic metabolism, and lack of drug-drug interactions but can cause behavioral side effects.

94. **Define "status epilepticus."**
Continuous seizure activity or intermittent seizure activity without regaining normal consciousness between spells lasting > 5 minutes. Status epilepticus is a neurologic emergency.

95. **How should status epilepticus be managed?**
First, focus on basic resuscitation principles—protect airway, apply oxygen, establish IV access. Fingerstick glucose should be obtained, and basic laboratory work including AED levels, if the patient is known to be taking any, should be sent. IV lorazepam should be administered. In adults, 2 mg is the typical first dose, followed by additional doses of 2 mg at 2-minute intervals up to 8 mg total. IV fosphenytoin is then loaded at 20 mg/kg given at 100 mg/min. If seizures continue or the patient remains unresponsive, transfer to the intensive care unit with EEG monitoring if indicated. Phenobarbitol at 20 mg/kg is a typical next step. This is followed by infusion therapy with midazolam, propofol, or pentobarbital. Other AEDs such as levetiracetam, valproic acid, or lacosamide are typically loaded at this point as well.

MULTIPLE SCLEROSIS

96. **What causes MS?**
The short answer is, "we don't know," although MS is clearly an immune-mediated disease. Genetic risk factors for MS have been identified, and an association with geographic latitude has been demonstrated, but the etiology remains uncertain.

97. **How does MS present clinically?**
With multiple neurologic lesions and, in the most common form, multiple clinical "attacks" or exacerbations. Something has to be the first symptom of MS, however. Many MS patients

complain of fatigue, depression, or mild cognitive impairment, but these are very nonspecific. Numbness or paresthesias affecting one part of the body and lasting for weeks with resolution is a classic clinical syndrome. Monocular vision loss or myelopathy are other common presenting syndromes.

98. **Are there accepted diagnostic criteria for MS?**
    Yes, the McDonald criteria that were first issued in 2001 and revised in 2005. The classic description of MS as a process with lesions separated by time and space (i.e., anatomically distinct) still basically holds true, but the new criteria allow for the use of MRI findings to satisfy these requirements.

    Polman CH, Reingold SC, Edan G, et al: Diagnostic criteria for multiple sclerosis: 2005 revisions to the McDonald criteria, *Ann Neurol* 58:840–846, 2005.

99. **What treatments are available for MS?**
    Interferon therapy given by subcutaneous or intramuscular injection or glatiramer acetate are the standard disease-modifying therapies currently available for relapsing-remitting MS. All have been shown to have a modest but significant impact on both disease activity and progression to disability. Second-line therapies include natalizumab and mitoxantrone. High-dose steroids (e.g., 1000 mg of methylprednisolone/day for 3–5 days) are commonly used to treat acute exacerbations of MS and has been shown to reduce short-term symptoms and disability. The effect on long-term outcome is unknown. Low-dose oral prednisone (i.e., 1 mg/kg) has been shown to be ineffective for treatment of MS exacerbations. Limited evidence suggests that high-dose oral therapy (e.g., 1250 mg of prednisone daily) may be equivalent to IV therapy, but IV administration is more common. The US Food and Drug Administration (FDA) recently approved fingolimod for oral therapy for MS.

MOVEMENT DISORDERS

100. **How are movement disorders classified?**
     Most broadly, movement disorders are classified into **hyperkinetic** (causing excess involuntary movement) and **hypokinetic** (causing paucity of movement or difficulty initiating movement). Hyperkinetic movement disorders include tremor, dystonia, myoclouns, and chorea. The hypokinetic movement disorders comprise PD and other parkinsonian disorders.

101. **Describe the most common types of tremor.**
     Tremor is a regular rhythmic oscillatory movement. Tremors are divided into **action tremors** and **resting tremors.** Action tremors accentuate with voluntary movement such as pointing toward a target or holding a posture with the limbs. The most common action tremors are enhanced **physiologic tremor** and **essential tremor (ET).** Enhanced physiologic tremor is a low-amplitude, high-frequency action tremor that can be exacerbated by sleep deprivation, stimulant medication, and anxiety. If you ever stayed up all night studying for an examination and drinking large amounts of coffee, you may have experienced this. Multiple medications can cause or exacerbate tremor, and the medication list should always be reviewed when evaluating tremor. ET is a genetic condition, though a family history is absent in up to 40% of cases. ET produces a moderate-to-high frequency action tremor that can affect the head, voice, limbs, and trunk. Resting tremors emerge when a limb is not being used voluntarily. Patients will often complain that their hand will start shaking when they are watching television or reading and that they can make the tremor stop if they pay attention to it. Resting tremor most often represents PD. Some drugs (especially lithium), cerebellar lesions, and rubral lesions can also produce resting tremor.

102. **How is ET treated?**
Initially with propranolol and primidone. Medications that may be exacerbating tremor should be removed if possible. Second-line medications include topirimate, gabapentin, and benzodiazepines. For disabling, medically refractory ET, deep brain stimulation of the ventral intermediate (VIM) nucleus of the thalamus can be a highly effective intervention.

103. **What is the difference between parkinsonism and PD?**
Parkinsonism is a clinical phenotype consisting of bradykinesia and rigidity. Resting tremor can be part of parkinsonism but is not necessarily present. Postural instability may also be present. "Bradykinesia" refers not just to a slowness of movements but to difficulty initiating movements with a characteristic diminishing amplitude to repetitive movements. Parkinsonian rigidity worsens when the patient is distracted. Parkinsonism can be caused by neuroleptic exposure (drug-induced and tardive parkinsonism), cerebrovascular disease, and other neurodegenerative conditions. **PD** is an idiopathic neurodegenerative disorder producing parkinsonism as its cardinal manifestation.

104. **How is PD treated?**
By providing pharmacologic stimulation of dopaminergic pathways in the brain. Degeneration of dopaminergic nigrostriatal neurons is a pathologic hallmark of PD, and administration of exogenous dopamine (in the form of carbodopa/levodopa) or dopamine agonists has been shown to ameliorate the symptoms of the disease. Drugs that inhibit dopamine metabolism are also used. Anticholinergics are sometimes used for the amelioration of tremor, and amantadine can also provide symptomatic benefit. No drug therapy has been conclusively shown to alter the rate of progression of PD. Rehabilitation and maintenance of physical activity are important components to PD treatment. Deep brain stimulation can be beneficial in carefully selected candidates.

105. **Describe chorea and myoclonus**
Chorea is a flowing "dancelike" hyperkinetic movement that is characteristic of Huntington's disease. Chorea can also be seen in other neurodegenerative disorders and in tardive dyskinesia.
  Myoclonus is defined by very short, jerky involuntary contractions. Myoclonus is most often symptomatic of a metabolic derangement but can also be seen after anoxic brain injury and in several rare genetic disorders. Asterixis is a related phenomenon and is sometimes termed "negative myoclonus."

NEUROMUSCULAR DISORDERS

106. **Classify the causes of myopathy.**
   - **Rheumatic diseases:** polymyositis, dermatomyositis, polymyalgia rheumatica, Sjögren's syndrome, vasculitis
   - **Endocrine disorders:** hypothyroidism, hyperthyroidism, Cushing's disease, adrenal insufficiency, hyperaldosteronism
   - **Electrolyte disorders:** hypokalemia
   - **Malabsorption:** celiac sprue, vitamin D deficiency, vitamin E deficiency
   - **Medications:** glucocorticoids, lipid lowering drugs (statins and fibrates), colchicines, chloroquine, phenothiazines, nucleoside reverse transcriptase inhibitors (NRTIs), d-penicillamine
   - **Toxic exposure:** alcohol, cocaine
   - **Infections:** HIV, other viral infections
   - **Genetic disorders:** muscular dystrophies
   - **Paraneoplastic syndromes**

107. **How is myopathy diagnosed?**
By clinical evaluation, EMG, and muscle biopsy, if necessary. Clinically, myopathy typically presents as symmetrical proximal weakness. A thorough history, physical, and laboratory evaluation for disorders described earlier should be performed, and blood levels of muscle enzymes (creatine kinase and aldolase) should be obtained. Muscle biopsy can be very helpful when the cause of myopathy is not otherwise apparent and is useful in confirming the diagnosis of an inflammatory myopathy.

108. **How does myasthenia gravis (MG) present and how is it diagnosed?**
Frequently, with intermittent diplopia or fatigable ptosis or both. Generalized fatigable weakness may or may not be present on a careful examination. MG is an autoimmune disorder in which antibodies to the acetylcholine (ACh) receptors of the NMJ impair neuromuscular transmission. Commercial blood tests are available for acetylcholinesterase (AChE) receptor antibodies and for muscle specific kinase (Musk) antibodies, which are positive in a subset of patients who are negative for AChE antibodies. When positive, repetitive nerve stimulation studies (a specialized nerve conduction study) is highly specific. Single-fiber EMG is more sensitive but more difficult to perform and less widely available.

109. **How is MG treated?**
By administration of the peripheral cholinesterase inhibitor pyridostigmine and by immunosuppression. In purely ocular MG or in very mild cases, monotherapy with pyridostigmine may be appropriate, but in patients with generalized myasthenia, some form of immunosuppressive therapy is indicated to control the underlying disease. Prednisone is highly effective, though steroid-sparing treatment with azathioprine, mycofenolate mofetil, or other immunosuppressive therapies is commonly used to avoid long-term complications of prednisone therapy. In severe myasthenic exacerbations, plasma exchange provides the most rapid clinical improvement in symptoms. Intravenous immunoglobulin (IVIG) is also an effective therapy, but response is less rapid.

110. **Are there other disorders of the NMJ?**
Yes. The Lambert-Eaton myasthenic syndrome (LEMS) is an autoimmune or paraneoplastic disorder in which ACh release is inhibited by antibodies to the presynaptic voltage-gated calcium channel. LEMS produces proximal weakness and autonomic dysfunction. About 50% of cases are associated with small cell lung cancer. Botulism, whether from infection or iatrogenic, is another presynaptic disorder.

111. **Describe the clinical feature of polyneuropathy.**
Neuropathies present with sensory and/or motor dysfunction. Most polyneuropathies affect nerves in a length-dependent fashion such that the toes and feet are most affected.

112. **What are some usual causes of neuropathy?**
- **Abnormal glucose metabolism:** prediabetes and diabetes
- **Toxins and drugs:** chronic alcohol exposure, chemotherapeutic agents (taxanes, platin-based drugs, bevacizamub)
- **Infection:** HIV, Lyme disease, neurosyphilis, hepatitis virus
- **Endocrine disorders:** hypothyroidism
- **Deficiencies:** vitamin B_{12}
- **Rheumatic disorders:** rheumatoid arthritis, Sjögren's syndrome, vasculitis
- **Protein disorders**

An extensive list is available at: http://neuromuscular.wustl.edu/.

113. **What are the features of an unusual neuropathy?**
Most neuropathies are chronic and insidious in onset. The acute presentation of neuropathy should raise a red flag for toxic, inflammatory, or immune causes. Most neuropathies have widespread involvement. The acute presentation of multiple isolated neuropathies (mononeuritis multiplex) should raise a red flag for vasculitic processes.

114. **What is the routine work-up for polyneuropathy?**
NCSs and EMG are often helpful. They can differentiate between predominantly axonal and demyelinating neuropathies. Recommended laboratory tests for all patients with neuropathy include thyroid function tests, vitamin B_{12} levels (with methylmalonic acid and homocysteine or both, if indicated), fasting glucose, and serum protein electrophoresis. In selected patients, testing for autoimmune and inflammatory disorders should be considered. LP for analysis of CSF protein and serum testing for specific antibodies (e.g. MAG, GQ1b) may be helpful in the work-up of demyelinating neuropathies.

115. **How does Guillain-Barré syndrome (GBS) present?**
As rapidly (several hours to a few days) progressive weakness usually beginning in the lower extremities. GBS is often preceded or accompanied by paresthesias and sensory loss. Areflexia is the norm.

116. **How is GBS treated?**
With plasmapheresis and IVIG. Cardiac and respiratory monitoring is necessary acutely while symptoms are still progressing. Most patients make a good functional recovery, but this can take many months.

SLEEP DISORDERS

117. **How are sleep disorders classified?**
   - Insomnia
   - Sleep-related breathing disorders
   - Hypersomnia
   - Circadian rhythm disorders
   - Parasomnias
   - Sleep-related movement disorders

   American Academy of Sleep Medicine: *International Classification of Sleep Disorders*, ed 2, Diagnostic and Coding Manual. Westchester, IL, 2005, American Academy of Sleep Medicine.

118. **How common is sleep apnea?**
Prevalence is estimated at 3–7% of the general population. Key symptoms include excessive daytime sleepiness, loud snoring, and witnessed apneas.

   Punjabi NM: The epidemiology of adult obstructive sleep apnea, *Proc Am Thorac Soc* 5:136–143, 2008.

119. **Does continuous positive airway pressure (CPAP) help sleep apnea?**
Yes. Multiple randomized trials have demonstrated improvement in sleep parameters including oxygen desaturation, number of apneas, and daytime sleepiness with CPAP compared with sham CPAP. Some patients have a difficult time tolerating CPAP apparatus, and it is worth trying various commercially available masks to enhance tolerability. Whereas many experts believe that CPAP improves cardiovascular outcomes and mortality, this has not been proved prospectively.

120. **What is rapid eye movement behavioral disorder (RBD)?**
Loss of normal muscle atonia during rapid eye movement (REM) sleep accompanied by complex motor behaviors. Patients enact dreams and can engage in behavior that is harmful

to self and others. Clonazepam is highly effective anecdotally (though this has not been demonstrated in a randomized trial) and is the treatment of choice. RBD can be the harbinger of a neurodegenerative disorder—especially PD.

121. **How is narcolepsy diagnosed?**
With an overnight PSG followed by a multiple sleep latency test. A test consisting of multiple naps is essential in the work-up for narcolepsy. Intrusive REM sleep during naps in the absence of another significant sleep disorder documented by PSG is basically diagnostic of narcolepsy. CSF hypocretin levels are sometimes measured; low levels are felt to be specific but not sensitive. Narcolepsy should be suspected in the setting of excessive daytime sleepiness accompanied by a history of cataplexy (brief loss of muscle tone during wakefulness often precipitated by emotional trigger) or sleep paralysis (inability to move or speak upon awakening from sleep).

122. **What is the most common cause of excessive daytime somnolence?**
Voluntary sleep deprivation is the most common cause of excessive sleepiness.

NEOPLASTIC AND PARANEOPLASTIC DISEASE

123. **What are the most common intracranial malignancies?**
Metastatic disease, usually lung, breast, or melanoma.

124. **How are primary brain tumors classified?**
By presumed cell of origin. A complete listing of brain tumor types can be found at multiple places on the web. Glioblastoma multiforme (grade IV astrocytoma) is the most common primary brain malignancy in adults.

    http://neurosurgery.mgh.harvard.edu/newwhobt.htm

125. **What are paraneoplastic syndromes?**
Disorders caused by an autoimmune reaction to malignancy. Important paraneoplastic syndromes include the LEMS (usually associated with small cell lung cancer), paraneoplastic limbic encephalitis, cerebellitis, and sensory neuropathy. Serum and CSF assays for some paraneoplastic antibodies are commercially available.

WEBSITES

1. American Academy of Neurology: www.aan.org
2. National Institute of Neurological Disorders and Stroke: www.ninds.nih.gov
3. National Stroke Association: www.stroke.org

BIBLIOGRAPHY

1. Johnson RT, Griffin JW, McArthur JC, editors: *Current Therapy in Neurologic Disease*, ed 7, St. Louis, 2005, Mosby.
2. Posner JB, Saper CB, Schiff N, et al: *Plum and Posner's Diagnosis of Stupor and Coma*, ed 4, New York, 2007, Oxford University Press.
3. Ropper A, Samuels M: *Adams and Victor's Principles of Neurology*, ed 9, New York, 2009, McGraw-Hill.

CHAPTER 18

GERIATRICS

John Meuleman, M.D., and Henrique Elias Kallas, M.D., C.M.D.

It's like walking ten miles, a step at a time, living and breathing, one day at a time, one week at a time. Before you know it, you're a hundred years old. The body doesn't function, of course. You know, some young girls gave me a seat on the bus. I was flattered.

Abe Goldstein
From Ellis N: If I live to be 100. Available at: www.ifilivetobe100.com

1. **What changes in organ function occur in advanced age?**
   See Table 18-1.

2. **What are some common sensory disorders in older persons?**
   - Cataracts
   - Macular degeneration
   - High-frequency hearing loss
   - Diminished taste sensation
   - Diminished olfactory function

3. **How does change in body composition with aging affect drug treatment?**
   Some drugs may have an altered volume of distribution owing to a marked increase in fat mass and decrease in lean body mass associated with aging. Patients who appear trim may still have these changes. As a result, water-soluble (hydrophilic) drugs such as digoxin or lithium have higher concentrations owing to a lower volume of distribution. Fat-soluble (lipophilic) drugs such as benzodiazepines or thiopental have a higher volume of distribution and will have longer times for steady-state concentration and elimination.

4. **How does sleep change with aging?**
   Sleep latency (time to fall asleep) increases and **sleep efficiency** (time asleep divided by time in bed) decreases. Elder patients tend to have an earlier bedtime, earlier morning awakening, more nocturnal arousals, and more daytime napping. Sleep structure changes include a notable decline in stage N3 (deep sleep) and an increase in stages N1 (transitional sleep) and N2 (intermediate sleep).

ASSESSMENT OF OLDER PATIENTS

5. **What are the essential elements of an evaluation for an elderly patient with recurrent falls?**
   - **History:** focusing on the circumstances and associated symptoms
   - **Gait:** using the get-up and go test
   - **Balance:** tested by observing side-by-side, semitandem, and tandem stance
   - **Muscle strength:** including quadriceps, hip flexors and extensors, and foot dorsiflexion
   - **Vision**

TABLE 18-1.   CHANGES IN ORGAN SYSTEM WITH AGING AND THEIR CONSEQUENCES

System	Aging-Related Change	Consequence of this Change
Skin	Xerosis (dry skin)	Frequent, diffuse pruritus.
Cardiovascular	Decreased LV compliance and relaxation	Elevated LV end-diastolic pressures, greatly increased prevalence of heart failure.
Renal	With loss of muscle mass, decreased creatinine clearance not reflected in commensurate increase in serum creatinine	Underdiagnosis of renal insufficiency with concomitant overdosage of certain medications.
Renal	Decreased maximum urine osmolarity	Inappropriately high urine outputs in hypovolemic states increasing propensity for dehydration.
Pulmonary	Decreased forced vital capacity and forced expiratory volume, increased A-a oxygen gradient	Propensity for hypoxia in the setting of pneumonia or other pulmonary insults.
Pulmonary	Decreased cough reflex	Propensity for aspiration.
Skeletal muscle	Sarcopenia (aging-related loss of muscle mass)	Weakness.
Vision	Decreased pupillary dilatation and light sensitivity of retina	Poor night vision, affecting night driving and nocturnal ambulation.
Hearing	Decreased high-frequency perception	Impaired understanding of certain sounds; some prefixes or suffixes drop out from perception.
Immune	Decreased T-cell function	Propensity for infections
Nervous	Decreased neural connectivity	Slower recall even in the setting of preserved memory.

A-a = alveolar-arterial; LV = left ventricular.

- **Feet and footwear:** for any deformities
- **Orthostatic blood pressure measurement:** if vasovagal reaction suspected
- **Dix-Hallpike maneuver:** if positional vertigo suspected
- Consider home safety evaluation if appropriate

6. **What is the get-up and go test?**
   A maneuver to assess the ease with which the patient can:
   - Rise from a chair without using arm supports
   - Stand still momentarily

- Walk about a short distance (~10 feet)
- Turn around
- Walk back to the chair
- Turn around
- Sit down in the chair without using the arm supports

Mathias S, Nayak USL, Isaacs B: Balance in elderly patients: The "get-up and go" test, *Arch Phys Med Rehabil* 67:387–389, 1986.

7. **What is the Dix-Hallpike maneuver?**
   A procedure to reproduce positional vertigo. The physician supports the patient while the patient goes from a sitting to a supine position approximately 20° below shoulder level with the head turned 45° to one side. The eyes are observed for nystagmus and the patient is asked about reproduction of symptoms. The patient then returns to the sitting position and the maneuver is repeated on the opposite side.

8. **Describe the usefulness of an assessment of function and activities of daily living (ADLs).**
   Many older patients value quality of life over quantity of life. Assessment of function and ADLs provides insight into the symptomatic impact and current status of the patient's various health problems. This assessment allows the provider to monitor the trajectory of a patient's health and ensures attention is given to maximizing quality of life. Also, a change in function is often the first sign of decompensation of a medical problem.

9. **How is such a functional assessment performed?**
   By evaluating whether there are any recent changes in the patient's ability to perform ADLs or whether the patient now needs assistance or has difficulty with some ADLs. Some of these observations are best made by others.

10. **What are the essential aspects of evaluating driving safety in an older adult?**
    - **Vision:** including a formal eye examination
    - **Cognition:** using the clock drawing test
    - **Neuromuscular status:** including active range of motion of the feet, shoulders, hands, and neck
    - Referral to a driver rehabilitation specialist if indicated

11. **How can one assess driving safety in a patient with dementia?**
    The following may indicate higher risk of unsafe driving:
    - Clinical dementia rating score ≥ 2.0
    - Assessment by caregiver that patient's driving is unsafe
    - History of traffic citations
    - History of crashes
    - Voluntary reduction of driving mileage by patient
    - Voluntary avoidance of certain situations by patient
    - Mini-Mental State Examination (MMSE) score ≤ 24
    - Aggressive or impulsive personality characteristics

Iverson DJ, Gronseth GS, Roger MA, et al: Practice parameter update: Evaluation and management of driving risk in dementia. Report of the Quality Standards Subcommittee of the American Academy of Neurology, *Neurology* 74:1316–1324, 2010.

Morris JC: The clinical dementia rating (CDR): Current version and scoring rules, *Neurology* 43:2412–2414, 1993.

Tombaugh TN, McIntyre NJ: The Mini-Mental State Examination: A comprehensive review, *J Am Geriatr Soc* 40:922–935, 1992.

NUTRITION

12. **A patient with severe dementia has recurrent admissions with pneumonia, likely due to aspiration. Will gastrostomy tube placement prevent further pneumonias?**
No. Aspiration is considered an expected consequence of advanced dementia. Oral secretions are often aspirated even in patients not fed by mouth. There is currently no evidence that a gastrostomy tube prevents aspiration or pneumonias. Caregivers should be instructed on techniques to help reduce the risk of aspiration such as sitting up at 90° when eating and tipping the chin forward.

13. **Is megestrol useful and effective in increasing lean body mass in underweight older patients?**
No, because of numerous side effects. Although megestrol often increases appetite, the weight gain is due to an increase in fat mass with decline of skeletal muscle mass in many patients. Megestrol can also blunt the beneficial effects of resistance exercise on strength. In addition, megestrol causes a decline in testosterone concentration in men to castrated levels and has catabolic effects from its glucocorticoid properties. Other side effects include Cushing's syndrome, adrenal suppression, hyperglycemia, and thromboembolism.

14. **For most oral supplements and enteral feeding tube products, how many calories are there in each milliliter?**
Most supplement and enteral products have around 1 cal/mL. As a result, most cans of oral supplement, which are usually 8 ounces in volume, contain roughly 250 calories. Patients subsisting just on enteral feeds will typically require 1400–2000 mL of enteral feeding per day to meet their caloric needs. Calorically dense products containing 2 cal/mL are available.

METABOLIC AND RENAL DISORDERS

15. **What are the physiologic changes that predispose older people to dehydration?**
   - Diminution of thirst perception in response to volume depletion or hyperosmolality
   - Decline in basal and stimulated renin levels with reduction in aldosterone secretion
   - Reduced renal responsiveness to antidiuretic hormone (ADH)
   - Impaired sodium conservation by kidneys when salt intake is restricted

16. **What laboratory tests best determine dehydration?**
Blood urea nitrogen (BUN), which is usually elevated. Other indicators include a BUN-to-creatinine ratio > 20 or a BUN greater than twice the baseline BUN.

17. **Why do frail, elderly patients sometimes present with severe hypernatremia?**
Because hypernatremia is a sign of severe dehydration. In mobile patients, hypernatremia induces the thirst response that leads to increased fluid intake. Frail elders may have inadequate intake of free water owing to immobility or cognitive impairment, leading to more severe hypernatremia. An elder with severe hypernatremia may be neglected, and the physician should look for other signs or symptoms or elder abuse or neglect.

18. **Does serum creatinine accurately reflect changes in glomerular filtration rate (GFR) in the elderly?**
No. The aging process is accompanied by a significant deterioration of the renal function. The GFR declines by ~8 mL/min/1.73 m^2 per decade after the fourth decade of life. The age-related reduction in creatinine clearance is accompanied by a reduction in the daily urinary creatinine excretion owing to reduced muscle mass. Accordingly, the relationship

between serum creatinine and creatinine clearance changes. The net effect is near-constancy of serum creatinine (S_{Cr}) where true GFR (and creatinine clearance) declines, and consequently, substantial reduction of GFR despite a relatively normal S_{Cr} level occurs.

Pompei P: Preoperative assessment and perioperative care. In Cassel C, Leipzig R, Cohen H, et al, editors: *Geriatric Medicine: An Evidence-based Approach*, ed 4, New York, 2003, Springer-Verlag, pp 213–227.

MUSCULOSKELETAL DISORDERS

See also Chapter 2, General Medicine and Ambulatory Care, Chapter 10, Rheumatology, and Chapter 16, Endocrinology.

19. **What are "red flag" symptoms that should raise suspicion for malignancy in an older patient with back pain?**
    - Unexplained weight loss
    - >1 month duration of symptoms
    - Pain not relieved by lying down (suggesting cancer or infection)
    - History of cancer
    - Focal neurologic deficit.

20. **How is an acute vertebral compression fracture managed?**
    With pain management and bed rest. Symptomatic acute vertebral fractures are a common problem for osteoporotic patients. Pain at the site of the fracture is often severe and requires initial bed rest and occasionally even hospitalization. Pain control is normally achieved with nonopioid analgesics, opioids, and nasal calcitonin spray. Imaging studies should be obtained if neurologic examination suggests the presence of fracture fragments in the spinal canal or if malignancy is suspected. Older patients with uncontrolled focal back pain related to a nonmalignant vertebral compression fracture may benefit from balloon kyphoplasty or vertebroplasty; however, these procedures are invasive and should be reserved for older patients who did not respond well to conservative management.

21. **If temporal arteritis is suspected, how soon must one perform a temporal artery biopsy?**
    The pathologic changes of temporal arteritis remain present for at least 2 weeks even with corticosteroid treatment. Corticosteroid treatment should be initiated immediately when temporal arteritis is suspected, and the biopsy can be scheduled when convenient.

22. **How long do most temporal arteritis patients require drug treatment?**
    One to 2 years. Patients receiving corticosteroids for this lengthy period benefit from bisphosphonate therapy to prevent osteoporosis. Because prolonged corticosteroid therapy is associated with significant risks and side effects, the diagnosis of temporal arteritis should be confirmed to avoid unnecessary treatment.

23. **Does Medicare routinely cover screening bone mineral density scans for older men and women?**
    Yes, every 2 years for women 65 years and older. Bone mineral density scans are covered for older men only if there is an underlying suspicion for osteoporosis such as vertebral abnormalities on x-ray or treatment with corticosteroids for over 3 months.

24. **What is a T score?**
    The number of standard deviations the patient's bone density is above or below the average value for a young adult of the same sex. Osteoporosis is defined by the World Health Organization as a T score < −2.5.

25. **What is sarcopenia? How can it be prevented?**
Loss of muscle mass related to aging and physiologic changes seen with muscle disuse. Sarcopenia significantly contributes to disability in the elderly and can be prevented with physical activity, especially moderate–to–high-intensity resistance exercise.

26. **What laboratory test measures vitamin D levels in the body?**
25-hydroxy vitamin D (25-OH vitamin D). According to a recent Institute of Medicine report, levels > 20 ng/ml are adequate for bone health.

   IOM (Institute of Medicine): Dietary Reference Intakes for Calcium and Vitamin D. Washington DC, 2011, The National Academies Press.

27. **Why is vitamin D deficiency important to diagnose in older adults?**
Vitamin D deficiency is common in elders and can contribute to osteoporosis, fractures, muscle weakness, and falls. Active people get most of their vitamin D from sun exposure, because few foods contain or are fortified with vitamin D. Many older adults who get little skin exposure to the sun have insufficient vitamin D levels.

28. **What are the recommended daily allowances for calcium and vitamin D in older adults?**
1200 mg of calcium/day in adults older than 50 years and 800 IU of vitamin D/day for adults older than 71 years. Most experts think that older adults require approximately 1000 IU vitamin D/day.

29. **Does calcium supplementation affect the absorption of other medications?**
Yes. Supplements such as calcium and iron (which are divalent cations) can reduce the absorption of commonly used medications such as levothyroxine and some quinolone antibiotics. Patients taking such medications should take the medications and supplements at least 2 hours apart.

30. **Why is lumbar spinal stenosis (LSS) sometimes misdiagnosed as claudication associated with peripheral vascular disease?**
Because spinal stenosis symptoms of leg pain increase with walking (neurogenic claudication) as do those of vascular claudication. LSS in older adults is most commonly caused by degenerative bone disease and is a common cause of disability. Treatment may involve spine surgery. Typical symptoms of LSS include pain in the legs associated with sensory loss and weakness. Many patients also have associated low back pain. Symptoms tend to increase with walking, standing, and back extension and tend to improve with lying, sitting, and back flexion. Vascular claudication is usually described as calf tightness and cramps on exertion that typically resolve immediately after rest. Neurogenic claudication symptoms are relieved only within minutes of sitting/lying but persist with standing erect.

31. **What are common causes of back pain in older people?**
Most common:
   - LSS
   - Degenerative disc disease with spinal instability
   - Vertebral compression fractures
   - Sciatica
Less common:
   - Cancer
   - Osteomyelitis
   - Ruptured or inflammatory abdominal aortic aneurysm

CARDIOVASCULAR DISORDERS

32. **In an older patient with chronic atrial fibrillation (AF), is "rate control" or "rhythm control" preferable?**

Randomized trials have shown that outcomes with a "rhythm control" strategy are no better than with a "rate control" strategy, and in some aspects, outcomes are inferior. For rhythm control, one attempts to convert the rhythm to sinus. For rate control, the rhythm remains AF, but the ventricular rate is controlled to a resting rate of 60–70 beats per minute (bpm) with beta blockers and calcium channel blockers. Unless a patient has significant symptoms, such as bothersome palpitations or exercise intolerance, treatment should focus on controlling ventricular rate both at rest and with exertion.

33. **Elderly people often fall every few months. Is warfarin use for AF contraindicated in such patients?**

No. Advanced age is considered one of the major risk factors for thromboembolic events in patients with AF. Studies comparing the protective effect of warfarin versus antiplatelet therapy in elderly patients with AF have shown significantly higher risk reduction of cardioembolic events with warfarin. Advanced age is also considered a risk factor for bleeding with anticoagulation therapy, and therefore, older patients should have a risk of bleeding assessment before initiation of therapy. Elderly people tend to have multiple episodes of falls, but studies have shown only a small risk for intracranial hemorrhages with the use of anticoagulation. As a general rule, warfarin use is not contraindicated in elderly people who fall.

> Mant J, Hobbs FD, Fletcher K, et al: Warfarin versus aspirin for stroke prevention in an elderly community population with atrial fibrillation (The Birmingham Atrial Fibrillation Treatment of the Aged Study, BAFTA): A randomized controlled trial, *Lancet* 370:493–503, 2007.
>
> Hart RG, Pearce LA, Aguilar MI: Adjusted-dose warfarin versus aspirin for preventing stroke in patients with atrial fibrillation, *Ann Intern Med* 147:590–592, 2007.
>
> Man-Son-Hing M, Laupacis A: Anticoagulant-related bleeding in older persons with atrial fibrillation: Physicians' fears often unfounded, *Arch Intern Med* 163:1580–1586, 2003.

34. **What tests should and should not be routinely ordered as part of a syncope work-up in an older adult?**

Indicated tests:
- Orthostatic blood pressure measurements
- Electrocardiogram (ECG)
- Echocardiogram (if unknown history of heart disease)
- Stress testing (if unknown history of heart disease)
- Tilt table testing (if cardiac work-up negative)

Not routinely indicated (unless dictated by clinical presentation):
- Electrophysiologic studies
- Computed tomography (CT) scan or magnetic resonance imaging (MRI) of head
- Electroencephalogram (EEG)
- Noninvasive carotid examination (NICE)

The most common causes of syncope in the elderly include neurally mediated syndromes, orthostatic hypotension, cardiac disease, and the presence of multiple abnormalities (including polypharmacy and acute or chronic medical problems in the setting of age-related physiologic impairments). A syncope work-up in an older adult should start with a complete history and physical examination, including an evaluation for orthostatic hypotension. A detailed history and physical examination and an ECG will generally suffice to identify the causes of syncope in the majority of patients. Older patients with known heart disease should be evaluated for arrhythmic syncope. Older patients without known heart disease who present with unexplained syncope should undergo further cardiac assessment to include echocardiogram and stress testing.

Physicians should try to identify and treat all factors contributing to syncope before ordering more invasive tests, such as electrophysiologic studies. Patients with a normal cardiac work-up may benefit from an upright tilt table test to look for signs of neurocardiogenic syncope. Further diagnostic tests can be ordered as dictated by this initial assessment. Unless clinically indicated, imaging studies of the head, lumbar puncture, EEG, and carotid vascular studies should not be part of the syncope work-up.

35. **Because systolic blood pressure increases with age, what level of systolic hypertension should be treated in the elderly?**
More than 160 mmHg. According to randomized trials, patients older than 80 years with sustained systolic blood pressure > 160 mmHg benefit from treatment. Evidence is less clear for treating elderly patients with systolic pressure between 140 and 160 mmHg unless they have an additional indication such as chronic kidney disease or heart failure. Patients with coronary artery disease should maintain the diastolic blood pressure > 70 mmHg.

   Beckett NS, Peter R, Fletcher AE, et al: Treatment of hypertension in patients 80 years of age or older, *N Engl J Med* 358:1887–1898, 2008.

36. **Does a normal echocardiogram rule out congestive heart failure (CHF) as a cause of dyspnea on exertion?**
No. In older patients with CHF almost 50% have diastolic heart failure (DHF) as the cause of CHF symptoms. DHF is also called "heart failure with normal ejection fraction (HFNEF)." Diastolic dysfunction occurs with stiffened ventricular walls owing to hypertension and other aging-related changes that lead to elevated left ventricular end-diastolic pressure and the symptoms of CHF. Systolic CHF is typically considered a "pumping" abnormality and DHF is considered a "filling" abnormality.

37. **Is metalazone uniquely synergistic with furosemide in diuresis of older patients with refractory CHF?**
No. Although metalazone is usually added to loop diuretic treatment in patients with refractory heart failure, other thiazide-type diuretics used in full dosage are also highly effective. Metalazone has an elimination half-life of 2 days, making dose titration difficult and leading to excessive diuresis in some patients.

38. **What factors contribute to orthostatic hypotension in older patients?**
Autonomic dysfunction frequently leads to orthostatic hypotension, even in patients with chronic hypertension. Hypertension can lead to reduced arterial wall compliance. Bed rest in frail elderly patients also contributes to orthostasis because of autonomic dysfunction and plasma volume loss. Nitrates, vasodilators, and tricyclic antidepressants accentuate orthostasis. Chronic antihypertensive therapy rarely leads to orthostatic hypotension.

39. **How are orthostatic blood pressure changes measured properly?**
   - Patient reclines for 5 minutes.
   - Measure blood pressure and pulse.
   - Patient stands quietly for 3 minutes.
   - Measure blood pressure and pulse.
   - If there is no change and clinical suspicion of orthostasis remains high, patient remains standing for several more minutes with repeat blood pressure and pulse measurement.
   - Repeat this process at different times during the day to fully document the presence or absence of orthostasis.

40. **What nonpharmacologic approaches reduce orthostatic hypotension?**
   - Discontinue medications that cause orthostatic hypotension.
   - Minimize bed rest.

- Elevate the head of the bed when sleeping.
- Liberalize dietary salt and water, if appropriate.
- Use compression gradient stockings with a pressure at least 20 mmHg when out of bed.

41. **What are the side effects of medications used to treat orthostatic hypotension?**
    - **Fludrocortisone** (mineralocorticoid): supine hypertension, fluid retention, hypokalemia
    - **Midodrine** (alpha$_1$ adrenergic agonist): supine hypertension, piloerection, urinary retention, pruritus
    - **Pyridostigmine** (acetylcholinesterase inhibitor): diarrhea, urinary urgency, bradycardia

NEUROLOGY

42. **What are potential pitfalls to avoid when performing an MMSE?**
    The MMSE lacks sensitivity for diagnosing mild cognitive impairment, especially in the highly educated. The English version is valid only in patients who are fluent in English and has not been well validated for patients who have completed less than 8 years of education. In assessing serial 7s, tell the patient to "keep going" but do not repeat your directions after each answer.

43. **What symptoms and signs suggest a cause for dementia other than Alzheimer's disease (AD)?**
    Variable progression (either stepwise or gradual) of symptoms and cortical findings such as prominent aphasia or motor weakness can suggest vascular dementia. Subcortical vascular dementias often disrupt frontal lobe function and present with mild memory deficits but prominent personality changes such as passivity, abulia, and psychomotor retardation. Subcortical vascular dementia is often undiagnosed and misperceived as depression or apathy. Patients lack internal drive and, therefore, require consistent external cueing. Lewy body dementia presents with parkinsonian signs, fluctuating mental status, and visual hallucinations and can be often misdiagnosed as Parkinson's disease or primary psychosis. Patients typically respond poorly to antipsychotic medications, with prominent extrapyramidal symptoms.

44. **What are treatable or reversible causes of cognitive impairment in older people?**
    - **Metabolic disorders:** vitamin B_{12} deficiency; electrolyte disturbances (hypercalcemia, hyponatremia); thyroid, renal or hepatic dysfunction
    - **Drug-induced:** neuroleptics, sedative hypnotics, antidepressants, anticholinergics, analgesics, muscle relaxants, steroids
    - **Alcohol** intoxication and withdrawal
    - **Depression**
    - **Neurologic disorders:** meningitis, subdural hematomas, normal-pressure hydrocephalus (NPH), tumors

45. **How prevalent is dementia in older people?**
    At age 65, the prevalence is approximately 1–2% but increases each year thereafter, approaching 20–25% by age 85.

46. **When a demented patient has behavioral problems, what nonpharmacologic approaches are helpful?**
    - Reduce the patient's frustration.
    - Remove challenges from the environment.
    - Simplify required tasks.

- Explain activities before asking the patient to perform them.
- Provide a predictable routine.
- Avoid corrections unless absolutely necessary.
- Distract the patient from an undesirable activity and redirect when possible.
- Encourage daily exercise.
- Encourage restful sleep.
- Consider pet therapy.

47. **What medications are potentially useful for treating dementia?**
Cholinesterase inhibitors such as tacrine, donepezil, rivastagmine, and galantamine in general have minimal benefit in reversing dementia but are often given with the hope of slowing progression. Memantine is an *N*-methyl-D-aspartate (NMDA) receptor antagonist that has modest benefit in moderate-to-severe dementia and may be combined with a cholinesterase inhibitor. Patients with mild-to-moderate dementia should be assessed for depression and treated appropriately. Severe agitation with delusions or hallucinations warrants a trial of an antipsychotic but adverse effects are common. Severe sleep disturbance that has not responded to nonpharmacologic measures warrants a trial of a nonbenzodiazepine hypnotic. Avoid use of anticholinergic medications because these can worsen dementia.

48. **How does one differentiate pseudodementia and dementia?**
Depression is commonly associated with cognitive difficulties (pseudodementia) and many patients in early stages of dementia become depressed. The differentiation of pseudodementia from true dementia can be a clinical challenge. Clues that depression is the cause of cognitive difficulties include decline over weeks to months rather than years and whether the patient has overt concern for their memory loss. Referral for complete neuropsychological testing can be helpful in elucidating the diagnosis in many cases. Treatment with antidepressants will significantly improve cognitive function in patients with pseudodementia, whereas truly demented patients may see improvements in overall function but will continue to have cognitive impairment.

49. **How can one prevent the development of AD?**
To date, modifiable risk factors for AD have not been identified. There are no currently available pharmaceutical agents or dietary supplements that prevent cognitive impairment or AD. Current research, though, focuses on antihypertensive agents, omega-3 fatty acids, physical activity, and cognitive activities as possibly effective.

Daviglus ML, Bell CC, Berrettini W, et al: NIH State-of-the-Science Conference Statement: Preventing Alzheimer's disease and cognitive decline. *NIH Consens State Sci Statements* 27, 2010 [Epub ahead of print]. Available at: www.ncbi.nlm.nih.gov/pubmed/20445638?dopt=Abstractplus

50. **How do you distinguish an essential tremor (ET) from the tremor associated with Parkinson's disease?**
See Table 18-2.

51. **What presenting features can lead to underdiagnosis or overdiagnosis of Parkinson's disease?**
The diagnosis of Parkinson's disease relies entirely on clinical impression. There are no blood tests or imaging studies for confirming the diagnosis, and other medical conditions present with similar features. For this reason, clinicians can easily underdiagnose or overdiagnose Parkinson's disease, especially at early stages. Presenting features leading to underdiagnosis include:

- Absence of resting tremor on initial presentation that occurs in 25% of patients with early Parkinson's disease.

TABLE 18-2. TREMOR CHARACTERISTICS OF ESSENTIAL TREMOR AND PARKINSON'S DISEASE		
Characteristic	Parkinson's Disease	Essential Tremor
Symmetry	Usually asymmetrical	Usually symmetrical
Occurrence	At rest	Postural or kinetic
Frequency (Hz)	4–6	4–10
Parts of the body affected	Hands, legs, tongue, and chin	Hand, arms, trunk, head, and voice

- Attribution of stooped posture, gait unsteadiness, and loss of facial expression to aging.
- Attribution of postural instability and bradykinesia to cerebrovascular disease.
  Presenting features leading to overdiagnosis include:
- Tremor related to other causes (e.g., ET).
- Bradykinesia and loss of facial expression due to hypothyroidism or depression.

52. **How is ET treated?**
Several drugs can be used for the treatment of ET. The most commonly used are nonselective beta blockers (such as propanolol) and primidone. Other useful drugs are phenobarbital and benzodiazepines. Surgical procedures may be tried in patients who had an unsatisfactory response to drug therapy, and after carefully weighing the benefit-to-risk ratio. Available surgical procedures include thalamotomy or placement of electrodes for high-frequency stimulation of the thalamus.

53. **Why is restless leg syndrome commonly undiagnosed? How is it treated?**
Many patients fail to mention restless legs, periodic limb movements, or nocturnal myoclonus unless specifically questioned, and only describe "poor sleep." The bed partner frequently provides a more specific history of nocturnal movement disorders. Evening treatment with a dopaminergic medication such as ropinirole is highly effective in many patients.

54. **What is the most effective treatment for patients who feel dizzy when they turn their head or roll over?**
Repositioning of the particles in the semicircular canals (e.g., Epley's and Semont's maneuvers). Benign paroxysmal positional vertigo (BPPV) is the most common cause of positional vertigo affecting older adults. This condition is attributed to the presence of free-floating calcium debris (dislodged from the utriculus) within the posterior semicircular canal. Some BPPV cases are associated with a history of head trauma, Ménière's disease, vestibular neuronitis, and cerebrovascular accident. The diagnosis is confirmed by the Dix-Hallpike maneuver, which provokes similar symptoms and a typical nystagmus. Particle repositioning maneuvers are the most effective treatment for BPPV. The maneuvers encourage the migration of calcium debris from semicircular canals back to the utriculus.

55. **An elderly hospital patient is acting oddly. What are the diagnostic criteria to determine whether it is delirium?**
- Presence of disturbance of consciousness with reduced ability to focus, sustain, or shift attention.
- A change in cognition that is not better accounted for by an evolving dementia.

- Rapid development of the disturbance over hours to days with fluctuation during the course of the day.

    Diagnostic and Statistical Manual of Mental Disorders, ed 4, Text Revision (DSM-IV-TR), Arlington, VA, 2000, American Psychiatric Publishing.

56. **What are the most common risk factors and causes of delirium?**

    RISK FACTORS

    Advanced age
    Dementia
    Male sex
    Sensory impairment
    Impaired function
    Comorbidities
    Chronic alcoholism
    Pain

    CAUSES

    Medications
    Infection
    Dehydration
    Metabolic disturbance
    Urinary retention
    Indwelling devices
    Bed rest
    Restraints
    Fecal impaction

57. **In an elderly patient who is incapable of giving even a decent medical history, how can one differentiate dementia and delirium?**
    See Table 18-3. Interviewing family members or friends is also helpful in obtaining an accurate history in a confused patient.

TABLE 18-3.	DIFFERENTIATION BETWEEN DELIRIUM AND DEMENTIA	
Characteristic	**Delirium**	**Dementia**
Onset	Abrupt	Insidious
Duration	Hours to days	Months to years
Attention	Impaired	Normal unless severe
Speech	Incoherent, disorganized	Ordered, anomic/aphasic
Consciousness	Fluctuating, reduced	Clear

GENITOURINARY DISORDERS

58. **What percentage of older adults are sexually active?**
    Among adults aged 57–64 years, 74% report sexual activity, declining to 26% among those aged 75–85 years.

59. **What sexual problems are most prevalent in older adults?**
    See Table 18-4.

60. **What are the common types of urinary incontinence in older adults?**
    - **Stress:** urinary leakage with increased abdominal pressure
    - **Urge or detrusor instability:** involuntary bladder contraction at a modest volume
    - **Overflow:** urinary leakage out of a distended bladder due to bladder outlet obstruction or a very weak detrusor muscle that does not empty the bladder

TABLE 18-4.   SEXUAL DYSFUNCTION SYMPTOMS AMONG OLDER MEN AND WOMEN

Symptom	Frequency (%)	
	Men	Women
Low desire	—	43
Erectile dysfunction	37	—
Inability to climax	—	34
Difficulty with vaginal lubrication	—	39
Climaxing too quickly	28	—
Finding sex not pleasurable	—	23
Pain	—	17
Performance anxiety	27	—

From Lindau ST, Schumm LP, Laumann EO, et al: A study of sexuality and health among older adults in the United States. N Engl J Med 357:762–777, 2007.

- **Functional:** failure to reach the toilet in a timely manner owing to physical or cognitive debility or both
  There may be overlap among the types of incontinence.

61. **What is the innervation of the urethral sphincter and detrusor muscle?**
    The urethral sphincter is activated by alpha$_1$ receptors in the sympathetic nervous system. The detrusor muscle is inhibited by the sympathetic nervous system and activated by the parasympathetic system, largely through M2 and M3 muscarinic (cholinergic) receptors.

62. **How does this innervation affect the choice of pharmacologic treatments for urinary incontinence?**
    For men with prostatic hypertrophy and a tendency to urinary retention, resting urethral sphincter pressure is usually high so **alpha$_1$ receptor blockers** are used to reduce sphincter tone and facilitate emptying of the bladder. For patients with urge incontinence, **anticholinergic** medications with activity in blocking the M2 and M3 receptors are used to relax the bladder.

KEY POINTS: CAUSES OF URINARY INCONTINENCE ✓

1. **D**elirium

2. **R**estricted mobility, retention

3. **I**nfection, inflammation, impaction (fecal)

4. **P**olyuria, pharmaceuticals

63. **What is a postvoid residual (PVR) measurement and why is it so helpful in assessing the patient with urinary incontinence?**
    The quantity of urine left in the bladder after an attempt at complete emptying. The PVR can be measured by in-and-out catheterization or noninvasively with a bladder ultrasound scanner. In

most patients with incontinence, it is diagnostically useful to measure the residual to determine whether urinary retention is occurring. The residual should be measured before bladder relaxant drugs are given because they are contraindicated if the residual volume > 200 mL.

64. **What are the risks of and indications for an indwelling catheter?**
The most significant risk is urinary tract infection (UTI) if the catheter remains for a week or two. Within 30 days of catheterization, infection is almost universal. Besides infection risk, patients attached to an indwelling catheter remain in bed more than usual, which is highly detrimental in older patients. The indications for an indwelling catheter are urinary retention, severe pressure ulcers where healing is compromised by incontinence, or for hemodynamically unstable patients whose urinary output must be closely monitored.

65. **Is it true that clamping a Foley catheter before pulling it out helps "train the bladder"?**
No, most geriatricians do not think this is true. When an indwelling catheter is no longer needed, it should be removed. There is no advantage to intermittently clamping the catheter for a day or two before removal.

66. **Can medications improve the symptoms of benign prostatic hypertrophy (BPH)?**
Yes. Several medicines are currently approved by the U.S. Food and Drug Administration (FDA) for the control of BPH symptoms. The alpha$_1$ adrenergic antagonists improve bladder outlet obstruction by acting in the prostatic urethra, bladder neck, and prostate. These drugs provide immediate therapeutic benefits and are considered first-line therapy for symptomatic BPH. The nonselective alpha$_1$ adrenergic antagonists (such as terazosin and doxazosin) also have antihypertensive effects and are useful agents for patients who suffer from BPH and hypertension. Tamsulosin and alfuzosin are selective alpha$_1$ adrenergic antagonists and have less effect on blood pressure. The 5-alpha reductase inhibitors (finasteride and dutasteride) work by reducing the size of the prostate over time. They work better for larger prostates (>40 g) and provide symptomatic improvement only after 6–12 months of therapy. The alpha$_1$ adrenergic antagonists and 5-alpha reductase inhibitors can be used together for optimal results in patients with larger prostates. Specialty referral is indicated when BPH symptoms are not relieved by the use of available medicines. Consultation with an urologist is recommended for men who develop complications such as hydronephrosis, renal dysfunction, recurrent UTIs, urinary incontinence, or bladder stones.

Roehrborn CB, Siami P, Barkin J, et al: The effects of dutasteride, tamsulosin and combination therapy on lower urinary tract symptoms in men with benign prostatic hyperplasia and prostatic enlargement: 2-year results from the CombAT study, *J Urol* 179:616–621, 2008.

67. **Should asymptomatic UTIs > 100,000 colonies in older women be treated with a brief course of antibiotics?**
Asymptomatic bacteriuria is common in older women. Studies show that treating it does not improve clinical outcomes. In a large proportion of patients who receive treatment, the bacteriuria recurs within a few months.

68. **Why do men with symptomatic UTIs require longer antibiotic treatment than women?**
Because the prostate gland complicates UTI treatment. Quite often, the prostate gland harbors bacteria even if prostatitis is not overt. Because antibiotics penetrate the prostate poorly and because in older men the prostate often contains prostatic calculi, short-course antibiotic treatment of UTI in men is associated with a high recurrence rate. In addition, many times older men with UTI have a high residual volume because of prostatic hypertrophy and this urinary stasis is an additional risk factor for recurrence with short-course therapy. Usually, UTI in men is treated with 14 days of antibiotics.

69. **What are the clinical manifestations and prevalence of testosterone deficiency in older men?**
Decreased libido and sexual dysfunction, fatigue, muscle weakness, and memory impairment. The aging process in men is accompanied by a gradual decline in serum testosterone levels. Approximately 50% of men in their 80s have total testosterone levels in the hypogonadal range. Physical examination may reveal significant decreases in muscle mass and strength. Testosterone-deficient men are also more prone to faster declines in bone mineral density.

Harmann SM, Metter EJ, Tobin JD, et al: Longitudinal effects of aging on serum total and free testosterone levels in healthy men. Baltimore Longitudinal Study of Aging, *J Clin Endocrinol Metab* 86:724–731, 2001.

70. **What are the contraindications to testosterone replacement in older men?**
Testosterone-dependent diseases such as prostate cancer and severe BPH. There is no proven benefit of testosterone supplementation for age-related declines in testicular function at this time. However, testosterone supplementation is commonly prescribed for symptomatic elderly men with serum concentrations < 200 ng/dL. Special caution is recommended for patients who suffer from sleep apnea, hyperlipidemia, and erythrocytosis, because testosterone supplementation may worsen these conditions. Patients should be screened for the presence of prostate cancer and evaluated for signs of the other mentioned conditions at the time of treatment initiation and periodically thereafter.

71. **Why is nocturia so common in older people?**
Because of age-related physiologic changes. Nocturia is defined as either excessive nocturnal urine output or increased nocturnal frequency. Age-related physiologic changes can alter the regular circadian pattern of urine excretion and lead to increased nocturnal urine formation. In addition, aging is associated with changes of the urinary tract itself that predispose to urinary frequency. These changes include reduced bladder capacity and lowered threshold for urination. Detrusor muscle contractions become less effective and PVR volumes are larger with aging. Some medical problems that typically affect older people such as BPH, fecal impaction, and recurrent UTIs can also predispose to nocturia.

Resnick NM: Voiding dysfunction in the elderly. In Yalla SV, McGuire EJ, Elbadauwi A, et al, editors: *Neurology and Urodynamics: Principles and Practice*, New York, 1988, Macmillan, pp 303–330.

INFECTIOUS DISEASES

72. **If pneumonia is suspected to be secondary to aspiration, should the antibiotics chosen provide full coverage for anaerobic bacteria?**
Not necessarily. Treatment with specific anaerobic coverage is required only if the aspiration was large in volume and contained food or if there is a cavitary infiltrate on chest x-ray. Virtually all pneumonia is secondary to some degree of aspiration of oral secretions. Most older patients with suspected aspiration pneumonia have gram-negative organisms, especially if the pneumonia was hospital acquired or acquired in a nursing home.

73. **How does aging affect tuberculosis skin testing?**
Delayed hypersensitivity from latent tuberculosis may wane with age, causing a nonreactive tuberculin skin test in patients with latent tuberculosis. If a second skin test is placed days to months later, booster phenomenon can occur with a resultant positive skin test. The second skin test can be falsely interpreted as a recent conversion. Patients who will undergo annual testing such as in nursing homes should undergo two-step testing on initial evaluation.

74. **What immunizations are recommended for older persons?**
   - Tetanus and diphtheria toxoid every 10 years.
   - Herpes zoster vaccine after age 60.

- Pneumococcal vaccine at age 65.
- Influenza vaccine every fall. In 2010, a high-dose inactivated influenza vaccine was licensed specifically for persons aged ≥ 65 years to try to increase antibody titers after vaccination. At this time, the ACIP (Advisory Committee on Immunizations Practices) has not yet expressed a preference for this vaccine for older persons.

   Licensure of a high-dose inactivated influenza vaccine for persons aged > years (Fluzone High-Dose) and Guidance for Use—United States, 2010. *MMWR Morb Mortal Wkly Rep* 59:485–486, 2010.

75. **When do older patients need revaccination with pneumococcal vaccine?**
    If they were vaccinated more than 5 years previously and were younger than 65 years at the time of primary vaccination, one-time revaccination is indicated.

76. **Why are there excess deaths from cardiovascular disease during influenza outbreaks?**
    Because influenza is a major physiologic stress on an older patient and frequently causes cardiovascular decompensation in patients with ischemic heart disease or CHF.

DERMATOLOGY

77. **Where are pressure ulcers most likely to develop?**
    - Sacrum
    - Posterior heels
    - Trochanteric areas

78. **What are the principles to follow in treating pressure ulcers?**
    - Avoid or minimize pressure on the wound.
    - Provide adequate pain control.
    - Correct nutritional deficiencies.
    - Perform chemical or surgical débridement of necrotic tissues.
    - Maintain a moist wound environment yet keep surrounding skin dry.
    - Intensify preventive measures such as frequent body repositioning and use of pressure-reducing products and special mattresses.
    - Stage and monitor pressure wounds very closely.

KEY POINTS: PRESSURE ULCER STAGING SYSTEM ✓

1. Stage I: Area of persistent redness (or red, blue, or purple discoloration in darker skin tones) in intact skin.

2. Stage II: Partial-thickness skin loss involving epidermis or dermis or both such as abrasion, blister, or shallow crater.

3. Stage III: Full-thickness skin loss that may extend to but not include the fascia such as deep crater.

4. Stage IV: Full-thickness skin loss with tissue necrosis and may involve muscle, bone, and adjacent structures.

5. Suspected deep tissue injury: Area of significant discoloration that may represent deeper tissue injury.

6. Ulcers covered with eschar cannot be staged.

79. **Why do older people have pruritus?**
Because the aging skin is associated with a decrease in eccrine and sebaceous gland function, as well as an increase in transepidermal water loss that predisposes to dryness. Xerosis (dry skin) is frequently seen in older people and is the most common cause of pruritus in the geriatric population. Xerosis can be easily treated or prevented by avoiding use of strong soaps and by regular use of topical emollients containing urea such as lactic acid 12% lotion (Lac-Hydrin) or occlusive preparations such as Eucerin cream or petroleum jelly.

HEMATOLOGY

80. **What are the common clinical manifestations of multiple myeloma?**
   - Fatigue
   - Unexplained anemia
   - Hypercalcemia
   - Renal failure
   - Osteoporosis
   - Lytic bone lesions on skeletal films
   - Increased total serum protein concentration
   - Presence of urine or serum monoclonal protein

81. **Does hemoglobin normally decrease with aging?**
No. There is a modest increase in prevalence of anemia, particularly in men older than 75 years. The mechanism probably relates at least partially to reduced sensitivity to erythropoietin because of decline in testosterone concentration. In mild anemia (hemoglobin > 12 g/dL) among elderly patients, a comprehensive work-up often fails to identify a cause. Anemia of chronic disease becomes increasingly common with aging and is typified by very low serum iron, low transferrin saturation, low total iron-binding capacity, and normal to increased ferritin.

82. **Should the normal range for erythrocyte sedimentation rate (ESR) be adjusted for age and gender?**
Yes. ESR is a common hematology test, which is a nonspecific measure of inflammation that is useful for diagnosing diseases such as temporal arteritis, polymyalgia rheumatica, and various autoimmune diseases. The ESR can also be used to monitor therapeutic response. ESR values tend to rise with age and to be slightly higher in women. The formula to calculate normal maximum ESR values in adults is:

$$\text{ESR (mm/hr)} < \frac{[\text{Age (in years)} + 10 \text{ (if female)}]}{2}$$

Bottiger LE, Svedberg CA: Normal erythrocyte sedimentation rate and age, *Br Med J* 2:85–87, 1967.

Miller A, Green M, Robinson D: Simple rule for calculating normal erythrocyte sedimentation rate, *Br Med J (Clin Res Ed)* 286:266, 1983.

83. **Why are patients with chronic lymphocytic leukemia (CLL) not always immediately treated?**
Because survival with CLL does not improve with early treatment. CLL is the most common form of leukemia and occurs mainly in older patients. The diagnosis is often made incidentally when a blood count reveals a lymphocyte count > 5000/μL. In these asymptomatic patients, many years may go by without disease progression. There is little evidence that early treatment improves survival or that CLL can be cured with present standard treatment. Therapy is recommended for the following:
   - Disease-related symptoms such as fever, weight loss, or night sweats
   - Significant anemia (hemoglobin < 10 g/dL) or thrombocytopenia (platelet count < 100,000/μL)

- Autoimmune hemolytic anemia or thrombocytopenia that is poorly responsive to corticosteroids
- Rapidly progressive disease, as manifested by lymphocyte count doubling in $<$ 6 months or rapidly enlarging lymph nodes, spleen, and liver

84. **What are the common clinical manifestations of vitamin B_{12} deficiency?**
Hematologic:
   - Megaloblastic anemia
   - Hypersegmented neutrophils on peripheral blood smear
   - Leukopenia (severe deficiency)
   - Thrombocytopenia (severe deficiency)
Neurologic:
   - Symmetrical peripheral neuropathy
   - Cognitive impairment
   - Ataxia

85. **If a patient presents with pancytopenia, what other diagnoses should be considered in addition to vitamin B_{12} deficiency?**
Aplastic anemia, myelodysplastic syndrome, and acute myeloid leukemia.

86. **Why does subacute combined degeneration of the spinal cord occur with vitamin B_{12} deficiency?**
Because of a defect in myelin formation due to cobalamin deficiency. This life-threatening neurologic complication may be reversed with an aggressive vitamin B_{12} supplementation over a period of several months.

87. **How prevalent is vitamin B_{12} deficiency in older people and what is the major cause?**
Ten to 20%. The major cause is food source cobalamin malabsorption related to gastric atrophy and achlorhydria and loss of intrinsic factor (pernicious anemia).

88. **In a patient with vitamin B_{12} deficiency, does replacement have to be given by intramuscular injection?**
No. Although, vitamin B_{12} deficiency is typically treated with frequent intramuscular injections for several weeks, followed by a monthly injection for maintenance, recent studies support the efficacy of alternative forms of administration such as oral and nasal. Oral and nasal treatments require high doses owing to erratic absorption and greater patient compliance for optimal results.

   Slot WB, Merkus FW, Van Deventer SJ, et al: Normalization of plasma vitamin B_{12} concentration by intranasal hydroxocobalamin in vitamin B_{12}–deficient patients, *Gastroenterology* 113:430–433, 1997.

   Hathcock JN, Troendle GH: Oral cobalamin for the treatment of pernicious anemia, *JAMA* 265:96–97, 1991.

MEDICATION USE

89. **Among the tricyclic antidepressants, is amitriptyline especially effective for neuropathic pain?**
No. All the tricyclic antidepressants have similar efficacy for treatment of neuropathic pain. Amitriptyline should be avoided in older patients because it has the most anticholinergic activity and frequently causes orthostatic hypotension.

90. **What body systems are adversely affected by anticholinergic medications?**
   - **Genitourinary:** weakness of bladder muscle contractions
   - **Gastrointestinal:** constipation, dry mouth
   - **Central nervous system:** impaired cognition

91. **What medications have significant anticholinergic properties?**
    - Antihistamines (diphenhydramine, chlorpheniramine, and hydroxyzine)
    - Tricyclic antidepressants
    - Cyclobenzaprine
    - Scopolamine and meclizine
    - Promethazine

92. **Some of my older patients do not know why they are taking many of their pills. Do pharmacists routinely write the medication indication on the pill bottle label?**
    No, because there may be multiple indications for the same medications. For example, hydrochlorothiazide can be taken for edema or for hypertension. To improve patient understanding and compliance with medication regimens, providers should always write the indication on the prescription (e.g., "HCTZ, take 1 daily for HTN").

93. **Patients often do not admit they are not taking their medications. How can one inquire about medication compliance?**
    Try asking the question about compliance in several ways. When reviewing the patient's medication list, ask:
    - Are you taking all your medications?
    - Have you missed any pills in the past week?
    - Are any of your pills causing you problems?

94. **What over-the-counter medications greatly increase or decrease the International Normalized Ratio (INR) by affecting liver metabolism of warfarin?**
    Cimetidine (increased INR) and St. John's wort (decreased INR).

95. **What common medications are renally excreted and require dose reduction in older patients, even those with serum creatinine in the "normal" range?**

Fluoroquinolones	Ceftriaxone
Colchicine	Digoxin
Glyburide	Gabapentin
Low-molecular-weight heparin	Lithium

    Because muscle mass is reduced in many older patients, reduced renal function is not reflected by a commensurate increase in serum creatinine.

PREVENTION

See also Chapter 2, General Medicine and Ambulatory Care.

96. **Should certain older adults be screened for abdominal aortic aneurysms (AAAs)?**
    Yes. AAA rupture is a common cause of death in older adults. The most important risk factors for AAA are advanced age, male sex, and smoking. Several organizations recommend one-time screening for AAA in men between ages 65–75 who have ever smoked. Men in this age group who have a first-degree relative who required repair of an AAA are also considered for screening.

97. **How is such screening performed?**
    With abdominal ultrasonography, a noninvasive test with a high sensitivity and specificity for diagnosing AAA. Medicare currently reimburses for AAA screening within the first 6 months of Medicare enrollment as part of the "Welcome to Medicare" physical for:
    - Men aged 65–75 who have smoked at least 100 cigarettes during their lifetime, and
    - Men and women who have a family history of AAA.

    Screening for abdominal aortic aneurysm: Recommendation statement, *Ann Intern Med* 142:198, 2005.

Fleming C, Whitlock EP, Beil TL, et al: Screening for abdominal aortic aneurysm: A best-evidence systematic review for the U.S. Preventive Services Task Force, *Ann Intern Med* 142:203–211, 2005.

Salo JA, Soisalon-Soininen S, Bondestam S, et al: Familial occurrence of abdominal aortic aneurysm, *Ann Intern Med* 130:637–642, 1999.

HEALTH SYSTEMS

98. **Which elderly patients qualify for home care services and what services are covered by Medicare?**
Those who need skilled services on an intermittent rather than a continuous basis **and** are homebound. **Skilled services** are defined as those provided by nursing (including teaching self-care skills, performing skilled procedures, and assessing changing or fluctuating medical conditions), physical therapy, speech therapy, and occupational therapy. **Homebound** is defined as leaving home infrequently, but only with assistance and considerable effort. Neither 24-hour nor personal care is provided if assistance is the only care needed.

99. **Does Medicare part D provide at least partial coverage for all medications?**
No. Part D plans are required to cover medications in all of the major therapeutic categories but are not required to cover every medication in each category. Each plan utilizes a unique formulary. In addition, coverage in many plans includes a "donut hole." This means payment for medications are covered up to a certain amount but then coverage ceases for further expenditures until the patient finally exceeds a certain yearly expenditure, at which point coverage resumes.

100. **When is an occupational or physical therapy referral appropriate?**
Occupational therapy referrals are appropriate if the patient needs assistance in ADLs, needs adaptive equipment, needs splint or orthotic fabrication, or requires a home safety assessment. Most occupational therapy focuses on optimizing use of the upper extremities. Physical therapy referrals are appropriate if the patient has significant balance or gait disturbance, needs an ambulatory aid, has mobility or transfer difficulty, or has range of motion or strength impairment.

101. **What percentage of American adults aged 65 and older lives in a nursing home?**
Approximately 7.5%. The number of older adults living in nursing homes has been declining over the past few years

102. **What is an older American's lifetime chance of spending at least some time residing in a nursing home?**
Over 40% after age 65. Many of these nursing home admissions are for post–acute care and patients have short stays for rehabilitation after hospital discharge.

WEBSITE

1. www.americangeriatrics.org

BIBLIOGRAPHY

1. Cassel CK, Leipzig R, Cohen HJ, et al, editors: *Geriatric Medicine: An Evidence-Based Approach*, ed 4, New York, 2007, Springer.

2. Hatler J, Ouslander J, Tinetti M, et al, editors: *Hazzard's Geriatric Medicine & Gerontology*, ed 6, New York, 2009, McGraw Hill Medical.

3. Pompei P, Murphy JB, editors. *Geriatrics Review Syllabus: A Core Curriculum in Geriatric Medicine*, ed 6, New York, 2006, American Geriatrics Society.

4. Reuben DB, Herr KA, Pacala JT, et al, *Geriatrics at Your Fingertips*, ed 12, New York, 2010, American Geriatrics Society.

CHAPTER 19

PALLIATIVE MEDICINE

Leslye C. Pennypacker, M.D.

GENERAL ISSUES

1. **What is palliative medicine?**
    A multidisciplinary medical specialty focused on pain relief and other symptoms in patients with serious and/or life-limiting illnesses. In contrast to the traditional disease model of medical care that emphasizes cure, the goals of palliative care include:
    - **Pain and symptom management**
    - **Establishment of care goals** (advance planning) based on patient and family preferences
    - **Functional optimization**
    - **Psychological and spiritual support** to patient and family
    - **Care coordination and delivery** in a setting appropriate to the patient's needs

2. **What is hospice care?**
    A subset of palliative care that provides multidisciplinary, noncurative care to patients with a life expectancy of 6 months or less. Most hospice patients decline all aggressive interventions that are not directed toward pain and symptom management. Hospice care is frequently the final phase of palliative care (Fig. 19-1).

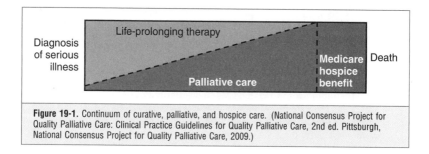

Figure 19-1. Continuum of curative, palliative, and hospice care. (National Consensus Project for Quality Palliative Care: Clinical Practice Guidelines for Quality Palliative Care, 2nd ed. Pittsburgh, National Consensus Project for Quality Palliative Care, 2009.)

3. **Which patients should be considered for palliative care?**
    All patients with serious and life-limiting illness. Palliative care may be provided anytime during a person's illness, even from the time of diagnosis.

4. **Which patients should be considered for hospice care?**
    Patients with a serious illness who have a life expectancy of 6 months or less.

5. **Where do most patients receive end-of-life care? Why?**
    Over 80% of patients in the United States die in either an acute care or a nursing home setting. Unfortunately, many patients do not receive adequate supportive care and symptom management at the end of life because health professionals and facilities do not always encourage a transition of care from curative to comfort-oriented goals in these specific care settings.

6. **If a patient on hospice improves, do they leave hospice care and return to palliative or curative care?**
Yes. Patients can "graduate" from hospice care if their illness improves unexpectedly. Also, some patients may opt to discontinue hospice care if a new or promising treatment becomes available, but they can re-enroll if they subsequently decline.

7. **What percentage of patients in the United States access hospice/palliative care at the end of life?**
Approximately 15%, with an average duration of hospice care of 3 weeks.

8. **Who pays for end-of-life care in the United States?**
Medicare and Medicaid programs. In addition, some third-party and health maintenance organization (HMO) insurance carriers also provide coverage but programs and covered benefits may vary. In general, veterans in the United States can receive coverage for end-of-life care via their basic benefits program if they are enrolled in the Veterans Administration (VA) Health Care System.

KEY POINTS: END OF LIFE CARE ✓

1. Physicians should begin discussions of end-of-life preferences early in the course of a terminal illness.

2. Medicare now provides coverage for end-of-life discussions between physicians and patients during the annual physical exam beginning in 2011. This discussion can include designation of surrogate decision makers and expressed wishes for end-of-life care. (See also Chapter 1, Medical Ethics.)

3. Patients approaching the end of life should participate in most of the decisions regarding their care, either through previous directives or continued active participation.

9. **Who is eligible for the Hospice Medicare Benefit?**
Patients with Medicare Part A (hospital insurance) and a diagnosis of a terminal illness with a probable life expectancy of 6 months or less. The patient's doctor and the hospice medical director must certify the limited life expectancy.

10. **What does the Hospice Medicare Benefit cover?**
   - Physician services
   - Nursing care
   - Medical equipment (e.g., wheelchairs, walkers, and hospital beds)
   - Medical supplies (e.g., bandages and catheters)
   - Medications for symptom control and pain relief
   - Short-term care in the hospital, including respite care
   - Home health aide and homemaker services
   - Physical and occupational therapy
   - Speech therapy
   - Social worker services
   - Dietary counseling
   - Family grief counseling

11. **When can nursing home patients receive hospice/palliative care?**
    When they develop a serious or life-limiting illness and choose to focus on symptom relief instead of cure. Hospice eligibility depends on the goals of care, not the site of care. Hospice/palliative care can be provided in the nursing home and home setting in addition to some other residential care facilities.

12. **Can patients on hospice receive treatment in the hospital for an acute illness?**
    Yes, but the patient may need to withdraw from hospice care during the hospitalization period. If appropriate, hospice services can be resumed at the time of discharge.

13. **Can hospice patients request cardiopulmonary resuscitation?**
    Yes. Hospice programs cannot require that the patient or family request no resuscitation in order to receive services, but the majority of hospice patients do not want aggressive interventions of likely low benefit. Once enrolled in hospice, many patients who initially requested resuscitation later ask for no resuscitation. They are assured that pain relief and symptom management will continue.

14. **What percentage of hospice patients die at home in the United States?**
    Approximately 66–75%. In-home death, though, requires the availability of family and caregivers who agree to support the patient during the dying process.

15. **What is the most common fear that prevents patients from accepting hospice care?**
    Inadequate pain management. Many patients fear that if they accept hospice care, then they will be "giving up and accepting death" and that they may not receive adequate pain and symptom management. Ironically, patients cared for by hospice programs generally report improved pain and symptom management, and many recent studies have shown that survival after admission to hospice programs may be longer than in those cared for in the standard models of care.

SYMPTOM MANAGEMENT: PAIN

16. **Do most patients experience pain at the end of life?**
    Yes, in nearly 85% of cancer patients and 67% of noncancer patients.

17. **How can the physician assess the severity of a patient's pain?**
    Several pain scales are available to help quantitative assessment of pain (Fig. 19-2).

18. **What medications are commonly used for severe pain in hospice/palliative care patients?**
    Opioid analgesics. Dosing should be tailored to the individual patient at the initiation of treatment and throughout the course of therapy. There are no absolute limitations on initial or maintenance doses because tolerance, metabolism, and response to treatment can vary widely between patients and within a given patient over time.

19. **What opioids are useful for treatment of mild-to-moderate pain?**
    See Table 19-1.

20. **What opioids are useful for treatment for moderate-to-severe pain?**
    See Table 19-2.

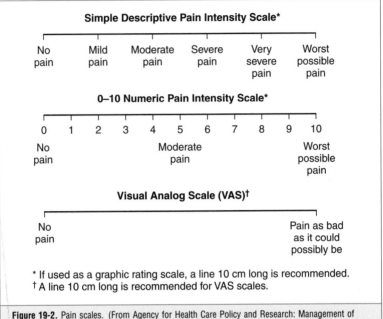

Figure 19-2. Pain scales. (From Agency for Health Care Policy and Research: Management of Cancer Pain: Adults. Rockville, MD: U.S. Department of Health and Human Services, Public Health Services, 1994.)

TABLE 19-1. OPIOIDS FOR MILD-TO-MODERATE PAIN

Drug	Route	Equianalgesic Dose (mg)*	Peak Effect (hr)	Duration of Effect (hr)	Comments
Codeine	PO	200	0.5	3–6	Ceiling for analgesia reached at doses > 240 mg/day PO
	IV/IM	130	0.5	3–6	
Oxycodone	PO	20–30	0.5	3–6	No ceiling dose if given without fixed combinations; parenteral formulation not available

(continued)

TABLE 19-1.   OPIOIDS FOR MILD-TO-MODERATE PAIN—*(continued)*

Drug	Route	Equianalgesic Dose (mg)*	Peak Effect (hr)	Duration of Effect (hr)	Comments
Hydrocodone	PO	30	0.5	4–6	Only available as fixed combination with acetaminophen or aspirin

IM = intramuscular; IV = intravenous; NA = not available; PO = oral.
*Approximate potency relative to 10 mg of parenteral morphine.
From Grossman SA, Nesbit S: Cancer pain. In Abeloff MA, Armitage JO, Niederhuber JE, et al (eds): Abeloff's Clinical Oncology, 4th ed. Philadelphia, Churchill Livingstone, 2008.

TABLE 19-2.   STRONG OPIATES FOR MODERATE-TO-SEVERE CANCER PAIN

Drug	Route	Equianalgesic Dose (mg)*	Duration of Effect (hr)	Comments
Oxycodone	PO	20–30	3–6	No ceiling dose if given without fixed combinations; parenteral formulations not available.
	PO (SR)		12	
Morphine	PO	30	4–6	Many PO formulations for individual patient needs.
	PO (SR)		8–12	
	IV/IM	10	3–5	
Hydromorphone	PO	7.5	3–4	Good choice for SC due to potency.
	PR	(?)	Unknown	
	IV/IM	1.5	3–4	

(continued)

TABLE 19-2. STRONG OPIATES FOR MODERATE-TO-SEVERE CANCER PAIN—
(continued)

Drug	Route	Equianalgesic Dose (mg)*	Duration of Effect (hr)	Comments
Meperidine	PO	300	3–6	Not preferred due to CNS toxic metabolite that accumulates in renal failure.
	IV/IM	75	2–3	
Levorphanol	PO	4.0	6–8	Long $T_{1/2}$ (11 hr) necessitates slow dose titration; drug accumulation may occur.
	IV/IM	2.0	6–8	
Fentanyl	TD	(?)	≥12	Short $T_{1/2}$ (<1 hr); TD dose titration difficult with depot in SC adipose tissue; TD fentanyl 25 μg/hr ~45 mg/day PO morphine.
	IV/IM	0.1	0.5–1.0	
Methadone†	PO	10	6–8	Despite long $T_{1/2}$ (15–>150 hr), duration of analgesia is not prolonged; however, drug accumulation can result in toxicities Caution is warranted when converting to methadone in patients with high opioid tolerance.
Oxymorphone	PO	10	7–9	Now available as immediate-release formulations.

(continued)

TABLE 19-2. STRONG OPIATES FOR MODERATE-TO-SEVERE CANCER PAIN—
(continued)

Drug	Route	Equianalgesic Dose (mg)*	Duration of Effect (hr)	Comments
	PO (SR)		12	
	IV	1	7–9	

CNS = central nervous system; IM = intramuscular; IV = intravenous; PO = oral; SC = subcutaneous; SR = slow-release formulation; TD = transdermal; (?) = unknown.
*Approximate potency relative to 10 mg of parental morphine.
†Ripamonti C, Groff L, Brunelli C, et al: Switching from morphine to oral methadone in treating cancer pain: What is the equianalgesic dose ratio? J Clin Oncol 16:3216–3221, 1998; Moryl N, Santiago-Palma J, Kornick C, et al: Pitfalls of opioid rotation: substituting another opioid for methadone in patients with cancer pain. Pain 96:325–328, 2002; Bruera E, Neumann CM: Role of methadone in the management of pain in cancer patients. Oncology 13:1275–1282, 1999; Pereira J, Lawlor P, Vigano E, et al: Equianalgesic dose ratios for opioids: a critical review of proposals for long term dosing. J Pain Symptom Manage 22:672–687, 2001; Bruera E, Sweeny C: Methadone use in cancer patients with pain: a review. J Pall Med 5:127–138, 2002.
From Grossman SA, Nesbit S: Cancer pain. In Abeloff MA, Armitage JO, Niederhuber JE, et al (eds): Abeloff's Clinical Oncology, 4th ed. Philadelphia, Churchill Livingstone, 2008.

21. **How is methadone used?**
For continuous pain management. Methadone has a long half-life and can lead to sedation and respiratory depression if not carefully and slowly titrated. For patients with appropriate life expectancy and end-of-life care goals, the electrocardiogram (ECG) may need to be monitored to detect a prolonged QT interval since methadone can lead to torsades de pointes. Methadone may also be helpful for neuropathic pain.

Gazelle G, Fine PG: Methadone for the treatment of pain. In *Fast Facts and Concepts*, ed 2, 2006. Available at: www.eperc.mcw.edu/fastfact/ff_075.htm.

22. **What are the most common side effects of opioid therapy?**
- Constipation
- Mild sedation
- Nausea

23. **How is sedation due to opioid use managed?**
Stimulants such as caffeine, methylphenidate, dexmethylphenidate, and dextroamphetamine may be helpful, as are newer stimulants such as modafinil and armodafinil. However, modafinil and armodafinil have been primarily studied in patients with nonmalignant pain.

24. **Should the concern for respiratory depression preclude the use of opioids in frail patients nearing the end of life?**
No. Opioids, if dosed carefully and monitored appropriately, should not be withheld in patients nearing the end of life for fear of decreasing respiratory drive. In fact, most palliative care providers agree that opioids are considered the preferred medication for patients with air hunger and dyspnea. Often, patients will have an improvement in effective ventilation if their pain is well controlled.

25. **In addition to opioids, what other treatment modalities can be used for pain management at the end of life?**
    - **Tricyclic antidepressants (TCAs)**
    - **Anticonvulsants** (clonazepam, gabapentin)
    - **Topical lidocaine** (available as a patch or gel)
    - **Biphosphonates** (for bone pain)
    - **Corticosteroids** (for inflammatory related pain)
    - **Capsaicin** (topical cream made from chili peppers)

26. **How are nonsteroidal anti-inflammatory medications (NSAIDs) used for pain?**
    Although effective pain relievers, the numerous side effects and risks of NSAIDs frequently outweigh the benefits of these medications in patients at the end of life with multiple organ dysfunction. The complications of NSAIDs use include dyspepsia, gastric bleeding and ulcers, nephrotoxicity, hepatotoxicty, and excessive bleeding owing to decreased platelet aggregation. For many patients at the end of life, particularly elderly patients, opioids are safer therapies.

27. **In addition to pain, what other common symptoms occur at the end of life?**
    See Table 19-3.

TABLE 19-3. SYMPTOMS AT THE END OF LIFE: CANCER VERSUS OTHER CAUSES OF DEATH

Symptom	Cause of Death	
	Cancer (%)	Other (%)
Pain	84	67
Trouble breathing	47	49
Nausea and vomiting	51	27
Sleeplessness	51	36
Confusion	33	38
Depression	38	36
Loss of appetite	71	38
Constipation	47	32
Bedsores	28	14
Incontinence	37	33

Adapted from Seale C, Cartwright A: The Year Before Death, Aldershot, UK, Avebury, 1994.

SYMPTOM MANAGEMENT: GASTROINTESTINAL

28. **What are some management strategies for treatment of constipation?**
    Patients receiving chronic opioid therapy should be encouraged to drink plenty of fluids, maintain regular physical activity as appropriate, and develop regular toileting habits. In addition, routine doses of stool softeners, laxatives, or both should be prescribed concurrently with the initiation of opioid therapy. Docusate (100 mg daily) and senna (2–8 tablets at bedtime) are frequently used in combination. Osmotic laxatives (lactulose or polyethylene

glycol) can be used both for acute relief of constipation and on a daily basis for patients who do not respond to stool softeners or mild laxatives, but some patients at the end of life may find the sweet taste unpleasant. More recently, subcutaneous methylnaltrexone was approved for treatment of opioid induced constipation and can be used long term.

Thomas J, Karver S, Cooney GA, et al: Methylnaltrexone for opioid-induced constipation in advanced illness, *N Engl J Med* 258:2332–2343, 2008.

29. **List the most common causes of nausea and vomiting in palliative care patients.**
    - **V**estibular
    - **O**bstruction of bowel by constipation
    - Dys**M**otility of upper gastrointestinal tract
    - **I**nfection, **I**nflammation
    - **T**oxins stimulating the chemoreceptor trigger zone in the brain (e.g., opioids)
    These causes can be remembered by the acronym VOMIT.

    Hallenbeck J: The causes of nausea and vomiting (V.O.M.I.T.). In *Fast Facts and Concepts*, ed 2, 2005. Available at: www.eperc.mcw.edu/factfact/ff_005.htm.

30. **What are some nonpharmacologic interventions to consider in patients with nausea and vomiting?**
    - Provide a peaceful, quiet environment.
    - Minimize odors, if possible.
    - Only offer requested foods.
    - Offer smaller food portions more frequently.
    - Consider the possibility of constipation as contributing factor to nausea, even in patients with minimal oral intake.

31. **What medications are helpful for the treatment of nausea and vomiting?**
    For vestibular causes, scopolamine (as a patch) or promethazine may be helpful. Promethazine is also helpful for labyrinthitis seen in inflammation. Metoclopramide is helpful for upper intestinal dysmotility but can cause tardive dyskinesia and worsen depression symptoms. Prochloroperazine is helpful for opioid-induced nausea. Ondansetron is specifically indicated for chemotherapy induced nausea and vomiting but also may be helpful in other settings.

32. **Are there nonpharmacologic approaches to the treatment of bowel obstruction that should be considered?**
    Yes. Enteral tubes may be used as suction. Procedures such as a decompressing ostomy are also helpful.

33. **What are the most common causes of diarrhea in palliative care patients?**
    - **Impaction** with resultant diarrhea around the impaction
    - **Medication side effects,** most commonly antibiotics
    - **Malabsorption,** particularly if the patient is receiving tube feedings
    - **Infection** such as *Clostridium difficile*
    - **Bowel or pancreatic malignancy**

34. **How should diarrhea be evaluated?**
    - History and physical examination
    - Limited laboratory and microbiologic testing
    - Reviewing medications for possible causes

35. **How can diarrhea be treated?**
    - Small sips of clear liquids to maintain hydration with parenteral hydration if needed and appropriate with end-of-life care goals.
    - Avoidance of lactose products.
    - Kaolin and pectin preparations for bulk formation, but these may take up to 48 hours to be effective.
    - Loperamide.
    - Aspirin and cholestyramine for radiation-induced enteritis.
    - Pancreatic enzymes if pancreatic insufficiency present.
    - Octreotide for severe secretory diarrhea (as seen in human immunodeficiency virus [HIV] infection).
    - Antibiotic treatment for possible infectious diarrhea.
    - Appropriate measures to prevent pressure ulcers due to diarrhea.

    Cherny NI: Evaluation and management of treatment-related diarrhea in patients with advanced cancer: A review, *J Pain Symptom Manage* 36:413–423, 2008.

    Ippoliti C: Antidiarrheal agents for the management of treatment-related diarrhea in cancer patients, *Am J Health Syst Pharm* 55:1573–1580, 1998.

36. **Should all oral food and fluids be withheld from patients with impaired swallowing at the end of life?**
    No. As a general rule, these patients can still be offered small bites of soft food and sips of fluids that they want for pleasure and taste. When unable to manage even these forms of alimentation, the patient's mouth and lips can be moistened with topical moistened swabs.

37. **What are some of the causes of hiccups in terminally ill patients?**
    Liver disease, gastroesophageal reflux disease (GERD), diaphragmatic irritation, central nervous system (CNS) tumor, and medication side effects (i.e., steroids).

38. **What medications are helpful for treatment of hiccups?**
    Although at times nearly intractable, the antipsychotic chlorpromazine is U.S. Food and Drug Administration (FDA)–approved for hiccup treatment. Baclofen and gabapentine have also been found to be effective in trials.

    Hernandez JL, Pajarón M, García-Regata O, et al: Gabapentin for intractable hiccup, *Am J Med* 117:279–281, 2004.

    Ramirez FC, Graham DY: Treatment of intractable hiccup with baclofen: Results of a double-blind, randomized, controlled, cross-over study, *Am J Gastroenterol* 87:1789–1791, 1992.

SYMPTOM MANAGEMENT: DYSPNEA

39. **What are the most common causes of dyspnea at the end of life?**

Chronic obstructive pulmonary disease (COPD)	Pleural effusion	Ascites
	Pulmonary embolism	Pain
	Pneumothorax	Anxiety
Pneumonia	Excessive airway secretions	
Congestive heart failure (CHF)	Anemia	

40. **Does supplemental oxygen help patients with dyspnea?**
    Sometimes. If the oxygen is delivered by face mask, the patient may feel more short of breath and claustrophobic. Nasal cannulae are usually better tolerated even if lower oxygen flow rates are achieved.

41. **What medications are most helpful in end-of-life patients with dyspnea?**
   - **Opioids** (generally most effective)
   - **Diuretics** for fluid overload
   - **Antibiotics** for pneumonia, if consistent with the patient's end-of-life care requests

42. **What nonpharmacologic interventions are helpful in relieving dyspnea?**
   - **Repositioning**
   - **Fans**
   - **Gentle postural drainage**
   - **Therapeutic thoracentesis** (with or without pleurodesis)
   - **Paracentesis** (if ascites prominent)

43. **What medications can help persistent cough?**
   The best treatment is to treat the underlying disorder causing the cough, if possible. Oxygen, frequent suctioning, and increasing humidity can also help. Coughs due to infections may benefit from antibiotics for symptom relief. Opioids and steroids may also be helpful. Lozenges and over-the-counter preparations such as dextromethorphan can be tried in combination with opioids if necessary.

SYMPTOM MANAGEMENT: GENERAL

44. **How should depression be assessed at the end of life?**
   Because many of the physical symptoms of depression (low energy, sleep disorders, change in appetite or weight, psychomotor retardation) are also seen as part of the terminal illness, the mood symptoms of depression are important for assessment. These symptoms include feelings of hopelessness, guilt, helplessness, and sustained thoughts of suicide.

   Block SD: Assessing and managing depression in the terminally ill, *Ann Intern Med* 132:209–217, 2000.

45. **What medications are used for depression treatment?**
   - **Selective serotonin reuptake inhibitors (SSRIs):** Fluoxetine, fluvoxamine, paroxetine, sertraline, citalopram. May have the best tolerated side effect profile.
   - **TCAs:** Amitryptyline, imipramine, desipramine, nortriptyline.
   - **Serotonin norepinephrine reuptake inhibitor (SNRI):** Venlafaxine.
   - **Norepinephrine dopamine modulators:** Buproprion.
   - **Serotonin and norepinephrine uptake inhibitor:** Desvenlafaxine.
   - **Psychostimulants:** Dextroamphetamine, methylphenidate, modafinil, and armodafinil.

46. **How can pressure ulcers be prevented in palliative care/hospice patients?**
   By use of a pressure-reducing mattress surface and regularly turning the patient (if bed-bound) to avoid prolonged pressure on one area. The skin should be inspected regularly and treatment started for early-stage ulcers or at-risk skin area.

WEBSITES

1. American Academy of Hospice and Palliative Medicine: www.aahpm.org

2. Education for Physicians on End-of-life Care (EPEC): www.epec.net

3. End of Life/Palliative Education Resource Center (EPEREC): www.eperc.mcv.edu

BIBLIOGRAPHY

1. Quill T, Hollway RG, Shah MS, editors: *Primer of Palliative Care*, ed 5, Glenview, IL, 2010, American Academy of Hospice and Palliative Medicine.
2. Walsh D, Caraceni AT, Fainsinger R, et al, editors: *Palliative Medicine*, Philadelphia, 2008, Saunders.

INDEX

Note: Page numbers followed by *f* indicate figures and *t* indicate tables.

Arterial gas embolism, 153
Arterial hypoxemia, 124–125
Arteriolar dilators, congestive heart failure and, 93
Arthritis, 254, 273, 274. *See also* Infectious arthritis
Arthrocentesis, 250
Arthus reaction, 318, 319
Ascitic fluid cell counts, 179
Aseptic meningitis, 364
Aspergilloma, 353
Aspergillus species, 353
Aspirin, 259, 426
 acute coronary syndrome and, 80
 aspirin-exacerbated respiratory disease, 323, 324
 gastrointestinal bleeding and, 2
 termination of and surgery, 56
Asplenia, immunizations and, 38
Asplenic patients, 4, 366–367
Assent, 11
Asthma, 132–136, 321–325
 aspirin-exacerbated respiratory disease, 323, 324
 asthma-related death, 136
 bacterial infections and, 321
 beta agonist therapy and, 322
 chronic obstructive pulmonary disease and,
  130, 130*t*
 classification of, 134*t*
 comorbid conditions and, 134
 corticosteroids and, 322
 definition of, 132–133
 diagnosis of, 133
 differential diagnosis and, 133
 exacerbation levels and, 135–136
 exercise-induced asthma, 136, 323
 gastroesophageal reflux disease and, 322
 hospital admittance and, 135–136
 infections and, 321
 management steps and, 133
 medications and, 135*t*
 nocturnal asthma, 322, 323
 pregnancy and, 136
 severity of, 321
 stepwise approach and, 135*t*
 theophylline treatment of, 322
Asymptomatic bacteriuria, 578
Asymptomatic hyperparathyroidism, 528–529
Asymptomatic urinary abnormalities, 196
Ataxia, 6, 552
Atherosclerotic renal artery stenosis, 218*t*
Atonic bladder, 211
Atopic (allergic) diseases, 308–310
Atorvastatin, 88–89, 107
Atovaquone, 389
Atrial fibrillation, 66–67, 67*t*
 anticoagulation and, 25, 97
 causes of, 25
 diagnosis of, 96
 treatment of, 96
Atrial flutter, 67, 67*t*
Atrial gallop, 60

Atrial infarction, 66
Atrial myxoma, 105
Atrial septal defects, 59–60, 101
Atrial tachycardia, 67
Atrioventricular block, 68
Atrophic vaginitis, 32
Atypical lymphocytosis, 358
Atypical squamous cells of uncertain insignificance, 32
Autoimmune hemolytic anemia, 413
Autonomy, 7
Autosomal dominant polycystic kidney disease, 217*t*
Autosomal recessive polycystic kidney disease, 217*t*
Avascular necrosis of bone, 289
Azathioprine, 215
Azoles, 361
Azotemia, 201

B
B lymphocytes (B cells), 294, 302–307
B-type natriuretic peptide, 96
Bacillary dysentery, 174
Back pain
 older adults and, 570
Bacterial conjunctivitis, 43*t*
Bacterial infection, 194–195
Bacterial meningitis, 224
Bacterial overgrowth, small bowel, 185
Balloon angioplasty, 85
Barrett's esophagus, 180, 181
Bartholin's cyst, 372
Bartonella-related diseases, 347–348
Bartter's syndrome, 231
Baseline functional status, preoperative interview
 and, 50
Basophils, 292
Bayes' theorem, 70–74
Behçet's disease, 111, 245
Bell's palsy, 551
Beneficence, 7
Benign (paroxysmal) positional vertigo, 549
Benign primary hepatic lesions, 179
Benign prostatic hypertrophy, 578
Berger's disease, 198
Best interest, 12
Beta blockers
 angina pectoris and, 89–90
 asthma patients and, 4
 cardioselectivity and, 107–108
 congestive heart failure and, 93, 94
 hypertension and, 78
 intrinsic sympathomimetic activity and, 108
 perioperative cardiac risk and, 1
 perioperative period and, 54
 variant angina and, 79
Beta-human chorionic gonadotropin, 452
Beta-lactam antibiotics, 360
Beta-thalassemias, 419
Bethesda titer, 445
Bezoars, 186, 187